The Outcomes Mandate

Case Management in Health Care Today

The Outcomes Mandate

Case Management in Health Care Today

ELAINE L. COHEN, RN, EdD

Director of Case Management,
Co-director, Office of Clinical Practice,
Quality Management,
University Hospital,
University of Colorado Health Sciences Center;
Associate Professor,
University of Colorado School of Nursing
Denver, Colorado

VIVIEN De BACK, RN, PhD, FAAN

Nurse Consultant,
Empowering Change,
Franklin, Wisconsin

with 55 illustrations

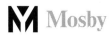 Mosby

St. Louis Baltimore Boston Carlsbad Chicago Minneapolis New York Philadelphia Portland
London Milan Sydney Tokyo Toronto

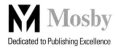
Mosby
Dedicated to Publishing Excellence

A Times Mirror
Company

Publisher: Nancy L. Coon
Managing Editor: Lisa Potts
Developmental Editor: Aimee E. Loewe
Project Manager: John Rogers
Production Editors: Steve Hetager/Jeanne Genz
Manufacturing Supervisor: Dave Graybill
Book Design: Renée Duenow
Cover Design: Brian Salisbury

Composition by The Clarinda Company
Printing/binding by R.R. Donnelly & Sons Company

Mosby, Inc.
11830 Westline Industrial Drive
St. Louis, Missouri 63146

Library of Congress Cataloging in Publication Data

Cohen, Elaine L. (Elaine Liebman)
    The outcomes mandate: case management in health care today/
Elaine L. Cohen, Vivien De Back.
        p.   cm.
    Includes index.
    ISBN 0-323-00277-3
    1. Nursing services—Evaluation.   2. Outcome assessment (Medical care)   3. Managed care plans (Medical care)   I. De Back, Vivien.
II. Title.
    [DNLM: 1. Case Management.   2. Nursing Care.   3. Outcome and Process Assessment (Health Care)   WY   100C678o   1998]
RT85.5.C64   1998
362.1'73'068—dc21
DNLM/DLC
for Library of Congress   98-37881
                                                              CIP

98 99 00 01 02 / 9 8 7 6 5 4 3 2 1

Contributors

Belinda J. Acosta, RN, BSN
Nurse Case Manager,
Parish Nurse,
Carondelet St. Mary's Hospital,
Tucson, Arizona

Carolyn E. Aydin, PhD
Research Scientist III,
Cedars-Sinai Medical Center,
Los Angeles, California

William G. Baker, Jr., MD
Vice President, Medical Services,
Piedmont Hospital,
Atlanta, Georgia

Robert J. Barnet, MD, MA
Clinical Professor of Medicine,
University of Nevada,
Reno, Nevada

Nancy M. Bennett, MD, MPH
Deputy Health Director,
Monroe County Health Department;
Clinical Associate Professor of Medicine and
    Community and Preventive Medicine,
University of Rochester,
Rochester, New York

Linda Burnes Bolton, RN, DrPH, FAAN
Chief Nursing Officer,
Cedars-Sinai Medical Center,
Los Angeles, California

Richard J. Botelho, BMedSci, BMBS, MRCGP
Associate Professor of Medicine and Psychiatry,
Director of Fellowship Training Program,
University of Rochester School of Medicine and
    Dentistry,
Rochester, New York

Nancy N. Boyer, RN, NP
Former Nurse Practitioner,
Vice President of Patient Care,
Fairport, New York

Carol Bradley, RN, MSN
Vice President of Patient Care Services,
Huntington Hospital,
Pasadena, California

Maggie L. Breckon, RN, RM, BAppSc, MN
Director of Nursing and Allied Health Services,
Angliss Health Service,
Melbourne, Victoria,
Australia

Bernadette M. Brennan, RN, DipAppSc, FR, CNA
Nurse Consultant,
Bernadette Brennan and Associates,
Burwood Heights, Victoria,
Australia

Bill Brodie, RN, MSHA
Administrative Leader,
Outcome Manager,
Brookwood Medical Center,
Birmingham, Alabama

Glenda Ethridge Brogden, RN, MSN
Chief Operating Officer,
Brookwood Medical Center,
Birmingham, Alabama

Pam L. Bromley, RN, MSM
Vice President of Patient Care Services,
Saint Alphonsus Regional Medical Center,
Boise, Idaho

Ann Marie T. Brooks, RN, DNSc, MBA, FAAN, FACHE
Vice President
Department of Nursing
King Faisal Specialist Hospital
Riyadh, Saudi Arabia

Sandra Schmidt Bunkers, RN, PhD
Associate Professor and Chair,
Department of Nursing
Augustana College,
Sioux Falls, South Dakota

Constance S. Burgess, RN, MS
President,
Connie Burgess and Associates,
Lakewood, California

Patricia Chiverton, RN, CS, EdD
Associate Dean,
Clinical Affairs,
University of Rochester School of Nursing,
Rochester, New York

Jon D. Christensen, RN, BSN
Nurse Manager,
LDS Hospital,
Salt Lake City, Utah

Bonnie L. Closson, RN, MSN, MRC
Clinical Nurse Specialist,
Mayo Medical Center,
Rochester, Minnesota

Elaine R. Colvin, RN, BSN, MEPD
Manager (Patient Service Representative),
Telephone Nurse Advisors,
Gundersen Lutheran
LaCrosse, Wisconsin

Roberta M. Conti, RN, PhD
Assistant Professor and Coordinator,
Masters Administration Program,
College of Nursing and Health Science,
George Mason University,
Fairfax, Virginia

Pam Cowart, RN, MSN, CCRN
Clinical Nurse Specialist,
Community Clinical Case Management,
Piedmont Hospital,
Atlanta, Georgia

Judith K. Crane, RN, MS
Deputy Director,
Sioux Falls Health Department,
Sioux Falls, South Dakota

Deborah Crist-Grundman, RN, BSN
Associate,
Van Slyck and Associates, Inc.,
Phoenix, Arizona

Grace McCormack Daly, RN, EdD, FNP, CS
Clinical Consultant,
Community Nursing Organization,
Visiting Nurse Service of New York,
Long Island City, New York

Phyllis E. Ethridge, RN, MSN, CNNA, FAAN
Consultant,
Carondelet Health Care Corporation,
Tucson, Arizona

Eleanor G. Ferguson-Marshalleck, RN, PhD
Professor,
Associate Chair,
Department of Nursing,
California State University,
Los Angeles, California

Donna Fosbinder, RN, DNSc
Professor,
College of Nursing,
Coordinator of Graduate Program in Health Care
    Systems Administration,
Brigham Young University,
Provo, Utah

Laurie Frahm, RN, BSN
Nurse Case Manager,
Immanuel-St. Joseph's Mayo Health System,
Mankato, Minnesota

Julie Frederick, RN, BSN, MBA
Nurse Manager
Immanuel-St. Joseph's Mayo Health System,
Mankato, Minnesota

Randi Friedl, RN, MPH
Parish Nurse Coordinator,
Gundersen Lutheran,
LaCrosse, Wisconsin

Susan C. Fry, RN, MEd, CNAA
Vice President, Patient Operations
ViaChristi Regional Medical Center
Wichita, Kansas

Kay W. Garcia, RMT, MBA
Change Management Consultant
Garcia and Associates
Boise, Idaho

Vicki M. George, RN, PhD(c)
Vice President,
Chief Nurse Executive,
St. Luke's Medical Center,
Milwaukee, Wisconsin

Linda F. Golodner
President,
National Consumers League,
Washington, D.C.

Linda Hertz, RN, BSN
Nurse Case Manager,
Immanuel-St. Joseph's Mayo Health System,
Mankato, Minnesota

Delma B. Huggins, RN, MS, FNP
Family Nurse Practitioner,
Carondelet Health Network;
Parish Nurse,
Carondelet St. Mary's Hospital,
Tucson, Arizona

Karen A. Ivantic-Doucette, MSN, FNP, ACRN
Faculty Member,
Family Nurse Practitioner/AIDS Specialist,
Marquette University College of Nursing,
Milwaukee, Wisconsin

Marjorie K. Jamieson, RN, MS, FAAN
Executive Director,
Living at Home/Block Nurse Program,
St. Paul, Minnesota

Gwenneth A. Jensen, RN, MN, CNS
Clinical Nurse Specialist,
Sioux Valley Hospital,
Sioux Falls, South Dakota

Stephen Jessup, CPA
Principal,
Jessup and Richmond, PC
Battle Creek, Michigan

Elizabeth Johnson, RN
Manager, Case Management
Cedars-Sinai Medical Center,
Los Angeles, California

Marion Johnson, RN, PhD
Associate Professor,
College of Nursing,
University of Iowa,
Iowa City, Iowa

Diane K. Josephson, RN, MA
Advanced Practice Nurse,
Augustana College,
Sioux Falls, South Dakota

Dianne F. Kaseman, RN, PhD
Coordinator of Special Projects,
Center for Health Policy,
College of Nursing and Health Science,
George Mason University,
Fairfax, Virginia

Jane Marie Kirschling, RN, DNS
Associate Dean for Academic Affairs,
University of Rochester School of Nursing,
Rochester, New York

JoEllen Goertz Koerner, RN, PhD, FAAN
Senior Partner
JoEllen Koerner & Associates
Sioux Falls, South Dakota

Mary Kay Kohles, RN, MSW
Transformation in Care Delivery Internal Consultant,
Piedmont Hospital,
Atlanta, Georgia

Bernardine M. Lacey, RN, EdD, FAAN
Director,
School of Nursing,
Western Michigan University,
Kalamazoo, Michigan

Maureen Laws, RN, MSc(App) (Nursing)
Nurse Consultant,
Wellington Hospital,
Wellington,
New Zealand

Cheryl Joy Leuning, RN, PhD
Associate Professor of Nursing,
Augustana College,
Sioux Falls, South Dakota

Patricia Hryzak Lind, RN, MS
Director, Health Management and Product Support
   for Preferred Care
Rochester, New York

Merian Litchfield, RN, PhD
Researcher,
Centre for Initiative in Nursing and Health Care,
Wellington,
New Zealand

Mary Ann Lough, RN, PhD
Assistant Professor,
Marquette University College of Nursing,
Milwaukee, Wisconsin

Karina Lovell, BA, MSc, PhD, RMN, ENB650, DpEd
Former Lecturer Practitioner,
Bethlem and Maudsley NHS Trust,
London,
England

Isela Luna, RN, PhD
Parish Nurse Specialist,
Carondelet St. Mary's Hospital,
Tucson, Arizona

Meridean L. Maas, RN, PhD, FAAN
Professor,
College of Nursing,
University of Iowa,
Iowa City, Iowa

Sr. Genovefa Maashao, PHN
Community Health Nurse-Midwife,
Diocese of Mombasa,
Mombasa,
Kenya

Julie MacDonald, RN, MS
Senior Vice President of Patient Care Services,
St. Joseph Mercy Hospital,
Ann Arbor, Michigan

Deborah B. Mangan, RN, MS, CS
Clinical Nurse Specialist,
Mayo Medical Center,
Rochester, Minnesota

Sharon Mass, PhD
Director of Case Management,
Cedars-Sinai Medical Center,
Los Angeles, California

Catherine Michaels, RN, PhD, FAAN
Director of Community Outreach,
Carondelet Health Network,
Tucson, Arizona

Jewel Moseley-Howard, RN, EdD
Individual Consultant,
Baltimore, Maryland

Elizabeth Luna Mourning, BS
Fellow,
Healthcare Forum;
Consultant,
Community Benefit;
Consultant,
New Healthcare Foundation,
Saratoga, California

Mary H. Mundt, RN, PhD
Dean,
Professor,
School of Nursing,
University of Louisville,
Louisville, Kentucky

Ellen K. Murphy, MS, JD, FAAN
Professor,
School of Nursing,
University of Wisconsin,
Milwaukee, Wisconsin

Margaret M. Murphy, RN, PhD
Nurse Consultant,
Empowering Change,
Wauwatosa, Wisconsin

Margot L. Nelson, RNC, PhD
Associate Professor of Nursing,
Augustana College,
Sioux Falls, South Dakota

Jean Newsome, RN, DSN
Operations Leader,
Brookwood Medical Center,
Birmingham, Alabama

Judith Papenhausen, RN, PhD
Chairperson,
Professor,
Department of Nursing,
California State University,
Los Angeles, California

Marjorie Peck, RN, PhD
Associate Professor (Clinical),
College of Nursing,
University of Utah,
Salt Lake City, Utah

Tim Porter-O'Grady, EdD, PhD, FAAN
Senior Partner,
Porter-O'Grady Associates, Inc;
Senior Consultant,
Affiliated Dynamics, Inc;
Assistant Professor,
Emory University,
Atlanta, Georgia

Karen A. Prussing, RN, MS, CS(ANP), CNN
Director of Regional Renal Services and Apheresis,
St. Alexius Medical Center,
Bismarck, North Dakota

Marilyn J. Rantz, RN, PhD, FAAN, NHA
Associate Professor,
Sinclair School of Nursing,
University of Missouri,
Columbia, Missouri

Sheila A. Ryan, RN, PhD, FAAN
Dean and Professor,
School of Nursing,
Director, Medical Center Nursing,
University of Rochester School of Nursing,
Rochester, New York

Marita MacKinnon Schifalacqua, RN, MSN
Project Coordinator of Case Management,
St. Luke's Medical Center,
Milwaukee, Wisconsin

Madeline H. Schmitt, RN, PhD, FAAN
Professor of Nursing,
University of Rochester School of Nursing,
Rochester, New York

Jill Scott, RN, PhD
Assistant Professor
Director of Professional and Portfolio Development
School of Nursing
University of Colorado Health Sciences Center
Denver, Colorado

Christine R. Shaw, RN, PhD, CS, FNP
Clinical Associate Professor,
Marquette University College of Nursing,
Milwaukee, Wisconsin

Roy L. Simpson, RN(C), FNAP, FAAN
Executive Director of Nursing Affairs,
HBOC and Company,
Atlanta, Georgia

Toni C. Smith, RN, EdD
Program Director of Nursing Support Operations,
University of Rochester Medical Center,
Strong Memorial Hospital,
Rochester, New York

Debora S. Snarr, RN, MS, CANP
Nurse Practitioner,
Winchester Medical Center,
Valley Health System,
Winchester, Virginia

Derek T. Spellman, RN, MSN
Chief Nursing Officer,
Brookwood Medical Center,
Birmingham, Alabama

Janice L. Stone, RN, MS, CS
Clinical Nurse Specialist,
Mayo Medical Center,
Rochester, Minnesota

Judith Lloyd Storfjell, RN, PhD
President,
Storfjell Associates,
Berrien Springs, Michigan;
Assistant Professor of Public Health Nursing,
University of Illinois,
Chicago, Illinois

Jane W. Swanson, BSN, MS
Associate Director of Nursing,
National Naval Medical Center,
Bethesda, Maryland

Sr. Carol Taylor, RN, PhD, CSFN
Assistant Professor,
Consulting Healthcare Ethicist,
Georgetown University,
Washington, D.C.

Ben Thomas, BSc (Hons), MSc, RMN, RGN, DipN, RNT, FRCN
Chief Nurse Advisor,
Director of Clinical Services,
Bethlem and Maudsley NHS Trust,
London,
England

Donna Tortoretti, RN, BS
Director, Clinical Operations
Community Nursing Center
University of Rochester School of Nursing
Rochester, New York

Ann Van Slyck, RN, MS, CNAA, FAAN
President,
Van Slyck and Associates, Inc.,
Phoenix, Arizona

Madeline Wake, RN, PhD, FAAN
Dean,
Marquette University College of Nursing,
Milwaukee, Wisconsin

Patricia Hinton Walker, RN, PhD, FAAN
Dean and Professor
University of Colorado Health Sciences Center
School of Nursing
Denver, Colorado

Julie Webster, RN, MN, CANP
Adult Nurse Practitioner,
Community Clinical Case Management,
Piedmont Hospital,
Atlanta, Georgia

Alice P. Weydt, RN, BSN
Director of Patient Care Services,
Immanual-St. Joseph's Mayo Health System,
Mankato, Minnesota

Jo Ann Whitaker, RN, MS
Education Program Coordinator,
Cedars-Sinai Medical Center,
Los Angeles, California

Lisa M. Zerull, RN, MSN
Program Director of Case Management,
Valley Health System,
Winchester, Virginia

To the collective genius of our many learning communities
and the great individuals who occupy its sacred space.
We are forever grateful for the opportunity to walk with you
and share in your spirit and life's work.

Foreword

The Outcomes Mandate: Case Management in Health Care Today is an unsettling book and is meant to be so. In this book some of the nursing profession's most creative thinkers and doers begin raising questions about current economic models of managed care. These models are primarily designed to reduce the cost of health care to employers by changing health care practices. As we move toward the final stages of the current managed care marketplace, these nurses begin asking the following difficult questions: Do what? Why? What will be the models for care delivery in the next millennium?

While the meaning of outcomes, the scope and parameters of new roles, the testing of boundaries within the health care field, and the characteristics of new relationships are meticulously explored in many chapters, the authors approach and address these topics from very different perspectives. This diversity encourages you to reread sections from earlier chapters in the book and then consider how the differing views may relate to each other. As a result, you are not likely to read this book straight through; rather you will find yourself skipping from one idea to another.

A number of themes arise, such as partnership and collaboration, technology and its meaning, the ethics of the marketplace, and the "connectedness" of everything. As *The Outcomes Mandate* leaps from the linear to the quantum and the mechanistic to the organic, you will gain comfort from this "chaos" and discover an underlying sense of order.

The concepts of partnership found throughout this book do not speak of the historic mentoring relationships, networking, or political influence; rather, this notion of partnership addresses the skills needed to structure and sustain learning relationships and communities over time. Within such relationships, the partners themselves are changed.

Many of the authors tackle the challenges of technology (e.g., telemedicine management, use of computer applications for clinical decision support, use of physiological methodologies). Because there are always unintended consequences of technology, the questions raised throughout this book call on us to re-commit as the discipline of nursing to acknowledge those unintended consequences and design future models of care, thus embracing the technology that enables us to care for patients as whole persons and reduce the growing chasm between patient and caregiver.

Also addressed in these chapters is the importance of understanding the ethics of the marketplace. With these discussions, questions such as the following arise: Should quality cost less? Can we render care without considering the costs? Can nurses help patients conserve physical, psychological, spiritual, and financial resources while not withholding necessary care?

One of the most pervasive concepts found in this book is the theme of the connectedness of all things: between patient and caregiver; between nursing and medicine; between church and state; between community and institution; between academic and service organizations; among business, education, and the arts; across the nations of the earth; and among the peoples and families of those nations.

Perhaps the most powerful of the chapters are the stories out of Africa. Scholars suggest that in this day of television and soundbites, we need to recall our human capacity to understand in a way that goes *beyond* the linear word. The African stories of case management literally lift us out of the literate to the postliterate society—a future society with the power of storytelling, enlisting the power of the word to evoke human understanding and action.

The Outcomes Mandate is certainly not an end unto itself. It winds from the quantum future back to the human history of storytellers. And it begins—just barely—to connect full circle. I predict that you will not find the answers in this volume, but I promise you will be intrigued by the questions.

Judith A. Ryan, RN, PhD
President and CEO
Evangelical Luthern Good Samaritan Society
Sioux Falls, SD

Preface

A Look Through the Kaleidoscope

Coming out of the tailspin of health care reform, most of us are still experiencing the effects of vertigo as we move to the next challenge of shaping an effective and humane health care system. Service integration, innovative partnerships, strategic alliances, healthy communities, and outcomes management are the latest buzzwords for how the nation and the world envision the future of health care management and delivery.

Major emphasis has been placed on the structural and support aspects of meeting challenges in today's health care environment. Dramatic improvements in quality, productivity, and "the bottom line" have been attained through restructured and reengineered approaches. Millions of dollars have been spent in defining appropriate models of patient care delivery, advancing integrated networks, supporting education and training, developing new technology and information systems, reconstituting management, and trimming the proverbial organizational fat.

Though few would argue with the inherent principles of cohesiveness, efficiency, and quality that these structural and support systems appear to endorse, little consideration has been given to the added value these methods have for the populations served. Many fundamental questions remain. Is the integration of services really efficient? What is the effectiveness of multiple providers in a single setting? What actually happens as a result of partnering? (Or more strongly stated, how is the quality of life of clients improved because of the interdisciplinary team?) How are the differences between the integrated environment and managed care defined, and what are their relationships to each other? What is the value of a product from the perspectives of the consumer and the community?

These questions attempt to get at the next important step, which moves from the safety net and familiarity of structure and support systems to the murky realm of outcome evaluation. Although nurse case management continues to provide appropriate, effective care in a variety of settings, information is needed about the contribution of case management to the total health care environment. This more global perspective is the major focus of *The Outcomes Mandate: Case Management in Health Care Today.* The book provides a more descriptive look at nursing's work with others, its important contributions, and the results of partnership. Interdisciplinary in nature, the contributors take a results-oriented approach by exploring the determinants and outcomes necessary to create healthy populations and improve the quality of life.

As the title implies, this book takes a hard look at outcomes. The literature is filled with descriptions of outcomes as a product. Our history in this country of focusing on cure has given us a mind set that there is always an end point (i.e., product) rather than a number of reference points along a process. We, and the many contributors to this book, think of outcomes in terms of anniversaries or markers throughout a process that are used to evaluate, take stock of the situation, review where we have been, and, more important, look at where we are going.

Outcomes in this book can be seen as a collection of works in progress. Every author is determined to discover the method that will best describe the success (or lack of success) in the programs that they have designed, implemented, and evaluated. Some authors disagree with others about approaches to care, theoretical underpinnings, or concepts that direct and guide the managed care phenomenon. We specifically sought this diversity. We looked for professionals who are reorganizing health care, and we invited people who were struggling with the outcomes to describe their struggles.

None of the authors of this book will tell you that they have the answer or the solution, because, as we have come to realize, there is no one right answer! Instead there are many answers, many methods, many theories, many processes. Some work more effectively than others, but none can be applied to *all* people at *all* times. That is probably the real insight one gains from reading these chapters. Health care deals with the human condition, and the human condition depends on

the population, the health conditions, the environment, the culture, and a host of other variables. Some
will argue that for these reasons outcomes cannot be
defined. But we take the view that these reasons offer
the basis on which criteria for outcome attainment can
be developed.

We think of this book as a kaleidoscope. Each chapter can be thought of as a brightly colored prism, expressing variations in thought, concepts, and theory.
When this book's content is looked at through these
diverse mirrors, different views emerge. Each time a
kaleidoscope is turned, a new perspective is achieved.
So too with this book; one prism or chapter provides a
new basis on which to read or interpret another. In this
book, managed care can be seen through the eyes of
the ethicist, the practitioner, the philanthropist, or the
entrepreneur. The variety that characterizes the national and international experts who have contributed
to the book provides us with the opportunity to learn
from the leaders and experience the kaleidoscope of
wisdom they offer.

Acknowledgments

Because we believe there is no single way to look at
health care, we realized early on that no one person
could write a book of this magnitude alone. This
book's strength emanates from the fact that many contributors entered the process with us. We are therefore
deeply indebted for the richness and depth their contributions lend.

The interdisciplinary nature of this book demonstrates a togetherness of purpose. We are proud to
present the strong and diverse perspectives of the contributors. They are perspectives worth hearing and
stories worth telling amidst the chaos and rancor of
our present health care system. Their voices are bold,
courageous, and full with the spirit of discovery. The
collective wisdom of their contributions helps stimulate dialogue, cultivating a new reality for all of us.

Much gratitude is also extended to the following
individuals who embarked on this journey with us:

To Dr. Judith Ryan, for her most spirited and visionary foreword. We applaud her foresight and
wisdom.

To the reviewers, Drs. Margaret (Margie) Murphy
and Alice Longman, whose insightful and clear
feedback helped keep us focused on the task at
hand.

To Yvonne Alexopoulos and Kimberly Netterville,
Lisa Potts and Aimee Loewe, and the staff of
Nursing Editorial at Mosby, who through their
own professional struggles, stayed committed to
and supportive of the vision of this book. In addition to the editorial guidance provided, their
consistent inquiry helped frame the views we
sought to get across.

To Steve Hetager, Jeanne Genz, and the production
staff. Their efficiency and expeditiousness produce true miracles.

We must also express loving thanks to our families
and friends. Their support for what we do and who
we are inspires us.

The process of writing this book also invited reflection on ourselves. It stretched us to think in different
ways and validated our belief that diverse views are
not divisive but necessary for continued growth. The
book's overriding humanistic theme of sustaining relationships intertwined almost every aspect of our
work as we built on long-standing relationships, created partnerships, and formed new friendships. It
challenged us to remain authentic and passionate
about embracing multiple perspectives, as well as reaffirmed the work's stewardship and professional integrity as we guided and mentored the contributors.
And it humbled us as we came to realize the power
and beauty of the written word.

Elaine L. Cohen and Vivien De Back

Contents

PART TWO   # New Roles
Restructuring the System

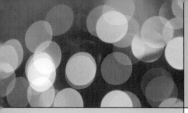

PART ONE

Basics

The Meaning of Outcomes in Today's Health Care Environment

The fit between the system's outcomes and purpose becomes the way the system measures its viability.

TIM PORTER-O'GRADY

PART ONE OFFERS A BASIC UNDERSTANDING of the health care environment at a time of incredible change—why the system is in flux, its component parts, its language, and its potential for the future. Multiple concepts are presented that will be helpful in delineating differences in expectations and behavior between the former Industrial Age and the emerging Quantum Age. Outcomes as definable and measurable components of health care are addressed, and methods to evaluate the results of care are described. A view of case management through the eyes of a financial manager offers an understanding of the cost of care juxtaposed with clinical management for quality. The consumer focus in this section addresses these same issues from the perspective of the customers who purchase health care. Validation that leaders will have to embrace a new set of skills and refocus their priorities to thrive in today's health care arena and in future health care arenas rounds off this section. ▲

CHAPTER 1

Sustainable Partnerships

The Journey Toward Health Care Integration

TIM PORTER-O'GRADY, EdD, PhD, FAAN

OVERVIEW

No discipline can ever again define solely for itself what its obligations, requisites, and services will be out of the context of its relationship with other disciplines.

Much is mutable in health care. The changes being experienced are a subset of a much larger framework affecting all human activities on the globe. Placed within this context, the experiences of reformatting health services make more sense. Articulating the nurse's role within the transitioning format for health care is the major activity of the time. It calls all nurses to discern the expectations and emerging role demands for nurses within a new paradigm for health service provision. All the parameters and processes of service delivery are subject to analysis. The emerging characteristics and content of the new health system call for a different way of seeing and doing. Nurses must now anticipate what these "signposts" are indicating and reconfigure their responses to these signposts. Review of these signposts and of the categories of change is essential to sorting through the health system reorganization and renewing nurses' commitment to health care within a much broader context for it. ▲

Transformation

We are in the midst of major global, sociopolitical, economic, and technological transformation. Indeed, the world is undergoing an age change. We are moving, essentially, out of the Industrial Age and are, perhaps, the last generation of the Industrial Age. As a result, we have a significant obligation to bring closure to the Industrial Age and usher in the initial stages of what the cultural sociologists are calling the Sociotechnical Age (Beneveniste, 1994).

This shift out of the Industrial Age and into a quantum age has tremendous implications for health care. Indeed, many of the technological innovations and miracles that have become commonplace in health care have been a part of the processes that have been leading us into the quantum age (Cleveland, 1993). As health care becomes more technologically driven, it becomes more portable, less institutional, less invasive, and much more mobile. As a result, the past focus on institutionalization, patient days, bed-based services, and high levels of intense intervention is no longer the framework for much of the delivery of health care service. In fact, much of health care service is becoming less invasive, less institutional, less bed-based, and more flexible, fluid, and mobile. This major shift in the orientation of health care has created increasing levels of trauma for health professionals, especially those whose practice and work have been historically dependent on predominantly bed-based, institutional, high-intensity, and highly invasive activities (Beckham, 1996).

Shifting Nursing

Nursing is one of the professional groups significantly impacted by this transformation in health care. Historically, nursing's role has been predominantly the care of the sick. Although there have been important community and health-driven roles for nursing, the predominant functions and activities of nursing historically have been in institutions where sick, infirm, or disadvantaged people have been resident. As this becomes less the paradigm for the delivery of health care services and since most nurses are located there, a major crisis in orientation, service, and location has resulted for the nursing profession (Barter, Furmidge, 1996).

The journey for nursing is out of predominantly institutional, residential, and bed-based service activities. The move to a stronger health orientation, more mobility and fluidity and flexibility in the delivery of service, and less intensity in the interventions required to address patients' needs has created the conditions and circumstances that now define the general influences on the future of nursing practice. The challenge associated with this shift has created a significant level of trauma for nursing professionals as they begin to consider individual and professional roles in a significantly altered health care delivery system (Hadley, 1996). Some of the challenges relate to the following:

- 60% of nurses practice in bed-based institutionally related activities (the good news: this is down from 68% only a decade ago).
- Job security and old traditional roles that were once firm now appear fleeting.
- The skill sets that nurses have in the care of the ill and those in need of residential services are no longer a part of the significant demand base for nursing professionals.
- New skill sets will be required in order to practice the profession within a different context and in different locations along the health care service continuum.
- The preparation of nurses for practice now requires a markedly different mix of learning activities and content than that provided in the last 30 years.
- Synthesis skills are now more greatly valued than analysis skills in a more integrated and fluid health care delivery system. Nurses have learned analysis well, but have not learned synthesis so well.
- Integration of services now becomes the predominant requirement for the health care system. Nurses are good at coordinating nonintegrated functions. Integration now creates problems with initiating the relationships nurses and other disciplines have failed to develop with each other throughout the past 30 years.

Principles for a Quantum Age

The contextual and conceptual foundations for the quantum age are fundamentally altered from those which defined the Industrial Age. Much of the principle of development and technological advancement in the Industrial Age was driven by Newtonian concepts: linear, reductionistic, analysis-based, and highly functional in their orientation (Drucker, 1995). As we move into the quantum age, much of the foundation and framework for it is defined better in quantum mechanics than in Newtonian concepts. The quantum processes begin by looking at whole systems requiring synthesis rather than analysis, and recognizing that any component of a system or set of orders is intimately related to another component (Zohar, Marshall, 1994). Substantial progress in sustainability depends on the degree of integration that is realized and applied.

Without understanding the elements of synthesis and integration and the principles that guide it, no discipline, including nursing, can create the conditions for its own thriving. No single element, function, group, or process can, in and of itself, define its future or its activities or its meaning out of the context of its relationship with other components, processes, or disciplines.

This realization creates significant difficulties for many of the health professions. Although the health professions are committed to the same purposes, most of the work, relationships, and functions of each profession have been defined by each group in isolation from their relationships to other groups. Indeed, much of the relationship with other groups has been narcissistic, competitive, compartmentalized, and segmented. In fact, many of the standards, policies, practices, principles, and politics of each discipline have been uniquely defined by the discipline through relationship and contact with its own members. Very rarely has there been contact with other disciplines and members of other professional groups, incorporating their insight into the position and policy statements of any other discipline. Indeed, professional exclusion and elitism have been the rule. As a result, this compartmentalization of relationships has created alienation, segmentation, and separate agendas for each of the professions in providing care and services to patients.

The problem with this has been the accommodation of the professions to this particular modus operandi for behavior in the old Industrial Age framework. Accommodation, adaptation, and adjustment to these kinds of patterns of relationship and behavior have become the norm. Isolated practices, behaviors, and interactions have been a reflection of this norm. The challenge now is that such patterns of behavior are no longer viable and do not create the conditions of either professional viability or service sustainability (Porter-O'Grady, 1994).

Along with the context of a quantum age comes a new set of principles that guide behavior, interactions, and relationships within the quantum age. These new principles articulate a different orientation to relationship and to functional proficiency. The ability to thrive in the quantum age represents a unique set of variables not currently understood or fully implemented by any discipline on its journey toward thriving in an age that has a different set of conditions. The challenge for the profession of nursing, as with other professions, will be the application of these principles in the nurse's own practices and processes and the undertaking of work sufficient to see that these principles act in a broader frame of reference.

The four principles that underlie the movement into the quantum age are partnership, equity, accountability, and ownership. Each of these principles relates to the others; each principle is unique in its application to the requirement for behavioral shift on the part of all professionals in health care. Although the principles apply specifically to each component of the major social and cultural shifts to a quantum age, they are also universal (Porter-O'Grady, Krueger-Wilson, 1995). They have specific implications for health care that are unique to the relationships that must be established in health care to create sustainability and service effectiveness within the health care system. The manifestation of these principles in health care creates a unique set of variables to which the profession and the professional must accommodate in order to create the conditions of sustainability and of contribution across organizational systems and, ultimately, across the continuum of care.

PARTNERSHIP

All change is local. In 1993 President Clinton proposed a nationally driven, integrated approach to changing the health care system, making it more accountable and effective. His proposals suggested broad and sweeping changes in the health care system that would ultimately shift the locus of control, the character of service, and the mechanism of paying for health care over the long term. However, the plan failed. A federally driven and mandated, single integrated health care system was anathema to the consciousness of the American political agenda and the population as a whole. Economic, political, and social reaction to the plan was of such breadth that it was not long before it was no longer a viable and meaningful approach to changing the health care system.

That did not stop change, however. Many of the changes proposed in 1993 have been subsequently implemented in an incremental, nonaligned, and nongovernmental way. The health care revolution and resulting transformation have occurred in spite of the collapse of the approach suggested in 1993. Since that time huge amounts of alteration, adjustment, and change have occurred in the health care system, such that a whole new range of rules apply.

The United States is not a social democracy. Social democracies are represented by such countries as Canada, Great Britain, and the other European democracies. Through their parliamentary systems and social mandates, the requirement of government to provide health service in support to its citizens has been clearly and legislatively articulated. Not so with the American Constitution. Indeed, much of the American Constitution was written in reaction to government's control and direction of individuals' lives. Threading through it is support of the free enterprise system and the right of citizens to be free to pursue their own goals. Indeed, the United States as a nation was formed in economic reaction to what was considered as inappropriate, heavy-handed behavior of the British government and its taxation policies (thus the Boston Tea Party). Therefore the American Constitution almost precludes the interest of its citizens to have government take care of anything that the individual could undertake for himself or herself. Although this does not necessarily create a permanent set of conditions, it does create a functioning and operational milieu in the American political and social structure that does not enamor its citizens of government control, intervention, or operation of any of the elements of life that can be better controlled (it is assumed, in America) by citizens through their own efforts and means.

This dynamic has created a strong marketplace orientation to any kind of structural, political, and social change in the United States. Although social change clearly occurs, it is driven by a different mix of activities than often is represented in other national entities. Currently, the major impetus of technology and the application of that technology to every aspect of our lives have created the conditions through which the process of change takes form. Many of the demands of technology and its impact on sociopolitical, economic, and technological processes have created a frame of reference that has generated the need for significant change. As a result, the changes that have occurred have had an impact on every aspect of American life. The marketplace has created tremendous changes in relational, political, social, and economic, as well as technological, activities of every American citizen (Brown, 1995). Some examples of this set of circumstances are as follows:

- The predominant characteristic of this market change has been the increasing integration, mergers, alliances, networks, and other formal arrangements that represent changing notions of partnership.
- Technology makes it possible to build partnership across political, cultural, and social landscapes because the infrastructure creates the conditions for a boundaryless world.
- Institutional models are collapsing into system configurations, resulting in an altered milieu for business, service, work, and relationships.
- The information infrastructure is becoming the new architecture for health care. The system will build its future around the construction of the information system and the infrastructure necessary to sustain it and the work of health care.
- New kinds of partnerships will emerge along the continuum of service, requiring the formation of unique and variable relationships between a range of entities to position the system to provide a broader range of comprehensive services to the system's members and clients.
- Leadership models will move away from command-and-control approaches and unilateral notions and styles of decision making to those models that are inclusive, engaging, and empowering, and invest the stakeholders in process and outcome.

EQUITY

In the Industrial Age, especially in the past 30 to 40 years (following Lyndon Johnson's "Great Society" initiatives), many of the goals of health care have centered around providing and expanding access and opportunity to utilize service (Cavenaugh, 1996). Indeed, the very way of funding and paying for health care created the conditions that resulted in unlimited access and increasing levels of duplication of services in an increasing number of service sites. Hospitals and health care services have proliferated across the country in ways that not only have provided opportunities for access but also have increased the amount of duplication of function, service, and technology across the nation.

Much of this supergrowth in health care has been driven at some level by debt economics. Indeed, much of the expenditure of dollars for the health care system has moved at a 10% to 12% growth rate. As a result, the percentage of dollars provided for social services in the United States, assumed by the health care system, has grown at an untenable rate over the past 30 years such that what began as $100 billion health care system has now become a $1.4 trillion health care system, and still continues to grow to this date (Johnson, 1995). There is much that must be done to return to a more equitable set of values and ways of doing business in health care:

- Controlling costs must include a different way of providing health service, not simply playing with the mechanics of the present service structure.
- In the past 30 years health care has funded its unparalleled growth with tomorrow's dollars, ignoring the fact that tomorrow would one day arrive and the bill would come due. That time has arrived.
- Money talks but it does not think. Simply controlling dollars and advancing the viability of the balance sheet will not create sustainable health care. Just ask Richard Scott, formerly of Columbia HCA, who advanced the company's profitability at the expense of long-term stability. There is much more to good health care than a healthy bottom line.
- Equity is about value. It is now time to move away from unilateral and poorly formed notions of "best" health care to more rational and measurable factors associated with "wise" health care services. Providers have learned to provide best care without thought to its price; now they must provide thoughtful and measurable health service in a wise way with a tight relationship between what one does (process) and what one achieves (outcomes).
- Sustainability in a system depends on the balance the system can bring between cost, quality, and work, recognizing that none of these alone can sufficiently act to sustain the viability of the system.

The value equation now drives the constructs of the formation of the health care system. Value is represented in a dynamic equation that is cybernetic and continuous in its flow and application. The elements of the value equation (therefore, the elements of equity) are cost, quality, and work (Figure 1-1). The value equation is the best representation of equity that is available. What the value equation suggests is that no one element of value is the driving force in creating sustainability. Indeed, in order to create sustainability, the value equation must consistently and dynamically remain in balance. This suggests that controlling costs alone does not create sustainability, but then neither does ensuring quality alone ensure viability. Furthermore, altering the work activities without a consideration of their impact on cost and quality does not create the context for success. It is only when all of the actions and elements of the value equation are considered (i.e., cost, quality, and work), and their consistent and constant impact on and interaction with

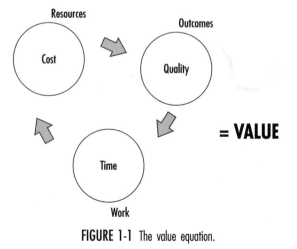

FIGURE 1-1 The value equation.

each other, that the conditions of sustainability are created.

Equity suggests then that there is balance between each element of the value equation, and that every role, process, function, activity, and construct in the system works together to ensure that those values are continuously promulgated and advanced in any service system.

ACCOUNTABILITY

In the Industrial Age, responsibility-driven constructs were the rule for defining work and relationships. In the quantum age the shift away from responsibility (individuated and functional constructs) and toward accountability is perhaps one of the most significant functional and role shifts in the delivery system. In the Industrial Age "control" was perhaps the clearest indicator of the structural integrity of an organization. In the quantum age it is "relationship" that is the driving force toward system integrity. Relationship becomes a critical factor in ensuring the viability and effectiveness of the system. Building relationship, and all of the intersections, interactions, and collaborations necessary to ensure it, is the major work of leadership in the current time. Some of the key issues around accountability are as follows:

- Accountability is not responsibility. It requires ownership investment and application at the individual level. Unlike responsibility, it is not "owned" by the system, manager, or group, nor can it be externally generated or mandated—it always comes from within the person (Box 1-1).

BOX 1-1	
Differentiating Responsibility and Accountability	
Responsibility	**Accountability**
Functional	Results focused
Task driven	Integrated
Process oriented	Outcome oriented
Hierarchical	Partnership based
Fixed skill set	Fluid skill set
Finite	Mobile

- Accountability focuses on outcome, not process. Sustainable expression of accountability can be evidenced in the tightness-of-fit between process and outcome, not simply the validation of each out of context with the other.
- Accountability must be owned by those who express it. This means that decisions must be made where they arise and by those who own them. It is essential that individuals buy into the contribution of their own work.

Since sustainability depends on the interface, relatedness, and interactional confluence of the activities of team members around a common purpose, it becomes important for the organization and the system to begin to focus on the relatedness between all of the players and the convergence of their activities as they impact the achievement of sustainable outcomes.

Systems are membership communities. Service systems agree in their contract with members to provide the full range of health care services needed in order to attain or maintain health. The focus of the system changes from providing late-engagement, illness-based services to early-engagement, health-driven services. This move to early engagement is not driven simply by the good intentions or high moral character of health care leaders. It is essentially a requirement of a cost-determined and priced-fixed system in advance of providing sustainable service. This requires that every member be fully accountable for his or her contribution.

Accountability, unlike responsibility, requires that each contributing member join together in the aggregate of service processes that are essential to create viable and replicable outcomes. Each member of the service team has an impact on both process and the resulting outcomes. Therefore the issue of fit between each member's process and the comprehensive outcome becomes a critical operating variable of the effectiveness of the health care system and its services. The system, therefore, must promulgate and promote the relationship between the various disciplines and the team members, and the interaction between the team members' work and the outcome to which they are all committed (Box 1-2).

Because of the requirements of partnership, accountability becomes an essential condition of the

---

BOX 1-2

Industrial Organization Versus Quantum System

Functional Organization	Systems Structure
Process oriented	Outcome oriented
Task driven	Protocol driven
Hierarchical	Partnered
Responsibility based	Accountability based
Institutional	Multidimensional
Individual focused	Team focused
Vertical control	Horizontal integration
Process driven	Relationship driven

---

relationship. The relationship between and among the providers now becomes critical to the achievement of value in the system. Value becomes the essential variable around which the health system can ensure its sustainability. The intersection and interrelatedness between these variables create the conditions for viable health service in the marketplace today. Furthermore, they create the demand for change in the relationship between and among providers as they begin to establish the team foundation for their functional activities and their clinical outcomes. The following elements in the formation of that relationship become critical to its success:

- No discipline can ever again define solely for itself what its obligations, requisites, and services will be out of the context of its relationship with other disciplines.
- All disciplines will have to intersect their clinical practices and protocols with each other, negotiating the resulting functional interface in order to create consistent clinical practices.
- Variable leadership of the team will have to be incorporated into its design. Teams should be led on the basis of the role of the players, the purpose of the team, the stage of the continuum within which the team is working, the predominant priority of the team at any given time, the issues of concern to the consumer having an impact on the function of the team, and the ultimate outcome of the team in exercising its obligation.

- All roles in the team are negotiated between and among the members of the team. No role is predetermined or ascendant without the concerted assent of the team members.
- Behavior becomes a serious concern to team development. Industrial model ascendant and vertically fixed behavior patterns now must give way to more fluid, interactional, and negotiated roles, representing a more horizontal behavioral pattern.
- Skill development around team-based activities will be as important as skill development around new clinical expectations. Simply forming relationships in a team because of the need for them does not ensure that the team has the skills necessary to behave as one.
- Performance expectation, functional delineation, performance evaluation, and outcome measures now must transition toward the team as a whole, away from simply looking at individual activities and functions. This movement from individual-based focus of organizations to team-based focus of systems will require considerable structural change, as well as the introduction of new processes and tools for focusing on team activities and outcomes.
- Outcomes drive all process. The negotiation and dialogue around consistent, replicable, and renewable outcomes will require considerable systems support. Renegotiating roles and relationships and functional intersections will be fraught with old role patterns, behavioral entrenchment, power positioning, and control practices. These must be identified for what they are, addressed directly, and incorporated into the challenge of building functional, accountable team processes.

OWNERSHIP

The principles of partnership, equity, and accountability drive us toward the fourth principle. None of the previous three principles can be fully invested and implemented without the ownership that is necessary to sustain them. Ownership is a recognition that every individual in a system plays an important role in the purposes and goals of the system.

Systems are membership communities. Systems demand that each member be clear about the con-

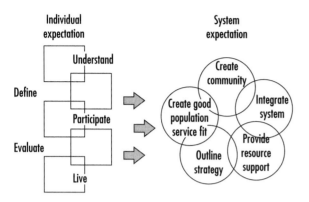

FIGURE 1-2 Differentiating roles.

tribution that he or she makes to the integrity of the system and to the fulfillment of its purposes. The fit between the system's outcomes and purpose becomes the way the system measures its viability. This notion of fit depends on the investment and commitment of the community of persons to the purposes of the system. The presumption of ownership threads through all principles and is the foundation on which thriving depends. The principle of ownership recognizes this quid pro quo relationship between individual and system. It is a functional symbiotic relationship that is essential to the advancement of both the individual and the system.

The intricate and intimate nature of the relationship between the two creates a substantial mutual obligation that advances the principle of ownership and the requirement for commitment. In any system the principle of ownership is reflected in the fit of individual expectations with those of the system. This interface is necessary to ensure congruence between the activities of the individual and the obligations of the system (Figure 1-2).

The Role of Nursing

The obligation and opportunity of the nursing discipline are in providing leadership in the creation of real partnership and advancing health systems toward integration. Nursing has a history of pulling together the many and disparate resources, players, and processes in health care around patients to ensure that they are obtaining what they need in the delivery of service. This skill in integrating the activities of many different disciplines, historically consonant with the role of the nurse, now provides an opportunity for leadership in integration, coordination, and facilitation of the health care team. In the development of team-based approaches, nursing can play a significant role in utilizing skills and resource management, in interdisciplinary interaction, and in planning the delivery of health care services. This effort incorporates the roles of other players in a way that now provides a skill base for team-based design and development.

Nursing's opportunity is in creating the continuum of linked and integrated services that is so much a part of its basic conceptual framework. Although, historically, nursing has been forced to operate in a nonaligned, compartmentalized, nonintegrated system, its fundamental, philosophical, and theoretical constructs always assume the need to link, integrate, and coordinate the whole range of services necessary to the patient's journey through his or her health care experience. It is the management of this journey that is specific and unique to nursing.

Nursing is perhaps the only profession whose focus is the patient's journey rather than any one given clinical event. There is virtually no other discipline in health care, with the partial exception of social work, where the focus of health service is on the patient's journey through the health experience rather than through any one given event of service. This focus and framework for the profession uniquely position it to facilitate the emerging continuum-of-care, integrated-delivery-system, whole-systems approaches, and the team-based constructs that will be necessary to promulgate health care in a capitated, advance-priced continuum-of-service system. The ability to focus on accountability and the outcomes to which it is directed encourages the profession of nursing to focus on those processes and activities which best fulfill the highest level of the relationship between disciplines and the consonant and converging activity of all disciplines around advancing patient care, facilitating the movement of patients through their health experience, and ensuring that meaningful and achievable outcomes can be obtained in the process. This is the exemplification and application of accountability in an efficient and effective health system.

Nursing Deconstruction: Building the Future

All of these elements create the foundations on which the future design of health care service will be built. The role of nursing is to provide leadership in the developmental and application process. Nursing, however, has itself much work to do in order to deconstruct many of the old barriers to building relationship and create the foundation on which new constructs can be built. New approaches to the following processes must be clearly undertaken:

- Nursing must move out of its reaction to the drama and the change of de-institutionalizing health care and de-debting health care services. Nurses must now advance the development of a health-based script and the service continuum that will reflect it.
- Nursing must join with other disciplines in the process of advocacy to ensure that what efficiencies, cost effectiveness, and service structures emerge are appropriately balanced, do not impede the ability to meet the needs of those who are served, and do not violate the mandate and commitment to provide quality services to those subscribers who look to the health care professions to act in their best interest.
- Nurses must move out of reaction and into design. Nurses should be at the design tables, influencing the creation of new models, new relationships, and new interdisciplinary compacts, and the negotiation of structural interrelationships between other players along the continuum of care. Without nurses present at the table, the application and implementation of clinical process will suffer and a renegotiation of roles will need to occur at a later stage, when it will be more expensive and more intensive and the process will be more volatile.
- The education and preparation of nurses from an illness-based model into a health-service and prescriptive model in a multitude of different settings becomes a priority for the development of the professional. Increasingly, focusing the professional on the continuum of linked services across the patient's journey and providing clinical opportunities to deliver service in that framework become the requisites of the developmental process for the nursing professional.
- Increasing focus on advanced preparation and preparing more baccalaureate and master's degree practitioners to position themselves well along the continuum of care to be decision makers and care providers in a decentralized, horizontally aligned, and integrated delivery structure will be critical to the viability of nursing over the long term. Team-based roles demand competence and articulation of professionals as members of the team. Increasingly, as other team members are prepared at the baccalaureate and master's levels, the credibility of the nursing profession within the context of the team will also include the comparability and consistency of its preparation and articulation with the team members at the level of function and interaction that can advance both the team and the profession's work.
- Focusing on coordinating, integrating, and facilitating the delivery of health care services across the continuum of care should be the predominant demand and requirement of the nursing profession. Changing its definitions, its advocacy, and its values statements to focus on the patient's journey and the management of the activities along the continuum should be the major thrust of policy and position changes for the profession of nursing for at least the next two decades. Focusing on recumbent, passive, intensity-based, bed-related advocacy and delivery service functions for the nurse is an antediluvian and recidivistic process that can only position nursing poorly to embrace and advance the health-based script unfolding over the next two decades.
- Nursing should provide much of the major leadership in moving from a late-engagement (sickness-based) system to an early-engagement (health-driven and prescriptive) health care system. Creating new models of health service driven by the technology that supports it, the sociopolitical demand for it, and the economic requisites that create the need for it will be an important function of the profession of nursing over the next two decades. Providing leadership in writing the

script for early-engagement systems positions nursing and nurses well to thrive in the emerging environment, lead its changes, and produce meaningful and viable, as well as sustainable, health outcomes.

Conclusion

In this chapter the four principles serve as the foundation for understanding the requisite partnerships that must emerge in the creation of the future health care system. Nurses' roles must now move from protecting and advocating for patients in a sickness-based system to advocating and representing the community in creating a much more comprehensive, consonant, and integrated health-based delivery system (Porter et al, 1996). The noise, challenge, pain, and process associated with moving from one system to another will create much anxiety, uncertainty, and challenge for the nursing profession and for each practitioner in the discipline (Paine, 1994). No one's role can remain the same. All roles will be transformed. Any nurse who wishes to remain precisely what he or she always was in the delivery of his or her service will pay a heavy price for nonengagement with the changes afoot. If nursing is to thrive, it must ensure that there is a tightness of fit between its response and the need to design an integrated, horizontally delineated, cost-effective, continuously linked, and health-driven system (Porter-O'Grady, 1995). The major work of the time is in the design, construction, and evaluation of processes that lead to just such a system. The major thrust of all of the activities of nursing for the foreseeable future must be based on these premises if the profession is to thrive.

References

Barter M, Furmidge M: Nursing's new frontier: reinventing our practice in a restructured health care system, *Advanced Practice Nursing Quarterly* 1(4):166-170, 1996.

Beckham D: Hearing the tidal wave, *Healthcare Forum Journal* 39(2):68-78, 1996.

Beneveniste G: *The twenty-first century organization*, San Francisco, 1994, Jossey-Bass.

Brown M: The economic era: now to the real change, *Health Care Management Review* 19(4):73-82, 1995.

Cavenaugh F: *The truth about the national debt*, Boston, 1996, Harvard Business School Press.

Cleveland H: *Birth of a new world*, San Francisco, 1993, Jossey-Bass.

Drucker P: *Managing in a time of great change*, New York, 1995, Truman Talley/Dutton.

Hadley E: Nursing in the political and economic marketplace: challenges for the 21st century, *Nursing Outlook* 44(1):6-10, 1996.

Johnson R: The economic era of health care, *Health Care Management Review* 19(4):64-72, 1995.

Paine L: Managing for organizational integrity, *Harvard Business Review* 72(2):106-117, 1994.

Porter A et al: Clinical integration: an interdisciplinary approach to a system priority, *Nursing Administration Quarterly* 20(2):65-73, 1996.

Porter-O'Grady T: Building partnerships in health care: creating whole systems change, *Nursing & Health Care* 15(1):34-38, 1994.

Porter-O'Grady T: Managing along the continuum: a new paradigm for the clinical manager, *Nursing Administration Quarterly* 19(3):1-12, 1995.

Porter-O'Grady T, Krueger-Wilson C: *The leadership revolution in healthcare: altering systems, changing behavior*, Gaithersburg, Md, 1995, Aspen.

Zohar D, Marshall I: *Quantum society*, New York, 1994, William Morrow.

CHAPTER 2

Managed Care

The Driving Force for Case Management

CONSTANCE S. BURGESS, RN, MS

OVERVIEW

Quality care and profitable bottom lines are not mutually exclusive, but the blending of these goals requires that all players who are ready to contribute and have the expertise to create better ways must come together, begin to understand and accept one another, and build a total system of care.

Much has been written about managed health care, the various types of plans, regional HMO penetrations, and the many relationships that have emerged. Less has been discussed about "how it is going" in different settings, what works, what does not work, and where and how some of the greatest impediments to implementation have arisen. The jury of consumers has not yet decided how well this is all working, and the philosophical differences and communication gaps between and among stakeholders do not appear to have closed in many marketplaces. When all that can be said has been said about the strengths and weaknesses of managed health care, the apparent and single most intrusive barrier to advancing the health care agenda, from both sides of the table, is trust. This chapter takes a pragmatic view of market-driven health care reform and some of the recurring beliefs and pitfalls surrounding the establishment of cost-effective, quality programs. ▲

Managed health care (MHC) has, if nothing else, stimulated thought, conversation, conflict, and ethical debates from all corners of the nation. Opinions have been formed and viewpoints have been given, often by individuals yet to experience their first managed care organization. In response to the new phenomena, health care providers both large and small across the nation have invested a great deal of time and money in restructuring, downsizing, right sizing, and developing internal case management systems, even before seeing their first HMO patient—not a bad strategy, given that managed care primarily cut its teeth in the west, worked out many of its inherent idiosyncrasies, and is now rapidly expanding to the east. For the rest of the nation this means that when the wave of MHC arrives, it will take hold in a fraction of the time it took in the west and southwest and organizations not currently developing alternatives will have very little time to thoughtfully respond.

The eastward migration of managed care organizations (MCOs) is one indication that the current cost-containment mechanisms are not, as some had hoped, disappearing. Consequently, the continued development of comprehensive managed care and case management programs is imperative for any provider organization to compete in today's market. However, before appropriate systems of case management can be established, the architects of these plans must first develop a new knowledge base and entertain different ways of thinking about care planning, cost accountability, management, and multidisciplinary professional roles. To prevent confusion and reduce poor and/or automatic decision making, the forces driving MHC must be understood.

Shifting Priorities and Incentives

Health care has shifted from a discipline-driven to a service-driven model, and so have the incentives and priorities. Dozens of interviews across the country with employers, payers, primary care physician (PCP) groups, consumers, health care executives and managers, and clinical staff have afforded me the opportunity to interact with multiple organizations struggling with transition and change. From that interaction, recurring observations and themes have emerged, which have been all too often ignored, misunderstood, or simply not be-

lieved to be important in designing and building a case management system. Among those recurring themes are the following:

- Employers are cutting their health care costs and driving the change.
- The MHC market is price driven, and quality must be redefined and agreed on by all the stakeholders, not just the provider.
- The consumer of services (the person served) is becoming a sophisticated participant interested in outcomes, value, and cost.
- The value of a provider to a payer rests in its ability to achieve the best outcome at the right time, in the right place, and with the right team and/or person at the right cost.
- The focus of health care system leadership is to save and expand the business, not a specific discipline. *Any* discipline's future is directly related to the value it brings to the patient, the payer, and the business.
- Although MHC looks different from one marketplace to the next, the basic cost-based principles do not dramatically change.
- Mature MHC organizations are directing major resources to prevention, early detection, and health maintenance.
- Industrial-strength solutions that include widespread downsizing and redesign without individualization of the institution's needs and identified use of specific talent required for future planning yield organizations that are stripped of the human resources needed for the change process.
- Managed care and therefore the business of health care will not be successful if, in addition to physicians, the people delivering and clinically managing the care are not fully involved in MHC program development.

Transitioning to Managed Care
MAKING A SUCCESSFUL TRANSITION

To prepare for and successfully transition into managed care, organizations must have a well-thought-out plan. Everyone, including clinical staff, must understand the managed care conversion process. There are no overnight conversions or quick fixes; rather, it is a planned event. Preparation for managed care is the time to redesign for future needs and not past practices and not the time to downsize first and then decide what is needed. Cheaper is not always better, and organizations need mentors and appropriate strategies. To eliminate the most costly personnel may also mean the loss of vital expertise and may well prove to be short sighted and fatal to the organization. A clinical staff made up primarily of new graduates, who barely have any life experience, much less clinical experience, to draw on, frequently faces difficulty in performing in an environment that demands creativity and improvization rather than routinized and prescriptive strategies. Cost containment is often implemented as a short-term "staff efficiency" model with little or no thought to the long-term costs or needs of the patient.

BARRIERS TO TRANSITION

Barriers to successful transition into managed care are to be expected, and several are universal nationally. Although many institutions are vigorously working to develop managed care or case management systems, many fail to recognize the importance of integrating their internal systems and talent toward creating comprehensive management programs. Contract information is often withheld from those developing the resource management approaches, such as clinical pathways or systems of case management. This results in costly, uncoordinated efforts that ultimately do not address the needs of the customer or the consumer. It is not uncommon for the Director of Managed Care to be unfamiliar with comprehensive case management principles and to define the process as the monitoring of resource utilization. Many health care executives seem to believe, and have expressed, that if physicians just "did their job right," there would be no need for case management at all. In the meantime, many nonphysician clinicians are so caught up in trying to control acute care medical practice that insufficient time is being devoted to developing the long-term goals of managed care, all of which take place beyond the hospital walls.

The reality is that changes in physician practices have positively affected resource utilization, and medical groups are managing those aspects themselves. However, the fact that the physician has become more efficient and cost conscious with procedures and medications does not necessarily mean that his or her newfound insight and effectiveness are automatically transferred to the patient. A recent example exemplifies what staff who are responsible for patient education and case management have known for years: just because the doctor ordered the medication does not mean the patient received it. A case in point is presented in Box 2-1.

The nonclinical managed care leader or the health care executive would not imagine the scenario presented in Box 2-1, and the physician was comfortable that he had acted appropriately. However, the case manager would view this as one of many situations patients face once they are home trying to manage their own care and health needs. Nobody was pulling it all together and factoring in the intervening social issues. Technically this patient's care met standards of practice, but the reality for him and many others is that "life's little nuances" frequently alter the best-laid plan. As long as each segment of the health care team works in isolation from the others, true integration and coordination of all aspects of care and maximizing of cost effectiveness will continue to be incomplete.

A major element that often keeps internal systems from collaborating with each other is a breakdown of communication and trust. Clinical staff have not grown up in the fiscal world and frequently do not understand what it takes for health

---

BOX 2-1
Exemplar of Perceived Patient Care Coordination

A cardiac patient was having increased trouble with heart failure even though he had recently seen his doctor. The physician could not understand why this man was having such difficulty, because the appropriate medication had been prescribed. Review of the patient's pharmacy profile revealed that in fact the patient had never received the medication. Follow-up uncovered that the medication had been too expensive but the patient had not wanted to say anything to the physician so he simply had not had the prescription filled.

systems to be successful as a business. However, the assumption that clinically based persons cannot learn about finance, and that fiscally oriented people cannot learn to appreciate and value the clinical contribution to managing costs, is wrong thinking. Without a meaningful dialogue, the strength of each of these groups will never be understood and incorporated into the long-term strategies. It is time for everyone to give up territories and labels (e.g., "bleeding-heart clinicians," "bean-counting executives"), get over biases, and get to the table. Without internal understandings and integration of all the available expertise, the next step of establishing those critical external relationships and successes will not be fully realized.

Equally important is the recognition of the issues that divide the payer and the provider in the early stages of their managed care relationship. First and foremost is that same issue of trust. The payer perceives the care delivery system to be overutilizing services, and the provider believes rationing of care is the motivating force behind most health plans. Getting beyond this barrier is often emotional and difficult. What clearly must be understood is that it is not in the best interest of either party for the other to fail. They need one another, and the sooner a common understanding can be established, the faster a mutually beneficial partnership can be reached.

Processes Surrounding Managed Care

Cutting costs, efficiency, innovation, and appropriate care are hallmarks of a managed health care system. The employer demands the change, the payer sets the conditions, the PCP accepts the risk, and the health care system accepts some risk, and adapts to provide service to the customer (employer), the purchaser (payer), and the consumer (patient). So what is it exactly that the health system must do to compete and serve? First and foremost is to accept the changes described here and throughout the managed care literature. Denial has possibly been the single greatest deterrent to change. Phrases such as "patients won't buy this," "no one's going to tell me how to practice," or "we won't let them into our community" all translate

into "I don't want to change." The evidence is undeniable; the tidal wave of managed care is coming, there are no protective domes over any community, and time is marching on.

Some would argue that they have moved well beyond this point and have implemented advanced practice models, shared governance, case management, and any number of other empowered, integrated approaches. Indeed, all of these important steps have moved many health care systems toward more cost-effective, integrated networks of service delivery with case management as part of the cost-reduction strategies. What must be examined, however, is the relationship of the case management system to the financial "risk" that has been assumed, or is about to be assumed, by the health care system. Have the newly developed cost management programs adequately factored in the type and level of reimbursement available to the patient being served, or are they generic solutions that will not hold up to scrutiny or cost accounting over time?

Initial investments in case management models or tools must be evaluated in light of changing reimbursement mechanisms. Many organizations continue to serve Medicare as their dominant payer and believe that gearing up for managed care will jeopardize the current revenue streams. At the same time, these same providers may have either established their case management systems without regard to available resources or used traditional utilization management to establish a generic cost-containment strategy. This approach continues to apply specific Medicare regulations related to bed assignments, lengths of stay, and eligibility requirements for skilled nursing and home health care to a customer who is not interested is such regulations, but rather is incentivized to move the patient much faster, to the least costly level of care, at the earliest possible moment. Organizations that have adopted the plan not to "change to managed care" until the last possible moment may not be actively positioning themselves to transition into this new market. This is a dangerous strategy that can be easily viewed by the payer community as naïve or unresponsive. Payers are actively seeking partnerships with health care systems that are sensitive to their needs and willing to negotiate, share risk, and build cost-effective and/or efficient health care delivery services.

Basic Managed Care

Although this chapter is not intended to be MHC 101, there are a few points that may assist the novice in thinking about managed care strategies. Preferred provider organizations (PPOs) are managed health plans that offer subscribers several choices from panels of physicians and hospitals, which are usually reimbursed by a fee-for-service (FFS) mechanism. Different plans offer various arrangements, but typically the patient will pay 10% to 20% of the total cost. PPOs are currently the dominant type of MHC plan in the marketplace. Health maintenance organizations (HMOs) offer prepaid physician and hospital services, members generally have fewer choices, and the out-of-pocket expense to patients is minimal. HMOs are growing at a rapid rate across the country, with penetration having increased most in large markets (population more than 1,000,000). An estimated 72% of all enrollment growth has occurred over the past three years (Hamer, 1997). Although HMOs have advanced slowly in some markets, businesses are particularly interested in moving in this direction because costs are more predictable and these plans are less expensive to the employer. HMOs are moving toward "open access," or more choice, for the subscriber to attract more members.

Related to aggressive managed care plans are the methods of reimbursement and the shifting of financial incentives and increased risk to medical groups and health care systems. Although PPOs tend to use fee-for-service reimbursement arrangements, HMOs use FFS and capitation as substitutes for each other (Hamer, 1997). PCP groups are entering into capitated relationships at a significantly faster rate than health care systems or medical specialists, which potentially puts all of them at odds with one another over referrals, utilization, and incentives. The desire and need for PCP groups is to establish relationships with health care partners who will share in the risk and participate in the behavior necessary to conserve resources.

Reimbursement Mechanisms and Incentives

The specific reimbursement methods that may be in place at one time are not difficult to understand, and knowledge of this information is essential to best provide for each patient's short-term clinical needs and long-term health management programs. Although attention must be paid to maintaining the security of important contract relationships, innovative ways to share information about patient benefits with treatment staff can be found. Providers of acute rehabilitation services have for years made specific benefit information available to the treatment team to assist them in focusing care planning and clinical treatment within the individual patient's allowable resources. This strategy gives the staff the information they need to prioritize care and to plan for the delivery of services, and the allocation of resources, across the continuum. The most common reimbursement arrangements are percent discount, per diem, and capitation and case rates.

PERCENT DISCOUNT

The first MHC reimbursement mechanism is a system of percent discount off of charges. Because this is used in a fee-for-service payment system, every procedure or test ordered is billed separately at the regular charge but is paid for at a prearranged percentage discounted rate. The incentives to the care provider include prolonged lengths of stay and high volumes of diagnostic tests and clinical procedures. This is not the arrangement of choice for most payers, as it is difficult to project and control costs over time. Insurance-based case management closely monitors the medical necessity for all orders in these cases.

PER DIEM

Per diem simply translates into a set daily amount that typically includes all nursing care, room and board, tests, procedures, and therapies in a single payment rate. Per diem rates are also fee-for-service arrangements, and the incentive to the provider is once again to keep the patient a few days longer. This is particularly true for complex cases in which the negotiated daily rate is the same for the entire stay. The cost of care for any given patient is typically the highest in the first few days of hospitalization or outpatient care. That is frequently the period for maximum intensity of involvement, including evaluations, tests, and early interventions. When the per diem rate is too low, there is a tendency on the part of the health care system to keep the patient a few days longer than medically necessary in order to recoup any losses. Additionally, when the provider system is utilizing a clinical pathway that calls for a longer length of stay than coverage allows, conflict and mistrust arise among the stakeholders. The payer case manager may control costs through allocation of days or length of stay.

To help mediate this issue, many per diem contracts now include graduated or "front-loaded" arrangements that allow for realistic cost-based care and step the rate down as the patient's condition improves. Architects of clinical pathways must be sensitive to the allowable benefits for specific conditions and/or procedures so that costs and pathways can be properly aligned.

CAPITATION AND CASE RATES

The third payment mechanism is cost based, and the incentive to the provider is now to conserve services so as not to use up all its financial reserves too soon. Capitation and case rates are the two most common cost-based methodologies, and are based on predetermined payment arrangements. Capitation, simply stated, is a negotiated fee that does not change, determined on a per-member-per-month formula for a group of subscribers over a specific period of time. The provider is responsible for all agreed-on care for the duration of the contract period. In the strictest sense, if the money runs out, there are no additional funds available and the provider remains responsible. Hence the concept of "risk." The incentives are now reversed. Every day in the hospital, every diagnostic test ordered, and every procedure performed take money out of the organization's risk pool. If the fee was established on inaccurate cost data, or staff delivering care have no idea about costs, the pool can be depleted before the contract period ends. Case rates are based on episodes of care, rather than on care over time; the same cost principles apply. Diagnosis-related groups (DRGs) are case rates, and many payers are now calling these specific commercial arrangements DRGs.

The cost-based incentive is the point where the clinical team becomes particularly stressed and distressed. Without previous experience with capitation or case rates, care planning often continues as usual without regard for the cost of the plan of care or the presence or lack of benefits available to a particular client. In addition, planning care for patients who share the same diagnosis but are represented by multiple payers with different levels of benefits can throw the clinical team into major conflict. This situation has been known to deteriorate further as the organization's financial reports indicate costs that are too high.

Cost-based strategies invite a different way of planning and delivering care. Unlike discounted and per diem rates, which provide a specific dollar target, cost-based plans take an average of all the projected needs and costs. Because these plans base treatment on specific patient need instead of the dollars available, some patients will use fewer resources while others will require more. Through the use of cost-progressive continuums, patients are moved to less costly care settings as soon as possible, where services formerly offered in a hospital environment may now be provided. Lack of a specific postacute program within a given health care system does not necessarily warrant a patient remaining in a more costly setting. A rule of thumb is that if a patient does not require 24-hour nursing care, then he or she does not need to be hospitalized, at any level of care. While some payers see the wisdom of continuity provided in a single system of care, others are not convinced. Given that there are always exceptions to the rule, it still holds that in large metropolitan areas, alternatives to inpatient stays are available in one health care system or another. If the first care setting does not have all parts of the care continuum, there may be an expectation that the patient will be moved to a less expensive setting as soon as possible, even if it belongs to a competitor.

Outcomes

When outcomes of care are considered, it is common to consider the use of HEDIS, UDS, SF-36, and various other commonly used measures. A particular measure used by MCOs to evaluate cost effectiveness is the number of days that patients are in hospital beds, which is expressed as bed days per 1000 lives. A drop in the number of days indicates that cost management strategies are working. Monitoring systems for bed days and many other activities are available, and national benchmarks have been established. The number of bed days has continued to drop in mature MHC markets, particularly when risk relationships exist. What is unclear is the degree to which clinical outcomes are sustained over time and whether the care and support delivered in postacute settings adequately meet the needs of those served. Most cost controls are targeted directly on acute care utilization in systems, which often lack integrated, well-developed care or case management programs in the community. The results of acute care cost containment raise the question "When is enough, enough?" How far can inpatient costs be reduced without comprehensive, sophisticated postacute services in place to monitor and support hospital intervention? Well-established community-based approaches can reduce the patient's risk for increased complications and consequences, and help hold the costs down if further care is required. However, the focus on physician practices and the reduction of bed days may have significantly stunted the growth of long-term, cost-effective community-based alternatives. For example, recently in a small medical center, 28 capitated patients were discharged and readmitted to the hospital in 30 days. The bed days in this institution fall below the national average, and every affiliated medical group is capitated. This readmission rate was so dramatic that the question of "have we gone too far" was raised. The good news was that the information system and a highly experienced case manager recognized the situation in real time, and the case manager was able to evaluate each circumstance immediately. One of the questions raised was the ability of PCPs to adequately manage acutely ill patients in the hospital. Early findings in the case cited here were that some waited too long before calling in the specialist, a decision that could cost them money.

Innovations

A recent innovation targeted at primary care provider productivity and quality of care issues is the role of the "hospitalist." These specialty-trained physicians provide all episodic care to patients while they are hospitalized. The PCP refers a patient for admission, and the care is turned over to the hospital specialist. At discharge the PCP resumes care accountability. For the patient who is uncomfortable with a complete lack of contact with the PCP, or who may wish to have his or her private physician participate in care management, flexible

alternatives ranging from "social rounds" to complete inpatient care can be negotiated. Nurse practitioners (NPs) are also managing specific inpatient populations, such as neonatal groups, while hospitalized. The positive effects of these arrangements include a reduction in travel and time required for rounds, which can save the PCP several hours a day to see patients in the office. The hospitalist, who may have multiple board certifications, and the NP who has specialized in a specific area are typically more experienced in working with large numbers of similar types of patients and diagnoses, and may be more current than the PCP with successful interventions. It is interesting to note that the case management staff evaluating the previously discussed 28 hospital readmissions expressed the view that a "hospitalist program probably would have helped" their situation.

Another innovation that makes incredible sense and reaches far beyond the acute care walls is "population-based risk identification" (risk ID). As groups assume more financial risk, they also identify the need to reduce the cost of care over time. For some time insurance carriers have identified their financial risk by reviewing their actuarial data for past experiences and by screening subscribers for risk factors.

In recent years similar strategies have been developed by provider organizations to determine the best utilization of staff and clinical resources and to identify the long-term health needs of groups of people. The approach developed by the National Chronic Care Consortium (NCCC) is population-based risk identification. "Risk ID is an ongoing process aimed at enabling health care providers to identify and manage the health risk of consumers and prevent disability or delay further deterioration. Risk identification can be comprehensive, spanning issues of health promotion and wellness, as well as chronic disease, illness, and disability. Risk identification can also be specific, identifying a person at risk of using high-cost acute and long term care services" (Paone, Iverson, 1995). It supports the management of resource allocation over time and allows for the prediction of care and costs over a period of years rather than months. Three levels of risk are identified in the strategy: primary, which is the prevention of disease and includes lifestyle choices such as smoking, diet, riding motorcycles, or cliff diving; secondary, which is defined

---

BOX 2-2
Levels of Risk

Primary
The prevention of disease, including lifestyle choices such as smoking, diet, riding motorcycles, or cliff diving

Secondary
Early detection, such as by mammograms, carotid artery angiograms, and diabetic screenings

Tertiary
The adequate management of an episode of care

---

as early detection such as by mammograms, carotid artery angiograms, and diabetic screenings; and tertiary, which is the acute management of an episode care.

Unlike many insurance methods, this model goes well beyond just the financial risk and includes an in-depth look at the accompanying clinical demands and opportunities for education and prevention. For the provider-based case management system, it provides the opportunity to align the skills of multidisciplinary staff with appropriate patients. Patients at high risk for medical issues clearly require the expertise of the nurse, while those with few medical problems but major social barriers can be effectively case managed by a social worker. This approach has enormous potential for bridging existing communication and relationship gaps between payers and providers. As provider organizations assume more risk, evaluation and adoption of this methodology should be considered.

Conclusion

This discussion has touched on a few of the issues surrounding managed care. The jury is still out on the long-term effects of MHC, and for some the verdict is uncertain. Many would suggest that a return to the "way we were" is the only course, some want to call in the law, and still others think the nation is on the right track. Legal opinions and legislative ac-

tion will focus attention on the issues but will not solve the problems. Many of the obvious, or at the very least probable, solutions have yet to be tried. In too many settings, the value that multidisciplinary professionals bring to the process is yet to be fully recognized and utilized, although gains are being made.

Whatever the reasons, the full potential of cost-managed health care, in an environment that still demands significant individual patient choice, remains untested. Opportunities to demonstrate just how powerful a system of care it can be, remain. Patient support programs like case management must include outcomes that go far beyond lengths of stay and bed days. Evidence-based outcomes that include not only cost information, but patient function, self-care capacity, access to services, recidivism, and service utilization outside the acute care setting must be captured.

Perhaps the single most important question that all the stakeholders need answered is, "Does everyone really care about what happens to the patient?" A difficult notion for many to reconcile when what they see before them is a focus on business rather than care. These are the roads yet to be traveled and the conversations waiting to unfold. Managed care is not going away. The early iterations of HMO and/or PPO implementation continue to be revised and fine tuned. Has everything been done to ensure that a comprehensive system of care is in place? Absolutely not! The process of change has just begun. It is now time to move beyond the MCO, the physician, and the hospital and to tap more fully into the other, multidisciplinary expertise available. Quality care and profitable bottom lines are not mutually exclusive, but the blending of these goals requires that all the players who are ready to contribute and have the expertise to create better ways come together, begin to understand and accept one another, and build a total system of care.

References

Hamer L: *The InterStudy competitive edge part III: regional market analysis 7.1*, St Paul, Minn, 1997, InterStudy.

Paone D, Iverson LH: *Risk identification: exploring a conceptual framework and identifying implementation issues*, Bloomington, Minn, 1995, National Chronic Care Consortium.

CHAPTER 3

Consumer Voice

From Whimper to Roar

LINDA F. GOLODNER

OVERVIEW

Although it may seem foreign to those with a restrictive scientific education, there is a need for subjective thinking to accept the consumer as part of decision making.

The voice consumers have in the health care system is shaped by a variety of forces. Today, a plethora of helpful information is available through technology as well as the popular press. In addition to traditional health care, consumers must be cognizant of health claims for alternative medication and nutrition. With data collection and improved electronic data interchange in the health care industry, the risk of violating a person's right to privacy increases. ▲

The expectation of any consumer is that the outcome of care will be excellent—that is, that the consumer will get better or feel better after a medical intervention. Unfortunately, achieving the desired outcome can be a harrowing experience. Consumers hope for a rosier future.

Few are spared the pain caused by trying to navigate today's health care system. Some, such as the elderly, the poor, and the disabled, often feel the pain more sharply. But we all pay for the system's problems by being completely frustrated with seemingly unnecessary administrative procedures, being the victim of an error or mistake, or feeling the sting of the heavy costs. Some in fact have to forgo medical care or give up wage increases to pay for the escalating costs of employer-provided health insurance. If consumers cannot pay for care or have to delay care, favorable outcomes are surely affected.

Managed care organizations are very aware that to operate in the black there are at least three variables to control—the benefits provided, the amount consumers pay, and the income providers receive—or a combination of all three. Managed care organizations can also control the amount of time a physician spends with each patient, institute a formulary for prescription medications, and limit the use of specialists and the number of visits per patient. It all works out very neatly on paper for the accountants and for those making bottom line decisions. But it can go awry when a consumer cannot get the medicine that works or is denied needed specialist care for a child or mother, resulting in an outcome that might be devastating for the patient. It is this system, or lack of a system, that can affect outcomes as much as a competent or incompetent health professional. But it is the "human factor" (i.e., a lack of adequate care for the patient) that forces the system to listen more carefully to the consumer voice.

How did we get to where we are in health care? What did our grandparents and our fathers and mothers do when they got sick? Before the 1930s, patients were cared for by family, often with the aid of the local family doctor. Consumers paid for care directly or went to a public hospital, charity hospital, or clinic. America's system of private insurance began in the 1930s. With the advent of World War II, unions could not bargain for strong wage increases in the face of government wage controls. They turned instead to employer-supported, nonwage benefit packages, including health benefit plans.

The Changing American Family

There has also been a change in the needs and expectations of the American family. For many years, the typical family was depicted as a father at work and a mother at home with the children. Today mothers of infants and toddlers make up the fastest-growing segment of the workforce. Eighty percent of working women are likely to become pregnant during their working lives, and half of those women will return to work within a year of childbirth (US Department of Labor, 1996). The issues of caring for children and ensuring health care coverage are workforce and family issues. These issues have also contributed to the change in the profile of the typical health care consumer—that is, someone who wants information and service fast and does not have time to deal with a system that is not responsive to the demand for quality, convenience, and affordable care.

A Plethora of Information

To a large extent, the consumer voice has traditionally been silent. The gatekeeper, who is most often the fee-for-service physician, liked it that way. The consumer also liked it that way. Today, there is a brand new playing field for both the consumer and the health care professional. A plethora of information (probably too much information) is available to help the consumers play their new role as responsible partners to ensure good health. This role, however, is not clearly defined, and certainly the responsibilities are not explicit to most consumers or health care providers.

Consumers obtain information on healthy lifestyles, diseases, conditions, and treatments through newspapers, magazines, radio, television, and the Internet, and even through lectures and seminars at the local community center, church or synagogue, or health club. Those who have the resources (i.e., time and money) are using interactive video, CD-ROM, and the Internet (i.e., surfing the more than 10,000 health-related web sites) to help make medical decisions. There are home monitoring devices to measure blood pressure and blood glucose level and to self-test for pregnancy or cholesterol level.

Companies are even pressuring the Food and Drug Administration (FDA) to switch lipid-lowering drugs from prescription to over-the-counter. Report cards are available on health plans, hospitals, and physicians and can help consumers make decisions. However, consumers must have good tools for good decision making. Some private purchasers are encouraging greater consumer responsibility for use of the system by offering more options, through cost sharing, and participation in choosing a plan. Choosing a health plan or deciding which doctor to visit is one thing, but are consumers going to be playing a greater role in the diagnosis and treatment of conditions? Are health care professionals receptive to this invasion into their territory? Are the traditional decision makers going to share the role?

The future direction of health care policy is bound to be forged by these current private sector initiatives, but policy also will be profoundly influenced by outside pressures such as the use of technology, the culture of media and commercial influence on decision-making, and new controls that consumers will insist on, such as protecting privacy and exercising freedom of choice. All will result in patients and health care providers jointly making health care decisions, including diagnosis and choosing the appropriate treatment plan.

Whether consumers are ready to have a voice in their own health care decisions does not seem to make a difference, at least for those in the pharmaceutical industry. Recently companies have advertised directly to the consumer in the daily newspaper, magazines, and the broadcast media. In August of 1997, the FDA issued a proposed guidance to clarify its rules on direct-to-consumer promotion in television and radio (Department of Health and Human Services, 1997). Why did the pharmaceutical industry spend $600 million in 1996, a number that may approach $1 billion in 1997, to reach out to a new customer (Ono, 1997)? Perhaps because it is the first to recognize that the consumer voice will help shape the future health care system.

Policy Consequences of Increased Consumer Participation

Managed care organizations are beginning to recognize that their customer is not the placid, dependent patient of yesteryear. The new customer comes armed with health care information, demands better service and open communication with health care professionals, and expects to be a member of the team, a team to "make me well under my terms." Consumers generally do not think caregivers provide enough information. They also do not feel that health care professionals involve them in decisions about care and that the system's gatekeepers set up too many barriers for them to be full partners. A 1996 report by the American Hospital Association and the Picker Institute (1996) says: "More than one in every five clinic or office patients (21%) said that they were not as involved in decisions about their care as they wanted to be; and at least one in every three hospital patients (36%) reported not having enough to say about their treatment."

Consumers often are not getting what they are paying for. There is a growing consensus that a significant proportion of medical care is inappropriate, excessive, and even harmful. This affects both the quality and the cost of medical care. What resources and information are currently available to consumers on health care quality? It is all there if you are educated, highly motivated, and have a lot of time. You have to know where to look, have access to resources, and stamina. But how many people know to look in the *Physician's Desk Reference* to check on medications they are taking? How many people read *JAMA* or the *New England Journal* weekly to find out the latest research findings? How many people even go to the doctor with a list of questions, and how many get them answered and get phone calls returned as a follow-up? How many people even know the questions to ask or know where to research the most qualified and compassionate physicians and the best hospitals and medical facilities, or even how to take medications or just what to expect when taking a new drug or trying a new therapy? How many sort through their insurance policies or the reams of paper sent to them by their managed care organizations to determine what is covered? How many sort through to determine what is *not* covered? Very few.

Unfortunately, most consumers get their information only from news reports, haphazardly from their pharmacists, or from medication labels or patient package inserts. They might glance at their health maintenance organization coverage when they first get it and probably when they need it, and most certainly when they are denied a claim. Colleagues, family, and friends tend to fill in the gaps when most consumers need advice or help.

There is no uniformity. There is no consistency. There is very little help in languages other than English or for those who have limited reading skills. What is the purpose of patient or consumer information on quality health care? Hopefully the answer is to improve health and outcomes of care.

These resources and information should do the following for consumers:

1. Information must empower consumers to make informed decisions about their own care. Empowerment must be for *all* consumers and not just those who can sort through reams of information. Patients should know enough to make informed choices in regard to medications, physicians, facilities, or refusing care.

2. Consumers should have as much information as they require for their individual needs. All alternatives should be explained.

3. There must be improved communication between consumers and health care professionals (e.g., physicians, nurses, pharmacists). The communication must be also be enhanced between those who administer health care plans and expect consumers to understand and use the plans effectively.

4. The simple transmission of information cannot be considered sufficient in itself. How the information is received and acted upon is integral to communication. Materials should be thoroughly tested for understanding on representative potential users, and refined.

5. Information must aid and encourage effective use of the system.

BOX 3-1
Comments From 1994 National Consumers League Focus Groups

- I want the information one-on-one, but then I want to read up on it later to help me to understand what's going on.
- I want to know the cost, what I am getting, that is, what the plan did not offer. I want to know how quick I can get an appointment. I want to know that everyone could go to any hospital to get the best of care from the finest of doctors. How easy is it to call them? Can I get through? Is a hotline for emergencies offered? Will the government have the compassion of the IRS and the efficiency of the post office?
- I am worried that rich people will have better services. I think we should have the same treatments and courtesy as a rich person.
- Make sure that all doctors use the same forms and that all the information is the same so we can compare the health plans. When it is too cumbersome, you just pick the plan that is less money. Then you aren't looking at the details. They should take complaints more seriously, even complaints about bedside manner.
- There should be one form. When I go to the hospital, they still go through the same paperwork over and over again.

- I would like to have a consumers report on the hospitals that report waiting time, quality of service, percentage of specialists, what kind of holistic feeling they have (i.e., whether they will have a philosophy about the whole person).
- What we are talking about is customer service. *You* need someone to be an advocate for you to be able to cut through the hidden agendas and the doctor's attitude.
- They have you when you have taken all your clothes off.
- It is really up to you. At the top, they talk the finest rhetoric in the world, and by the time it gets down to the street it is too convoluted and screwed up to understand.
- You should only have to take a day off from work to go to all the doctors. They should have the doctors all in one place for the tests and the examinations.
- Consumer information, consumer protection, and quality improvement programs must be accountable to the public, independent of providers and payers of health care, and free of potential conflicts of interest.

In 1994 the National Consumers League held several focus groups made up of old and young, professional and blue collar, racially and culturally diverse, some on Medicaid and others fee-for-service or in a managed care organization. The National Consumers League asked them, if they were in charge, what information consumers should have (Box 3-1).

If consumers are going to make informed choices, they need good, understandable information describing plan configurations, how the health care delivery system works, how to appeal a health care decision, how to resolve complaints, and how to contact a health ombudsman or counseling program.

Consumers also need to know the prices, benefits, and services of each plan option. The information should include descriptive and practical summaries presented in a comparative format. Armed with this information, consumers can then do their part in making an informed decision.

Privacy of Personal Health Care Data

With the emphasis on data collection and improved electronic data interchange in the health care industry, the risk of violating a person's right to privacy increases. Health care information contains extremely personal data about physical and mental medical history, conditions, and treatments. The collection, storage, handling, and transmission of individually identifiable health care data should in no way infringe upon a person's right to privacy.

What "privacy" is, and what it encompasses, is an individual concept. There may, in fact, be at least 250 million different notions of privacy in the United States alone. At least two types of invasion of privacy exist in regard to health care data collection and use—intrusion and misuse of personally identifiable information.

The first concept is rather easy to convey. Intrusion means violation of "the right to be let alone." This concept is very much a part of our national fabric. For example, the Bill of Rights limits the powers of the central government to certain clearly enunciated and defined areas of authority. Otherwise, the individual is left to his or her own devices or those of the state in which he or she resides. The myth of early America leans heavily on the pioneer

spirit, the notion that a family has to move on when it can see the smoke from a neighbor's chimney.

The other important form of invasion of privacy revolves around misuse of personally identifiable information, or "informational privacy" issues. This issue deals with the countless ways in which public and private organizations collect, store, use, and transfer to third parties the volumes of data pertaining to our finances, our persons, and our health. Although there are in fact no new issues in the right of individual privacy, there are emerging issues in the new technology currently on the market or poised for delivery, which give public and private organizations a tremendous "leg up" in their ability to collect, manipulate, and transfer data. Privacy concerns relate directly to the adaptation and use of that technology in databases containing personally identifiable information, including information about a person's health.

In defining the privacy issue, we rely on work done by the United States Privacy Protection Commission (1977) in the mid-1970s. The major concern, as stated by the Commission, is "information about individuals being collected for one purpose then used for another purpose without the knowledge and/or consent of the subject of that information." This can involve something as simple as the rental of mailing lists of people who have asthma to a company that has just received the go-ahead from the FDA to market a new medicine, or it can involve complex health care issues such as who should be made aware that an individual possesses a defective gene that may make him or her susceptible to cardiac disease and therefore likely not to live to full life expectancy. Does a drug company have a right to know who has asthma? Does an insurance company have a right to access personally identifiable information on genetic research?

What drives the privacy debate today is not just the arguments of privacy advocates versus those who demand a greater access to information. What also drives the debate is emerging technology and the dwindling power of the individual to curtail the flow of personal information. The nineteenth-century pioneer had only to pack up and move to cheap land farther west to maintain freedom from intrusion. Today's pioneer has no place to hide.

When the Privacy Protection Study Commission deliberated informational privacy issues in the mid-1970s, it envisioned a world in which computers would play a dominating role in our culture. It also predicted the emergence of the electronic smart card, which could be inserted into a machine anywhere in the world and reveal a person's health record. It envisioned a world in which complicated lists would become available to enable marketers to "target" likely purchasers of goods and services.

All of this has come about, and the Privacy Commission did not predict the half of it. Computer and telecommunications technology has advanced to the point where computers will do pretty much whatever we ask them to do. It is an age in which the ways in which we communicate with each other and about each other will profoundly affect the way we live and the way we understand our health care. Information can be transferred from a person's home in Montana to a physician in Idaho through the combination of high-density digital imagery and the person's own television monitor. A single microchip on a card can include an individual's entire credit record, medical history, educational background and achievements, and even faulty chromosomes.

The opportunities for misuse of the information contained in these so-called smart cards are difficult to quantify. One thing is clear: health care policy and outcomes of care will be in part driven by emerging technology. There is little we can do to stop it, and there little reason to try.

There are, of course, a host of legitimate uses for collecting, storing, and making data available to predict outcomes for a single patient or to decide what strategies work to produce favorable outcomes for several patients. Insurance companies would cease to insure if it were not possible to determine the best prospects for longevity and good health. However, invasion of personal privacy may curtail some of the legitimate uses and benefits. What is wrong with a pharmaceutical company knowing that you have asthma? The question is, whose business is it if you do?

This is the crux of the issue. Everyone acknowledges the need to collect data and use data for improved outcomes. The problem is that there is simply too much data out there, and it can get into the wrong hands. Public policy on privacy of one's own health records must be defined so that data are used to heal rather than harm the patient. The compromise lies not in trying to push back technological advance, but in taming the beast and making it work economically for all.

Improving Outcomes Does Not Depend Solely on Medical Interventions

Improving outcomes is dependent not only on a consumer's interaction with the health care system but also on what happens when the consumer leaves the hospital or the doctor's office and returns to work or back home. It means leading a healthy lifestyle through exercise, good nutrition habits, and controlling the use of substances that could lead to abuse. Americans do need change in their eating habits. Each year hundreds of thousands suffer from heart disease, stroke, or colon or breast cancer. People die prematurely and needlessly because they have consumed too much fat, sodium, or cholesterol, or have not had enough fiber. The scientific community has conducted hundreds of studies that link fat or salt or fiber to public health.

In response to the need for clear, comprehensive food labels to help consumers make appropriate choices in the supermarket, the most extensive food labeling proposal in U.S. history was passed by Congress in 1990. In January of 1993 the FDA (1993) published 3000 pages of regulations that affect virtually all foods sold in grocery stores, comprising more than 80,000 types of food and almost 300,000 food labels. Claims are permitted if there is scientific proof to back them up.

To marketers, "healthy" is a lucrative buzzword to lure consumers to try their products and services. Increasingly under fire for their often unfounded use of such nutritional claims as "light," "organic," "fresh," "low fat," and "cholesterol free," food processors turned to another adjective—"healthy." They put the word "healthy" on everything from soup to nuts to pizza.

"Healthy" is unique among nutrition descriptors and conveys a positive message about *all* of the key nutrients in a food product; its power as a marketing tool dwarfs all other individual nutrient content claims. The National Consumers League (1992) commissioned a national survey to determine just how this powerful word influenced consumers in making very important nutrition choices. It found that people do read labels. Eighty-eight percent reported that they read them at least some of the time; only 12% said they never do. Although a relatively small percentage said they specifically look for the term *healthy* on packaged food products, the survey showed that its presence on the label can nonetheless be a powerful motivator for consumers to buy the product. Nearly three out of five people (i.e., 59%) said they would be likely to choose one product over another simply because this word was on the box.

This survey confirmed that consumers often make purchasing decisions in response to messages that appear on labels or claims in advertisements seen in magazines and on television. Unfortunately, oftentimes free pamphlets, government public service announcements, and well-meaning warnings are overlooked by consumers. Consumers expect "someone" to be monitoring advertisements to ensure that they are not false and misleading. They expect "the government" to be looking out for the best interest of the public, to make sure that claims and labels are clear and truthful and understandable.

Understanding and Trying to Achieve Quality of Life for Every Patient

Health care practitioners many times confine their practice to objective criteria when reaching a diagnosis and prescribing care and providing treatment for a patient. Although it may seem foreign to those with a restrictive scientific education, there is a need for subjective thinking to accept the consumer as part of decision making. This includes understanding the perspective of the consumer, especially his or her quality of life. The quality of anyone's life is an individual perception. How to identify that quality cannot be found in textbooks or the scientific literature. It can be determined only by talking to the individual or a caregiver who is responsible for another person, such as a child, a disabled individual, or an elderly person. Only the patient can help health professionals understand that a certain therapy or medicine just does not fit into the work or family schedule. Only the individual can explain that surgery is just not an acceptable alternative or that chemotherapy is not wanted. Only the individual can make the determination whether an out-of-pocket cost for a specialist can be part of the family budget this year. Only the patient can make the decision to choose hospice instead of an alternative way of dying.

Some health professionals are trying to come up with questionnaires to measure quality of life. But according to Leplege and Hunt (1997), "Most of the currently used questionnaires do no more than force patients to address themselves to the concerns of physicians and/or social scientists and statisticians, and many require lay people to adopt professional artifices invested to fit particular theories." The authors recognize the difficulty of addressing cross-cultural issues with standard questionnaires. "Attempts to adapt questionnaires for use in more than one culture have, too often, paid scant attention to the subtleties of cultural diversity; such a failing is all the more accentuated if one considers that cultural diversity exists not solely between but also within countries" (Leplege, Hunt, 1997). Quality of life is a fragile issue that health professionals must address and that consumers themselves must address each time there is a change in their own health regimens.

The voice consumers have in shaping the health care system will be shaped by a variety of forces. Probably the greatest influence will be how quickly and willingly health professionals accept the consumer as a partner in care.

References

American Hospital Association, The Picker Institute: *Eye on patients: a report from the American Hospital Association and The Picker Institute,* American Hosp Assn, Chicago, 1996.

Food and Drug Administration: *Draft guidance for industry, consumer-directed broadcast advertisements, availability,* Washington, DC, (Docket No. 97D-0302), 1997, Department of Health and Human Services.

Food and Drug Administration: *Federal Register* (vol 58, no 3, CFR parts 5 and 101), January 1993, Department of Health and Human Services.

Leplege A, Hunt S: The problem of quality of life in medicine, *Journal of the American Medical Association* 278(1):47-50, 1997.

National Consumers League: *Consumer attitude toward the word "healthy" on food packaging,* Washington, DC, February 18, 1992, Penn & Schoen Associates, Inc.

Ono Y: Magazines spar with television over drug ads, *Wall Street Journal,* p B1, October 20, 1997.

US Department of Labor: *Characteristics of families,* Washington, DC, 1996, US Government Printing Office.

US Privacy Protection Commission: *Report to the President and the Congress,* Washington, DC, July 1977, US Government Printing Office.

CHAPTER 4

The Ethics of Case Management

The Quality/Cost Conundrum

Sr. CAROL TAYLOR, RN, PhD, CSFN, **and ROBERT J. BARNET**, MD, MA

OVERVIEW

An important element of ethical competence for health care professionals is the ability to critique changes in the way we design, deliver, and finance health care in light of their human consequences.

Many now suggest that what managed care is really about is managing costs, not care. Health care professionals increasingly worry that their integrity is being sacrificed in systems in which the commitment to quality is all but eroded. This chapter explores the case manager's ethical obligation to work to create a system of quality, affordable care that is accessible to all. It argues that the case manager's access to outcome data for specific population aggregates positions her or him uniquely to advocate for quality as costs are managed. The chapter challenges the assumptions that quality care is unaffordable in today's society and that quality and cost considerations are diametrically opposed. ▲

Hard as this may be to believe, it seems that the Wicked Witch of the West recently waved her wand over the American health care system while health care professionals and the public were all fast asleep in their beds. Nothing has been the same since. According to this popular fairytale, the wicked witch cast a horrible spell on all the competent and caring clinicians who once spared no financial or personal expense to secure valued patient outcomes. Suddenly clinicians were all pawns of an evil giant who cared nothing for patients and who had an insatiable hunger for gold. Patients, reclassified as "covered lives," were valued only to the extent that they generated revenues, "gold" for the giant. Time-honored health care services were quickly transformed into profitable product lines or terminated. Clinicians who resisted the giant were stomped out of existence, and those who survived sacrificed all notions of quality to the god of economics and cost analysis.

No competent health care analyst would accept the above fairytale as an accurate description of contemporary United States health care. There are far too many simplifications. Not all clinicians were competent, caring, and altruistic in the past, and certainly not all systems today are greedy and uncaring giants preoccupied with profit. Perhaps most important, today's negative changes were not forced upon us by a malicious being, and none of us can claim that we are not responsible, at least at some level, for the system being created. On the other hand, the recipients and providers of health care are concerned with good reason about the extent to which cost concerns are trumping quality concerns. According to a poll by the National Coalition on Health Care (1997), most Americans lack confidence in the "quality, cost and accessibility of medical care and the health care system overall." The telephone poll of 1011 households, conducted in December 1996 by International Communications Research, revealed the following:

1. Eight out of 10 Americans believe the quality of medical care is "being compromised in the interest of profit."
2. Seventy-nine percent of Americans believe quality care is unaffordable for average Americans.
3. Seventy-four percent of Americans believe hospitals "cut corners to save money."

4. Eighty percent of Americans believe that health insurers often compromise quality to "save money."

Only 4% of respondents expressed confidence that the health care system will take care of them, and only 15% have complete confidence in hospital care. To the extent that this survey is representative of the people we serve, our ethical mandate is clear.

The Quality/Cost Conundrum

In the not so distant past, it was taboo to introduce cost considerations into discussions about treatment options. Most health care professionals cannot remember ever learning about health care economics in their academic programs. We did learn that health is an essential good, necessary for the enjoyment of all other goods. It followed that no costs were too high when health was threatened. We came to believe, and successfully instructed the public to believe, that if a little health care was good, more was better. The reigning myth was that if health care professionals were only willing to work hard enough and to spend enough money, we could "fix" whatever "ailed" anyone. When you add to this picture a fee-for-service structure that financially rewarded doing more rather than less, an amazing lack of consensus (some would say "caprice and variability") about what ought to be considered appropriate intervention, and a sizable cohort of profiteers who were not adverse to fraudulently duping payers to reap exorbitant profits, it should surprise no one to find cost control central to reform efforts.

So why is it not only "OK" but even necessary for health care professionals today to be cost conscious? The most obvious reason is that the financial and other resources allocated to health care are limited, and we ought to be concerned about getting the best value for our dollar. Pressure to reform health care came from legislators trying to balance budgets and to fairly allocate spending for health care, education, defense, public safety, and other social goods. With health care spending consuming an ever greater percentage of the gross domestic product, it made sense to question unchecked health care spending and to demand greater accountability. The business sector similarly demanded reform as it watched a growing percentage of its revenues being committed to costly employee health benefits. As a consequence, health care systems committed to survival accepted the mandate of fiscal accountability. The problem for all is how to continue promoting quality in the midst of draconian budget cuts and bottom-line decision making. In other words, how do we keep the quality–cost control pendulum from swinging to the pole where quality is routinely and unquestioningly sacrificed for cost control? In a critical article on managed care, Zoloth-Dorfman and Rubin (1995) correctly, we believe, direct our attention to:

- Who is doing the managing?
- With what intention and goals (managed *care* versus managed *costs*)?
- Under whose authority?
- With what effect?

They write that the foundational questions we should all be asking are:

- How can people be assured that the quality of care they receive will not drop below a minimum quality of care and standard of safety?
- How can physicians, nurses, and other health care providers who work in managed care organizations be assured that their professional integrity will not be compromised by their being compelled to participate in care that they deem to be substandard?
- What incentives will managed care organizations have to maintain standards of quality care and safety when such standards may be expensive and such costs may be difficult to control?

Ethical Challenges for Case Managers

Case managers who take the questions listed in the previous section seriously face several key ethical challenges: challenging the new mind set, maintaining personal and professional integrity, and working smart to ensure quality outcomes. Strategies case managers can use to invite their colleagues to "own" and respond to these challenges accompany the following discussions.

CHALLENGING THE NEW MIND SET

An important element of ethical competence for health care professionals is the ability to critique changes in the way we design, deliver, and finance health care in light of their human consequences. While others use the lens of profit or liability or market advantage to evaluate decisions, health care professionals bring to decision-making tables the voices of the people who will be most directly influenced by the decisions being made. The lens we use is that of human well-being. Our obligation to secure the interests of those we have publicly professed to serve demands from us an untiring commitment to quality, affordable, accessible care. Thus, one of the first ethical challenges for case managers is questioning the conventional wisdom that reduces quality considerations to quaint, outdated, impractical concerns of idealistic individuals who somehow cannot "get the picture" that health care is a business today, a *big* business. Compare this attitude to that reflected in the Institute of Medicine's (1994) white paper, *America's Health in Transition: Protecting and Improving the Quality of Health and Health Care*, which issues a strong call for high standards of quality:

"As we try to provide adequate access to health care for all Americans and to reduce the future cost of care, we want also to ensure that we preserve and improve the quality of health care that the nation now enjoys. By enhancing the quality of health care we will also gain greater value for our health care expenditures. Quality-of-care concerns have often been set aside to tackle the seemingly more pressing problems of access and financing. The Council of the Institute of Medicine believes that quality-of-care matters must be given the same attention in policy and research as the other problems that have led us to the health care reform path on which the nation is now embarked. In fact, the quality of health care can be measured and quality measurement tools can be used to improve care and to help the health care transition succeed." (p. 1)

So how can case managers effectively nudge the "powers that be" within a system to make quality a high priority at all levels of decision making? At the very least, time and space must be created for everyone to reflect critically on the nature of health care and the moral obligations institutions and professionals assume when they make public promises. Unless we have a clear idea of what morally defensible health care looks like and a commitment to defend what we call "the nonnegotiables" of moral health care, it is easy to barter away the very goods that we have promised society and that legitimate our practice. Box 4-1 highlights what we take to be the nonnegotiables of moral health care. We invite readers to reflect on whether they would arrive at the same list of "nonnegotiables" and whether decision making in their institutions or systems is supportive of these elements. The next step is to create the time and space for dialogue about these concerns. The prevailing mind set that sacrifices quality for cost control will be successfully challenged when policies and decision making at all levels reflect a strong commitment to quality, affordable care for all.

Strategies for Case Managers

1. Instruct colleagues to make a list of the last five administrative decisions that have had the greatest impact on their practice. Invite them to analyze which of the following objectives were most likely behind these decisions:
   - To better serve the community
   - To improve quality of care
   - To enhance patient satisfaction
   - To increase revenues and/or decrease costs
   - To enhance efficiency
   - To affirm employee worth and express gratitude for services rendered

   Invite discussion on the following:
   - What does this reveal about the institution or system's values?
   - Is there a good match between the system's mission statement and everyday decision making?

BOX 4-1
Nonnegotiables of Moral Health Care

Just System of Health Care
- Views health care as an obligation of a moral society rather than a mere business commodity
- Ensures a basic, decent minimum of care for all
- Responsive to the needs of the most vulnerable members of society
- Distributes the benefits and burdens of care giving justly

"Patient-First" Orientation
- Commits system resources and professional competencies and will to an orientation that consistently puts patients first
- Demands the subordination of self-interest to the promotion of patient well-being when patient interests are at stake

Broad Notion of Health That Encompasses More Than Physiological Functioning
- Commitment to wholeness of being versus wholeness of body; to cure as *one* of the manifestations of care
- Commitment to quality of life that is multidimensional (i.e., physiological, emotional, social, and spiritual functioning) and subjective
- Range of therapeutic interventions to include more than the "technological fix," that is, com-

passionate presence, development of coping strategies that address problems related to life's meaning and purpose, and so on

Trusting Professional Relationships
Includes relationships among the health care system and the public-at-large; patients, families, and employees; and health care professionals and patients, families, and other health care professionals.

- Grounded in the system's and the health care professional's commitment to secure the patient's and/or society's health and well-being (i.e., fidelity to fiduciary responsibilities)
- Based on a respect for human dignity, which affirms the worth of everyone with whom one interacts
- Provide the individualized knowledge that guides collaborative efforts to achieve valued health outcomes

Clinical Competence
- Encompassing interpersonal, intellectual, technical, and ethical competencies
- Demonstrated ability to "work the system" to achieve valued health outcomes

- Do policies and decision making support the "nonnegotiables" of moral health care?
- Are you "comfortable" with the institution or system's values? If not, what do you plan to do about this?
- How can case managers as a group strategize to "transform the culture of care" within the institution or system?

2. Direct colleagues to list all the descriptors they can think of which they associate with being a *good* case manager. Next direct them to list the descriptors of a *successful* case manager in your institution or system. Then invite them to compare their lists, analyzing the values that underlie the descriptors they chose. Are there differences between what makes someone a "good" case manager and what makes one a "successful" case manager in your practice setting? If there is a discrepancy, how ought everyone respond?

MAINTAINING PERSONAL AND PROFESSIONAL INTEGRITY

Identifying and recommitting oneself to the nonnegotiables of moral practice will do little to assuage the guilt of case managers who find themselves practicing in systems that consistently make it impossible to offer quality care. In fact, this process will augment their guilt. The more clear one is about individual and collective professional moral obligations to the public, the more one's integrity is at risk if forces beyond one's control continually thwart quality initiatives. In the past it was suggested that integrity was impossible for nurses, social workers, and other nonphysician caregivers because they so frequently found themselves powerless to effect needed change. Today even physician integrity is threatened by a system that subjects physician decision making to payer review and approval. Philosopher Andrew Jameton (1993) terms the phenomenon of knowing the morally right course of action to take but being blocked from taking it by institutional structure and conflicts with other co-workers "moral distress." He counsels caregivers to be cautious about too quickly accepting a posture of powerlessness and recommends a series of reflection questions that we have slightly modified in the list that follows. Case managers who are finding it increasingly difficult to secure the quality outcomes to

which they are committed may find it helpful to reflect on the following questions:

- What is possible for me to do when I am troubled by deficient quality?
- Is trying to change bureaucratic practices an exercise in futility?
- If I invest time and energy, are large or even small changes possible?
- What is the extent of my responsibility?
- When do I have an obligation to challenge the status quo?
- Is there some way that I can collaborate with others to secure valued goals and needed change?
- Are there external resources we can tap to better ensure our success?
- Can our professional organizations provide valuable support or leadership?
- When others are not meeting their responsibilities, what is the extent of my/our responsibility to step in and to make up for their omissions?
- What personal risks are health professionals obligated to take for patients?
- Are we obligated to take career risks by speaking out for vulnerable populations?

There are two extreme responses to avoid when responding to these questions. One is to simply accept that one is powerless to effect necessary change, and the other is to assume unrealistic responsibility for outcomes that will never be effected. The first extreme perpetuates the status quo and mediocrity; the second leads quickly to burnout. Neither is capable of securing the type of quality care that the public both needs and wants. Case managers concerned about quality issues need to be careful not to concede the battle before it is begun: "Things have gone from bad to worse here and there is *nothing* we can do." One of our greatest challenges is nurturing the conviction that good, talented, and rightly motivated people *working together* can effect necessary changes. What is true is that the type of change that is needed will often be resistant to individual efforts. For this reason it is more crucial than ever before to collaborate with colleagues and to tap the resources of our professional organizations. Group discussion of problematic practice situations like those listed in strategy 2 (p. 32) will enable case managers as a group to evolve responsible courses of action. Ideally, actual practice scenarios can then be explored with the interdisciplinary team, management, and payers.

Strategies for Case Managers

1. Direct your colleagues to quickly write down the party or parties to whom they are primarily responsible. Then invite everyone to share their responses and explore the significance of the parties they identified: patients, families, community; employer (i.e., self, managed care organization, hospital, or other health care institution or system); health care team; self and family.
   - Does everyone identify the same parties, and do they rank these the same from most to least important?
   - Is there congruence between who they think deserves most of their time and energy and who is actually getting their time, energy, and best efforts?

   Use these findings as the springboard for a discussion about the conflicts they are experiencing as they attempt to meet their multiple responsibilities. Invite sharing of the strategies they have found useful as they attempt to do this. If the practice realities are such that more and more case managers are finding it impossible to meet their responsibilities to patients, or to themselves and their families, explore options to make the system responsive to their needs.

2. Use the following cases, or similar cases derived from your practice setting, to explore how case managers are responding when they experience conflicting demands. Focus on the interests of involved parties and the conflicts these interests create, their obligation to secure the interests of each party involved, and the variables that positively and negatively influence their ability to meet these obligations. "Walk through" different responses, and try to determine which course(s) of action best meet the needs of everyone. How can the team change to better support each case manager as she or he struggles with future conflicts? How should the system change to better facilitate the work of case managers?
   a. A case manager discovers that the managed care organization responsible for several children with cystic fibrosis is poorly equipped to manage the special treatment they and their families require. What are the responsibilities of the case manager? Does it matter if the case manager is an employee of the managed care organization or not?
   b. A hospital case manager learns that a young woman with AIDS who is well known to the hospital staff is being readmitted with new complications. The woman has requested to see her and to be admitted to a particular unit. The case manager, who is generally quite tolerant, "hates" this patient and has found each interaction with her in the past frustrating. She wants to protect the staff on the unit the woman requested because she likes this staff, believes they are already overburdened with their share of difficult patients, and has no desire to satisfy this woman's preferences. She is "sorely tempted" to have someone tell the woman she cannot meet her that afternoon and to ensure that she is admitted to a different unit.
   c. A community-based geriatric case manager is discovering that more and more of the older couples she meets are complaining about a new Medicare-managed care program. When they were recruited, they were promised that they would be eligible for the same services they were currently receiving under Medicare. Unfortunately, many are discovering that their requests for these services are being denied. These benefits exist on paper, but they have not been successful in securing them. Does the case manager have any obligations to these couples and to the community?
   d. At a regional meeting for geriatric case managers, discussion reveals widespread dissatisfaction with the services available for older adults. The hospital-based case managers are growing increasingly concerned with the diminishment of rehabilitation services that managed care organizations are allowing after a stroke. Case managers from the nursing homes are complaining that they also cannot get adequate coverage for the special treatment

needs of this population. "Government did something about women post-delivery and about mastectomy needs, but no one is going to bat for the elderly who are being deprived of necessary care." What do you consider to be an adequate professional response to this situation? Do the case managers have any obligations to the older adults in this community?

e. A managed care organization case manager visits a woman on her second postoperative day following removal of a grapefruit-sized abdominal tumor and orders her discharge because the woman is tolerating liquids and has been out of bed. The hospital case manager for this service has been briefed by the surgical attending that this woman needs an extended length of stay because the unusual size of the tumor and preexisting conditions place the woman at increased risk for postoperative complications. Unfortunately, the managed care organization is "not allowing exceptions."

f. A case manager from a university student health center is growing increasingly frustrated by the challenge of meeting the needs of a small group of students with serious mental health problems requiring frequent inpatient stays. The inpatient unit is complaining that they cannot get coverage for the inpatient treatment and monitoring that these students need and expects the student health center to "pick up the slack." The case manager believes these students to be at great risk for harm to themselves and others.

WORKING SMART TO ENSURE QUALITY OUTCOMES

The Institute of Medicine defines quality of care as the degree to which health services for individuals and populations increase the likelihood of desired health outcomes and are consistent with current professional knowledge (Lohr, 1990). It later identified three fundamental quality of care issues: use of unnecessary or inappropriate care; underuse of needed, effective, and appropriate care; and shortcomings in technical and interpersonal aspects of care (Institute of Medicine, 1994). We believe that case managers are obligated to play a vital role in addressing these issues and in securing valued quality outcomes for target populations. Case managers should routinely investigate the extent to which high-priority outcomes reflect a commitment to quality of life concerns. Quality of life experts continually remind us that quality of life judgments are multidimensional (incorporating physiological, mental, social, and spiritual functioning) and subjective. Their subjectivity (i.e., what constitutes a desirable or even acceptable quality of life can vary dramatically from one patient to the next) necessitates a great deal of flexibility in designing plans of care. Sadly, the current system is structured to meet the needs of hypothetical statistical persons ("this critical pathway will work for 90 percent of the people 90 percent of the time"), not real people who may in fact be outliers. Someone needs to question if outcomes are truly holistic and if they are responsive to the particular needs of individual patients. Case managers who take their ethical responsibilities to the public seriously understand that there is a profound ethical dimension to how health care outcomes are determined, funded, achieved, and evaluated.

Outcome Determination. Case managers ought to be concerned about who is determining valued structure, process, and patient outcomes, and about the process being used to determine these outcomes. Increasingly there are complaints that clinician input is undervalued and that some payers are actively seeking to limit clinician input. A related concern is the absence of consumer voices at the many tables where health outcomes are being deliberated and set. Equally troubling is the lack of consensus about the principles that should guide the deliberations about outcomes. In a collection of essays from *The Journal of the American Medical Association*, David Eddy (1996), senior advisor for health policy and management for Kaiser Permanente Southern California, recommended a set of 11 principles to guide debates over evidence and costs in organizations that must allocate shared or public resources to serve a defined population. His hope was that health care organizations would debate each of the following principles and either agree with them or develop better ones:

1. The financial resources available to provide health care to a population are limited.

2. Since financial resources are limited, when deciding about the appropriate use of treatments it is valid and important to consider the financial costs of the treatments.
3. Since financial costs are limited, it is necessary to set priorities.
4. A consequence of priority setting is that it will not be possible to cover from shared resources every treatment that might have some benefit.
5. The objective of health care is to maximize the health of the population served, subject to the available resources.
6. The priority a treatment should receive should not depend on whether the particular individuals who would receive the treatment are our personal patients.
7. Determining the priority of a treatment will require estimating the magnitudes of its benefits, harms, and costs.
8. To the greatest extent possible, estimates of benefits, harms, and costs should be based on empirical evidence. A corollary is that when empirical evidence contradicts subjective judgments, empirical evidence should take priority.
9. Before it should be promoted for use, a treatment should satisfy the following criteria:
   • There should be convincing evidence that, compared with no treatment, the treatment is effective in improving health outcomes.
   • Compared with no treatment, its beneficial effects on health outcomes should outweigh any harmful effects on health outcomes.
   • Compared with the next best alternative treatment, the treatment should represent a good use of resources in the sense that it satisfies principle No. 5.
10. Judgments about benefits, harms, and costs, to the greatest extent possible, should reflect the preferences of the individuals who will actually receive the treatments.
11. When determining whether a treatment satisfies the criteria of principle No. 9, the burden of proof should be on those who want to promote the use of the treatment.

More recently, Eddy (1997) proposed four ethical principles to apply in cost/quality trade-offs—fairness (equal consideration), equality (similar cases should be treated similarly), optimality (choice of treatments with best outcomes), and accountability (responsibility deriving from a promise or contract and requiring control/authority). We believe that the access case managers have to large population aggregates with complex and costly health needs enables them to play an important role in gathering the type of data that are necessary to make the types of judgments demanded in principles 7 through 11. This requires a commitment of case manager time and effort, but without this level of involvement we will never have the data to support quality-based outcomes.

Outcome Funding. The challenge for case managers here is to ensure that quality-based outcomes will be funded. This entails making the case that quality serves the bottom line. Reports are already coming in that short-sighted efforts to cut quality to generate a quick profit served programs poorly by increasing costly complications and by so lowering patient satisfaction that market share became compromised. If the only language that administration will hear is financial, health care professionals must be able to make the case for quality in financial terms. Although we still lack the type of data that would allow us to do this easily, these data are becoming available and case managers need to keep a portfolio that demonstrates all the benefits of quality.

Outcome Achievement. Unless the parties responsible for ensuring outcome achievement are designated, outcomes may exist only on paper. One of the responsibilities of case managers is working within the system to ensure that the right providers are all working together on valued outcomes. This often entails clarifying who is responsible for each outcome and developing mechanisms of accountability. All too frequently, no one assumes the coordination role. When Columbia Hospital in Milwaukee launched its Coordinated Care Program in 1993, it solved this problem by developing a *responsibility matrix* that not only provided a checklist of actions but also designated *primary responsibility* for each action. The responsibility matrix became an important educational tool as well as a communication tool that helped multidisciplinary teams understand the process of developing and implementing clinical pathways. An example of a coordinated care responsibility matrix may be found in the December 1996 *Journal of Nursing Care Quality* (Holst, 1996).

Outcome Evaluation. Quality reporting remains a challenge. Most managed care organizations continue to focus evaluation measures on cost, utilization, and member satisfaction. As late as 1995, a survey of 384 employers conducted for the Washington Business Group on Health revealed that only 29% of employers said they considered quality benchmarks when choosing a health plan for employees, compared with 97% who considered cost and 85% who considered service to employees. More recently, health care benefits managers appear to be losing faith in the ability of managed care companies, especially for-profit HMOs, to manage quality. In June of 1996 the Foundation for Accountability, a coalition of corporation and consumer groups, tried to move "an enormous trillion-dollar health care system in a more consumer- and patient-oriented direction." It endorsed a set of questions for health plans to answer that included things like the following (Freudenheim, 1996):

- How many breast cancer patients had no symptoms of cancer 5 years after diagnosis, and how many died?
- How many diabetics kept their blood sugar and cholesterol below unsafe levels, and how many avoided hospital stays?
- How many seriously depressed patients showed significant improvement within 6 months?

Case managers have a role to play in ensuring that both the recipients of care and health care benefits managers have available to them the type of quality benchmarks that allow wise decision making about care. Finally, case managers' commitment to continuous quality improvement must remain strong. Issuing a strong call for continuous quality improvement as an ideal in health care, Berwick (1989), a Harvard Community Health Plan physician, advocates the following:

1. Leaders must take the lead in quality improvement.
2. Investments in quality improvement must be substantial. In other industries, quality improvement has yielded high dividends in cost reductions, which may occur in health care as well.

3. Respect for the health care worker must be reestablished.
4. Dialogue between customers and suppliers of health care must be open and carefully maintained. Quality improves as those served and those serving take the time to listen to each other and to work out their inevitable misunderstandings.
5. Modern, technical, theoretically grounded tools for improving processes must be put to use in health care settings.
6. Health care institutions must "organize for quality." Furthermore, health care regulators must become more sensitive to the cost and ineffectiveness of relying on inspection to improve quality. In addition, professionals must take part in specifying preferred methods of care, but must avoid minimalistic "standards" of care. Quality-control engineers know that such floors rapidly become ceilings, and that a company that seeks merely to meet standards cannot achieve excellence (Berwick, 1989).

Strategies for Case Managers

1. Direct case managers to use the list below to check off what figures prominently in their reasoning as they plan care for a distinct population aggregate or individual. Instruct them to rank these in order of importance from most important (1) to least important (7).

   _____ Research clearly demonstrates that this is the best option for the condition(s) being treated

   _____ Availability of resources to execute this plan of care

   _____ Willingness of payers to reimburse for the proposed plan of care

   _____ Patient preferences dictate the plan of care

   _____ Convenience for providers dictates the plan of care

   _____ Experience demonstrates high level of patient and family satisfaction with this approach

   _____ Other: _____

Have case managers discuss with their colleagues whether what they actually do in practice is what they think they should be doing. If there are discrepancies, what do they plan to do about this?

2. The Institute of Medicine identified three fundamental quality of care issues: (1) use of unnecessary or inappropriate care; (2) underuse of needed, effective, and appropriate care; and (3) shortcomings in technical and interpersonal aspects of care. Have a meeting in which you invite case managers to do the following:

   a. Describe a recent patient situation in which you noted one or more of these problems.
   b. Think carefully about how you responded to your initial sense that something was wrong:
      - Tried to ignore your discomfort and pretend there is no problem.
      - Experienced the frustration of knowing that conditions are less than optimal but accepted that you are powerless to effect a solution.
      - Committed your best energies to attempting to bring about a resolution of the problem.
   c. Think through the consequences of the way you characteristically respond to problems with quality of care. Are your responses serving your patients well?
   d. Do you need to improve your response to problems with quality? If so, can you and your colleagues strategize about how best to do this?

Conclusion

Let us return to the fairytale that opened this chapter. It is certainly true that the public, with good reason, no longer trusts health care professionals to be committed to their well-being. Quality care is no longer the unquestioned goal of health care institutions and systems. But there is no magic wand or incantation forcing health care professionals to abandon their commitments to the people they have promised to serve. The choices case managers make in the context of each day's practice will play an important role in determining whether this tale will have a "happy ending." No competent case manager who values integrity can afford not to creatively challenge systems that are unresponsive to human need. Affordable quality care for all . . . fairytale or reality? The choice is ours.

References

Berwick DM: Continuous improvement as an ideal in health care, *The New England Journal of Medicine* 320(1):53-56, 1989.

Eddy DM: *Clinical decision making: from theory to practice*, Boston, 1996, Jones & Bartlett.

Eddy DM: Balancing cost and quality in fee-for-service versus managed care, *Health Affairs* 16(3):162-173, 1997.

Freudenheim M: The grading becomes stricter on H.M.O.'s, *The New York Times*, pp D1, D5, July 16, 1996.

Gold MR et al: *Cost effectiveness in health and medicine*, New York, 1996, Oxford.

Holst R: Responsibility matrix for clinical pathways, *Journal of Nursing Care Quality* 11(2):3-4, 1996.

Institute of Medicine: *America's health in transition: protecting and improving quality*, Washington, DC, 1994, National Academy Press.

Jameton A: Dilemmas of moral distress: moral responsibility and nursing practice, *AWHONN's Clinical Issues in Perinatal and Women's Health Nursing* 4(4):542-551, 1993.

Lohr KN, editor: *Medicare: a strategy for quality assurance*, Washington, DC, 1990, Institute of Medicine/National Academy Press.

National Coalition on Health Care: How Americans perceive the health care system: a report on a national survey, *Journal of Health Care Finance* 23(4):12-20, 1997.

Zoloth-Dorfman L, Rubin S: The patient as commodity: managed care and the question of ethics, *Journal of Clinical Ethics* 6(4):339-357, Winter 1995.

CHAPTER 5

Nursing-Sensitive Patient Outcomes

Development and Importance for Use in Assessing Health Care Effectiveness*

MARION JOHNSON, RN, PhD, **and MERIDEAN L. MAAS**, RN, PhD, FAAN

OVERVIEW

To facilitate continual quality improvement, information about patient outcomes should identify not only inadequate outcomes but also those that are marginal, adequate, or superior.

Patient outcomes have emerged as essential measures of health care quality in managed care systems. Although a number of patient outcome measures are now available, there has been minimal emphasis on the identification and measurement of outcomes for the evaluation of nursing interventions. Standardized, nursing-sensitive patient outcomes are important for assigning nursing accountability for the development of clinical information systems and knowledge development. The Nursing Outcomes Classification (NOC) provides a comprehensive taxonomy of standardized patient outcomes that is useful for evaluating the effects of nursing care in all settings and with all populations. ▲

*This research was funded by Sigma Theta Tau International and NIH, National Institute of Nursing Research, Grant No. 1R01 NR03437-01.

Political interest in patient outcomes and health care costs initiated a revolution in health care in the 1980s that has been labeled the "era of assessment and accountability" (Iezzoni, 1994). The result is increased pressure on health care providers to justify their practices and the effects on individual patients and national health (DeFriese, 1990). Thus, it is necessary for each health care discipline to identify and measure patient outcomes most influenced by its practice in order to foster the development of knowledge, ensure that standards of care evolve as knowledge increases, and demonstrate the effectiveness of its interventions. This chapter overviews current efforts to measure patient outcomes, highlights the significance of the development of outcomes that are sensitive to nursing interventions in the current environment, discusses the development of the Nursing Outcomes Classification (Iowa Outcomes Project, 1997), and explores the implications and future directions for NOC in assessing nursing effectiveness and for the development of nursing science.

Emphasis on Patient Outcomes

Rapidly escalating costs of health care during the 1970s and 1980s forced policymakers to seek ways to provide care more economically. Efforts at cost containment encouraged managed competition and new health care system configurations. Health maintenance and preferred provider organizations and integrated systems offering a continuum of care have evolved to meet current demands. With the increased emphasis on cost containment and competition and the evolution of health care systems, greater concerns about quality of care have emerged. Payers and consumers want to know what they are getting for their money. Basic questions raised are: Is the care provided by one organization or agency worth the expense relative to the care provided by other organizations or agencies? What are the benefits patients receive from health care? What is the quality, and is it adequate in light of what is being paid (Shaughnessy, Crisler, 1995)? What are the benefits to the health of the population as well as to individuals (Iezzoni, 1994)? What outcomes can be expected, given various patient characteristics and health states? If outcomes are not adequate, what needs to be changed to improve the outcome? If outcomes are adequate, can improvements still be achieved (Carey, Lloyd, 1995)?

Given this climate, health care providers, whether organizations or individuals, are increasingly accountable for the quality of care provided as determined by the outcomes achieved by their clientele. Although quality of care can be examined from the perspectives of structure, process, and outcome, outcomes are an essential component of quality evaluation and effectiveness research. "Outcomes are the changes, either favorable or adverse, in the actual or potential health status of persons, groups, or communities that can be attributed to prior or concurrent care" (Donabedian, 1985). Outcomes are the trigger for quality assurance programs since they answer the question, did the patient benefit or not benefit from the care provided (Shaughnessy, Crisler, 1995)?

To facilitate continual quality improvement, information about patient outcomes should identify not only inadequate outcomes but also those that are marginal, adequate, or superior. Identification of all outcomes allows providers to focus on system structure and delivery process changes that foster continual improvement in all patient outcomes and not just those that are inadequate.

Current Outcome Measures

Development of patient outcome measures has received increased attention since the late 1980s. As a result, a number of standardized tools and measures have been developed to evaluate managed care systems (National Committee for Quality Assurance, 1995), general health status (Ware, Sherbourne, 1992), disease-specific conditions (Health Outcomes Institute, 1993), or physician practice (Tarlov et al, 1989). Currently a number of different types of outcomes, as illustrated in Figure 5-1, are being developed and used to evaluate health care effectiveness.

Patient, system, and provider factors represent the health care delivery and individual patient factors that can influence outcomes achievement. Although much has been written about the effect of these factors on outcomes achievement, only recently has the influence of these factors been empirically investigated.

The core represents global or end outcomes, such as health status. These outcomes, which are multidisciplinary, measure general health status and patient satisfaction with their health and with care provided (Iowa Outcomes Project, 1997). These

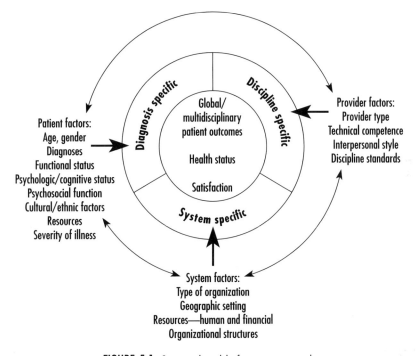

FIGURE 5-1 Conceptual model of outcomes research.

measures provide useful information for payers evaluating alternative health care plans, but are not specific enough to determine accountability for changes to improve outcomes and are not suitable for monitoring the health and treatment status of individual patients, particularly those with chronic diseases (McHorney, Tarlov, 1995).

The outer circle represents intermediate outcome measures in current use. These outcomes are specific to a particular medical diagnosis, system, or type of provider.

1. *Diagnosis-specific outcomes* are used in critical paths and in standardized evaluation instruments, such as those developed by the Health Outcomes Institute (1993). Outcomes in critical paths are often organization specific, and stated as multidisciplinary patient goals that are met or not met. Standardized instruments have captured primarily indicators of physician practice; some may include multidisciplinary outcomes.

2. *System-specific outcomes* include adverse factors such as medication errors, infection rates, and patient falls, and measures of organizational effectiveness such as cost and produc-

tivity. These measures are commonly found in benchmarking or total-quality management systems and emphasize multidisciplinary, system-wide outcomes.

3. *Discipline-specific outcomes* reflect the practice and standards of a health care discipline and are important for evaluating the performance and quality of that practice. To date, the focus of effectiveness research using discipline-specific outcomes primarily has been on physician practices or processes of care (Prescott, 1993). Each health care discipline, however, must identify and measure patient outcomes most influenced by its practice to foster the development of knowledge and ensure that standards of care evolve as knowledge increases in the discipline.

Need for Outcome Measures Influenced by Nursing

Although it is recognized that patient outcomes are influenced by a number of patient characteristics and organizational factors, and shared by all disciplines, it is also important to identify outcomes highly attributable to a specific discipline to establish effectiveness and assign accountability. For management of quality, it is necessary to delineate the accountability of each provider as well as that of the health care team. It is important also to identify the intermediate outcomes that influence the health and satisfaction of patients, the achievement of which may be the primary responsibility of one discipline. Intermediate outcomes are critical in an integrated health care system in which the patient receives care in a number of settings, as only intermediate outcomes may be achieved in any given setting before the patient is transferred to another setting.

ACCOUNTABILITY

Global measures and disease-specific measures that emphasize multidisciplinary outcomes provide needed information about the overall effects of health care on the patient's health status, but make it difficult to assign accountability for outcomes. Given that nursing care represents a majority of the hours of care provided in all settings except physician offices and clinics where nurses may practice as primary care providers (Aiken, Smith, Lake, 1994), it is essential that health care organizations and nursing practice settings be able to evaluate patient outcomes influenced by nursing care. For nurses to work effectively with managed care organizations to improve quality and reduce costs, nurses must be able to measure and document patient outcomes influenced by nursing care (Phoon, Corder, Barter, 1996). For example, the costs of decubitus ulcers are well documented, and prevention is largely a function of nursing care (Frantz, Bergquist, Specht, 1995); however, information about tissue integrity is not readily available in most global health care measures.

The need for information about patient outcomes influenced by nursing care has increased as organizations restructure to obtain greater efficiencies. Without these data, organizations have little information on which to adjust staff mix, determine the cost-effectiveness of various structural or process changes in the nursing care delivery system, or provide information about the quality of nursing care available in the organization. In a review of nurse staffing and hospital quality of care, the Institute of Medicine found that existing work in outcome measurement typically has not focused on isolating the contribution of nursing to overall hospital quality (Institute of Medicine, 1996). Such information will be vital for organizations if the quality of nursing care is one of the criteria used by payers and consumers when selecting health care organizations.

INTERMEDIATE OUTCOMES

Intermediate outcomes that facilitate or hinder the achievement of end outcomes, such as improved health status, must be measured to study their effect on end outcomes and to determine how organizational structures and care delivery processes affect the achievement of these intermediate outcomes. Many of the discipline-specific outcomes will be intermediate rather than end outcomes. If the discipline most concerned with the outcome has not identified the need to measure the outcome, important outcomes may be missing from critical paths, diagnosis-specific measures, and other measures used to evaluate health care effectiveness. For example, functional status may be hindered by tissue breakdown—an intermediate outcome of concern to nurses that might not be available for outcome analysis if not identified by nursing. In addition, patients are often discharged from one setting and one team of clinicians before the desired end outcomes are realized, making it important that subsequent providers know the patient's status in terms of the intermediate outcomes at the time of transfer.

Intermediate outcomes include measures that assess patient knowledge, attitudes, and behaviors; or outcomes that are important measures of the effects of nursing interventions directed at assisting the patient to modify behaviors to improve health status. If nursing does not measure these outcomes, the effectiveness of nursing interventions cannot be assessed and data to analyze the effects of changes in knowledge, attitude, and behavior on health status may be missing since other disciplines do not routinely measure these outcomes. Intermediate outcomes that measure wellness care effectiveness also are increasingly important as attention is directed to illness prevention and wellness care as well as illness care (Issel, Anderson, 1996). Wellness care—that is, care to improve the health status of individuals without an identified illness—traditionally has been provided by nursing, and attention to the measurement of the intermediate outcomes of wellness care is most likely to come from the nursing profession. With intermediate outcome data, nursing has the opportunity to demonstrate the value of longitudinal care, patient education, and physical and emotional support to the health of individuals and populations (Simpson, 1997).

Need for Standardized Nursing-Sensitive Outcome Measures

In addition to identifying discipline-specific patient outcome measures for nursing, it is equally important that these measures be standardized and validated. If the nursing profession is to become a full participant in clinical evaluation, it is essential that patient outcomes influenced by nursing care be measured in conjunction with outcomes important to other disciplines and, ultimately, to the patient. Furthermore, participation in clinical evaluation and policy making requires that standardized nursing data be included in integrated, computerized, clinical information systems.

USE IN UNIFORM DATA SETS

Several uniform data sets have been developed for the U.S. health care delivery system, for example, the Uniform Hospital Discharge Data Set (Health Information Policy Council, 1985), the Uniform Ambulatory Medical Care Minimum Data Set (National Committee on Vital and Health Statistics, 1981), and the Long Term Care Minimum Data Set (National Committee on Vital and Health Statistics, 1980). This type of data set "defines the central core of data needed on a routine basis by the majority of decision-makers about a given facet or dimension of the health care delivery system, and it establishes standard measurements, definitions, and classifications for this core" (Murnaghan, 1978). Although such data sets provide valuable information about systems and organizations, the paucity of information available to determine nursing care effectiveness hinders decision making and policy development relative to nursing practice. National health policy and health care management systems will

not accurately reflect health care delivery in this country until invisible nursing data are converted to visible useful data.

A structure for minimum data for nursing, the Nursing Minimum Data Set (NMDS), was described by Werley and colleagues (Werley, Devine, Zorn, 1990) a decade ago, but the standardized nursing nomenclatures to fully implement the NMDS are only now being developed. The NMDS contains four unique nursing care elements: nursing diagnoses, nursing interventions, nursing-sensitive patient outcomes, and intensity of nursing care. Comprehensive standardized nomenclatures describing nursing diagnoses, interventions, and outcomes have been developed by the North American Nursing Diagnosis Association (NANDA) (1997), the Iowa Intervention Project (1996) (Nursing Intervention Classification [NIC]), and the Iowa Outcomes Project (1997) (Nursing Outcomes Classification), respectively, and are recognized by the American Nurses' Association (ANA) as languages for informatics. Two community nomenclatures, the Omaha System (Martin, Scheet, 1992) and the Home Healthcare Classification (Saba et al, 1991), also have been recognized by the ANA. Intensity of nursing care has not been adequately defined and measured, although work is underway in this area (Prescott, Soeken, 1996). Efforts to standardize data sets for the NMDS are timely. Advances in computer technology and applications in health care maximize the quantity and efficiency of clinical data collection, storage, and retrieval. In addition, these efforts are responsive to current work to develop national standards to enable the electronic exchange of health information.

COMPUTERIZED CLINICAL INFORMATION SYSTEMS

Uniform data sets define a set of minimum specifications for the content of computerized information systems. Although the development of clinical information systems for health care has been rapid, there is little standardization of data in nursing information systems because of the lack of a common language and a standardized way to organize data. Computer technology will make a significant contribution to increasing nursing knowledge and thus nursing care quality if uniform, standardized data sets are used for nursing effectiveness research and management decisions. Computerized nursing information systems have the potential to improve nursing performance and productivity, maximize positive clinical outcomes, and provide information for strategic planning. Although the potential is great, few nursing information systems do more than automate what is currently documented, and their potential will not be realized until integrated nursing information systems are developed. Standardization and uniformity of data sets are one of the preconditions necessary for the development of integrated nursing information systems (McCormick, 1991).

EVALUATION OF NURSING CARE

Standardized patient outcome measures that reflect the quality of nursing care allow payers, accrediting programs, and consumers to compare service quality across organizations. Although outcomes responsive to nursing are not the only measures used by payers and consumers, it is vital information since consumer satisfaction is partially influenced by nursing care (Boscarino, 1992). Since standardized measures of nursing care quality are not currently available, this information is missing from regional and national data sets that evaluate the performance of health care systems and organizations. As a result, research to identify the contribution and effectiveness of nursing care is hindered and data in existing databases are not adequate for the comprehensive study of patient outcomes. Since direct measures of nursing care quality are not available, proxy measures, such as the frequency of incident reports, are used (Bostrom, Zimmerman, 1993), or traditional measures of multidisciplinary care, such as death, physiological complications, or readmission rates, are used (Ebener, Baugh, Formella, 1996).

KNOWLEDGE DEVELOPMENT

The development of nursing knowledge requires the use of patient outcome measures influenced by nursing to evaluate the effectiveness of a nursing intervention and the appropriateness of the decision-making process in selecting an intervention. Expanding this knowledge beyond the individual patient to patient populations requires adequate clinical data to study linkages between diagnoses, interventions, patient characteristics, and patient outcomes (Iowa Intervention Project, 1996; Blegen, Tripp-Reimer, 1997). Measuring the outcome is only one step; attributing a change in the outcome to nursing practice requires an understanding of the reason the practice influences the outcome and the way patient characteristics influence outcome achievement. Development of nursing databases that contain standardized information, including outcomes and interventions, will increase the rapidity with which knowledge can be expanded.

Nursing-Sensitive Patient Outcome Measures

Early work to identify and classify nursing-sensitive patient outcomes took place in the late 1970s. Outcomes used in nursing research to evaluate the effectiveness of nursing care were identified and categorized in the eighties (Lang, Clinton, 1984; Marek, 1989). Based on a review of the literature, three levels of patient outcomes are in current use for the evaluation of nursing practice. A number of broad categories have been developed without identifying specific measures, except for the work reported by Horn and Swain (1978). At the other extreme, a multitude of specific measures, often untested and not standardized, are used in clinical practice to evaluate patient outcomes related to specific nursing diagnoses and interventions. There also is an increasing number of outcomes at a middle level of abstraction, which are used in critical paths, nursing care plans, quality assurance programs, and clinical information systems to evaluate nursing or multidisciplinary outcomes. In general, the specific measures and intermediate-level outcomes used by nursing had not been tested, did not use standardized terminology or measures, and were not used within a conceptual framework or classified in a consistent manner until the Nursing Outcomes Classification was developed.

Recent work to standardize and test outcome measures for nursing has focused primarily on community settings. The Omaha System (Martin, Scheet, 1992) has a five-point rating scale for three outcomes: knowledge, status, and behavior. Each of these outcomes can be applied to the 44 problems identified in the problem classification. The Home Healthcare Classification (Saba et al, 1991) uses three discharge status measures as proxy measures of expected outcomes: improved, stabilized, and deteriorated. These discharge measures are assigned to each active problem. Both systems have limited outcome measures, and no further testing is reported in the literature. The Outcome-Based Quality Improvement System developed at the Center for Health Policy Research at the University of Colorado (Shaughnessy, Crisler, 1995) contains core measures that apply to all client groups and specific measures for specified client groups. All outcomes are measured on a scale specific to the outcome to determine if the patient has improved, stabilized, or other. Patient attributes that influence outcome attainment, often referred to as risk factors, have been specified in the work by Shaughnessy and Crisler (1995). Outcome measures in all of these systems are developed for home care and do not provide for evaluation of patient status across a continuum of care, a disadvantage in the developing integrated health care systems in which patients receive nursing assistance in several settings during a single episode of care (Head, Maas, Johnson, 1997).

Current efforts to standardize outcome measures in acute care settings have been recently reported. The Nursing Care Report Card (ANA, 1995) identifies adverse incidents and complications to be collected in acute care settings, but does not provide outcome measures for individuals. Incidents and complications, while collected at the individual level, are aggregated and reported as ratios or occurrence rates. The standardized patient outcomes developed for hospital settings by Ozbolt and colleagues (Ozbolt, Fruchtnight, Hayden, 1994) link outcomes with specific patient problems and thus do not provide a comprehensive spectrum of outcomes. The International Council of Nurses is developing an International Classification for Nursing Practice (ICNP) that will contain patient outcomes when complete; however the outcome portion of the classification is in the early stages of development. The ICNP is not research based, but recognized standardized languages, such as NANDA and NIC, have been considered in its development. Absence of risk adjustment factors, except in the

Outcome-Based Quality Improvement System, makes it extremely difficult to compare outcomes across multiple settings. Large, standardized data sets that include NIC interventions and NOC outcomes will make it possible to test risk adjustment factors that are important for assessing the effectiveness of nursing interventions.

The Nursing Outcomes Classification has been developed by a research team at the University of Iowa (Maas, Johnson, Moorhead, 1996; Iowa Outcomes Project, 1997). The classification is comprehensive and developed for use across the care continuum.

Nursing Outcomes Classification

Work to develop nursing-sensitive patient outcomes included in NOC is ongoing. To date, approximately 200 outcome measures with associated indicators have been developed, have been evaluated for content validity, and have undergone some pilot testing in clinical sites. NOC represents the most comprehensive attempt to standardize outcome terminology and measures for nursing practice and to develop a taxonomy of patient outcomes sensitive to nursing care.

DEVELOPMENT OF NURSING OUTCOMES CLASSIFICATION

The current classification was developed over a period of four years using inductive and deductive methodologies. Outcome statements, representing outcomes used by nurses in all clinical specialties and settings, and for patients of all age groups, were sampled from nursing literature and two clinical information systems.

Two hundred eighty-two (282) outcome labels were identified and subjected to concept analysis and expert clinician review. Following content validation, 190 outcomes with a label, definition, a set of indicators, a 5-point Likert scale to rate patient status and selected references used to develop the outcome were reported for clinical testing and were used by the clinical researchers. Table 5-1 provides an example of an NOC outcome. A detailed report of the methods used to develop the outcomes and indicators and validate their content is provided elsewhere (Iowa Outcomes Project, 1997).

TABLE 5-1
Example of NOC Outcome

Treatment regimen—Extent of understanding and skills conveyed about a specific treatment regimen

	NEVER	SLIGHT	MODERATE	SUBSTANTIAL	EXTENSIVE	N/A
Knowledge: Treatment	1	2	3	4	5	
INDICATORS:						
Describes prescribed diet	1	2	3	4	5	N/A
Describes prescribed medication	1	2	3	4	5	N/A
Describes prescribed activity	1	2	3	4	5	N/A
Describes prescribed exercise	1	2	3	4	5	N/A
Describes prescribed procedures	1	2	3	4	5	N/A
Describes rationale for treatment regimen	1	2	3	4	5	N/A
Describes self-care responsibilities for ongoing treatment	1	2	3	4	5	N/A
Describes self-care responsibilities for emergency situations	1	2	3	4	5	N/A
Describes expected effects of treatment	1	2	3	4	5	N/A
Demonstrates self-monitoring techniques	1	2	3	4	5	N/A
Other	1	2	3	4	5	N/A

    (Specify)

PILOT STUDIES

The NOC outcomes were piloted in three practice sites: a tertiary care center, a community hospital, and a nursing home. Data collected from each site were dependent on the method of implementation at the site. Table 5-2 presents the frequency with which NOC outcomes were selected for 23 patients on an orthopedic surgical unit in the tertiary care setting. The nursing outcome column indicates the outcome label used at the time the pilot was conducted, and the labels in parentheses indicate the current label name as modified following content validation and refinement.

    Overall, outcomes selected for this population reflect the nursing diagnoses and patient problems that nurses are concerned with in a population of patients with orthopedic surgery, many of whom are elderly and on bed rest for a period of time. Similar results were obtained with other patient populations, indicating the usefulness of the NOC outcomes for nursing practice.

DEVELOPMENT OF THE TAXONOMY

The NOC taxonomy provides a structure for organizing the outcomes at four levels of abstraction. The broadest level is the domain, the second level is the class, the third level is the outcome, and the fourth is the indicator level. The classification was developed in two steps using similarity-dissimilarity clustering and hierarchical analysis of the outcomes to form classes and of the classes to

TABLE 5-2
Frequency of Nursing Outcomes Chosen and Documented on an Orthopedic Unit

NURSING OUTCOME	NO. OF PATIENTS FOR WHOM OUTCOMES SELECTED	NO. OF TIMES OUTCOMES DOCUMENTED
Ambulation: walking performance (now called ambulation: walking)	2	2
Balance	5	7*
Bowel elimination	3	3
Cognition: orientation (now called cognitive orientation)	1	3*
Coping	1	1
Fatigue (now called endurance)	1	1
Nutritional status	1	1
Pain control (now called pain level)	1	1
Safety status: personal (now called safety behavior: personal)	1	3*
Tissue integrity: skin and mucous membranes	4	4
Transfer performance	6	9*
Urinary elimination	3	3
Wound healing	7	10*

*Outcomes charted on more frequently for a patient.

form domains. These analyses resulted in 25 classes and six domains, each of which was given a name and a definition. The outcomes were then coded for inclusion in computerized clinical information systems. Each level of the taxonomy, as well as each measurement scale, is coded. Thus, each outcome, indicator, or measurement scale has a unique code number for use in computerized systems.

Conclusion

Evaluation of the effects of patient characteristics, health care system factors, and nursing interventions requires the identification of measurable patient outcomes. To evaluate the effects of the organizational or nursing structure and the nursing and multidisciplinary processes in an organization on the quality of nursing care requires the identification and measurement of outcomes influenced by nursing practice.

The current health care environment requires that providers demonstrate the cost effectiveness of their interventions. Nurses are the largest group of health care providers, yet their interventions and outcomes are mostly invisible. Nursing's slowness to develop standardized nomenclatures describing patient problems addressed, interventions used, and patient outcomes influenced and the low priority for computerization of nursing data among decision makers are fundamental reasons for nursing's invisibility and the corresponding inability of nurse administrators and scientists to systematically assess the cost effectiveness of nursing interventions. Large database analysis is critically important for nursing outcomes effectiveness research, yet nursing databases will not be available and nursing data cannot be extracted for large national datasets if standardized nursing data are not included in computerized information systems. The development and clinical validation of outcome measures that are responsive to nursing interventions will enable exposition of the accountability of individual nurses and the collective of nurses for care that is delivered, as well as strengthen the contribution of nursing as a member of the interdisciplinary team. Thus the interdisciplinary team's accountability for cost-effective care will be more genuine and less distorted.

NOC outcomes, measured on a continuum rather than as goals, will facilitate the identification and analysis of outcomes that are achieved for specific populations. They also will facilitate the identification of patient and organizational characteristics that influence outcome attainment. Assessment of the level of outcomes over time provides much more useful information than just documenting whether outcomes are achieved. For example, patients can be aggregated by a nursing diagnosis and differences in level of outcome achievement analyzed by personal characteristics such as age, gender, and functional status, or by organizational characteristics such as staff mix, unit size, and ratio of registered nurses to patients. This information will help nurse managers and clinicians to develop realistic standards for specific patient populations. Standards can be consistent with achieved outcomes if the outcome level is satisfactory, or they can reflect desired, higher levels of achievement, in which case the nurse manager will have an understanding of the amount of improvement needed to attain such outcomes. This will be quite different from the usual practice of setting standards without adequate knowledge of whether the standard is actually achieved, is too low, or is too high. Development of outcomes as variables, however, also encourages the identification of specific goals for each patient. Nurses can specify the desired level of achievement for each patient on the basis of the initial assessment and then measure the actual level of achievement. Another important application of measuring outcomes as variables is that they are useful for evaluating the effects of nursing care over time; in other words, one can trace or graph a patient's status over a prolonged period within and across care settings.

Outcomes should be identified that are sensitive to the interventions of specific disciplines. If outcomes are identified only for the composite of interdisciplinary interventions, each discipline will be unable to judge the effects of its specific interventions. Furthermore, no one discipline can be held accountable. If interventions do not work, it will be difficult to determine what needs to be changed in order to meet the outcomes. However, there is an important need to identify outcomes that are used by more than one discipline and can be assessed across patient populations and settings. NOC will contribute to the standardization of outcomes needed for assessing the effectiveness of nursing, and some will likely be useful for multiple disciplines. The conceptual and methodological approaches used by the NOC team will facilitate consensus regarding how outcomes and indicators should be defined, structured, and measured for optimum database development and assessment of outcome effectiveness.

NOC will be available for inclusion in nursing clinical data sets in all settings and in large regional and national data sets. Before assessment of the reliability and validity of outcome measures using clinical field data, which is planned for the next phase of the NOC research, the repeated measurement of the outcomes can be used by clinicians to manage progress over time. Crude measurement may be better than no measurement of outcomes, provided users remain aware of limitations of the measures (Duggar et al, 1995). Following the development and psychometric evaluation of explicit measurement procedures, data from individual patients and various settings can be aggregated, while controlling for other factors that may influence the outcome, to determine the levels at which outcomes are most commonly achieved for patients with a specific medical or nursing diagnosis. Accumulation of this more detailed information about the effectiveness or lack of effectiveness of nursing interventions and the linkages among nursing diagnoses, interventions, and outcomes will add to nursing knowledge and allow nurses to identify areas of practice that need improvement. Furthermore, standardized outcomes and measures with demonstrated reliability and validity will be available for experimental research to test specific hypotheses derived from theories or descriptive studies needed to build the science of nursing.

The benefits of standardized languages and their contributions to quality care open up exciting possibilities for nursing science, education, and practice. Data from standardized nursing diagnoses, interventions, and outcomes will provide nurses with information only dreamed about in the past, will make nursing a visible and influential science and practice discipline, and will benefit clients through more informed health care policy and data-based practice.

References

Aiken LA, Smith HL, Lake ET: Lower Medicare mortality among a set of hospitals known for good nursing care, *Medical Care* 32:771-787, 1994.

American Nurses' Association: *Nursing care report card for acute care,* Washington, DC, 1995, American Nurses' Association.

Blegen MA, Tripp-Reimer T: Implications of nursing taxonomies for middle-range theory development, *Advances in Nursing Science* 19(3):37-49, 1997.

Boscarino JA: The public's perception of quality hospitals. II: Implications for patient surveys, *Hospital and Health Services Administration* 37(1):13-35, 1992.

Bostrom J, Zimmerman J: Restructuring nursing for a competitive health care environment, *Nursing Economics* 11(1):35-41, 54, 1993.

Carey RG, Lloyd RC: *Measuring quality improvement in healthcare: a guide to statistical process control applications,* New York, 1995, Quality Resources, A Division of the Kraus Organization Limited.

DeFriese DH: Measuring the effectiveness of medical interventions: new expectations of health services research [Editorial Preface], *Health Services Research* 25:697-708, 1990.

Donabedian A: *The methods and findings of quality assessment and monitoring: an illustrated analysis,* vol 3, Ann Arbor, Mich, 1985, Health Administration Press.

Duggar B, DeLozier J, Goldenberg D, Palmer RH, Lawthers AG, Banks NJ, Kurland D, Hargraves JL, Peterson L: *Understanding and choosing clinical performance measures for quality improvement: development of a typology,* Rockville, Md, 1985, Department of Health and Human Services, Public Health Service, Agency for Health Care Policy Research, contract No 282-92-0038, delivery order no 3.

Ebener MK, Baugh K, Formella NM: Proving that less is more: linking resources to outcomes, *Journal of Nursing Care Quality* 10(2):1-9, 1996.

Frantz RA, Bergquist S, Specht J: The cost of treating pressure ulcers following implementation of a research-based skin care protocol in a long-term care facility, *Advances in Wound Care* 8(1):36-45.

Head B, Maas M, Johnson M: Outcomes for home and community nursing in integrated delivery systems, *Caring* 16(1):50-56, 1997.

Health Information Policy Council: 1984 revision of the uniform hospital discharge data set, *Federal Register* 50(147):31038-31040, 1985.

Health Outcomes Institute: *Condition-specific type specifications,* Bloomington, Minn, 1993, The Institute.

Horn BJ, Swain MA: *Criterion measures of nursing care,* Hyattsville, Md, 1978, National Center for Health Services Research (DHEW publications no. PHS78-3187).

Iezzoni LI: Risk and outcomes. In Iezzoni LI, ed: *Risk adjustment for measuring health care outcomes,* Ann Arbor, Mich, 1994, Health Administration Press, pp 1-28.

Institute of Medicine, Wunderlich GS, Sloan FA, Davis CK, eds: *Nursing staff in hospitals and nursing homes: is it adequate,* Washington, DC, 1996, National Academy Press.

Iowa Intervention Project, McCloskey JC, Bulechek GM: *Nursing interventions classification,* ed 2, St Louis, 1996, Mosby.

Iowa Outcomes Project, Johnson M, Maas M, eds: *Nursing outcomes classification (NOC),* St Louis, 1997, Mosby.

Issel LM, Anderson RA: Take charge: managing six transformations in health care delivery, *Nursing Economics* 14, 78-84, 1996.

Lang NM, Clinton JF: Assessment of quality of nursing care. In Werley HH, Fitzpatrick JJ, eds: *Annual review of nursing research,* 2, New York, 1984, Springer, pp 135-163.

Maas ML, Johnson MR, Moorhead S: Classifying nursing-sensitive patient outcomes, *Image* 28(4):295-301, 1996.

Marek KD: Outcome measurement in nursing, *Journal of Nursing Quality Assurance* 4(1):27-34, 1989.

Martin KS, Scheet NJ: Problem rating scale for outcomes, *The Omaha System: applications for community health nursing,* Philadelphia, 1992, Harcourt Brace Jovanovich, pp 90-98.

McCormick K: Future data needs for quality care monitoring, DRG considerations, reimbursement and outcome measurement, *Image* 23(1):29-32, 1991.

McHorney CA, Tarlov AR: Individual-patient monitoring in clinical practice: are available health status surveys adequate? *Quality of Life Research* 4:293-307, 1995.

Murnaghan J: Uniform basic data sets for health statistical systems, *International Journal of Epidemiology* 7(3):263-269, 1978.

National Committee for Quality Assurance: *Health plan employer data and information set 2.1 (HEDIS 2.1),* Washington, DC, 1995, The Committee.

National Committee on Vital and Health Statistics: *Long-term health care: minimum data set,* Washington, DC, 1980, US Department of Health and Human Services, National Center for Health Statistics (DHHS publications No. PHS 80-1158).

National Committee on Vital and Health Statistics: *Uniform ambulatory medical care: minimum data set,* Washington, DC, 1981, US Department of Health and Human Services, National Center for Health Statistics (DHHS publications No. PHS 81-1161).

North American Nursing Diagnosis Association: *Nursing diagnoses: definitions & classification 1995-1996,* Philadelphia, 1994, The Association.

Ozbolt J, Fruchtnight J, Hayden J: Toward data standards for clinical nursing information, *Journal of the American Medical Informatics Association* 1(2):175-185, 1994.

Phoon J, Corder K, Barter M: Managed care and total quality management: a necessary integration, *Journal of Nursing Care Quality* 10(2):25-32, 1996.

Prescott PA: Nursing: an important component of hospital survival under a reformed health care system, *Nursing Economics* 11:192-199, 1993.

Prescott PA, Soeken KL: Measuring nursing intensity in ambulatory care. II: Developing and testing PINAC, *Nursing Economics* 14:86-91, 1996.

Saba VK, O'Hare PA, Zuckerman AE, Boondas J, Levine E, Oatway DM: A nursing intervention taxonomy for home health care, *Nursing & Health Care* 12(6):296-299, 1991.

Shaughnessy PW, Crisler KS: *Outcome-based quality improvement: a manual for home care agencies on how to use outcomes,* Washington, DC, 1995, National Association for Home Care.

Simpson R: Take advantage of managed care opportunities, *Nursing Management* 28(3):24-25, 1997.

Tarlov AR, Ware JE, Greenfield S, Nelson EC, Perrin E, Zubkoff M: The medical outcomes study: an application of methods for monitoring the results of medical care, *JAMA* 262:925-930, 1989.

Ware JE, Sherbourne CD: The MOS-36 item short-form health survey (SF-36), *Medical Care* 30(6):473-483, 1992.

Werley H, Devine E, Zorn C: The nursing minimum data set (NMDS): issues for the profession. In McCloskey JC, Grace HK, eds: *Current issues in nursing,* St Louis, 1990, Mosby, pp 64-70.

CHAPTER 6

The Economic and Financial Implications of Case Management

JUDITH LLOYD STORFJELL, RN, PhD, and STEPHEN JESSUP, CPA

OVERVIEW

When the true cost of achieving outcomes of care is known, case managers and care providers alike will be better able to make cost-benefit decisions for individual cases.

A primary purpose of case management is to improve the cost-effectiveness of health care services through coordination and management of service utilization. The case manager is responsible for integrating the financial and clinical aspects of care. To determine the financial impact of case management, it is necessary to understand the costs of providing case management services and the cost of purchased services (i.e., services provided by other providers). This is best achieved by determining the costs activities (e.g., case management, service delivery) and then identifying the way various types of clients utilize these activities. This type of information can thon be used to support critical decisions rogarding the utilization of case management as a cost-effective intervention and to improve operational efficiency. ▲

Although the concept of social and clinical case management has been around for some time, recent economic concerns have contributed significantly to current interest in nursing case management. Historically, case management was a by-product of the close relationship between clients and providers. However, as care has become more complex and the number of providers for each client has grown, management of clinical regimens has also become more difficult. Likewise, as the importance of controlling health care costs has increased, reimbursement strategies and approaches have proliferated (e.g., reduced fees, case rates, capitation), and payers have hired "case managers" to control health care utilization. Suddenly, there are a variety of individuals participating in planning and providing care to individuals, resulting in a system in which actual accountability for client results is fragmented. Coordinating this alignment of powerful (and frequently competing) economic, social, and clinical forces critical to achieving cost-effective outcomes of care has fostered the reemergence of nursing case management.

Nurse case managers are responsible for obtaining or providing cost-effective health care on either an episodic or a continuous basis. This means that they must integrate both the clinical and financial aspects of patient care. Because of their education and experience, nurses should be able to assess the clinical needs of patients and plan care that will produce desired clinical outcomes. However, understanding the financial implications of this care is more complex than it first appears.

For instance, case managers need to determine and manage the financial as well as the clinical impact of services—not only for services purchased from other providers but also for those delivered by the sponsoring organization. Costs of care are fairly easy to calculate when services are purchased in a fee-for-service system. However, when they are provided directly, it is more difficult to determine their actual cost. Also, there are times when an upfront investment (preventive services or education) will save health care costs at a later date by preventing or limiting need for other services. Therefore, to make good judgments about when to utilize these types of services, the case manager will need to understand the total potential costs of care. In addition, case management itself also has a cost,

TABLE 6-1 **Case Manager Activities and Costs**		
ACTIVITIES	PERCENT	ANNUAL COST
Assess clients	15%	$ 9,000
Plan/coordinate care	20%	$12,000
Counsel/teach clients	30%	$18,000
Document care	15%	$ 9,000
Travel	10%	$ 6,000
Manage external relationships	10%	$ 6,000
TOTALS	100%	$60,000

which needs to be included when the total costs of health care are determined.

Costs of Case Management

Let us first consider the costs of case management itself. The major expenses involved in case management are the time of the case manager and the space and supplies she or he uses. These expenses can be calculated fairly easily. However, it is more difficult to assign them to specific functions or types of clients. To determine whether the expense of case management is worth the investment by a payer or provider, it would be very useful to know what specific functions cost and/or which type of case management costs more. Therefore, it is useful to look at the specific activities a case manager does to understand costs associated with case management.

Actually, a case manager's time can be divided into five or six major activities. Obviously, these activities will vary according to the model of case management used. However, some potential activities could include: assess client needs, plan/coordinate care, counsel/teach, document care, travel, and manage external relations.

If the percentage of the case manager's time can be determined for each activity, the cost of each activity can be calculated by dividing the case manager's total compensation (wages and fringe benefit costs) by the activity percentages (Table 6-1).

Support costs can also be added to each activity or process area. For instance, the cost of the clinical forms, record storage space, and the time of any clinical records personnel can be added to "documentation" to calculate the total cost of clinical record management. Once the activity cost is calculated, a per case or PMPM (per member per month) cost can easily be determined by dividing the total number of clients or client months into the activity or process cost.

Huggins and Lehman (1997) determined costs per client for Carondelet's Nurse Case Manager Program using similar activities and separating the indirect activities (e.g., documentation, travel) from the direct service activities (e.g., assessment/monitoring, teaching/informing, supporting/sharing, direct care, exploring alternatives/goal setting, other interventions).

A capitated case management program also used this approach. Costs were determined for a number of case management processes. For instance, it was determined that each initial assessment cost the organization $81.41 and that reassessments cost $60.17 each. Ongoing case management (e.g., coordination, teaching, travel) cost $7.20 PMPM, while clinical record management cost $27.74 PMPM. In other words, clinical record costs were over three times more than the cost of providing continuing case management services. This type of information can be used for projecting client costs as well as to identify opportunities for cost reduction. Obviously, in this example, clinical record management became a process-improvement target.

Also, this type of information can be used to determine case management costs for different types of clients. For instance, it could be determined that chronic care clients take twice as much coordination activity as acute care clients, or that utilization of case manager services varies according to age or sex or ADL impairment. Therefore the activity-specific costs per client can be weighted according to actual practice, and the differing costs of providing case management services to a variety of client groups can be determined.

A number of attempts have been made to identify the costs of various models of case management. For instance, Demarest (1996) compared nonnursing broker-model case management costs with a care delivery model using nurse case managers.

Activities were separated for each, and costs were assigned to activities as suggested above. Direct costs were found to be higher per client for the nursing model when two different agencies were compared. However, it is difficult for generalizations to be made on such a small sample, especially when there was no attempt in this analysis to identify issues regarding differences in case mix, travel time, efficiency of internal processes, or the outcomes of the case management interventions.

Determining Service Costs per Case

Unless services are purchased for a set fee, the true costs of care are not easily understood. However, since managing the costs of care is a critical component of case management, it is important to know what the actual costs of care are. Fortunately, there are tools available.

Unfortunately, case managers usually have access only to information about charges for health care services, not costs, even in their own facilities. Frequently hospitals use charges as a surrogate for actual costs of care. For instance, after charges are set for certain procedures, costs are assumed to be a certain percentage of the charge (e.g., 50%). Although such assumptions may have been adequate in the past, it is generally recognized that this approach lacks considerable accuracy. To control the costs of care, it is helpful to have actual cost data. Fortunately, providers are beginning to recognize the need for more accurate cost-finding approaches, such as ABC, and are updating their former costing systems.

Actual costs of care are divided between labor and products (e.g., medication, equipment, tests). Here again, when services are provided directly either by the case manager or by other individuals in the same organization, labor costs are best understood by identifying the activities performed by the care providers and assigning the costs to them. Once the activity costs have been determined, the next step is to determine how each type of client or service utilizes each activity.

For example, one capitated case management program determined that Medicare-eligible clients younger than 65 years of age consumed three times

TABLE 6-2
PMPM Community Care Costs per Enrollee by Age

SERVICES	ENROLLEE AGE GROUPS				
	<65	65-74	75-84	85+	AVERAGE
Initial assessments	2.13	1.30	1.86	1.48	1.62
Case management	38.05	23.59	27.57	26.55	26.25
Home health care—nursing	22.50	5.86	15.24	25.71	14.14
Home health care—non-nursing	26.18	8.36	18.02	23.54	15.96
Personal care	-0-	13.83	9.09	15.00	11.55
Outpatient services	48.04	6.15	10.54	14.33	10.34
Other services	19.63	11.32	12.51	22.47	13.99
Total PMPM	156.54	70.41	94.83	129.08	147.18

as much outpatient service costs PMPM as other enrollees. It also determined that the overall community-based care costs increased with age (after age 65), especially for home health services (Table 6-2).

By calculating the costs of both case management and other services by client category, this program could make a number of strategic and operational decisions. First of all, which types of clients should it target for marketing purposes? Second, where should prevention strategies be employed? Which services should be targeted for rate renegotiation? Which processes are high priority for performance improvement initiatives?

An Explanation of Activity-Based Costing

The costing methods suggested here are based on a growing field of knowledge about cost analysis and cost management called activity-based costing (ABC). ABC has revolutionized traditional cost accounting by translating financial information according to work processes. Instead of categorizing expenses according to how bills are paid (e.g., wages, rent, supplies), ABC takes these same expenses and assigns them directly to work activities (e.g., documentation, assessment, coordination).

Activities can be seen as the basic unit of work. A group of related activities becomes a process (e.g., admission process composed of intake, payer authorization, assessment, etc.). Once the cost of an activity has been determined, it can be used to determine the cost of an entire process—even processes that cross disciplines and/or departments. Activity costs can also be used to determine costs of services to specific populations or groups on the basis of how much of the activity the group uses. In addition, activity costs can be assigned to different types of services to differentiate costs among services (e.g., HIV case management, diabetic case management). These recipients of activity costs are called cost objects. The number of potential cost objects is limited only by the number of cost-related questions asked (Storfjell, Jessup, 1996).

Managing Costs

As stated earlier, case managers need to manage two types of costs: (1) costs of their own case management services and (2) costs of other health care services. To do this, case managers need specific financial information, including service utilization costs and their own case management costs.

Here again, ABC can provide insight for controlling costs. Costs of specific case management activities or processes can be regularly compared with standards or benchmarks. For instance, if it was determined that the cost of the clinical record process needed to be reduced, an investigation into the components of the clinical record process could reveal targets for improvement and indicators that could be monitored over time.

Strategically, the case manager must determine which clients will benefit most from his or her services—which clients will bring the most return from the investment of the case manager's time. In addition, determining service cost trends for groups or categories of clients based on case mix categories could provide information for planning and ongoing management.

Most cost control systems are focused on reducing the utilization of services. This is often successful, but in certain instances the reduction of services can actually increase costs. For example, it is doubtful that you could find someone who would suggest that we try to reduce the cost of care for a diabetic by cutting insulin utilization by 50% to reduce pharmacy charges. The impact on clinical outcomes and ultimate cost of care is obvious. In many other situations, however, the options are not so clear. What is clear, though, is the need for knowing the cost of achieving specific outcomes. When the true cost of achieving outcomes of care is known, case managers and care providers alike will be better able to make cost-benefit decisions for individual cases.

Economic Impact of Case Management

Once the issue of determining the true costs of case management is settled, the second and probably most important question begs to be addressed: "Is case management cost-effective?" In other words, do case management services make a difference in reducing costs or in improving clinical outcomes? If so, when? Also, if we assume that a little case management is good—that it is successful in reducing overall costs—then can we assume that more is better? Or is there a "therapeutic dose" of case management above which it is not cost-effective? These questions have considerable policy and theoretical implications.

We will leave the discussion of the clinical impact of case management to others and focus on the determination of the economic impact of case man-

agement. Here again, Carondelet's experience has demonstrated some promising findings. Huggins and Lehman (1997) studied a sample of high-risk elderly patients receiving nursing case management services and determined that utilization of inpatient and emergency department services was reduced by more than 50%. This resulted in an estimated PMPM cost reduction of nearly 62%, including nurse case manager time.

Davis and Chesterman (1995) attempted to look at case management from an economic point of view. Their assumption was that if case management is an input, an investment, it should demonstrate results (in this case, decreased costs) as an outcome. They discovered that errors have been made in evaluating the cost-effectiveness of many case management programs, including the following: insufficient or excessive "doses or inputs" of case management have been used, the time period for evaluating the "outputs" or results has been insufficient, case management has been only part of the intervention, and/or combined costs of case management services and other services have not been adequately identified. In fact, in many cases inclusion of program start-up costs has adversely affected findings.

After studying a number of case management programs, Davis and Chesterman (1995) determined that intensive case management with complex cases is a process through time—that, in fact, while the expectation has often been that case management in the short run will lower the utilization of expensive institutional facilities in the longer run, in many cases the assessment and development of the best care package take time. This experience has also been demonstrated in the Visiting Nurse Service of New York's Community Nursing Organization (CNO) experience, in which the long-term relationship between the nurse case manager and the enrollee is seen to be the key therapeutic intervention (Storfjell, Mitchell, Daly, 1997).

However, both groups have determined that there is an intensive "set-up" period with each client, consisting of assessment and planning activities. This initial period is separate from the ongoing period of continuous case management. It is often the "set-up" period that is most costly, the costs of which must be recouped through lower service utilization over the long run. The key is to determine which types of clients are worth the investment—

what case mix attributes respond to varying amounts of both "set-up" and "continuation" case management interventions.

Here is a model that is amenable to analysis, because the costs of the "set-up" activities can be separated from the "continuation" activities. By determining the case management costs and service utilization costs of each period (i.e., set-up and continuation) for a variety of different client groups, the economic impact of case management services can be determined.

There is one more complicating factor in determining the cost-effectiveness of case management. That is that case management has both a direct and an indirect effect. The direct effect is the impact of case management as a single intervention. However, the very nature of case management—coordination—suggests that case management does not work in isolation. In fact, it may enhance or improve the outcomes of other interventions as well (e.g., physicians, social workers). Therefore, in assessing the economic impact of case management, it may be important to stratify cases according to the number or type of additional interventions involved (Davis, Chesterman, 1995).

The challenge is to demonstrate the long-term cost-effectiveness of case management services by, first, clearly identifying case management costs, and, second, comparing expected service utilization costs with actual costs.

Conclusion

An activity-based costing approach can be valuable in, first of all, identifying the costs of specific case management activities. These activity costs can then be assigned to a variety of questions or cost objects to accurately determine the costs of case management for different mixes of clients or situations. This cost information has an operational and a strategic value. Operationally, it will help managers identify performance improvement targets. Strategically, it will provide data to support critical decisions regarding the utilization of case management as a cost-effective intervention.

References

Davis B, Chesterman J: *The economics of case management: the relationships between case management costs, other costs, needs and outputs.* Paper presented at the annual meeting of the 1995 American Public Health Association.

Demarest P: Financial analysis: two methods of case management delivery, *Caring,* pp 64-67, July 1996.

Huggins D, Lehman K: Reducing costs through case management, *Nursing Management* 28(12):34-37, December 1997.

Storfjell JL, Jessup S: Bridging the gap between finance and clinical operations with activity-based cost management, *Journal of Nursing Administration* 26(12):12-17, December 1996.

Storfjell JL, Mitchell R, Daly GM: Nurse-managed healthcare: New York's community nursing organization, *Journal of Nursing Administration* 27(10):21-27, October 1997.

CHAPTER 7

Zen Leadership in a Time of Rapid Change

JANE W. SWANSON, BSN, MS

OVERVIEW

A leadership style that emphasizes team concepts and maximum involvement of all players, focusing on preventive care and health promotion rather than just treatment of illness in the hospital, is the ultimate goal.

Personal exemplars and examples from the literature are used in applying characteristics of leadership to today's health care system. Skills are described for leaders to use in surviving rapid changes in professional and personal lives and suggestions to facilitate enjoying the journey. ▲

If you want one year of prosperity, grow grain

If you want ten years of prosperity, grow trees

If you want one hundred years of prosperity, grow people

CHINESE PROVERB

Change can create turmoil and fear but also offers tremendous opportunities for leadership. Dramatic changes in health care have occurred over the last decade. The current turmoil may be "in-between" steps to new solutions that will occur in 5 to 10 years as managed care and integrated delivery networks are evaluated and other contemporary developments surface. Health care systems are exploring better ways to meet community and client health care needs, and also provide illness care, accident prevention, and health promotion services. Changing roles and expectations for the managed care provider, either primary care physician or advanced practice nurse, require new or a revision of leadership skill sets. A leadership style that emphasizes team concepts and maximum involvement of all players, focusing on preventive care and health promotion rather than just treatment of illness in the hospital, is the ultimate goal. This chapter will discuss traits required of the leader not only to survive the rapid changes in professional and personal life but to provide suggestions to facilitate enjoying the journey.

Margaret Wheatley (1992), in her book *Leadership and the New Science,* discusses self-renewing organizations, which avoid rigid or permanent structures and instead develop a capacity to respond with great flexibility to external and internal changes. When the need changes, so do the organizational structure and mission. However, for an organization to exist in such an open and fluid fashion, it must constantly be processing data with high levels of self-awareness and a strong capacity for reflection and leadership. A singular leader, or a leadership team, who is reflectively monitoring the organization's destination, can review changing information, determine what choices are available, and what resources to rally in response.

Merger, redesign, and cost reduction are recent changes in health care but are old news in the business world. Business and industries that report profits and growth have leaders who created an environment that embraced change not as a threat but an opportunity for improvements. Jack Welch, ap-pointed General Electric (GE) Company Chairman in 1981, is an example of visionary leadership, with the courage to change and a passion for teaching and involving others in the change. Welch felt that GE must improve its quality and profit margin or risk being trampled by the foreign competition that was producing higher-quality goods, faster and cheaper. Welch made drastic changes at GE at a time when company profits were rising; he felt these were short-term profits at the sacrifice of long-term gains which stressed conservatism over innovation. By 1986, the GE work force had been cut to 229,000 from 412,000, almost a 50% reduction. The business plan for GE moved to a decentralized management and massive cultural changes, with organizational layers being pared from 11 down to five. GE had, at the start of the 1980s, $25 billion in sales and profits of $1.5 billion. In 1993 the company had revenues of $60.6 billion and net earnings of $5.2 billion.

The radical change Welch employed was called restructuring. In the early 1980s, this was a new idea. Restructuring did not mean stripping away a little bureaucracy here or divesting a business there. It meant taking a realistic look at one's company, and then deciding what the primary mission was and reorganizing to accomplish that vision. As drastic as Welch's cuts were, they focused on his vision of GE being number one in an international market and keeping only products and services that fit within that vision and mission. Welch said, "Take a hard look at your overall business, and decide as early as possible what needs fixing, what needs to be nurtured, and what needs to be jettisoned" (Slater, 1994). Welch eliminated people and eliminated unnecessary work. Welch's leadership took redesign a step further by removing the various boundaries and barriers between functions and levels and bureaucratic waste. Instead of a hierarchy, there would be cross-functional teams. Instead of managers, there would be business leaders. Instead of workers being told what to do, workers would be empowered and given responsibility. Welch's view of the liberation of the work place: "If you want to get the benefit of everything employees have, you've got to free them—make everybody a participant. Everybody has to know everything, so they can make the right decisions by themselves" (Slater, 1994). In other words, let each individual function to his or maximum potential.

Health care leaders are scrambling to decide what needs to be fixed, nurtured, or jettisoned and how to best remove the boundaries to attain the desired outcomes. James (1996) asserts: "We are all confused and ambivalent, trying to get our bearings in a age of rapid change . . . we are experiencing epic shifts in the way we think, feel about ourselves and our jobs, about the way we live, and about the future itself. Leadership in such an environment requires courage, character and a broader perspective."

Leadership Characteristics

Review of Jack Welch's leadership style and other leadership literature reveals characteristics that are common to outstanding leaders who make the most of opportunities, change, and produce outcomes that make a difference. The attributes of these match what Tichy (1986) describes as the transformational leader: change agents, courageous individuals, believe in people, value driven, life-long learners, experts in dealing with complexity and ambiguity, and visionary. The leader judged to be outstanding or transformational in the present time of rapid change will also require expertise in building relationships, a commitment to self-renewal and reflection, and a commitment not only to learning but also to teaching of others. Outstanding leaders are willing to evaluate a situation as it exists now and lay out a plan to inspire and redesign to build a winning team and organization. Successful leaders are change agents who facilitate a new approach, risk takers, innovative and willing to challenge the process. This is difficult because evaluating a situation as it exists now requires an awareness of filters that may disguise discomfort with current shortcomings or painful reality. Facing realities is about awareness, acceptance, and a willingness to change and the ability to create this willingness in others. The successful leaders have an enthusiasm that positively infects others. They make the vision seem attainable and desirable to others. They are persistent and energetic and take the initiative for change. Tichy (1997) believes "outstanding leaders have teachable points and invest considerable time teaching with well defined methodologies, coaching techniques, frequently of personal stories which emphasize their point, a willingness to admit mistakes and show vulnerabilities

in order to serve as an effective role model for others." Zen leadership includes the transformational leadership characteristics, with a willingness to increase knowledge of self and others, broaden perspectives, deepen reflection, and live in the present moment.

COURAGEOUS INDIVIDUALS

Zen leaders are courageous. They have a tolerance for risk, a willingness to try new things, and a bias toward action directed at achieving the beliefs or vision. They take action, even when it means making errors. When they make errors, they learn from them. Zen leaders are not afraid to try the untried. They are early to see trends and new ideas and to articulate a new idea, even when it is unpopular and in the minority opinion. Zen leaders are individuals whose expectations are beyond the current realities and see the need for change. Leaders may find it lonely out on a top limb by themselves! But part of their courage is possessing a high level of stress tolerance, or "heartiness," being able to keep cool under fire, and keep their heads when others are losing theirs. Courageous leaders are able to maintain focus under strenuous conditions. Zen leaders have the courage to make hard choices and tough decisions. They have the "guts" to admit a mistake and show their vulnerabilities, frequently shared as stories to serve as an effective example for others.

For example, some of the risks I have taken as an ambulatory nurse administrator have flopped! Once I tried to institute a peer recognition award program modeled after one I had read about in a national publication. The peer recognition award program was an idea driven from the top and did not have "buy-in" from the participants. Slowly it was realized that only temporary or part-time employees had been selected for the award and the objective of rewarding outstanding accomplishments and ingenuity was not being met. The award program was scrapped.

BELIEVERS IN PEOPLE

Zen leaders, who are multidimensional and nonjudgmental, can mobilize diverse groups of individuals—community leaders, employers, patients, physicians, nurses, public policy makers, legislators, board members, health care executives, and employees—to work toward a common goal. Outstanding leaders can balance financial imperatives with the realities of health care clinical practice, while creatively resolving conflicts that arise between operations and finance. These leaders get beyond the narrow financial niche that focuses on cost and determine how long-term benefits can enhance an organization. Zen leaders' involvement with various civic groups enables them to learn the community view of their organizations and their effectiveness in the community, such as how managed care may be affecting local employers or providers. Leaders who believe in people believe that each person will perform and contribute to his or her maximum capabilities if you catch his or her interests and passions. Outstanding leaders are frequently high-energy people and enhance the positive emotional energy of others. They do this by sharing their enthusiasm, by stretching, stimulating, and giving energy to others. Hendricks and Ludeman (1996) believe that successful leaders have developed the ability to "let go of being right." Release of the attachment to one's own viewpoint allows them the flexibility to change and have increased openness to the possibilities.

VALUE DRIVEN

Zen leaders are considered value driven when they are perceived by themselves and others as having integrity and the capacity to generate and sustain trust by being candid, by communicating effectively, and by exhibiting constancy and caring. Leaders are role models when their words and actions are congruent. Doing what one says enhances the sense of commitment or reciprocity needed to encourage others to increase their own vulnerability and willingness to risk. Being trustworthy as an individual leader promotes trusting behavior from others. To develop trust and respect for individuals, including oneself, one must reflect on values held. Values are seldom discussed openly, but are widely shared throughout an organization. These boundaries form the basic underpinning of the organization system and adhere to the leader's beliefs. The Zen leader willingly discusses and clarifies values, usually by sharing stories and life experiences. Zen leaders exhibit integrity. Hendricks and Ludeman (1996) define integrity as "being authentic with yourself, being authentic with others and doing the things you said you would do."

LIFE-LONG LEARNERS AND TEACHERS

Zen leaders are active listeners, open to new ideas, continual learning, and teaching. Leaders learn about leadership through life and job experience. Leadership is nurtured with on-the-job education and through role model mentorship. People learn to be leaders through adversity. They learn through the pain and agony of having to come up with the hard answers, of being fired, of failing, of downsizing, of having to take over an inexperienced group of people. Leaders learn by reading of leadership success and failure of others in history or business and by being placed in situations from which they receive feedback from valued sources around them and learn from the experience. Zen leaders are always in the business of learning, teaching, and sharing.

For example, I have learned from mistakes and reflection. Although the staff award previously discussed was scrapped, positive outcomes were achieved. After teaching a series of lectures on diversity and conflict that used the analogy of carp (i.e., passive, positive behaviors), shark (i.e., aggressive, negative behaviors), and dolphin (i.e., flexible, positive behaviors), new phrases were overheard at work. "You are acting like a shark" or "You're such a dolphin" were sprinkled into conversation. Miniature dolphin pins and symbols were prominently displayed at work and given as gifts. Staff morale as measured by shared laughter, communication, and participation soared. Although the original idea of a peer recognition award had not met the designers' anticipated outcomes, the objectives of improving communication, trust, and team building were achieved . . . eventually. I learned a valuable lesson on listening, building relationships, and the difference between empowering and overpowering.

EXPERTS IN DEALING WITH COMPLEXITY, AMBIGUITY, AND UNCERTAINTY

Leaders have the tough job of being in a challenging and complex environment with many unknowns. They work within a system populated by individuals who are continually scrutinizing every decision and action. Carlson (1997) believes there is wisdom in not knowing. He suggests that the best way to solve a problem without an immediate solution is to tap into our creative process. He defines this creative process as "a flow of thoughts that emerge naturally as the mind is emptied of analytical thinking. This deeper free flowing thinking . . . provides a deeper level of understanding and the answer comes." Zen leadership is being willing to not know, having the humility to admit that analytical thinking is not providing the solution, a willingness to clear the mind, stay in the present, and slip into a free-flow mode of thinking. Zen leaders are confident in their abilities to attain a positive outcome and invite others to join them. Their self-confidence and flexibility are infectious and impart a degree of enthusiasm and optimism into the situation. Zen leadership motivates others to do what Heifetz (1994) calls "adaptive work." Adaptive work means clarifying a conflict or ambiguity, clarifying values, or bridging the gap between values that the leader believes in and the current existing conditions. Heifetz believes that when a problem or challenge has no technical remedy, a problem for which it will not help to look to an authority for answers . . . the answers are not there . . . that problem calls for adaptive work.

According to Rivers (1996) in *The Way of the Owl*, "Historians say that the inferior general is always fighting the last war. He learns one lesson and then reactively applies it to every situation he faces, forgetting that every fight and every enemy is unique. But the wise . . . leader . . . looks at each conflict with the fresh eyes of seasoned innocence . . . learns and adapts from the past, but doesn't give it more significance than it deserves. History may repeat itself, but it may fly off in a nonlinear, chaotic leap. Do not be a slave to a historical model. Fight today's fight today."

This is a warning that events or cycles may repeat themselves but that the experienced leader knows to anticipate the unexpected and to be flexible enough to adapt and try new approaches. James (1996) reminds us that there are patterns beneath the current chaos or rapid change. She cautions, "The trick is to develop an eye for bits of information [that] when assembled provide new and visible patterns or trends." The Zen leader develops the analytical and intuitive skills necessary to recognize these patterns so that he or she can anticipate change, not just follow it.

VISIONARIES

How does a leader rally individuals with different perspectives and areas of expertise toward a common goal? One approach is the leader's articulation of beliefs, vision, and strategic plan. The leader repeatedly communicates the vision clearly, compellingly, and consistently in memos, meetings, newsletters, videos, satellite broadcasts, and, most of all, eyeball to eyeball to establish consistency and conviction of purpose. The leader's vision must be anchored in organizational realities. To anchor the vision means interweaving it into everything that the leader does . . . recruiting, rewarding, decision making, policy making, and empowering. Successful leaders are avid learners. They update ideas and visions to keep current with changing circumstances and translate their visions into actions and achievable strategies. Successful leaders focus externally and are responsive to the market. They draw from their pasts and reflect on their experiences to develop distinctive visions of the future. They are decisive, broad-brush administrators who empower and build effective management teams; they are motivated to achieve and are not afraid to take chances. Outstanding leaders have the "big picture" and are prepared to take risks to better position their organizations for three to five years in the future. The leader's vision is grounded in an appreciation of the environment and ways in which it can be improved. Zen leaders dream and are able to describe their dreams and images so that other people can share and help achieve them.

A favorite leadership story is of two monks who traveled all day from one monastery to another after a rain storm. In a chance encounter the monks meet a lovely woman traveling on foot and dressed in a beautiful kimono; she has halted by a gigantic mud puddle blocking the path. One of the monks graciously wades through the water and carries the young woman safely across to dry footing on the other side. The two monks continue on their way. Much later in the day, the other monk questioned the actions of picking up the woman and carrying her, accusing him of violating his sacred vows prohibiting any contact with women. The helpful monk chastised his fellow monk for taking the situation out of context. Saying he had put that woman down hours ago, why was the other monk still carrying her around?

This admonishment shows that leadership requires a willingness to confront the dilemmas, reflect on past perceptions, meet challenges, embrace new realities, and, as appropriate, take analysis and risks to reach the destination of the vision. The Zen leader is willing to release what is no longer pertinent, useful, or required.

Health care redesign, like the Zen monks, requires a major analysis of the entire health care system to identify what remains pertinent and what can be released. What makes this so risky from previous health care redesign or changes? The answer is the speed of change in economics, financing, competition, and health practice standards. Health care systems struggling to provide care in a cost-effective manner are questioning the validity of certain past practices and health care staffing patterns and scopes of practice of various health care professionals. In the past, anecdotes about dissatisfied patients focused on overuse of tests, unnecessary treatment, greedy doctors, and a health care system riddled with waste and out-of-control costs. Now the anecdotes often feature denial of treatment, limits on hospitalization and choice of physicians, use of unlicensed assistive personnel instead of registered nurses, greedy health care plan executives, and a system that cuts corners to increase profits.

What is demanded of health care leaders during these turbulent times? Zen leaders possess the ability to build relationships based on trust, communication, commitment, and cooperation.

There is an ancient Chinese parable about an old man who knew he would soon die. Before he died, he wanted to know about the difference between healthy and unhealthy organizations . . . in his case heaven and hell. So he visited a wise man in his village to ask, "Can you tell me what heaven and hell are like?" The wise man invited him to take a walk with him and led him out of the village and down a strange path, deep into the countryside. Finally, they came to a large house with many rooms and went inside. Inside they found many people sitting on the floor under enormous shelves of food with an incredible array of food. Then the old man noticed a strange thing. The people in the house were all thin and hungry, but were each holding chopsticks 12 feet long. They tried to feed themselves, but of course they could not get the food to their mouths with such long chopsticks. "This is surely hell," said the old man. "Now will

you show me heaven?" The wise man led him out of the house, and they walked further along the same path. They reached another house, similar to the first, and again entered. The scene was very much the same, much food and many people, again with 12-foot chopsticks. But this time the people were happy and well fed. The old man could not understand. "These people are happy and well fed, but they too have 12-foot chopsticks. Please explain to me," said the old man. The wise man responded simply, "In heaven, people feed each other."

Healthy relationships may not be heaven, but healthy relationships do nurture healthy behaviors and deliver what they advertise. Zen leaders nurture people and help them to nurture each other by building relationships.

Building Relationships

In *The Quantum Society*, Zohar and Marshall (1994) discuss quantum reality, which is the relationship between "individual particles," located in fixed positions in time and space, and "wavelike particles," which are spread across all time and space and whose instantaneous effects are everywhere. This "wave-particle dualism" offers us a powerful new model for seeing ourselves as individuals, distinct and effective in our own right, and at the same time as members of wider groups through which we acquire further identity and a wider capacity for creative relationship. Our rapidly changing environment is poised constantly between order and chaos. In allowing ourselves new experiences, nonjudgmental attitudes, we seek many possibilities and our ability to thrive on change is drastically increased. This model offers the opportunity to live and function at the highest level of our potential. In the dynamics and systems approach of quantum reality, dialogue is a willingness to put our attitudes, beliefs, and plans "on hold." We are willing to listen creatively to our instincts and the other person and release familiar concepts and categories. The other person does the same. Through this process of dialogue a resynthesis occurs. Each learns new concepts and new categories. Each arrives at a new understanding and perhaps even a new position that neither one could have achieved individually. We do not necessarily agree at the end of dialogue or deep listening to the other's point of view, but we do, in the quantum sense already described, agree to disagree (Zohar, Marshall, 1994). The discussions and convergence of our differences is our consensus. Kritek (1994) believes that the negotiation of our differences can teach us compassion. She says, "If you listen closely to others, try to hear what they are saying and also what they are not saying, what they are feeling and what they are trying not to feel, you begin to know and understand the dimensions of their humanness: the fears that bind them and the courage they show despite the odds" (Kritek, 1994). Or another way of saying to walk a mile in someone else's shoes is to experience life from their perspective. For leaders to continue giving to others, they must be able to nurture self and others in life-giving ways. Koerner (1995) says, "The creative care leader has a reversed image of life and leadership. To transcend ourselves we must support, empower and learn from others. We must develop a reverence for the uniqueness of each individual, including ourselves. Understanding and honoring self and others are essential, leading to changes in attitudes and behaviors that radically transform outcomes for all. From the vantage point of mutual valuing we move out of a pattern of domination and control toward connection of the heart, soul and mind. Leaders open the door to power, sharing it through creation of true partnership with mutual responsibility" (Koerner, 1995).

TEAMWORK AND COLLABORATION

What is the underpinning of teamwork and collaboration? Chrislip and Larson (1994) define collaboration as "a mutually beneficial relationship between two or more parties who work toward common goals by sharing responsibilities, authority, and accountability for achieving results." According to Chrislip and Larson (1994), "Collaboration is more than the communication of sharing knowledge and information and more than a cooperation which helps each party achieve its own goals. The purpose of collaboration is to create a shared vision and joint strategies to address concerns that go beyond the purview of any particular party." This combination provides the synergy of a whole that is better than the parts.

Chrislip (1994) believes the following four common areas cause difficulty for collaboration or team-building efforts: failure to manage conflict effectively, incomplete sharing of information, ineffi-

cient use of technology, and interpersonal relationship issues. First, and most common, is the failure to manage conflict effectively. Many individuals have never learned that an honest difference of opinion is okay and that confrontation can be anything except violent. Second is sharing of information. Functional teams and organizations require accurate and timely information that is shared. In our information-dependent culture, convoluted transmission patterns and distorted communications are bound to have an impact on efficiency, productivity, and harmony. Third is taking advantage of new technology to become more efficient and productive and making work easier. It also means improving our use of people resources, the human system. The bottom line of working smart with teams is the focus of one's time, energy, and resources. Fourth is building and maintaining relationships. Managing conflict, communicating and sharing information, and working smart all affect the quality of one's relationships with co-workers and colleagues.

Key aspects relevant to relationships are intimacy and commitment. Intimacy means openness and a willingness to share, to both give to and receive from others. Commitment is demonstrated by dependability and reliability, a sense of obligation and accountability. Chrislip and Larson believe intimacy and commitment are the foundation on which relationships are built and the cement that holds them together and maintains them. Intimacy and commitment are essential to teamwork and cooperation. Cooperation and teamwork require enough openness and sharing to nurture mutual confidence. Confidence that co-workers will share the work load fairly, that each will carry out his or her responsibilities reliably, and that each is accountable to the others and to their product.

In 1995, I participated in an action learning group composed of nursing experts, who were reflecting on their leadership styles and habits as change agents and transformational leaders. The first afternoon together, participants were asked to briefly tell a true story and a false story about themselves. The group members would then decide which story they believed to be true and why. The facilitators of the group had allocated about 90 minutes for 25 quick vignettes. Instead over three hours were spent weaving fascinating and revealing stories, which formed a strong foundation for openness, rapport, mutual respect, and trust for the group's activities and learning.

This exercise supports Kouzes' theory that the best way to show your trust in others is through openness and self-disclosure. "When you let others know things about yourself and you make yourself vulnerable by telling them about your own uncertainties and doubts, they are more likely to be open with you. This mutual openness is fundamental to trust" (Kouzes, Posner, 1987). Carlson (1997). Carlson relates that in ". . . healthy relationships there is a feeling of being at ease." He calls this feeling of ease "rapport" and defines it as ". . . the lubricant in virtually every social and meaningful interaction. With rapport we are in the present . . . light hearted, warm and respectful towards others. In a lack of rapport there are feelings of tension, fear, discomfort, and insecurity."

With collaboration, and trust and rapport, individuals are ready to work with one another to make extraordinary things happen. By strengthening others and giving power away, the Zen leader turns this readiness into action. Delegation is fundamentally a component of trust. One indicates trust in someone when one delegates authority to that person. Trust is also developed when people feel safe. When one's thoughts and ideas are ridiculed, one quickly realizes that the climate is neither safe nor conducive to making oneself vulnerable or to a willingness to open oneself up and place trust in another person. To create a climate of trust, leaders can be open about their own mistakes and vulnerabilities. Leaders may have a reluctance to admit mistakes for fear they will lose their power to influence. Letting others see one's humanness is one of the best ways to enhance one's credibility.

NETWORKING

A few years ago one rarely heard "network" used as a verb, but that usage has spread widely. Networking describes an increasingly necessary function: the process of creating or maintaining a pattern of informal linkages among individuals or organizations. Gardner (1993) explains the necessity of networking in a swiftly changing environment, because "established and formal linkages may no longer serve, or may have been disrupted. New and flexible interconnections become necessary." Gardner recommends that leaders should be skilled in creating or recreating the linkages neces-

sary to establish extensive networks in order to get goals and visions accomplished.

MENTORING

Mentoring is another way to increase our skills. Huang and Lynch (1995) define mentoring as "a two way opportunity for us to experience both giving and receiving wisdom without limitations and fears." Their mentoring model depicts giving and receiving knowledge that incorporates both ancient Taoist wisdom of self-reflection, simplicity, and openness and new insights gained from cultivating relationships with a willingness to learn and grow. Tao mentoring is a process of learning in which the reward is not only in reaching one's goals but also in the very process of guiding and growing together. When two parties enter into Tao mentoring, they create a safe environment where truth and wisdom can be discovered by both. This nonthreatening, uncritical exchange enables each partner to admit to not knowing, which at times may seem uncomfortable or threatening. Tao mentoring gives permission to face our vulnerabilities and insecurities. Profound growth and change can come to one who is willing to let go and admit not knowing. The admission of not knowing creates enormous internal strength and freedom to be open to learning or wisdom. The willingness and shared openness enable one to participate in a cycle of learning, teaching, and sharing. By mentoring others, one becomes aware of the gaps in one's own knowledge. This constant exchange is mutually accepted. The essence of mentoring is admitting that one needs help on the journey of learning and living. Huang and Lynch (1995) believe effective mentors "guide in an atmosphere of inspiration, trust, courage, and harmony, where independence and personal strength are created and individuals grow and become more aware of their inner selves as well as the greatness and inner selves in others."

My definition of mentoring has changed from a one-directional coaching to a reciprocal exchange of learning, teaching, and sharing. Many of my own mentoring experiences started with an admiration of a colleague or acquaintance's skill. Sometimes over time a mentoring relationship developed if we both perceived value and a willingness to give and take from the relationship. I slowly realized that reciprocal relationships are dependent on this mutual respect and the courage to admit one does not know or understand.

Carlson and Bailey (1997) offer the following suggestions to enhance mentoring relationships:

- Each party is respectful and works to establish rapport.
- Each party listens without interruption and seems to draw the other person out.
- The sharing comes from the heart . . . free-flowing thinking . . . in a spontaneous manner.
- Both participate in the intimacy, and the exchange is usually memorable

Building Relationships with Self: Self-Renewal and Nurturing

McGee-Cooper's (1993) research showed that children, geniuses, and exceptional leaders all have the common traits of intense passion and the ability to have fun without the pressures of following rules, fulfilling expectations, keeping score, or judging one's performance. Passion nourishes our soul and creativity if we are open to the events of life. This means, without sufficient rest and relaxation, even if we love our work and are renewed and energized by it, we can fall into unhealthy traps that can block our passion, self-nurturing, and creativity.

As a child, I remember that on Saturdays, my mother would give me permission to go play when all weekly chores were completed. As an adult with a sense of responsibility and obligations, I have found that there is always more work to accomplish and usually no one encouraging or giving permission to go.

Distorted Perspectives

One can become so involved in work that certain relationships, such as marriage, friendships, families, and self, are taken for granted. One can miss out on the richness of the diversity of experiences. By getting caught up in the daily tasks of work performance and commuting, it can become easy to overlook simple treasures such as nurturing children and mates and participating in their life events. Then the day comes when one realizes it is too late to participate.

One's ego can also become fused with one's work. This can result in a feeling of worthlessness if one is not constantly accomplishing. Individuals are not their work. A danger of this lifestyle is becoming one dimensional and having no other outlets if one is abruptly severed from the job. Having a balanced set of values and joys provides a safety net that can improve the quality of one's life and work.

One can become better at work than at interpersonal relationships, so relationships are avoided. Work can be highly rewarding, but the more prestige one has, the more vulnerable one can be to external trappings. Successful leaders may find themselves "too busy to deal with family issues," not realizing that, deep down, they do not like the anxiety of uncertainty caused by inability to solve family problems the way they control work situations. So they conveniently stay too busy to deal with issues in areas where they are not succeeding. Losing a marriage, alienating a child, or loss of self-respect is a high price to pay for living out of balance.

Enjoying the euphoria of achieving difficult goals and winning big successes can be addictive. One may become single-focused and unwilling to expose oneself to situations in which one is not the expert or in control. One tries new adventure or participates less and less out of fear of not excelling. Pretty soon one's life consists of only work. One's life can become terribly out of balance without even noticing.

One Halloween, for work I dressed in a clown costume instead of the standard military uniform. The responses and courtesies customarily provided a senior officer in a military facility were not automatically given. The experience provided a learning opportunity regarding customer-focused care and increased my awareness of humility. It also stirred memories of the evening I snapped at my husband, inquiring about dinner plans and asking what he had been doing all day . . . other than taking care of a 2-year-old. He reminded me that his role and obligations were not to snap to attention and salute when I walked through the door. Reflections on priorities and balance are important.

Living in simultaneous waves of change, one can easily get caught in one of these traps and be thrown out of balance. The light bulb is a visual symbol for balance. The light bulb's capacity is thousands of hours, so it can shine brightly for months. But eventually it is going to burn out, especially if it is left on all the time. Human burnout can be a gradual dimming of what once was bright.

One experiences burnout when one loses the excitement and energy once felt for a job, a passionate cause, or a way of life. Avoiding burnout is like installing a new light bulb or turning the switch off periodically. Think about ways to renew and regenerate life passions, and take time for reflection. Maintaining balance in our personal and professional lives in these chaotic times is difficult. However, this is an age-old challenge. In Zen philosophy, Buddha explained that the good ox driver knew how much the ox could carry and kept the ox from being overloaded. The Zen philosophy of prevention corresponds to a state of staying in the present and being mindful. Huang and Lynch (1995) describe mindfulness, a state of relaxed consciousness, as "the process of becoming aware and acting in accordance with what the leader knows to be right. It is a harmony created . . . (by attention to) subtle details. As a practice of awareness, it requires being conscious of the implications of all actions . . . mindfulness is the letting go of preconceived notions and the tendency to fix problems and judge, it is the willingness to discover, explore and appreciate what is with centered, trustful attention" (Huang, Lynch, 1995). When one is in the present and practicing mindfulness, one is practicing Zen leadership at the zenith. Mindfulness is the aware, balanced acceptance of present experience. It is open to the present moment, pleasant or unpleasant, just as it is. Thich Nhat Hanh reminds us, "Every morning, when we wake up, we have 24 brand new hours to live . . . and a capacity to live in a way that will bring peace, joy, and happiness to ourselves and others . . . planning for the future is part of life but planning can only take place in the present moment." Carlson and Bailey (1997) warns, "Life is what's happening while we are busy making other plans," or in other words, we need to live in the present to our fullest capacity.

Conclusion

Zen leaders are distinguished in this time of rapid change by their clarity and persuasiveness of ideas, the depth of commitment, openness to continually learning and teaching, and ongoing struggle to live life in the moment. In the process of change and chaos, outstanding or "ZEN" leaders realize they do not always "have the answer." But they have the humility to admit they do not know, are open to

the moment, seek balance and self-renewal, and are continuously building relationships with self and others so that the desired outcomes can be developed and achieved. Wheatley and Kellner-Rogers' (1996), in the book *A Simpler Way,* describe a leader in rapid change leading with integrity, taking care of the present, and listening to self and others:

There is a simpler way to organize human endeavors. It requires a new way of being in the world. It requires being in the world without fear. Being in a world with play and creativity. Seeking after what's possible. Being willing to learn and be surprised . . . This simpler way summons forth the best in us . . . It asks us to understand human nature differently, more optimistically. It identifies us as creative. It acknowledges that we seek meaning. It asks us to be less serious, yet more purposeful about our work and our lives. It does not separate play from the nature of being . . . As we change our ways . . . we welcome back ourselves.

References

Carlson R, Bailey J: *Slowing down to the speed of life,* San Francisco, 1997, Harper Collins.

Chrislip D, Larson C: *Collaborative leadership: how citizens and civic leaders can make a difference,* San Francisco, 1994, Jossey-Bass.

Gardner J: *On leadership:* New York, 1993, Free Press.

Heifetz R: *Leadership without easy answers,* Cambridge, 1994, Belknap Press.

Hendricks G, Ludeman K: *The corporate mystic: a guidebook for visionaries with their feet on the ground,* San Francisco, 1996, Harper Collins.

Huang C, Lynch J: *Mentoring: The Tao of giving and receiving wisdom,* San Francisco, 1995, Harper Collins.

James J: *Thinking in the future tense,* New York, 1996, Simon and Schuster.

Kouzes J, Posner B: *The leadership challenge: how to get extraordinary things done in organizations,* San Francisco, 1987, Jossey-Bass.

Koerner J: The power of place: career transformation through stability, *Nursing Administration Quarterly* 19(4):44-53, 1995.

Kritek P: *Negotiating at an uneven table; developing moral courage in resolving our conflicts,* San Francisco, 1994, Jossey-Bass.

McGee-Cooper A: *You don't have to go home from work exhausted,* New York, 1992, Bantam.

Rivers F: *The way of the owl: succeeding with integrity in a conflicted world,* San Francisco, 1996, Harper Collins.

Slater R: *Get better or get beaten! 31 leadership secrets from GE's Jack Welch,* New York, 1994, Irwin Publishing.

Thich Nhat Hanh: *Peace is every step: the path of mindfulness in everyday life,* New York, 1991, Bantam.

Tichy N: *The leadership engine: how winning companies build leaders at every level,* San Francisco, 1997, Harper Collins.

Tichy N, Devanna M: *The transformational leader,* New York, 1986, Wiley & Sons.

Wheatley M: *Leadership and the new science: learning about organization from the orderly universe,* San Francisco, 1992, Berrett-Koehler.

Wheatley, M. & Kellner-Rogers, M. *A Simpler Way.* San Francisco, Barrett-Koehler, 1996.

Zohar D, Marshall I: *The quantum society: mind, physics, and the new vision,* New York, 1994, Morrow and Company.

CHAPTER 8

Transformational Leadership in a Changing World

SUSAN C. FRY, RN, MEd, CNAA

OVERVIEW

We should have high expectations for those who lead us. Their personal conduct and public conduct should be one and the same.

This chapter discusses the challenges in moving from a management focus to a leadership focus in the rapidly changing times in health care. One is challenged to examine the core beliefs and practices that lead to making the right decision, not just in doing the right things but in rethinking some previously accepted practices to journey toward a transformation. ▲

Covey (1989), in his best seller *7 Habits of Highly Effective People*, graphically illustrates the difference between managers and leaders when he describes "a group of producers cutting their way through the jungle with machetes." He tells of the producers cutting the undergrowth, the managers "writing the policy and procedure manuals," while the leader climbs a tree, surveys the situation, and yells down, "Wrong jungle!" Then he asks, "But how do the busy, efficient producers and managers often respond? 'Shut up! We're making progress.' " During times of rapid, radical change, it is very easy to get caught up in making change (because everyone is doing it) and not utilizing good leadership skills to determine if we are changing in the right direction and areas.

What is the difference between leadership skills and management skills? For several decades now, American business has focused on identifying, quantifying, and building management skills, and only recently has begun to acknowledge that there is a difference between management skills and leadership skills and that exercising these skills independently of each other leads to very different outcomes. Management "manages" doing things the right way; leadership "leads" to doing the right thing. How does one become a leader when the recent past has focused on learning management?

The Path to Leadership

Nair (1994) became intrigued with Gandhi's impact on India and the world, and set about to determine how someone who never really held a policy making position could have so much impact on a nation and the world. Nair's first observation, and challenge, speaks to individual responsibility. He observed that personal principles and values need to be the basis for actions, rather than policies or rules. We should have high expectations for those who lead us and their personal conduct and public conduct should be one and the same. Only by having high expectations do we have good leaders and leadership. Nair's exploration of Gandhi's life and the leadership principles identified hold great meaning in light of the events happening in today's health care arena.

"Striving toward an ideal requires commitment" (Nair, 1994). The basis for personal responsibility is to identify and commit to those values (absolute truths) that, no matter what, you will not violate. Gandhi's truths, as Nair explains, were truth telling at all times and to treat each person with dignity and respect. Both of these absolute values were great challenges for Gandhi in India at that time, where the class system was an accepted way of life and the untouchable class an accepted aspect of Hindu life. Gandhi then began to translate these beliefs into actions, realizing that there was the need for continuous self-improvement, based on self-reflection.

What are those core values, those absolute truths that, no matter what, we in health care are unwilling to violate? It is important to understand that living up to these values is not without risk. As a nurse, is not "patient first" an honorable value? What is the risk then in a policy-driven organization when the policy does not support "patient first"? It is not uncommon in today's cost-conscious environment for there to be more concern and discussion about the cost than there is about what is the right thing to do for a particular patient and family. The nurse is frequently the closest to the situation, and without his or her voice asking the all-important question "Is this the right thing to do?" the business side of health care can overshadow the right provision of service. What about the manager who believes truth telling is a core value and then is asked directly about something that his or her supervisor wants "kept secret"? The current focus on the business aspects of health care challenge many of the traditional values that we have held and may not have had to examine during our careers.

Many organizations today have published value statements so that all employees, patients, families, and other customers have access to the corporate values. These statements do not, however, replace the need for personal values, but need to be used for self-reflection about how the corporate values can and do support personal values. When there is great disparity between the organizational values and personal values, it may mean that some difficult employment decisions may have to be made. Depending on the values in question, it is not always possible to remain true to personal values, when the mission and values of the organization are clear and practiced. For example, an OB nurse who is prochoice, and who works in a Catholic health care center, will encounter conflict between her or his personal value system and the firm values of the organization.

Once one identifies one's personal values, it becomes a journey to apply them to one's public and private life. One needs to continuously evaluate how well these values are being utilized and what improvements are needed to continue to move toward fulfilling one's commitment to oneself. Self-reflection requires setting aside time for open and honest internal communication. Even though one's time for self-reflection is limited, one needs to devote some time daily for self-review to stay true to self and to assess how one's actions are supporting one's personal values. Nair (1994) points out very clearly that Gandhi felt that working toward personal truth was a lifetime journey and not something that you adopted completely in a short period of time. Given the major changes that have taken place and those yet to come in health care, allocating time for personal reflection is no longer optional. One busy managed care executive, who is a nurse, sets aside one day a month for "planning." She tells only her secretary where to reach her, and to do so only in an emergency, and uses the time for study and self-reflection to center herself for the work ahead of her. Her staff respects this work habit because she returns with ideas and a more energized approach. She states, however, that it has taken discipline to use the time wisely and not feel guilty that tasks do not get done during her "planning."

SERVICE ORIENTATION

Covey (1989) and Nair (1994) speak to the importance of devoting one's life to service, not to obtaining positions or income. Once one focuses on a life of service, it becomes unimportant what title one holds or which office one occupies. This may be one of the most important points as we move into the twenty-first century. With the rapid change and reorganizations yet to come, the focus will be on outcomes and skills to obtain those outcomes, making titles and organizational charts meaningless. If one's focus is on service, then outcomes become important and the skills to accomplish those outcomes become important and one can be fulfilled by accomplishing the work and not being focused on the title or office. A life of service, not one devoted to self-service, is the hallmark of a true leader. It mat-

ters not what position one holds, or what income one makes; if service is a personal value, those around you recognize that and will support the service being provided. When there is a focus on self-service, associates and peers recognize that the "work" supports an individual, which probably, in the long run, will benefit one person or only a few. Morale is affected. It is under these circumstances that one feels that one has been used to further someone else's career, and not for the good of the whole. Self-servicing leadership gives rise to feelings of disempowerment and ultimately low morale within work teams. The self-serving person does not need to be the formal positional leader for this effect to take place. This phenomenon is frequently seen within work groups that feel that "everyone is not pulling their weight." It is at this point that the formal leader needs to intervene and work with the self-serving member or members to help them refocus on service. If that is not obtainable, it may be necessary to move or remove the self-serving person for the good of the whole. Working toward a new standard is not without challenges!

Nair (1994) speaks of the importance of using the privileges of the position to further the work (objectives) of the organization and not as a right of the position. This focus should also help leaders to evaluate what is really important and contributing to the good of the organization and not just the good of the individual, an important concept when one is focusing on controlling costs and building teams. Who, according to the goals of the organization, should have reserved parking places? Who should have company cars? Who needs to travel first class and why? If the reason is for prestige or a feeling that the person deserves these things, then a true leader focused on service will forgo these privileges for the good of the organization. "We cannot expect to reach a higher standard of leadership if we do not recognize that meeting our responsibilities should be a way of life, not a way of gaining rewards," writes Nair (1994).

BUILDING TRUST

Management is about formal position power, ability to allocate resources, and implementing policy; it is about control. Leadership is internally driven and is about vision, service, values, and personal commitment. Leadership is the ability to influence and does not need to be directly tied to a formal position. Obviously, if one has both a formal position of power and leadership skills, one potentiates the other, but there are plenty of people who are very influential but do not hold formal management positions. It would be unusual for any nurse with experience not to have met a ward clerk, nursing assistant, or staff nurse who could influence an entire work team, no matter what management wanted to accomplish. An office environment is no different.

Influence is about trust. We will do things for people we trust that we will not do for anyone else. When our private and public values are in alignment and we focus on service and being trustworthy, we build trust and, ultimately, influence. "By balancing control with service, the leader can experience decision-making authority without diminishing the personal power of the individual" (Nair, 1994). In times of rapid and major change, it is important that the personal power of the individual be acknowledged and maximized, if one wants the change to be accepted and internalized. If the power of the individual is not acknowledged, then the change becomes the program of the moment, and once management moves onto something else, old ways will reemerge. "The key issues facing today's manager-leaders are no longer task and structure; they're questions of spirit" (Hawley, 1993).

CREATING SPIRIT

What is spirit? How do we build spirit in the workplace? Why do we need to build spirit? In times of radical change such as we are facing in today's world, the old answers no longer apply and the new answers have not been found. Spirit: "It's a call of purpose, meaning, and character in life and business life," writes Hawley (1993). Spirituality is not religion (that is the path). Spirituality is the goal; it is "the transition from uncertainty to clarity," writes Hawley (1993). In such uncertain times, is it any wonder that there is a need for spirit in the work place? Hawley challenges us to move our organizations to "revering," to develop a "deep caring for others—a respect so intense it becomes reverence" (Hawley, 1993). Then to repower ourselves and finally to "recharacter . . . live by one's inner truth" (Hawley, 1993).

When there is spirit in the employees in an organization, there is energy "and energy—organiza-

tional or personal—is strength" (Hawley, 1993). Energy is what will fuel the organization for maximum beneficial change; spirit grounds the employees in doing the right thing when there are no longer policies and procedures that apply to the new problems. Many of us may have experienced this spirit and energy in retail experiences, health care experiences, and other personal experiences. It is the feeling that something is different about the place. One feels that one wants to return and experience it again, that one was helped beyond the norm. How do leaders create that difference?

CREATING REVERENCE

Hawley gives a wonderful explanation of "the reverence continuum in organizations" (1993). He explains that in organizations, there is a plan of civility below which is uncivilized behavior and above which is politeness, moving onto caring, then respect, and then reverence. Many health care workers have probably experienced uncivilized behavior, although most, if not all, organizations have policies and procedures to deal with the uncivilized. Application fairly to all parties may be an issue, especially if the uncivilized behavior belongs to a very position-powerful person. If there is uncivilized behavior tolerated, there are probably also some attempts to manage to politeness, but most recognize it is surface politeness and can revert to uncivility at any time. Working in this environment requires energy to be used just to make it through the day (or shift, or week) without tempers erupting. Energy is used for self-protection and is not available for creativity or organizational or personal improvements.

There has been an emphasis on caring in health care, a period of time when many health care organizations made very public with advertising and employee "We Care" campaigns. For many, that was the program of the year. How many have continued on to respect and ended with an environment of reverence? James Autry (1991) tells a wonderful story about Bob Burnett, in the acknowledgments section of his book *Love & Profit*. Bob Burnett became the president and chief executive officer of Meredith Corporation, publishers of *Ladies Home Journal, Better Homes & Gardens,* and dozens of other magazines. Autry explains that Bob was the "first man I ever heard use the word *love* as an attribute of someone in business" (Autry, 1991). Considering that was more than 25 years ago now, Burnett was certainly ahead of his time. How many health care leaders are so brave, when the business is about caring? If we are to move our organizations, our work teams, ourselves, to an environment of reverence, where do we start?

PUTTING THOUGHT INTO ACTIONS

Once we have identified our core values, those absolute truths beyond which we are not willing to go, we must then translate those beliefs into our consciousness and then into action. The very foundation of our thoughts is our language. Hearing and speaking consistent messages drive much of what we do and think. There is considerable everyday language that is accepted and mentored but if examined with reverence, would probably not pass and should be changed. Do nurses have daily "assignments" instead of patients "to care for"? Are patients asked their preferences for first or last names? The word *patient* should describe a relationship and not a person. One group of ICU nurses calls admissions "hits," as in "I had two hits today." Is it any wonder that they feel overworked and unappreciated? What would some simple language changes do to their mental health and ultimately to the unit atmosphere, if reverent language were used?

Thoughts translated into language drive the beliefs that guide us and ultimately create the environment in which we find ourselves. Leaders, in times of rapid change, need to be creating an environment of reverence so that positive energy can be produced to create more positive energy. Energy creates energy, which drives the work and workers. If energy is negative, it produces negative results. Positive energy produces positive results. It is the work of leaders to create positive energy and then of managers to channel and direct that energy.

One very successful CFO always made it a point to call the long-term babies in the neonatal intensive care unit by their first names when discussing their cases. This created an environment of respect for them as people and, he stated, assisted him in remembering to ask if financial decisions he was making regarding these babies "were the right thing to do." Personalizing them with names created a personal relationship, and kept him centered, even though he never saw them or knew them directly.

Success in the New World

Blanchard (1997) succinctly identifies the following three key points for success in the new world:

1. Success in organizations is all about creative use of untapped human energy.
2. The way to tap this energy is to make people your partners.
3. The way to make people your partners is to meaningfully engage them in either improving the present operations or creating the organization's future.

Blanchard's book is not directed at health care, but at business in general. How poignant that the three points speak to the very issues current in health care today: partnerships, operational improvement, and creating a new future. Perhaps the redesigns and reorganizations that non–health care businesses have experienced over the past decade have moved non–health care businesses further along the reverence continuum than some health care organizations. Nordstrom's, the large West Coast retail establishment, prides itself on its service and the minimum number of policies it needs in order to "manage" its workforce. Certainly it has discovered how to bring spirit into the workplace and empower "associates" to meet the vision and mission of the organization. Granted, health care is more complex than retail sales (or so we think), but we are dealing with a high percentage of professionals who have received advanced education within their professions, as well as some exposure to a professional orientation to "protect the public good," as the basis of a profession. The challenge is how to harness all that knowledge and dedication, to create spirit and reverence to move our organizations to a different place, a new future, so that the work is meaningful and the care received by our patients is continuously improving.

Hickman notes that "most executives find themselves confronted with an escalating conflict and schism between managerial and leadership requirements of organizations. An 'either/or' mentality dominates at a time when organizations most desperately need the best of both" (1992). He further explains that he is saying that "the new balance needed by organizations today requires the full deployment of both managers and leaders. . . . Such balance comes not from within one person, but through the effective, open and empowered interaction of different people who would otherwise succumb to counterproductive conflict." There is always tension between the two, "a natural phenomenon," he points out, and the challenge is "What combination works best?" (1992)

The common theme in business publications today is to create an organization driven by vision and mission. An organization in which leadership is recognized and nurtured, and management is supported to harness and guide the creativity that is produced. One where there is recognition and valuing of what each entity contributes toward attainment of mutual goals. There is a wonderful story about a dietary worker in a hospital cafeteria, who offers a free second helping to a visitor who compliments him on the rice pudding. When asked by the visitor how he would dare to give away the cafeteria food, the dietary worker explains that it is his responsibility to "delight the customer" and see that people return. When he gives second helpings as reward for customers' compliments, he sees his actions as a small investment toward this goal. This is surely an empowered employee who can articulate the goals of his work area and then produce an action to demonstrate his understanding. The ending to the story: the visitor was so impressed with the service that he chose to return to the cafeteria for each meal during his family's hospital stay. Many customers returning to Nordstrom's will tell the same kinds of stories about the service they have received. Should health care organizations deliver any less?

Florence Nightingale in her *Notes on Nursing* offers this advice: "Let who ever is in charge keep this simple question in her head (*not*, how can I always do this right thing myself, but) how can I provide for this right thing to always be done?" (Ulrich, 1992) Empowerment and partnerships were not common concepts during Miss Nightingale's time, but clearly she grasped their meaning and importance when she offered this advice over 100 years ago.

A True Story of Tomorrow

A very rural section of a Midwestern state recognized in the early 1990s that the managed care con-

cepts of coordination of the continuum of care, reduction of costs, and focus on wellness would probably not come to their area for years, if at all. The visionary county leadership initiated a county health assessment and then has been able to coordinate all the services needed to improve meeting the identified health needs of its citizens by designing partnerships between agencies and "managing" the health of its citizens through effective provision of services, rather than through an insurance plan. The theme that continuously comes out is "we want to do what's best for our citizens." The hospital, nursing homes, county ambulance, county health department, schools, and churches are all aligned for the provision of services to address the health needs of the citizens of the county. The project has taken years and has not always been smooth, but the vision and the focus on what is the right thing to do have guided the leadership to develop a model that is unique for its time and place. The health outcomes of the population are being measured and initiatives developed to address identified areas, all of which is being done very quietly because of the focus on service and not seeking the limelight.

Conclusion

Leadership is a journey, a transformation both personally and professionally. The journey starts with personal values identified and lived and then expectations created for our leaders and ourselves. Our thoughts about our expectations, together with a service orientation, form a belief structure that guides us, both privately and publicly. The beliefs form the framework of our vision—our vision about what we want to be and also a vision about what we want our practice and work to be. If the beliefs are positive, the vision will be positive. Positive people are surrounded by positive people. Energy is created when people come together to accomplish a common goal. Positive energy creates more positive energy, which leads to creative problem solving, thinking outside the box, and instilling hope that solutions can be found. It is this transformation that is needed in health care today. This is a time of many questions and few answers, a time to draw out the best in the providers in the system while, all around them, there is chaos and confusion. It is only with hope and positive expectations that the recipient of our services, the patient, will benefit.

Non–health care businesses seem to have arrived at an understanding that there is a difference between management and leadership, and that leadership to transform is critical for survival. The literature on transformational leadership began to appear in the business world in the early 1990s. It has only recently begun to appear in health care literature. Is this a trend from which health care can learn and avoid some of the trials and failures of other businesses? Or is the health care environment so chaotic that it is closed to learning from other industries?

Since leadership is a journey, it is never too late to begin, for one's own benefit as well as for the benefit of those with whom we work and those to whom we provide care. In times of stress and change, do we not deserve positive and hopeful leadership as well as spirit and reverence in our daily environment? Do we have leaders who will tell us "Wrong Jungle!" and empowered employees who will holler back "We know, we'll help you find the right one!"?

References

Autry JA: *Love & profit: the art of caring leadership,* New York, 1991, William Morrow & Co.

Blanchard K, Waghorn T: *Mission possible: becoming a world-class organization while there's still time,* New York, 1997, McGraw-Hill.

Blanchard K, Zigarmi P, Zigarmi D: *Leadership and the one minute manager,* New York, 1985, William Morrow & Co.

Bridges W: *Managing transitions: making the most of change,* Reading, Mass, 1991, Addison-Wesley.

Champy J: *Reengineering management: the mandate for new leadership,* New York, 1995, Harper Business.

Cohen WA: *The art of the leader,* Englewood Cliffs, NJ, 1990, Prentice Hall.

Cooper RK, Sawaf A; *Executive EQ: emotional intelligence in leadership and organization,* New York, 1997, Grosset/Putnam.

Covey SR: *7 habits of highly effective people: powerful lessons in personal change,* New York, 1989, Simon & Schuster.

Covey SR: *Principled-centered leadership,* New York, 1991, Simon & Schuster.

Hammerschlag CA: *The theft of the spirit,* New York, 1993, Simon & Schuster.

Hancock H, Bezold C: Possible futures, preferable futures, *Healthcare Forum Journal,* pp 23-29, March/April 1994.

Hawley JA: *Reawakening the spirit in work: the power of Dharmic management,* San Francisco, 1993, Berrett-Koehler.

Hickman CR: *Mind of a manager, soul of a leader,* New York, 1992, John Wiley & Sons.

Kanungo RN, Mendonca M: *Ethical dimensions of leadership,* Thousand Oaks, Calif, 1996, Sage Publications.

Lee B: *The power principle: influence with honor,* New York, 1997, Simon & Schuster.

Leonard-Barton D: *Wellsprings of knowledge: building and sustaining the sources of innovation,* Boston, 1995, Harvard Business School Press.

Miller KL: Keeping the care in nursing care: our biggest challenge, *Journal of Nursing Administration* 25(11):29-32, 1995.

Moore JD Jr: Medical Mecca, *Modern Healthcare,* pp 30-37, June 1997.

Morgan G: *Imaginization: the art of creative management,* Newbury Park, Calif, 1993, Sage Publications.

Nair K: *A higher standard of leadership: lessons from the life of Gandhi,* San Francisco, 1994, Berrett-Koehler.

Reynolds J: *Out front leadership: discovering, developing, and delivering your potential,* Austin, Texas, 1994, Mott & Carlisle.

Senge PM: *The fifth discipline: the art and practice of the learning organization,* New York, 1990, Doubleday.

Toffler A: *Future shock,* New York, 1970, Random House.

Toffler A: *Powershift: knowledge, wealth, and violence at the edge of the 21st century,* New York, 1990, Bantam Books.

Ulrich BT: *Leadership and management according to Florence Nightingale,* Norwalk, Conn, 1992, Appleton & Lange.

Wheatley MJ: *Leadership and the new science: learning about organization from an orderly universe,* San Francisco, 1992, Berrett-Koehler.

CHAPTER 9

The Role of Health Care Philanthropy in Community Health Outcomes

ELIZABETH LUNA MOURNING, BS

OVERVIEW

Health is being defined not by hospitals or even health care professionals, but by communities, and that definition does not revolve around the local hospital's services. Health is being defined as quality of life.

"Healthy communities" is a popular theme and one that deserves to be more than just a health care delivery fad. To sustain these programs over the long term, how will they be funded? The author suggests that a transformation in the purpose of hospital and health care philanthropy can accomplish this goal. In fact, it is a return to the original mission of health care. ▲

It started around 1658 in the city of New Amsterdam, New York, when the concept of a hospital began to take shape as a central place to care for the poor. Those more fortunate were treated in their homes. At that time, charity was a mainstay for hospitals and took the form of people giving essentials (e.g., food, blankets). It was in 1751 when the first formal organization of a hospital was chartered in Pennsylvania. This also began the first formal organization of charitable giving to a hospital. The chief fundraiser for this newly chartered hospital was none other than Benjamin Franklin.

After 1926, tax-supported hospitals grew because so many of them were established for the purpose of helping the neediest of citizens. Favorable tax treatment by the government acknowledged hospitals as being organized and operated for a charitable purpose and designated them as qualified not-for-profit organizations (IRC Section 170). In exchange, not-for-profit hospitals assumed a social obligation to provide community service in the public interest.

Over time hospitals began to meet a variety of needs in their communities. They became centers where medicine progressed and some of the greatest minds developed complex technologies and made profound discoveries, making diagnosis of disease extremely accurate and treatment very effective. Equipment that literally saved lives became indispensable. Hospitals no longer cared just for charity cases. If you wanted the best care for a medical problem, you went to a hospital.

These changes revolutionized much about health care. Hospitals charged fees so that they could meet their increasing and complex needs. In recent years, hospitals became overtly competitive businesses and engaged in marketing warfare. We referred to patients as customers. We used radio, television, billboards, and other media to advertise that we were the best. Along the way, for many, the true historical mission of hospitals got lost. Hospitals acted like big business, and that is exactly how the public now views us.

In the late 1970s charity to support hospitals became much more sophisticated. Separately controlled "foundations" with their own not-for-profit status and governing boards were formed by hospitals to avoid Medicare's attempt to force hospitals to use up their charitable dollars before they could bill Medicare for services provided. That attempt eventually changed, but the organization of foundations remained. Having a separate arm of the organization that did the fund-raising seemed to work.

Over time hospitals began an ever-increasing aggressiveness to improve the bottom line and purchased the latest technology available. When more money was needed, fees and charges for hospitalization and hospital services would rise so that those with insurance could make up the difference. There was a clear understanding that this rise in charges was to pay for the charity care being provided to those who could not pay for their care. Instead of focusing on prevention to help those without care, we just raised the fees charged those who could pay their bills. Eventually businesses and corporations rebelled over the constant increases in the cost of providing health insurance to their employees.

As cost reduction became a driving force, health care experienced mergers, acquisitions, buy-outs, hospital failures, and a dramatic increase in the number and success of for-profit hospitals.

We have come a long, long way from the original definition of a hospital, with its charitable purposes.

The Community Steps In

Health is being redefined not by hospitals or even health care professionals, but by communities, and that definition does not revolve around the local hospital's services. Health is being defined as quality of life. Having less crime, better education for our children, and clean air and water and being able to take a walk at night without fear often dominate the public's perception of a healthy community.

In addition, legislators have been pressured to look at the real purpose of not-for-profit hospitals. Some states have passed community benefit laws that require hospitals to prove, quantitatively, through programs and services for the entire community, including the needy, that they indeed should continue to merit their not-for-profit-status.

In California, community benefit is defined by state law (SB 697) as "a hospital's activities that are intended to address community needs and priorities primarily through disease prevention and improvement of health care status, including but not limited to, health care services rendered to vulnerable populations . . . cost containment . . . en-

hancement of access . . . services that help maintain a person's health."

Return to the Purpose of Charity

At Camino Healthcare (formerly an integrated delivery system located on the San Francisco Bay Area's Peninsula) we used the passage of the Community Benefit legislation to change the focus and
mission of our foundation, the fundraising arm of
the organization. The foundation, being a significant bridge between the community and the health
care system, became the focal point for creating and
implementing the community benefit concept.

From a mission that was focused inward and
based on the needs of the hospital ("bricks and
mortar"), the foundation's mission became "creating a healthier community through philanthropy,
volunteerism, and community partnerships." This
complemented the integrated delivery system's
mission "to be an innovative, locally integrated
health care organization which provides quality
services to improve the health and well-being of
our community."

Across the Country

Not only in our communities, but across the country, people are redefining what good health really
means. In several important national studies both
the Healthcare Forum (*What Creates Health? Individuals and Communities Respond*) and the California
Wellness Foundation (published by the California
Center for Health Improvement, entitled *Getting Involved*) have reported that Americans define health
not in terms of their local hospital's equipment and
hotel-like amenities but in terms of a cleaner environment, safer streets, and reduced violence. This
definition has shaped our views, in a new way, toward our responsibility as a health care foundation.

The following is quoted from the Healthcare Forum's *What Creates Health? Individuals and Communities Respond:*

The public has a new concept of what creates health and
healthy communities. Americans are moving away from a
narrow concept of health as the absence of disease, to a
broader definition that encompasses quality of life issues.
Today, the passive approach to health is being supplanted
by an emphasis on actively "creating" health. This trend
is built on several values that Americans have come to
embrace in recent years:

- Individuals can influence their own health through
  behavioral and lifestyle changes. These changes
  should be linked to disease and illness prevention
  strategies such as check-ups, immunizations and
  diagnostic screening.
- One's own health and well-being includes numerous quality of life factors, like family, safety and the
  quality of our environment, that impact everyone
  in the community.

Responding to the Community

OUR MISSION

Camino Healthcare and Camino Healthcare Foundation, each a separate charitable not-for-profit corporation, came together to collaborate on the development and sustainability of community benefit
activities.

The Camino Healthcare Foundation created a vision that embodied the value of volunteerism and
philanthropy to sustain community benefit. Its new
mission was "to create a healthier community
through philanthropy, volunteerism and community partnership." The Foundation managed both
the fund-raising and the community outreach efforts on behalf of Camino Healthcare and took the
lead in monitoring our responsibilities to fulfill the
mandates of state law SB 697.

Camino Healthcare, the parent organization,
operated an acute care hospital and a broad spectrum of outpatient services, educational programs,
and clinical care. The system's mission was "to be
an innovative, locally integrated health care organization which provides quality services to improve
the health and well-being of our community." The
system committed up to $1.5 million, each year
for 5 years, to underwrite the purpose and implementation of Community Benefits. The Foundation
board likewise made a commitment of 5 million
dollars over 5 years that would be raised to create
or sustain programs to improve the community's
health.

OUR VISION

Peter Senge (1990), in his book *The Fifth Discipline*,
says, "Few if any forces in human affairs are as
powerful as shared vision." He is right. The force of
our vision for a new health care foundation was as
powerful as anything I have ever experienced.

Our vision emerged from a transformation from doing our work as we had in the past to doing what was right for our community. Rather than the hospital determining what was best for the community, as health care professionals we asked the community how we could help. How could we be a better partner to those we served? We had to throw away our rules and orthodoxy. We had to join the community in its new definition of health. We had to learn a new way to lead and to be led by the people we served—person to person, neighbor to neighbor.

We had a strong community hospital, which had always provided a comfortable, supportive, healthy environment with superior professional expertise and technological resources. We combined that expertise with our newly found obligation to the broader definition of health, which the community defined as safe streets, good education, a clean environment, and a productive economy. In addition, we found ourselves funding programs that we had never considered before, but that were worthy of our donors' generosity.

Through their commitment to Community Benefit, Camino Healthcare and the Foundation contributed to the health of their community by joining with community-based organizations that provided services to their communities. Our first planning task force included community volunteers, a lawyer committed to the underserved, the local community services agency, a county health department representative, the Chamber of Commerce, the City Manager's office, the local school district nurse, our hospital auxiliary, representatives from the existing clinic for the underserved, doctors, and health care professionals from our hospital. As a result of bringing this diverse group together, we created a free clinic for the working poor in partnership with the Mountain View Rotary. We learned much about each other and about the community's needs and assets. By having a better understanding of what was truly needed, we found ourselves funding a nurse to loan to local schools and the local community health clinic, which was sorely understaffed. In essence, our nurse belonged to the community and the most pressing health needs of the underserved.

Our greatest lesson was learning to be collaborative, to join and partner and not take over. We could not force our vision on our partners. We had to

share, together with our community, our collective successes.

A New Foundation for Community Benefit

Every new vision or new concept comes with its problems and mistakes. The transformation was powerful for our institution and the community. We realized that an important part of our success depended not on the sophistication of our equipment, buildings, and services but on our outcomes, and the health status of the people we served.

The changes the Foundation initiated included the following:

- The Foundation
- A new department within the Foundation
- An expanding definition of hospital volunteerism
- New services appearing in the Foundation structure

THE FOUNDATION

This 501 (c) (3) structure had been in place for many years, and it was time to increase the value of its existence. We established a Division of Philanthropy and Community Benefit, from and including our existing hospital foundation, to serve as an umbrella for all of the hospital's programs dedicated to community benefit, volunteerism, and philanthropy. Our goal was to create a more effective, efficient coordination for using the hospital's resources to help the community. Intentionally these efforts did not automatically become part of the marketing department's efforts. Thus we made a statement that what we were doing was genuine and not just aimed at our marketing goals.

The Division transformed the philosophy of fund-raising. For decades, we had been asking each other, "How much money did the Foundation raise this year?" But the real question, the more important question, should be, "Through the money raised by the Foundation, what impact did we have on the community and its well-being?" The outcomes and the sustainability of health care organizations are what matters, not the number of dollars raised in the philanthropic process. Success should be determined by the number of people we were able to help with the generosity of our donors. Charity is about helping others, not about how much money you can raise. A Foundation's responsibility should not be to keep the doors of the hospital open in defiance of marketplace realities, but to provide leadership and resources to help fulfill the organization's charitable purposes. Not-for-profit hospitals have made a promise—they have a social contract, so to speak—by seeking and accepting their not-for-profit status. That obligation must be fulfilled for the sake and well-being of our communities. In addition, the Foundation is one way of helping to fulfil the goal.

I have always been troubled by the budgeting process for foundations. Each year the foundation had to show what percentage increase it was going to achieve in raising money. Although this is important, it never truly allowed a foundation to reach its full potential. My board and I never found lasting inspiration in just increasing our fund raising goals, but we were greatly inspired to increase the quality of life for individuals. How much more meaningful it would have been if we had given more importance to the value of the program rather than increasing fundraising goals.

Hospitals are seen as big business nowadays. The chaos surrounding the definition and delivery of health care has forever changed health care philanthropy. Philanthropy for hospitals has suffered in more ways than fundraising results. Foundations must take an intense look at their reason for being and adjust their vision to ways they can truly make a difference in their communities.

A NEW DEPARTMENT

A new department within the Foundation was created, called the *Community Benefits Department*. We hired a Community Benefits manager, two bilingual nurses, and a bilingual social service worker. Our next effort was to hire someone from the community that we were serving. We knew that building trust within the community being served would be a key success factor in the future.

The function of this department was to develop relationships with community-based organizations and assist the health care system in fulfilling its responsibilities to enhance the health and well-being of the community. This department also helped to comply with the mandates of SB 697 by conducting community health assessments every three years, developing a community benefit plan with annual updates, and promoting collaborative working relationships with community-based health and human services organizations. Our goal was to develop and maintain true partnerships with social service agencies, neighborhood groups, schools, churches, senior centers, and local governments.

The department served as the focal point for hospital employees and departments to identify how each could participate in the organization's overall community benefit commitment. We were encouraged by the tremendous response. We had given our employees at all levels of the organization an opportunity to make their reasons for being in the health care profession in the first place truly come alive. Our focus was to help those in need. We did not require paperwork, strategic initiatives, budgeting, or so many of the other things that the big business of hospitals requires of our managers and employees.

EXPANDING THE DEFINITION OF HOSPITAL VOLUNTEERISM

It became increasingly clear that just having more money was not going to solve our community's health problems or sustain well-intentioned and important programs. Although certainly not a new concept, volunteerism became the key to sustaining programs we implemented. With the goodness of people and the gift of their time and involvement, we felt confident that whatever was started in the community could continue, even if cutbacks in funding were necessary in the future.

It was the role of this department to work closely with the traditional volunteers who served our hospital in so many meaningful ways, and to work cooperatively with them to expand volunteerism out into the community. It was difficult at first, but through building trust and a common vision, we created a wonderful synergy with our auxiliary. The traditional boundaries and mind set of what it meant to be a hospital volunteer were expanded, providing opportunities for a new group of committed people in our community with rich and rewarding experiences.

One of the most fulfilling components of establishing an expanded volunteer program was putting together opportunities for employees and physicians to join us. The department encouraged and helped hospital employees and physicians to be a part of the community through volunteerism. Without the generosity of our employees, nurses, and doctors we would not have been successful.

NEW SERVICES IN THE FOUNDATION STRUCTURE

We began adding existing services and programs that were defined as community benefit. These included our Older Adult Resource Center and the Chaplaincy service. We became responsible both financially and operationally for the future of these programs. They were dependent upon the foundation to raise the necessary funds to keep them operating. It was my responsibility to create an organizational structure and operation that could be sustained in correlation with the funds we were raising and trying to raise for future years. This type of accountability energized our fundraising and our obligation to success. No longer did the staff or the foundation board work in a vacuum. We had accountability, responsibility, and visibility in a very meaningful way.

Learning What Was Important From Our Community

At the onset of our transformation, we did several things to be better able to respond to those we served, and to better understand the real passions in the hearts of our donors.

WE ASSESSED THE COMMUNITY NEED

The foundation began its efforts by sponsoring a series of focus groups, interviews, and a half-day conference to determine what the community wanted from its hospital. The questions asked of the participants are found in Box 9-1. Survey respondents included social service professionals, community leaders, police and fire officials, seniors, and school children. Each of these groups included a rich blend of our community's ethnic diversity.

The results pinpointed some serious concerns.

> **BOX 9-1**
> ## The Questions Asked
>
> - How do you decide where to go for health care?
> - Where do you go for health care?
> - What medical needs are not being met for you or your family?
> - What are the most important health care needs in our community at the present time?
> - When you think about health care in our community, what concerns you the most?
> - What community health care resources do you find helpful?

Social service professionals in particular told us that the less fortunate see the health care system as unresponsive, impersonal, and out of reach.

Rather than placing importance on the technical quality and breadth of our services, as we might have thought, respondents expressed an urgent need for basic services. The community did not need any new services; what it needed was access to what already existed. This assessment process propelled us to shift to what the community needed and wanted, and was the beginning of the Foundation's transformation to a new purpose and mission.

The Participants. Participants for the focus groups were selected in the following categories:

- Seventeen meetings were held with organized groups of senior citizens, with a mixture of low income, middle income, very low income, and those who receive adequate pensions and are well insured.
- Three focus groups with non-English speaking people were conducted. In our locality they included Spanish-, Vietnamese-, and Chinese-speaking people. Two groups of students were represented: high-school-aged and middle-school-aged participants.
- Twenty-three interviews were conducted with social service providers: community service professionals, corporate benefits admin-

istrators, hospital administrators, educators, hospital and clinic board members, law en forcement officers, community leaders, and activists. In addition, 50 participants from these groups joined us in an assessment day to pinpoint more precisely what the compelling needs were in our community.

The agencies that participated with us included school districts, the Council on Aging, the United Way, Community TV, private practice physicians, the police department, city council members, the Chamber of Commerce, industry, the League of Women Voters, the Junior League, churches, the community clinic, and home health care and community service associations.

The Three Main Themes that Emerged. Three themes emerged from our work: to improve access to service, to provide more preventive care, and to provide better information and coordination of services in our community.

Health Care Concerns by Defined Population. Although these findings represent the needs in our community, I have found that these concerns are not unlike what is often articulated in communities across the county. When our groups talked about health care, their concerns did not extend to technical quality or range of medical services. They expressed a need for access to services. They lacked information about what was already available, and they had difficulty getting to the places where services are provided. There was a very important lesson for all of us participating in this study: there was no lack of services for our community—just a lack of information about them and how to access them. We learned the following from our study:

- *Children*, ranging from infants to preteens, need preventive care (low-cost periodic examinations, immunizations, and health education), school-based clinics, and transportation to health care facilities when their parents are not available.
- *Teens* need preventive care, access to confidential counseling (including pregnancy counseling and care), health education (healthy lifestyles, drug and alcohol abuse prevention, HIV and STD prevention and treatment, and reproductive health), and

school-based clinics. In addition, teens at risk need integrated services (provided by the school, health care agencies, and police), drug and alcohol treatment facilities, and protection from violence, including gun control.

- *Young adults* who are no longer living with their parents need affordable health insurance, drug and alcohol treatment facilities, and HIV and STD prevention and treat ment.
- *Senior citizens* need "advice nurse" services or others who can answer questions about their health that do not require a doctor's attention, health education, better physical access to health care, such as health care at locations they frequent (such as senior center, in-home care when they cannot leave the house, and transportation to health care facilities), and primary health care for people with dementia.
- *Families* need general preventive care, domestic violence services (prevention and response), and school-based family health clinics.
- *Low-income families*, in addition to the care provided to all families, need maternal and infant care, prenatal care, medical care as a component of rotating shelters already in operation, and transportation to health care facilities.
- *Homeless people* also need medical care as a component of rotating shelters already in operation and mental health care.
- *Non-English speaking people* need health care providers nearby who speak their own languages and are sensitive to their cultural differences.
- *Medicare patients* need convalescent care at home after they have left a hospital, follow-up care to emergency treatment, and new technologies used to monitor in-home patients more efficiently.
- *Caregivers*, who take care of ill family members, need professional support, networking, and information about available support.
- *Professional health care providers* need help in primary care giving, better education about current prescription drugs, and information about available community resources that can support their efforts.

- *Small businesses* need affordable health care for all employees.

WE SURVEYED OUR DONORS

We asked community leaders and our philanthropists what they wanted from their foundation and if they would support us in developing programs that reached beyond the hospital's walls. Some respondents continue to see the greatest value for their contribution in the traditional sense of enhancing "bricks and mortar" or equipment. However the majority of the respondents favored our new vision. In fact, the uncertainty about the financial future of hospitals gave the community-based concept of giving more appeal.

What We Learned from Our Donors. People feel positive about supporting community benefit initiatives with their gifts. Donors are willing to change from giving for "bricks and mortar" and equipment to supporting community benefit programs. They encouraged the hospital to form collaborative partnerships with other service agencies in the community. Many said, however, that they wanted to support programs that were led by the hospital rather than have it be a "pass-through" foundation to simply fund community activities. In a world where hospital loyalty is being lost, one way to develop and maintain loyalty is through community benefit programs and services. They are something donors can hold onto as hospitals become large, complex, and confusing systems. We learned that if a hospital is not already highly regarded by the community and the donor, creating loyalty and maintaining credibility during very confusing times will be difficult.

Giving by corporations and private foundations played a particularly important role in helping us define our charitable responsibilities to the community. These "institutional donors" wholeheartedly supported our concepts and changes, and had envisioned this move for us long before we did! For them it was about time.

THE COLLABORATIVE LEADERSHIP PROCESS

There was a transformation of leadership styles toward collaboration. However, being veterans of health care competition, we found it difficult at first to embrace this new style and begin collaborating with our competitors. To motivate collaboration, the entire employee performance evaluation process must be changed. Your staff must be evaluated on the total success of the organization and not just on their own individual accomplishments, what they have contributed to making a healthier community. When value is placed in joint success rather than individual performance, you are giving freedoms and permission to share and work together. You as the leader become completely responsible for making this work. It is your attitude, your dialogue, and how you reward that will instill the passion for collaboration and joint successes. Once learned, it is a powerful force in doing good and purposeful work for your community. We learned the great joy of shared successes that may not advance the immediate marketing goals of our hospital, but do indeed serve the community. Our leadership position in the community enabled us to build bridges, partnerships, and collaborative relationships. We could bring leaders, providers, and users together to begin developing a community agenda for a healthier community. We could take our assessments and, with the help of the community, build upon them to create effective action plans.

PHYSICIANS AS VOLUNTEERS

We found that community health has a particular appeal to family practitioners, pediatricians, gerontologists, and physicians whose ethnic backgrounds matched those of the underserved community. Our renewed focus on community created a passion for many of our physicians by giving them an opportunity to practice medicine in the manner that motivated them to become doctors in the first place. We provided experiences that did not sweep them up in paperwork, regulations, and corporate meetings. Importantly, our retired physicians, who make up such an important part of our community, were able to reignite their own passions for helping others by volunteering in our free clinics.

We assisted our physicians in developing a meaningful process to review requests from the community for their services. Physicians are a vital component of any healthy community (or community benefit) initiative if it is to be successful. They were a vital component of the partnerships being developed. No community can afford to be without the voluntary help of its doctors and other health care professionals in improving health status.

WE STARTED A GRANT-MAKING PROGRAM

Across the country many hospital foundations are finding themselves in the new role of giving money to agencies other than the hospital. There are many inherent problems with this process. Our approach was to find real solutions by gathering the community together to solve problems rather than just throwing large sums of money at the problems we identified.

When a nearby school district, a city government, and a major local employer formed a partnership to build a new community center, they approached us to help fund a health clinic as part of the project. In helping them look realistically at the proposal, we discovered a far simpler, less costly alternative. Years earlier, budget cuts had eliminated the traditional school nurse. By agreeing to fill that key position, we helped meet a community need with relatively minimal financial resources.

We could not have raised all the dollars needed for a health clinic, but we could raise the money needed to pay for a school nurse, and we knew that it was a goal we could reach year after year. It is crucial that when we start a program for the community, there will always be resources to keep the program operating. Otherwise, we hurt the very people we were trying to serve by having to suspend a program they learn to count on for services. We need to promote partnerships, collaboration, and pooling of community resources. One funding source cannot meet all of the needs of an important community service. Success is achievable by focusing activities on supporting those projects that most closely meet established criteria and the most pressing needs in the community.

The donor survey, mentioned earlier, pointed out that leaders mentioned the many community agencies already at work in human and social services. They cautioned against duplication of services. They want to see collaboration in the community. Resources simply are too scarce for several agencies to be doing similar work. One of the Foundation's initiatives was to lead the way in working together and maximizing resources for the good of the community. This was exemplified when we brought our first community benefit task force together, representing numerous agencies. Our discussions revolved around helping each other, sharing resources, facilities, computer knowledge, and other things that would bring mutual success to what we were doing.

The Granting Guidelines

Some of the nation's biggest foundations are not just funding singular initiatives of a single organization or agency, but looking at grant requests that are based on agencies working together to solve the needs of the community.

The criteria established that ultimately would serve as our guide to collaboration and partnerships include the following:

- Enhance the health status of people in our community.
- Make sure that the need is clearly and thoroughly demonstrated and does not unnecessarily duplicate programs and services available elsewhere in the community.
- Increase awareness and understanding of health care resources that already exist.
- Promote collaborative relationships among other agencies in the community, and encourage the use of volunteers.
- Contribute in an innovative way to the efficiency, cost effectiveness, and quality of patient-focused care, providing timely and appropriate intervention.
- Address the health problems of minorities, the poor, and other vulnerable populations, and consider the multicultural and multigenerational populations in our communities. It is nondiscriminatory.
- Structure management to ensure quality control and optimal outcomes.
- Clearly state goals, objectives, and the criteria for measurable success.
- Use funds directly for services, care, and self-sufficiency.
- Involve the stakeholders affected by the project in its development.

Money is not always the solution! We must try other means of creating a healthier community.

Conclusion

We must find simple, sustainable solutions to health care problems within our communities. Large, expansive, grandiose plans have no place in our future because they will not be sustainable. To propose and pursue such goals is a disservice to our communities. Through partnerships and sharing of resources, we can help our communities obtain what they really need and want and advance our own purposes in the process.

The people we are trying to serve are changing the definition of health care. To them it is so much more than our hospitals having the latest piece of equipment. Health is about the quality and dignity of life. People all across the country are challenging health care leaders to build better visions and models of care in their communities. They are saying "don't wait for us to get sick!" and "help us stay healthy" in all respects of the word. For our communities, health is a great deal more than what happens within the walls of our hospitals.

We were ready to go back to blankets and food and to touch the spirit of human beings. We believe that healing does not happen in a hospital alone, but in sincere partnerships with families and neighborhoods and through compassion, respect, and love for our fellow human beings.

References

Community authorship: *Community health care assessment,* El Camino Hospital, Mountain View, CA, September 29, 1993.

Dickman E, Mourning EL, Sutherst G: *Three year community benefit plan,* California, 1996, Camino Healthcare Foundation.

The Healthcare Forum: *What creates health?: individuals and communities respond* (a national study), California, 1994, The Healthcare Forum.

Mourning EL: Managed care, healthy communities and the new healthcare foundation, *Fundraising Management,* pp 24-31, September 1996.

Risley M: *House of healing: the story of the hospital,* New York, 1961, Doubleday.

Senge PM: *The fifth discipline: the art and practice of the learning organization,* New York, 1990, Currency Doubleday.

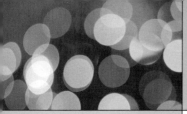

PART TWO

New Roles
Restructuring the System

Health is not given to people but is generated by them.

C.P. TRESOLINI and THE PEW-FETZER TASK FORCE, 1994

IN A "BEST-CASE" SCENARIO, health care system redesign will result in competent, caring practitioners who work in supportive settings that provide seamless and coordinated services to individuals in the community. High-level wellness will be the guiding principle. A goal of this type requires all participants in health care, including consumers, to take on new roles and responsibilities. Part Two includes several discussions of systems working to develop those new roles and evaluate their effectiveness with the population being served. Each role design focuses on a better way to provide care, serve a particular population, or lead the change toward an improved system. Whether it is a parish nursing program in mid-America or case management in the United Kingdom, the authors in Part Two focus on the role changes needed for organizations and communities, as well as for the providers and recipients of care. ▲

CHAPTER 10

Emerging Competencies for Nurse Case Managers

Blending the Strengths from the Past

MARY H. MUNDT, RN, PhD, **and ELAINE L. COHEN,** RN, EdD

OVERVIEW

Whether it be the consumer, service provider, or payer, the emphasis on outcomes evaluation portends universal changes in health care and addresses the practice requirements necessary for the evolutionary success of case management.

The challenge of today's health care environment is to build a more effective and humane system for the future. In this chapter the authors argue that the nursing profession has essential expertise to lead the search for new clinical practice paradigms. They explore the history and traditions of nursing that demonstrate the profession's early and continuing tradition of comprehensive management of care. Building on the themes of the past, recognizing the challenges of the present and the opportunities of the future, the authors propose a list of emerging competencies for nurse case managers in the re-designed world of health care. ▲

Many opportunities await case management as the nation moves into the challenge of shaping an effective and humane health care system. Service integration, integrated delivery networks, innovative partnerships, strategic alliances, and healthy communities are the latest national attempts at envisioning the future of health care delivery and management.

To meet the new challenges and continue to provide appropriate, effective care in diverse settings, attention must now be paid to the added value that the results of case management interventions have for the client population served. Whether it be the consumer, service provider, or payer, the emphasis on outcomes evaluation portends universal changes in health care and addresses the practice requirements necessary for the evolutionary success of case management.

While future opportunities abound, they are surrounded by uncertainty as new systems are developed. The future role and competencies for nurse case managers are unclear as these redesigned systems emerge. In exploring the future, we believe that it is important to examine the past and the strengths that the nursing profession brings to the challenges of care coordination and integration of services.

In this chapter, four points are presented as central to the discussion of future roles for nurse case managers in a reorganized health system. First, we argue that the core element of future health care design is clinical integration. Second, we describe nursing expertise in clinical integration as a consistent historical theme in practice and education. Third, we propose that the nursing profession recognize these historical continuities in building new clinical practice paradigms. Fourth, we propose a selected list of emerging competencies for nurse case managers of the future that blend the strengths of the past with the vision of the future.

Clinical Integration

The dramatic evolution of American health care escalates the need to ensure competent clinical model development in a redesigned system. In emerging, integrated delivery systems, the essential component of the model is clinical integration, "the extent to which patient care services are coordinated across people, functions, activities, and sites so as to maximize the value of services delivered to patients" (Shortell, 1996). Expertise in clinical integration is a hallmark of nurse case management and an essential value in the nursing profession.

One of the current crises in managed care is the control of clinical integration by nonclinical design teams driven by financial rather than client-centered objectives. When this occurs, care is defined as linear and hierarchical, and there is a poor understanding of how to operationalize a continuum of care. In these situations, care continuity can be compromised, with a risk of negative outcomes for both clients and providers. It is essential that nurse case managers influence the process of clinical integration and call on the history and tradition of nursing as a resource in designing care.

Nursing History and Traditions of Practice: Themes of Clinical Integration

The fundamental concepts of clinical integration linked to managed care and integrated health care systems are consistent with the history and tradition of the nursing profession. For example, concepts such as population-based assessment and community health care services are hallmarks of public health nursing. Continuity of care across settings, family-centered care, and community-based primary care are all found in the history of nursing, from the Henry Street Settlement in New York to the early Visiting Nurse Associations to the Frontier Nursing Service in Kentucky, to the present-day Nursing Centers. For more than 100 years, nurses have seen clients in homes, schools, work places, clinics, and hospitals. Nurses have served as advocates for patients and families, established links with community resources, and assumed responsibility for the outcomes of care. First Lady Eleanor Roosevelt (1934) lauded these characteristics of nursing in an address to the biennial convention of the national nursing organizations. She praised the work of nurses in the Henry Street Settlement and called for a nurse in every community to coordinate preventive care and health education efforts.

When clinical intervention is effective, positive health outcomes result. The concept of health care outcomes is very familiar to nursing. Florence Nightingale urged the use of statistics to demonstrate the influence of good nursing care on health outcomes. The influence of visiting nurses on improving health outcomes of immigrant populations, teaching prevention and instituting programs to reduce infant and child mortality, is well documented. As early as 1939, the nurse's role in coordinating care was described in the *Manual of Public Health Nursing*. Public health nursing was defined with an expanded role, beyond caring for the sick in their homes, as follows: ". . . it is the additional responsibility of the public health nurse to assist in analyzing health problems and related social problems of families and individuals; to help them, with the aid of other community resources, to formulate an acceptable plan for the protection and promotion of their own health; and to encourage them to carry out this plan" (National Organization for Public Health Nursing, 1939). It is clear from this statement that nurses were expected to address the issues of population assessment, coordination with community resources, and development of health promotion, protection, and prevention plans and interventions essential to today's managed care environment.

Nursing Education: Evidence of Clinical Integration Themes

To further verify the strength of tradition in professional nursing that supports managed and integrated care systems are statements from the national curriculum guides for nursing in the earlier part of the century. In 1932, Isabel Stewart, a strong nursing leader, stated: " . . . our position is that 'health' nursing is just as fundamental as 'sick' nursing and the prevention of disease at least as important a function of the nurse as the care and treatment of the sick. Indeed these functions cannot be separated" (*A Curriculum for Schools of Nursing*, 1932, p. 11). This statement supports the nurse's role in responsibility for the continuum of care and an integrated and holistic approach to care delivery. Even more resounding are three of the objectives for nursing education listed in the 1937 *A Curriculum for Schools of Nursing* (*Note:* we have numbered these objectives for purposes of comparison with future competencies listed later in the chapter):

1. All professional nurses should be capable of taking part in the promotion of health and the prevention of disease.

2. All professional nurses should possess the essential knowledge and ability to teach measures to conserve and restore health.

3. All professional nurses should be able to cooperate effectively with the family, hospital personnel, and health and social service agencies in the interests of patient and community. (p. 24)

Each of these objectives, written for the profession more than 60 years ago, echoes the types of competencies required for today's practice in managed care and integrated health networks.

It can also be demonstrated that these 1937 objectives have been continuously present in nursing curricula and foremost in today's educational thinking. For example, the 1996 position statement of the American Association of Colleges of Nursing (*Nursing Education's Agenda for the 21st Century*) states: "Advanced nursing practice requires graduate preparation, which may focus on primary health care, case management, specialization, education, or administration across health care settings. Preparation for the entry level professional nurse now requires a greater orientation to community-based primary health care, and an emphasis on health promotion, maintenance and cost-effective coordinated care that responds to the needs of increasingly culturally diverse groups and underserved populations in all settings."

Still another historical truism is the continuing contribution of nurse leaders in shaping the way in which nursing practice and education develop. Examples abound, but we have chosen Virginia Henderson as an excellent model of a visionary leader, who was a member of the curriculum committee that developed the 1937 *A Curriculum Guide for Schools of Nursing*. Henderson wrote a key article in 1982 critiquing the nursing profession's use of the nursing process as the defining feature of nursing practice. She argued that although nurses use a problem-solving process in decision making, it is only one component of practice. To fully understand the richness of clinical practice, it is essential to include clinical judgment, experience, intuition, and interaction with patients and other professionals. Her clarity of vision and understanding of the complexity of clinical practice contribute to understanding the history of the profession as a "clinical discipline" and linking it to the future requirements for nurse case management.

Themes of Continuity for the Future

Having reviewed the historical traditions of nursing practice and education serves the purpose of establishing a sense of continuity with our professional past. The relationship of this past to emerging competencies in new systems can be helpful if we build on the continuity of the past to interpret the reality of the present and the hope of the future. The anthropologist Mary Catherine Bateson (1989, 1994) has written two books reflecting on the concept of continuity as a way of interpreting and creating meaning during times of social and personal change. She states, "Even in completely new situations response depends on recognizing continuity." Her thesis is that only by recognizing the familiar in strange situations can we forge ahead and create new meaning and purpose in unfamiliar situations.

Another theme she shares in her book *Composing a Life* (1989) is the art of improvisation. In entering new and ever-challenging situations, one can develop a confident sense of "making things work" by piecing together responses that draw on experience and knowledge in new and different ways. The challenge for nurses is to recognize and appreciate the continuities of the past and share them with each other as a way of developing confidence and direction as they deal with increasingly diverse audiences. In addition, they can take comfort in risk taking in newly improvised solutions to the challenges of the future because of their connections to the past. Because of their connections to the past, nurses who use their historical strength and knowledge can emerge as strong players in the evolving, integrated health care systems of the future.

How then will the future role and competencies of advanced-practice nurse case managers be determined? The urgent need for future role determination is to systematically and strategically position nursing in key health care organizations. The political agenda of the profession must be to resurrect the strengths of the profession that blend with the agenda of managed care organizations, capture and disseminate descriptions of expert practitioners, and negotiate for inclusion in models of care.

It is more than unfortunate that nursing has been invisible in many areas of health policy and health system design, even though the traditions of practice and leadership are abundant. In a recent analysis of books on health policy and health reform (Mundt, 1997), it was found that of 35 books written during 1994 and 1995, only three books contained a substantive discussion of nursing in the health care system. When nursing was mentioned, it was most likely to be in relation to nurses in conflict with physicians, shortage and supply issues, and nurses as substitutes for physicians. This continuing stereotype of nursing as a large, dependent, and conflicted group ignores the strengths and contributions of the profession and negates more than 100 years of clinical practice, care coordination, and partnering with other professions. The degree to which nursing is ignored and discounted by decision makers in health care signifies an ethical problem in ensuring the highest quality of care for customers.

The argument for inclusion of nursing in redesigning health care systems emphasizes the perspective that clients will be underserved if they do not have access to excellent nurse case management and that outcomes will be compromised. Nurses can and do demonstrate that quality care can be achieved only in systems with a strong role for nursing. Finally, we in professional nursing have a responsibility to educate ourselves and other nurses that what history has taught us is true: nurses are "connectors" of health care for consumers and providers.

Future Competencies for Nurse Case Managers

Reviewing the past and recognizing the present offer us a springboard to identify nursing's potential future. The practice elements presented here are representative of an exhaustive list of currently emerging and evolving parameters of case management practices worldwide. They call for nothing less than resocialization of health care professionals to understand and address the consumer's needs. In addition, they expect from the professional nurse consumer advocacy and civic responsibility that will have a profound impact on the improvement of service delivery outcomes, health status, and eventually the revitalization of our health care system. Finally, these twenty-first-century abilities can be clearly seen as "connected" to our historical roots as we pair them with the 1937 objectives for nursing education described earlier:

- *Active engagement with consumers* and ability to demonstrate increased responsiveness to their health care needs will be the hallmark of the advanced practitioner of case management. This is best accomplished through collaborative and integrative alliances with other providers and recipients of health care services. By redefining our partnership, the determinants and outcomes necessary to create health and quality of life can be defined, evaluated, and achieved (1937 objective 3).
- *Integration of broader, increasingly global perspectives into healing approaches* and cultural and spiritual beliefs and the capacity to embrace tolerance and accept change will help the practitioner assimilate into diverse work groups and teams. They will also aid in developing a belief ethic that is grounded in a more soulful practice and infuse the practitioner with the sensitivity, strength, and confidence needed in the process of reinventing the country's health care system (1937 objective 1).
- *Reframing leadership to ask the unpopular questions* and seek the solutions that will assist in the establishment of benchmarks for quality care and further improvements in health outcomes. This stewardship is greatly needed to promote civic responsibility and societal accountability in our attempts to formulate a combined, socially based health care policy (1937 objective 3).
- *Practice that is rooted in ethical principles and values* that support human dignity and self-actualization will form the core of professional socialization and competency standards for the advanced practitioner in case management. The heightening of these beliefs beyond the individual level to the community, nation, and world will help focus our energies to deal with the global issues that challenge humankind (1937 objective 3).
- *Mastery of information technology and communication* will ease the practitioner's journey through the virtual community. This education and knowledge will be crucial in evaluating the appropriateness and usefulness of outcome data to consumers, providers, and purchasers. It will also help develop an outcomes-based practice as we begin to link and share information networks with communities to provide health care services (1937 objective 2).
- *Political savvy, system know-how, and conflict resolution* will play prominent roles as the case manager negotiates between various health care arenas and settings (1937 objectives 1 and 3).

Conclusion

A historical perspective lends richness, depth, and balance by blending the stability of the past with the challenges that futuristic vistas hold. This balance weaves many strong and life-sustaining threads as nurses prepare themselves for full partnership in health care delivery. Holding a sense of their heritage and honoring its traditions will empower nurses to co-create their new reality rather than wait for recipes of what the future will look like.

Becoming multidisciplinary partners in reshaping the health care system means reestablishing the basic connections with society that revere multiple perspectives and ways of knowing. It means recommitting to the values that the constituencies expect and demand. It means embracing the principles of leadership that respect diversity of opinion and reflection. It means restoring those precepts of power that inspire humility, authenticity, and integrity. To achieve positive outcomes of care through nurse case management, nurse educators are challenged to create learning and assessment experiences that result in nurse graduates who are adept at these competencies for the future.

References

American Association of Colleges of Nursing: *Nursing education's agenda for the 21st century*, Washington, DC, 1996, American Association of Colleges of Nursing.

Bateson MC: *Composing a life*, New York, 1989, Atlantic Monthly Press.

Bateson MC: *Peripheral visions*, New York, 1994, Harper Collins.

Henderson V: The nursing process—is the title right? *Journal of Advanced Nursing* pp 103-107, 1982.

Mundt MH: Books on health policy and health reform: how is nursing represented? *Journal of Professional Nursing* 13(1):19-27, 1997.

National League of Nursing Education: *A curriculum for schools of nursing*, p. 11, 1932.

National League of Nursing Education: *A curriculum for schools of nursing*, p. 24, 1937.

National Organization for Public Health Nursing: *Manual of public health nursing*, ed 3, New York, 1939, Macmillan.

Roosevelt E: What does the public expect from nursing? *American Journal of Nursing* 34(7), 1934.

Shortell SM et al: *Remaking health care in America*, San Francisco, 1996, Jossey-Bass.

CHAPTER 11

The Health Action Model
*Academia's Partnership With the Community**

SANDRA SCHMIDT BUNKERS, RN, PhD, **MARGOT L. NELSON,** RNC, PhD,
CHERYL JOY LEUNING, RN, PhD, **JUDITH K. CRANE,** RN, MS, **and DIANE K. JOSEPHSON,** RN, MA

OVERVIEW

Academia's partnership with the community may be a new way of living health.

Community is living in relationship. The Health Action Model for Partnership in Community (HAMPIC) is a futuristic, collaborative nursing practice model addressing the connections and disconnections existing in human relationship. Augustana College Department of Nursing and six site communities within Sioux Falls, SD, are addressing the lived experience of connection-disconnection for homeless and low-income people who are challenged with access to health care along with a lack of economic, social, and interpersonal resources.

The HAMPIC is an advanced practice nursing model based on nurse theorist Rosemarie Rizzo Parse's human becoming school of thought. This school of thought focuses on the primacy of the nurse's presence with others and conceptualizes health as human becoming—the pattern of the whole of one's life. The focus of the nurse-person-community health process is quality of life from the person-community's perspective. Quality of life, which is the central concept in the model, is elaborated on in the conceptualizations of health as human becoming, community interconnectedness, and voices of the person-community. Advanced practice nurses, a steering committee, and six site communities are moving together in seeking mutual understanding while holding as important the unique perspectives presented by individuals and groups in complex health situations. ▲

*The authors wish to acknowledge the following funding sources for The Health Action Model: Augustana College; Sioux Falls Area Foundation; Sioux Valley Hospital Community Fund; Sioux Falls School District Head Start Program, Sioux Falls, SD; and Sioux Empire United Way, Sioux Falls, SD.

The Health Action Model: A Community Focus

Community is living in relationship. The Health Action Model for Partnership in Community (HAMPIC) is about health care professionals living in relationship with people in community. It is a futuristic, collaborative nursing practice model addressing the connections and disconnections existing in human relationship. This model is based on Parse's human becoming school of thought and focuses on the primacy of the nurse's presence with others. Transformation of the community occurs when nurses in research and practice "live the belief that unitary humans know the way, structure a personal reality, and coauthor their health freely with situation" (Parse, 1997b). As such, this philosophy serves as a guidepost for the development of nursing practice in community. "To participate with presence in the nurse-person-community health process is . . . nursing's opportunity" (Bunkers, Michaels, Ethridge, 1997).

Through HAMPIC, Augustana College's Department of Nursing is seizing the opportunity to co-create a new paradigm in community nursing practice in partnership with the Sioux Falls, SD, community. This new paradigm "involves designing health care delivery systems responsive to health care cost, creating nursing practice models addressing quality of care and quality of life issues, and being responsive to the rights consumers have in decisions concerning their health and health care" (Bunkers, Michaels, Ethridge, 1997).

A NEW PARADIGM OF CO-CREATING CONNECTIONS

Research findings indicate that people struggling on the edge of economic sufficiency and homelessness experience critical disconnections from adequate income, homes, health care services, schools, and families (Bauman, 1993; Bunkers, 1996; Francis, 1992). In a descriptive study of eight homeless families, Francis (1992) identified the central organizing theme in those families as disconnection-connection. Families experienced moving from violations and disconnections to private temporary connections, to public temporary connections, to a rebuilding of connections with community. Bauman (1993), in a study of homeless families with children, used the metaphor of "a whirlpool of poverty and powerlessness" to describe the experience of homelessness.

Bunkers (1996) studied the meaning of "considering tomorrow" with 10 homeless women and uncovered two significant core concepts dealing with a sense of connection-disconnection in their lives. The first core concept was intimate alliances with isolating distance. This concept depicted these women's day-to-day struggles in relationships. Feelings of connectedness to those loved were coupled with a sense of alienation from others in community. This paradoxical pattern of engaging and disengaging from others was a dominant theme in their lives. The second core concept was resilient endurance amid disturbing unsureness. The women in Bunkers' study described unique ways of moving and surviving on the streets (i.e., "resilient endurance"). At the same time, however, they talked about a disturbing unsureness, not knowing what tomorrow would bring or whether they would live to see tomorrow (Bunkers, 1996).

HAMPIC addresses this lived experience of connection-disconnection for homeless and low-income people who are challenged with the lack of economic, social, and interpersonal resources. Adrian van Kaam (1985), in *Living Creatively*, posits that in today's world two matters seem to oppose one another—the need to live by the customs of society and the need to make these customs personal by living them in one's own way. van Kaam (1985) suggests that we must share certain customs with fellow humans yet go beyond them. HAMPIC seeks to go beyond present-day nursing practice customs and base nursing practice in the community on Parse's unitary, human-science perspective in which relationship in true presence is integral to the nurse-person-community-health process. Through the working components of HAMPIC (i.e., advanced practice nurses, a steering committee, and site communities), HAMPIC addresses the issues of establishing connections and relationships with health care providers and the larger community. It is a collaborative community that responds to the health concerns of low-income and homeless families. The model seeks to address in an original way the relational connection-disconnection issues of those underserved by health and human resources in society by working with selected site communities in developing this prototype model.

The Cornerstone: Nursing Theory–Guided Model Development

HAMPIC's conceptual framework is the guide for working with others in community. Quality of life, the central concept, is elaborated upon in the conceptualizations of health as human becoming, community interconnectedness, and voices of the person-community (Figure 11-1). This advanced practice nursing model is an alternative to the present-day customs of health care experts diagnosing, prescribing, and providing what *they* see as needed services to those disadvantaged in a community. HAMPIC is grounded in the formation of collaborative relationships with persons, families, and groups who are living the experience of marginalization and disenfranchisement. The purpose of the model is to respond in a new way to nursing's social mandate to care for the health of society by gaining an understanding of what is wanted from those living these health experiences. "Since persons choose and live their values, only they can change their health and quality of life. Changing one's health patterns only happens when one is personally committed to change; essentially, the choice to change is up to the person, not the health professional" (Pilkington, 1997).

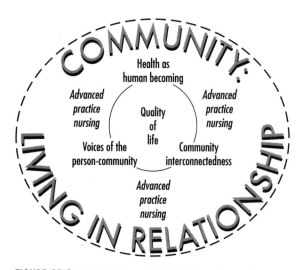

FIGURE 11-1 The Health Action Model for Partnership in Community. Model based on Parse's human becoming school of thought. (From Augustana College, Sioux Falls, SD)

HEALTH AS HUMAN BECOMING

Health as human becoming involves the belief that health is a personal commitment to a lived value system; it is the process of living one's value priorities (Parse, 1992). The health process involves making choices about what is important. Advanced practice nurses, in believing that health is the process of choosing how one lives, respect and honor the choices people-communities make toward changing health patterns. Parse's nursing theory of human becoming emphasizes the value of the meaning of lived experiences of health and is "grounded in the belief that humans coauthor their becoming in mutual process with the universe, cocreating distinguishable patterns which specify the uniqueness of both humans and the universe" (Parse, 1995). Persons and families are asked what their hopes are for the future; thus, personal health descriptions and health action plans are based on what the individual, family, group, or community feels is important for quality of life (Box 11-1).

QUALITY OF LIFE

Quality of life, from the human becoming perspective, is how a person-community lives health. Parse (1994) writes the following concerning quality of life:

The very word quality comes from the Latin *qual* meaning what and *qualities* meaning whatness. Whatness is the stuff or essence of something, in this case, the essence of life, the core substance that makes a life different and uniquely irreplaceable. The whatness or essence for one person differs from that of another. Thus, the answer to the question "Who can judge a person's quality of life?" is: only the person living the life.

In HAMPIC, advanced practice nurses work with persons and groups in the site communities in creating a prototype of collaboration in addressing issues concerning quality of life.

COMMUNITY INTERCONNECTEDNESS

Community interconnectedness involves the interrelationship of persons, ideas, places, and events. Community, in its most abstract sense, is viewed as " . . . the universe, the galaxy of human connectedness" (Parse, 1996a). The interconnectedness of community involves relationship that tran-

BOX 11-1
Case Study   Heidi's Story*

"Ever since I was a young girl, I have wanted to be a missionary, but everyone has kept telling me that I couldn't, so I don't think I can." This was Heidi's first statement when I asked her to tell me about her hopes for the future. I met Heidi at the soup kitchen where I spend each Thursday as one of the nurses working with HAMPIC site communities. Heidi is a 41-year-old, single woman who lives alone in low-income, subsidized housing in the city. Heidi and I continued to meet at the soup kitchen, where she indicated that she wanted to discuss a personal health description and health action plan.

In describing her health, Heidi stated, "I probably need to get more exercise, but I've been working for a veterinarian for almost a year now walking dogs and taking care of animals. I get tired of walking all the dogs, so I don't exercise as much as I should. My teeth need some fixing, but right now I'm saving my money to buy new furniture. I want my apartment to be right. After that I'll save money to fix my teeth. I have a desk and lamp that are important to me, and I want my whole apartment to go with them. My place is real important to me, and right now I don't have a couch in the living room."

Heidi then focused on the relationships in her life. She continued, "I get short with people. I don't have much patience. I think I'm pretty gruff with people. I also get stressed easily so I tend to stay away from people, but I know that isn't always what is best for me. I would like to be more social.

I need to work on dealing with people because that might help my stress. Sometimes I feel very alone."

Heidi then identified the health concerns she wanted recorded in her personal health description; they included relationships with people, money to buy furniture and fix her teeth, and dealing with her stress.

With Heidi focusing on these issues, the following health action plan developed:

1. Meet weekly with the advanced practice nurse about concerns involving relationships and stress, and explore ways of getting more involved with people.
2. Develop a plan to save money to buy furniture, and then save for dental work.
3. Continue to explore the possibility of becoming a missionary.

At this writing, Heidi has now saved enough money to buy a couch and a bed for her apartment. The last time we met, Heidi said to me with a smile, "I've saved almost $900.00 for this furniture. I did it! Now the church group I belong to is going to help me get it to the apartment." She continued, "Something else I want to tell you. Since I talked with you about being a missionary I have hope again that some day I can do that. It might take me a couple of years to get ready and to save the money I would need, but I still wouldn't be too old to do it. I have hope again."

*Written by Diane Josephson.

scends separating differences. There is no lack of spoken and written words about persons experiencing the separating differences of living with little or no money and no place to call home. What is missing in community is an intentional listening to the sound of these voices speaking and writing about their own hopes and meanings. To embrace separating differences involves listening and understanding others. The nurse-person-community-health process involves being truly present with others with a listening

receptivity to differing values. Nurses practicing in this model understand that community as process entails a moving together in seeking mutual understanding while holding as important the unique perspectives presented by individuals and groups in complex health situations. Moving together in seeking mutual understanding calls for a type of listening to one another in which both nurse and person-community engage in contributing to expanding choices for living health.

VOICES OF THE PERSON-COMMUNITY

Listening to the voices of others requires being with others in true presence. Listening to how others experience their world and the meaning of their lived experience is foundational to nursing practice based on the human becoming school of thought. Parse (1996b) denotes that the focus of practice is quality of life from the person's perspective. Since what constitutes quality of life differs from one person to another, the nurse living Parse's theory respects each individual's or family's own view of quality, and "the person is appreciated as the captain of his or her own ship, as one knowing the way." Similarly to Parse's position, Chittister (1990) in *Wisdom Distilled From the Daily* writes, " . . . To be unable to listen is to be unable to give as well. It is easy to know what is good for someone else. It is difficult to listen and let them define themselves." It is through careful, reflective listening in true presence that advanced practice nurses hear the voices of the person-community. "It takes a lot of listening to hear the needs of those around us before they even speak them" (Chittister, 1990). Parse's human becoming nursing practice methodology requires an attentive, reflective listening as the person-community illuminates meaning by explicating what is going on in its lived experiences, synchronizes rhythms by dwelling with what is happening, and mobilizes transcendence by moving on with changing patterns of health. It is in this process of illuminating meaning, synchronizing rhythms, and mobilizing transcendence that person-communities do define themselves. HAMPIC responds to the definitions the person-community brings forward. "The content of a nurse-person or nurse-family process emerges through true presence and may lead to planning for changing health patterns" (Parse, 1996).

Co-Authoring Health: Originating New Roles and Relationships

HAMPIC consists of three simultaneous integrating components—advanced practice nursing, the steering committee, and site communities. They are described separately to provide clarity in understanding the dynamics of the project.

ADVANCED PRACTICE NURSING

Advanced practice nursing in HAMPIC supports the notion of theory-guided, individualized, participatory nursing practice in the nurse-person-community health process. Nursing practice in this model is committed to "individualized care that respects the wishes and choices of people served" (Mitchell, 1997). Advanced practice nurses, guided by this perspective, listen in true presence to others as they describe what is important to them and what their plans and hopes are for the future. Parse (1992) identifies true presence with others as "a special way of 'being with' in which the nurse bears witness to another's living of value priorities." The true presence of the nurse with others is the way in which the human becoming theory of nursing is lived in community nursing practice. Regarding true presence, Parse (1997a) writes, "The person at all realms of his or her universe experiences the intent of the nurse, which is to bear witness to changing health patterns. The intent of the nurse is languaged in his or her whole being, in the subtle knowings of the messages given and taken at all realms of the universe, so words are not necessary to live true presence in the nurse-person process."

The intent of advanced practice nurses in the HAMPIC is to connect in true presence with persons and communities and to understand their health experiences with connections-disconnections and their hopes for changing patterns of health. Advanced practice nurses work with persons and groups in the identified site communities in co-creating collaboration among site communities and health care agencies in addressing quality of life.

The project director is a PhD-prepared nurse who directs and coordinates the work with the site communities, advanced practice nurses, a steering committee, a medical consultant, and a health professional education field coordinator. The project director is involved in all aspects of program development, implementation, and evaluation.

Advanced practice nurses in the model work with individuals, families, and "site" communities in creating personal health descriptions and health action plans. Box 11-2 describes the protocol used in identifying health issues. It is in this process of identifying a health action plan that the nurse explores how she or he can work with the person-

The personal health descriptions are written in the words of the person, family, or community.
- What life is like for me now . . .
- My health concerns are . . .
- What is most important for me now . . .
- My hopes for the future are . . .
- My plans for the future are . . .
- How I can carry out my plans . . .
- My specific health action plan is . . .

community in changing patterns of health (see Box 11-1).

The health professional education field coordinator's role is to develop undergraduate and graduate level nursing student experiences within the model. The focus of the master's program in nursing at Augustana is very congruent with the aims of this project. The master's program is entitled *Advanced Nursing Practice in Emerging Health Systems* and is designed to prepare nurses for community-focused practice with special emphasis on the health care needs of the underserved. The contributions of the master's in nursing to the model are: (1) development of advanced practice nurses with expertise in community-focused nursing practice and (2) creative innovation and change in the health care system. Future plans include the involvement of medical students and other health professional students in the educational process.

The medical consultant serves on the steering committee and is a liaison with the medical community. The medical consultant is a key link in working with care providers in the Sioux Falls area in creating new health services.

THE STEERING COMMITTEE

A group of community leaders came together to brainstorm and develop the plan for HAMPIC. This group remains active in the project and takes on the role of steering committee. Representation on the committee includes nursing leaders from Sioux Valley Hospital, Sioux River Valley Community Health

Center, and Augustana College Department of Nursing. Other members of the committee include individuals who are experiencing economic marginalization and homelessness and who are active in the Health Action Model, the Director of the Sioux Falls School System Alternative Youth Program, Director of The Banquet, Director of County Welfare, Director of the Sioux Falls Area Foundation, Director of Heartland House, Executive Director of Interlakes Community Action, a physician from Sioux River Valley Community Health Center, two physicians from the University of South Dakota's School of Medicine, a local pastor, Director of Planned Giving from Sioux Valley Health Systems, and Supervisor of Health Services for the Sioux Falls School District. All members of the steering committee are active within other political organizations and institutions and are known for being where things happen in the community.

The steering committee meets quarterly to listen to the voices of persons-communities. These leaders have strong beliefs that community interconnectedness occurs when everyone involved has a voice. It is important to note two important guiding principles of this steering committee: (1) the conceptual framework of HAMPIC serves as a guide in decision making and (2) community participant interaction and decision making go beyond the normative client participation in suggesting and discussing to a deeper involvement in charting the direction of the project (i.e., all documentation forms were developed with the input of those served). Those served by the model are viewed as experts in their own lives, and they voice their choices regarding personal health patterns. In creating their personal health descriptions, person-communities may work on a health goal that seems a lesser priority to others typically viewed as "the experts," but it is a greater priority to the person-community. The steering committee models the principle of HAMPIC, that the person is expert in his or her own life, in communications with those in the community who believe that "educated experts" know what is best for other people concerning matters of health. This is a priority for the steering committee, along with seeking expanded sources of funding for the model and creating new and unique linkages of care without creating new administrative structures. Jennifer James (1996) writes in *Thinking in the Future Tense* that true partnership in community includes the ability to do more with less.

SITE COMMUNITIES

The following site communities are partners with Augustana College Department of Nursing in the Health Action Model and are critical in co-creating connections (Figure 11-2).

- Inter-Lakes Community Action Program, Inc., began a transitional housing project for families who are homeless at Heartland House in 1996. The Heartland House Project is designed to provide housing and other supportive services (e.g., education assistance, job search, living skills, family case management) for a maximum of 24 months, with the goal of fostering family self-sufficiency.
- The Good Shepherd Family Center provides a combination of services, such as individual and family counseling services, through the Catholic diocese, and serves as a drop-in center for families.
- The Banquet provides meals for those needing sustenance.

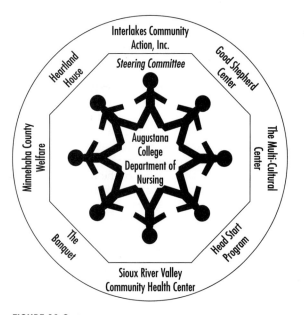

FIGURE 11-2 Creating connections in community: site communities. (From Augustana College, Sioux Falls, SD)

- Minnehaha County welfare system provides financial assistance and residential facilities for individuals and families economically marginalized. A downtown motel and a set of duplex apartments are used for the latter purpose.
- The Multi-Cultural Center provides education and referral services to many immigrants and refugees in the Sioux Falls area as well as providing culturally sensitive responses to minority groups' human needs.
- Sioux River Valley Community Health Center, a federally and state funded community health center, provides health care for low-income and indigent persons and those with limited access to health care.
- Head Start programs in Sioux Falls are operated by Inter-Lakes Community Action Program, Inc., and the Sioux Falls Public School System. The project will begin with the Head Start Programs and will expand to work with other classes in the Sioux Falls school system.

These collaborating agencies have identified a shared interest in the health and well-being of underserved populations in the Sioux Falls community. Representing different disciplines and areas of interest and expertise (public and private entities, health care and social action, and education), all are committed to the creation and implementation of the model.

Evaluation Process: Responsibilities of Creating Connections

There are four overarching objectives for the Health Action Model, all of which involve connecting with new ways of identifying health issues of populations and co-creating health services. The objectives and progress made with them in the first 6 months of bringing up the model are delineated as follows:

1. Creating a model to guide provision of health services based on Parse's human becoming school of thought within the discipline of nursing for families experiencing economic marginalization and homelessness.
   a. A conceptual framework for guiding the work of the model has been developed.

b. Specific documentation forms to identify the various health issues of individuals, families, groups, and site communities have been developed.

c. Six site communities have been identified, and a collaborative working relationship with Augustana's Department of Nursing has been established. Agency staff and persons served by the site are involved in developing HAMPIC.

2. Utilizing HAMPIC to address health issues of site communities.

a. Advanced practice nurses have begun meeting with individuals, families, and groups in all of the site communities. Personal health descriptions and health action plans are being created.

b. Steering committee members are meeting quarterly with the project staff to discuss emerging health issues and attend to the further development of the model.

c. A steering committee member, along with one of the advanced practice nurses, was instrumental in creating a new child care service for families at Heartland House so that parents can attend tenant meetings. The need for additional alternative child care for single-parent families is a critical health issue.

d. A Health Discussion Group for guests at The Banquet is offered on Thursday evenings after the soup kitchen meal is served. An advanced practice nurse facilitates the group discussion of health issues the guests identify as important to them. This is emerging as a place where referrals to other health resources will occur.

e. A Family Health Program in alliance with the Sioux Falls Public School System has been developed within HAMPIC. This program began by addressing the issue of chronic infestation with head lice among Head Start children. An advanced practice nurse and a family mentor work with families who request assistance with following the procedures for head lice eradication. Other health issues of families are beginning to emerge.

f. Women living at Heartland House identified the need for an exercise program as a way of dealing with their stress and weight control issues. However, the issue of cost and child care in becoming involved in an exercise program was prohibitive. A Water Walking Aerobics Program is being established for them at the local YWCA, addressing cost and child care issues.

3. Providing culturally sensitive educational experiences for health professional students.

a. Undergraduate Augustana nursing majors are assigned community health nursing experience at Heartland House. Students work with families who are residents of this site community.

b. Undergraduate Augustana nursing majors are involved in clinical learning at the site community of Sioux River Valley Community Health Center. The focus of this experience is to understand the lived experiences of those who are struggling with economic marginalization, homelessness, and access to health care.

c. Augustana graduate nursing students, as part of their clinical course work, become involved with individuals and families at the site communities of Heartland House and The Banquet.

d. HAMPIC was presented to occupational therapy students at the Multi-Cultural Center in Sioux Falls. The focus of the educational panel was on the importance of understanding the diversity within and among cultures in the community.

4. Extending HAMPIC beyond the local area to the surrounding region, and sharing it as a prototype for health care regionally, nationally, and internationally.

a. Current publication of the model will provide both national and international sharing of the prototype.

b. HAMPIC was presented at an International Qualitative Research Conference held at Loyola University Chicago, November 1997. The presentation focused on the utility of qualitative research in providing insight for creating this practice model.

c. HAMPIC was presented at a nursing theory conference entitled *Nursing in Com-*

munity: A Human Becoming Perspective, held May 7, 1997; in Sioux Falls.

d. Plans are underway for international collaborative educational experiences in working with HAMPIC, a master's in nursing program in Toronto, Canada, and a large Toronto-based health care system.

e. Requests from other teaching institutions and health care systems have been received for use of the documentation forms developed by the model.

Other evaluative processes to be developed in the model include:

- Researching personal stories of lived experiences of health
- Identifying new understandings emerging from the work of the steering committee
- Noting modifications and innovations made in health care delivery systems
- Analyzing cost savings related to the model
- Identifying changes in the nature of collaborative relationships among members of the steering committee
- Describing quality of life from the person-community perspective

Conclusion

In these changing times filled with ambiguity and inequity in health care access, there is a call for a new way of caring for the health of the community. Hattie, a 51-year-old woman who struggles with living homeless, describes her response to HAMPIC's new way of partnering with the community around issues of health as follows (personal communication, July 1997):

I have never experienced anything like this before. You've actually listened to what I had to say. It feels like what I have to say is important. So many people won't even talk to me. My son died of AIDS and people wouldn't even help . . . I've never heard before that health is a personal choice about the way a person lives their life. I believe that's true and there are some things I want to do differently and can do differently. I have so many things to do and I need to stay strong and healthy to be able to do them. When you are on the street, a person

needs to be strong. I can tell you what will help me to stay strong.

Academia's partnership with the community may be a new way of living health.

References

Bauman S: The meaning of being homeless, *Scholarly Inquiry for Nursing Practice: An International Journal* 7(1):59-70, 1993.

Bunkers SS: *Considering tomorrow: Parse's theory-guided research.* An unpublished dissertation, 1996, Loyola University Chicago, Chicago, Illinois.

Bunkers SS, Michaels C, Ethridge P: Advanced practice nursing in community: nursing's opportunity, *Advanced Practice Nursing Quarterly* 2(4):79-84, 1997.

Chittister J: *Wisdom distilled from the daily,* San Francisco, 1990, Harper Collins.

Francis M: Eight homeless mothers' tales, *Image: The Journal of Professional Nursing* 24(2):111-114, 1992.

James J: *Thinking in the future tense,* New York, 1996, Simon & Schuster.

Mitchell G: Questioning evidence-based practice for nursing, *Nursing Science Quarterly* 10:154-155, 1997.

Parse RR: Human becoming: Parse's theory of nursing, *Nursing Science Quarterly* 5:35-41, 1992.

Parse RR: Quality of life: sciencing and living the art of human becoming, *Nursing Science Quarterly* 7:16-20, 1994.

Parse RR: The human becoming theory. In Parse RR, ed: *Illuminations: the human becoming theory in practice and research,* New York, 1995, National League for Nursing, pp 5-8.

Parse RR: Community: a human becoming perspective, *Illuminations: The Newsletter of the International Consortium of Parse Scholars,* Spring 1996a, p 4.

Parse RR: The human becoming theory: challenges in practice and research, *Nursing Science Quarterly* 9:55-60, 1996b.

Parse RR: The human becoming theory: the was, is, and will be, *Nursing Science Quarterly* 10:32-38, 1997a.

Parse RR: Transforming research and practice with the human becoming theory, *Nursing Science Quarterly* 10:171-174, 1997b.

Pilkington FB: Knowledge and evidence: do they change patterns of health? *Nursing Science Quarterly* 10:156-157, 1997.

van Kaam A: *Living creatively,* New York, 1985, University Press of America.

CHAPTER 12

Clinical Nurse Specialists in Clinical Case Management

Evolution of a Model in a Large Tertiary Medical Center

DEBORAH B. MANGAN, RN, MS, CS, **†BONNIE L. CLOSSON**, RN, MSN, MRC, **JANICE L. STONE**, RN, MS, CS

OVERVIEW

In all case management programs, a combination of patient-centered and resource-utilization outcomes is crucial for comprehensive outcome measurement related to the success of the program.

Increased chronic illness, expansion of technology, shorter lengths of hospital stay, and complexity of care have resulted in changes for health care delivery. The rising cost of health care, purchaser demand to control cost, and changes in reimbursement in the United States from a fee-for-service to a prospective pay and capitated fee system necessitate provision of the most cost-effective quality care. These changes translate into a need for better coordination of patient care across disciplines and health care settings, especially for high-risk groups of patients. An advanced practice role, such as the clinical nurse specialist (CNS), can facilitate health care in meeting the demand for serving patients with increasingly complex needs, as well as cost-containment goals. At the Mayo Medical Center, a large tertiary care center, clinical case management (CCM) focuses on the care of high-risk, complex patients. In this chapter the authors define CCM, share a chronic illness model that supports the definition, describe the development process for the CCM program, discuss a patient care process for CCM, describe the application of standardized nursing language to support the practice, explore three different clinical applications of the CCM model, and discuss the evolution process from inception to expansion for the CCM program. Potential implications for practice, opportunities for research, and factors considered for successful development and implementation of CCM are integrated throughout the chapter. ▲

---

†Deceased.

Establishment of Need for Case Management

The incentive to develop clinical case management (CCM) at the Mayo Medical Center originated from the study of various disease management strategies and changes in health care systems. Tools for practice management such as clinical pathways and practice guidelines were in place in some clinical areas, but they did not adequately address the issues related to managing the high-risk, complex population of patients who did not have predictable patterns of care. Institutional and national data were used to identify populations that might have increased resource use in terms of hospital length of stay, readmission, length of stay when readmitted, and visits to the emergency trauma unit. Development of the practice started by identifying subsets of these populations that consisted of patients who were at higher risk for complex care and extensive use of services and who might benefit from CCM.

The definition of CCM in the Department of Nursing at MMC focuses on coordination and management of the clinical course for high-risk patients (Box 12-1). Four clinical specialty groups were identified as having populations amenable to nursing case management. Experienced clinical nurse specialists (CNSs) from these areas were selected for a work group with the charge to design and implement case management. Use of the CNS in the CCM role added specificity to an already valued role and was supported by the American Nurses' Association (ANA) *Scope and Standards for Advanced Practice Registered Nursing*. Specifically, Standard VI, "Case Management/Coordination of Care," states: "The advanced practice registered nurse provides comprehensive clinical coordination of care and case management" (ANA, 1996). Table 12-1 describes the advantages of utilizing CNSs as case managers for high-risk, complex patients.

FOUNDATION FOR CLINICAL CASE MANAGEMENT

Based on the defined goal to coordinate and manage the clinical course, a patient model was developed for the CCM of patients with chronic illness. The Patient Chronic Illness Model (Figure 12-1) incorporates concepts related to illness trajectory, crisis theory, chronic illness, and normalization theory (Aguilera, Messick, 1990; Lazarus, Folkman, 1984;

BOX 12-1
Definition of Nursing Clinical Case Management

Clinical case management is a care strategy in which an advanced practice nurse, such as a clinical nurse specialist, provides direct patient care for select high-risk patients/families with a complex, chronic, and/or debilitating illness. A clinical case manager:

- Uses advanced practice assessment, nursing therapeutics, care coordination, outcomes measurement, and data trending to facilitate continuous improvement in patient care
- Functions collaboratively within a multidisciplinary team to manage individual and/or group health services during the entire episode of illness, crossing all settings in which a patient receives care
- Focuses on utilization of appropriate resources to achieve optimal patient care outcomes within effective time frames

---

Strauss, 1984). Key terms for the model are defined in Box 12-2. The primary effort of CCM focuses on the crisis-to-acute, stable-to-unstable core of the model. Throughout the illness trajectory, interventions focus on the context and course of illness for the patient. This model identifies comprehensive foci for advanced practice intervention. Healthy living while managing chronic illness is the desired outcome. Driven by the model, the following four overall advanced practice intervention goals for CCM emerge:

1. Prevent crises, and therefore decrease hospital readmission and/or decrease patient acuity on admission, and length of hospitalization.
2. Facilitate management of the health care regimen and management of problems related to carrying out the regimen, thereby reducing recidivism.
3. Intervene to facilitate patient and family adjustment to the illness and the treatment regimen.

TABLE 12-1

Advantages of Clinical Nurse Specialists as Case Managers for High-Risk, Complex Patients

FUNCTION	CNS AS CASE MANAGER
Identifying population	Identifies high-risk patients with unpredictable patterns of care; analyzes data to identify subsets of populations
Screening	Adapts screening processes and tool to specialty; determines eligibility for case management
Assessment	Advanced physical assessment skills required (i.e., specialty-focused comprehensive assessment); utilizes NIC domains and classes as assessment framework
Critical analysis	Analyzes data from health and illness perspectives to identify comprehensive, holistic interventions; anticipates patterns of illness trajectories
Interventions	Interventions are highly individualized and include independent advanced practice interventions; focus is across the continuum
Evaluation	Seeks and synthesizes data to trend and determine treatment and program development options
Discharge planning	Modifies knowledge to help patient adapt to home environment; incorporates plan for use of community resources
Synthesis	Evaluation for trends and patterns in patient populations and care delivery; communication of the relationship among nursing diagnoses, interventions, and outcomes
Research/continuous improvement (CI)	Research agendas and CI projects evolve from data analysis

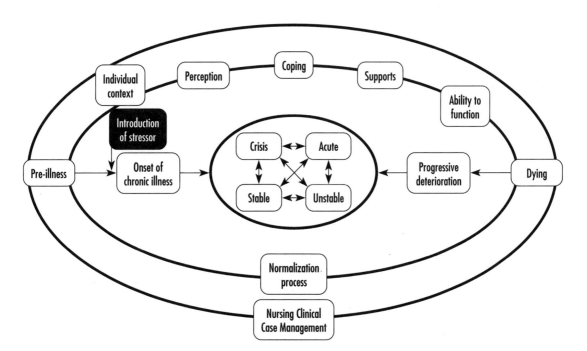

FIGURE 12-1 A patient model for nursing clinical case management of a patient with chronic illness (By permission of Mayo Foundation.)

BOX 12-2
Patient Chronic Illness Model Definitions

Illness Trajectory
The physiological, social, and spiritual aspects of an illness faced by an individual and/or family living with a chronic illness (Strauss, 1984).

Normalization
The process of an individual redefining bio-psycho-social-spiritual status in response to a chronic illness. During this process an individual may experience anger, denial, bargaining, depression, and acceptance.

Individual Context
An individual's personality, experience(s), and sociocultural makeup. Sociocultural makeup includes attitudes, values, beliefs, and role(s).

Perception
Cognitive representation or subjective meaning attached to an event. This event may be perceived

as harm, threat, challenge, or loss, depending on an individual's appraisal of the situation (Aguilera, 1990; Lazarus, Folkman, 1984).

Coping
Cognitive, behavioral, and/or physiological responses to change a circumstance that occurs in response to biological, psychological, social, and/or spiritual stressors.

Supports
Resources available in the environment that can be depended on to help solve or prevent a difficult situation (Aguilera, Messick, 1990).

Ability to Function
The ability to meet one's own bio-psycho-social-spiritual needs.

---

4. Facilitate patient referral for and/or utilization of appropriate resources necessary to manage and adjust to the illness.

Initial Development

With the foundation established for the context of chronic illness, the process of implementing CCM began through a study of various approaches to patient care management. Clinical experience and the review of previous research relating to patients with chronic congestive heart failure facilitated development of the context, components, and specifics of the CCM program. In a 3-year study of 50 patients with chronic cardiomyopathy, Frost et al (1994) identified factors that may influence psychosocial adjustment to cardiomyopathy. Factors identified in this study as significant predictors of less effective patient adjustment included a more negative appraisal of the situation, greater number and degree of changes related to interpersonal relationships, needed environmental changes, and symptoms. Statistics based on multiple-regression analy-

sis identified a combination of these variables as predictors of less effective adjustment, accounting for 65% of the variance in psychosocial adjustment to illness. These results were instrumental in establishing intervention foci for CCM practice. Valentine, Stiles, and Mangan (1995) did a qualitative study with 98 nurses and 33 patients and their families. This study provided input about patient and family values and expectations related to nursing care, and contrasted beliefs about caring between nursing and patients. Another study, by Rich and colleagues (1995), identified independent predictors of readmission of elderly patients with congestive heart failure, which included blood urea nitrogen, systolic blood pressure, serum sodium, diabetes mellitus, and assignment to a multidisciplinary treatment intervention. This information served to identify screening criteria for high-risk patients who may benefit from clinical case management.

Congestive heart failure (CHF) is a complex, chronic, debilitating disease that has tremendous impact on the use of health care resources and an individual's quality of life. Although case management of CHF patients has been associated with cost-effective use of health care resources, research related to the influence of case management on patient-centered outcomes is limited. To further measure the impact of case management on patient outcomes, the cardiovascular CNS initiated an outcomes study entitled *Evaluation of a Nursing Clinical Case Management Program for Patients with Chronic Congestive Heart Failure.* This study evaluated a clinical case management model, specifically addressing the impact of CCM on a patient population with chronic, debilitating cardiovascular illness. In the study the CNS provided consultation

and intervention during hospitalization and in outpatient follow-up. In addition to standard care, the experimental group of patients had outpatient follow-up by phone at approximately 1, 4, 8, and 12 weeks after discharge. Additional visits with the CNS were based on patient status and availability.

The findings of this research-based outcomes-evaluation study were impressive (Box 12-3). Consequently they were disseminated to key groups within the medical center. The goal of these presentations was to gain support for the development of specialty-based CCM that includes the identification of high-risk patients through screening and assessment processes.

Clinical Case Management Demonstration Project

To extend beyond the CHF population, the demonstration project for CCM was implemented over a 2-year period in four specialty practice areas utilizing the CNSs in a practice that covers the continuum of care. The key goal of this project was to operationalize the direct patient care aspect of CCM, while enhancing care coordination. An additional goal was to develop systems designed to:

1. Synthesize existing patient data along with cost and care outcome data
2. Document care and patient outcomes
3. Evaluate the potential quality and organizational effect of the CCM model

CONTEXT

The focus of the CCM Work Group expanded well beyond discussion of roles and role implementation and included consideration of key principles that provide a context for CCM. Guidance for the context of this practice was provided by the department's mission, vision, and core values. These principles served as a guide in transforming the vision of case management into a practice model. The CCM model strongly supports the core values, which are R.N. accountability for patient care, a professional practice environment, and continuity of patient care.

Prior to the implementation of case management, the Department of Nursing Service had restructured role functions and processes into a framework of collaborative practice. The CCM work group was committed to support the principles of this collaborative practice. These include support for specialty-based research-driven practice, progressive development of care delivery, and advanced practice nursing resource at the point of patient care delivery.

The context for data and outcome management was based on commitment to a common language. This allowed for evaluation of the efficacy of CCM-based synthesis and comparison of data. Three of the standardized classifications of nursing language, NANDA (*Nursing Diagnosis: Definition and Classification 1997-1998,* North American Nursing Diagnosis Association, 1996), University of Iowa Nursing Interventions Classification (NIC) (McCloskey, Bulechek, 1996), and Nursing Outcomes Classification (NOC) (Johnson, Maas, 1997), were embraced as the standardized nursing language to represent advanced practice diagnosing, intervention, and outcomes. The possibility of measuring patient outcomes, using NOC, as they relate to specific nursing interventions (NIC) and classified nursing problems (NANDA) was a key driver for this decision. The CCM uses standardized nursing language and links the classification systems to describe the CCM process, the breadth and complexity of the care delivered by the advanced practice nurse, and patient outcomes. This includes the type of patient in the designated populations, priority types of interventions used, the practice styles of the practitioner and specialty, and desired clinical outcomes. The particular linkage of classification systems was easily understood by the CNS, since it flows naturally and easily from the nursing care process and allows for more accurate communication of care needs and desired intervention.

CNS MODEL FOR CCM

Prior to implementation of any case management process, it is critical to evaluate patient needs, resources and programs available to meet those needs, and the system of health care delivery. Assessment of the above factors clearly indicated variation in each of the four clinical areas in the demonstration project. Despite this variation, a core system-level process for CCM evolved. This is best represented as input, process, and outcome elements that interact and impact each other. These

factors can be applied to multiple patient populations and care delivery systems, and focus on various levels of influence. However, individual patient needs remain the core of the "input."

The challenge in case managing lies in having input processes that can predict patients who would benefit from CCM. Databases can facilitate the identification of high-risk diagnostic-related groups (DRGs) of patients and other characteristics that are predictive of individuals who may use extensive services (Figure 12-2). This is the first level of data analysis to identify high-risk patients from the entire population.

A target population can be further defined using additional nursing and specialty-based screening, the second level of data analysis. Screening categories include physical, psychosocial, and discharge criteria as well as previous use of resources. Specialty-specific screening indicators may also be added. Examples of these indicators include the New York Heart Association Class for the CHF population, the Functional Independence Measure for the rehabilitation population, and the Hamilton Depression Scale for the psychiatric population.

The process phase of CCM begins with a complex nursing assessment. The domains and classes from the Iowa Nursing Intervention Classification taxonomy provide a framework for a comprehensive nursing assessment. A benefit is that this taxonomy is inclusive and can also be applied across the continuum of care: intensive care, acute care, primary care, outpatient and community setting. The process phase of the model continues to utilize standardized nursing language with the identification of NANDA nursing diagnoses (1994). For each nursing diagnosis, one or more outcomes from the NOC system and one or more nursing interventions from the NIC system are selected and entered into the plan of care (Johnson, Maas, 1997; McCloskey, Bulechek, 1996). Using standardized nursing language that links a diagnosis with interventions and outcomes strengthens the data base and the potential ability to derive a cause-and-effect relationship. In all case management programs, a combination of patient-centered and resource-utilization outcomes is crucial for comprehensive outcome measurement related to the success of the program. Success of this case management model will lie in the fact that patient-centered outcomes are considered to be as important as outcomes that measure

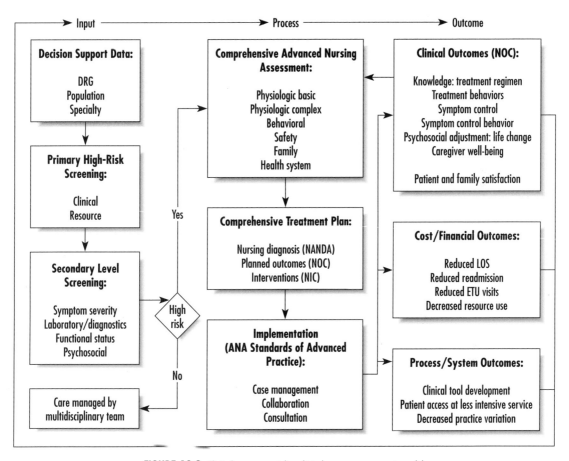

FIGURE 12-2 Clinical nurse specialist clinical case management model.

the use of resources. Early identification of key practice outcomes a key for CCM use was a major point to consider in the development process for the project. These include a set of core nursing clinical outcomes, cost/financial resource outcomes, and process/system outcomes (see Figure 12-2). A nursing CCM database was developed that includes screening criteria and process information with NANDA, NIC, and NOC data (NANDA, 1994; McCloskey, Bulechek, 1996; Johnson, Maas, 1997). To facilitate acquiring higher numbers of patients for data analysis and aggregation of data, all case managers are encouraged to use at least five core nursing clinical outcomes for each patient in the CCM program (see Figure 12-2). Additional NOC outcomes measured are those which the case manager identifies as being related to a specific patient,

along with their NANDA diagnoses. These might include an NOC outcome such as Tissue Integrity: Skin and Mucous Membranes, for the individual who is at high risk for skin breakdown.

Another set of outcomes relate to resource utilization, such as financial outcome (see Figure 12-2). The resource outcomes are analyzed by using existing institutional data bases, as much as possible. These include information such as admission unit, demographics, severity for DRG, and patient access to the health care facility. The ability to aggregate data within and across specialty practices will be key in assessing resource use, developing tools such as practice protocols and guidelines, and evaluating the effectiveness of a case management intervention. Since the CNS can apply critical thinking and data analysis, it is also hoped that specific research agendas will evolve out of the existing system for CCM.

Specialty Application of Clinical Case Management

CARDIOVASCULAR

CCM of patients with chronic CHF is an example of a population-focused application of CCM. This population was selected from DRG data. When a patient is admitted to the hospital, the staff RN does a learning needs assessment for the patient within 24 hours of admission and initiates a cardiac rehabilitation referral. This referral includes the identification of patients who are high-risk, complex patients admitted with a CHF diagnosis who need to be evaluated by the cardiovascular CNS for the CCM program. The majority of the referrals for the CCM Program come from the staff RN Additional referral sources are other interdisciplinary team members, such as physicians, cardiac rehabilitation coordinators, and social workers, and regional practice professionals such as nurse practitioners.

The CNS screens the patient for high-risk, complex needs indicators. Examples of these for the CHF patient include such factors as significant decrease in cardiac function as evidenced by a heart ejection fraction less than 35%, New York Heart Association class, diabetes, compromised kidney function, other co-morbidities, and ineffective coping. The CNS reviews the patient's chart and conducts an advanced assessment in addition to the staff RN's and other interdisciplinary team members' assessments and interventions. Examples of expanded assessment include:

- Assessing the patient's perception of his or her illness as a major harm, threat, or loss
- Assessing coping mechanisms and identification of the utilization of planful problem solving and distancing versus avoidance
- Assessing how the patient and family mobilize supports such as family, spirituality, and resources
- Assessing patient and family needs related to maximizing quality of life

Intervention is patient focused and determined by patient needs, staff RN abilities and time available, and availability of inpatient and outpatient resources to meet the patient and family needs. The CNS as case manager works very closely with all of the interdisciplinary team members, especially the primary RN, who always remains a pivotal professional in the interdisciplinary process.

Advanced practice interventions flow from the assessment and diagnoses. These may focus on cognitive restructuring to support the patient and family's viewing their situation as realistically as possible. Additional interventions include values clarification, counseling, complex discharge planning, guided imagery, and stress management to facilitate maximum functional status. An example of a case with complex discharge planning is a patient going home on an IV dobutamine drip and oxygen for symptom control. The CNS may work with the staff RN and the patient to expand the plan of care and/or may follow up with the patient in the hospital and after dismissal for four visits. Patients are followed in the hospital and after dismissal at approximately 1, 4, 8, and 12 weeks as necessary. Patients and families are also given the phone number of the case manager and told to call with any questions and concerns between visits. The focus of this follow-up is on symptom control, management of the treatment regimen, and adjustment to the illness. Follow-up may be by phone, home visits as necessary (if the patient is from the local area), or office visits. The major overall goal is to support continuity of care from hospital to home or another health care facility and intervention by the advanced practice nurse. The CCM does not replace home health care. The majority of outpatient follow-up is accomplished by phone.

CNS interventions during hospitalization are documented in the Patient Plan of Care, the Patient Education Flowsheet, and Multidisciplinary Integrated Patient Progress Notes. Postdismissal CNS patient interventions are documented through outpatient clinical notes, which are part of the permanent patient record. Major changes in patient status or a need for additional physician follow-up is communicated directly to the primary care physician or cardiologist as appropriate. When a patient is dismissed from the hospital, a dismissal summary is typed, with the following identified on the summary: referring physician; primary care physician; cardiologist; home health care agency or public health nursing facility, as appropriate; and CNS NCCM. All of these individuals receive a copy of the dismissal summary, and one is sent home with the patient. Follow-up in the CCM program by the CNS is also included in the "Patient Follow-up and Appointments" section of the dismissal summary.

REHABILITATION

In the rehabilitation specialty, the CNS assumes an active role in a partnership relationship with the registered nurse by coaching and mentoring the primary RN in identifying high-risk patients. This is accomplished by performing a physical assessment using the NIC domain and class framework previously described, selecting the appropriate nursing diagnoses and interventions, and being responsible for outcomes of a high-risk population. As the RN develops in his or her role, the CNS continues to provide support to the registered nurse, but also continues to intervene in the more complex aspects of a case, which include interventions that are considered advanced practice in scope. For example, in case managing a morbidly obese patient with a new cervical spinal cord injury, the staff nurse may have responsibility for routine interventions such as assistance with activities of daily living, skin surveillance, and urinary catheterization. In contrast, the CNS may assume responsibility for nutritional counseling, coping enhancement, and hope instillation.

In discharge planning, the CNS addresses the home environment and provides caregiver support, while the staff nurse teaches psychomotor skills to the caregiver. Continuity is facilitated by ongoing interdisciplinary collaboration, especially through patient care conferences. Throughout the process the CNS maintains a role as coach and mentor for the staff nurse, and continues informal teaching to expand the staff nurse's knowledge of nursing interventions and the CCM process for complex patient populations.

PSYCHIATRY

In some populations, a majority of patients are high risk and complex. In medical psychiatry, a clinical population of dementia patients was identified, the majority of whom were high risk and complex. De-

mentia patients are generally at risk because of the deteriorating nature of dementia as well as the existence of multiple co-morbid conditions. Data supported this general statement in terms of multiple co-morbid conditions (more than five per patient) and extended length of stay (more than 10 days) as high-risk indicators for patients with dementia. Initially the CNS case manager worked with a multidisciplinary group as well as with a group of primary RNs who focused on nursing care and patient and family education issues. The work with these groups involved a thorough assessment of issues in practice, such as dementia-specific assessment, learning needs of staff related to specific approaches for patients with dementia, family and caregiver needs, and referral processes to extended-care facilities. Education and practice changes involved all members of the multidisciplinary team with an intensified focus on nursing care interventions, on reducing practice variation at the point of assessment, and on improving transition in care.

This broader approach to case management was applied because of the following:

- The specificity of interventions for all patients with this diagnosis
- The existence of a cohesive multidisciplinary team invested in making care improvements
- The benefit of decreasing practice variation to decrease length of stay, resource use, and care coordination for this complex illness
- The benefit of care coordination improvements to caregivers and referring agencies

Core case management concepts, such as caregiver strategies for managing a complex illness, crisis management, and care coordination, were applied to all patients in this population.

This process has helped the team to more clearly identify patients who may be at risk for extended stays or readmission or who may have difficulty with treatment management. The care of this population continues to evolve toward a more individualized application of CCM across the continuum of care. The primary RN and the social worker both complete postdischarge follow-up phone calls to the patient, caregivers, or care agency. From information gained in these contacts, a referral will be made to the CNS for CCM if complications of treatment or concern about patient behaviors is present. The CNS will then assess the patient for further need of nursing care and/or work with the caregivers to revise the treatment plan.

Expansion

Throughout the development process the potential for flexible application of the CCM model according to specialty-practice patterns surfaced as a valuable asset. This flexibility could serve to support cohesiveness of the multidisciplinary team and provide for consideration of risk factors in a specialty-based patient population. These strengths, along with support for primary nursing and collaboration with all disciplines, were identified as key factors for success of the implementation of the CCM program in different specialties and settings. All of these factors enhanced the perception of the benefits of the CCM process.

In this cost-conscious health care environment, the decision to use a CNS as case manager is not an easy decision for an organization to make. However, this approach was supported by the positive outcomes reported in Box 12-2 and the expertise the CNS brings to the care of the complex, high-risk patient population (see Table 12-1). Therefore the Department of Nursing supported the inclusion of CCM as a role component for all CNSs. The CCM Demonstration Project succeeded in establishing the nature of the CCM practice and the systems to support and evaluate the practice. The challenge was to disseminate this information to all CNSs in the system. In this section the effort to expand the practice to all CNSs and develop necessary supports to sustain the practice over time are described. The initial CCM work group began the process by facilitating several discussions with the Department of Nursing administrative team to gain commitment on the nature of the CCM practice and its interface with care delivery, the desirability of utilizing advanced practice CNSs in the care of complex patients, and the need to maintain support for the CCM process by educating all nursing leadership on the goals and expectations. This also allowed an opportunity to discuss the impact of this work load on other aspects of the CNS role and on the work load for other resource and staff roles. In addition, it was essential for the members of the Department of Nursing to provide education throughout the department and develop processes to sustain directions for use of outcome-focused clinical processes, including implementation of standardized nursing language. The CCM Work Group and the administrative team worked together to gain the commitment critical to supporting the collaboration and negotiation related to work load changes as a result of increased CNS time in CCM, the CNS crossing the continuum of care, the assessment of processes to sustain continuity of care, and the resources for the learning and documentation of outcomes of this practice.

CNS EDUCATION

The process for CNSs to implement the practice of CCM for a high-risk patient population began with the development of a needs assessment, which was administered to all of the CNSs. The education and professional development objectives were achieved through formal and informal didactic, as well as computer lab, time to facilitate learning of the CCM database. The sequence of the process was as follows:

- Integration of CCM into institutional goals and objectives
- CCM as a role component of the CNS role
- Integration of standardized nursing language into clinical decision making
- Utilization of the nursing CCM database
- Evaluation of practice patterns through data synthesis
- Analysis of CCM process and outcomes for improvement opportunities

The total time for the educational sessions was approximately 32 hours per CNS over a one and one-half year period. This time line allowed both assimilation of concrete information and application to specialty practice.

Conclusion

The CHF CCM provides evidence of the link between research and improved clinical model implementation. The success of the CHF model has facilitated development of CCM in other specialty-practice areas. The CCM program described in this chapter has many implications for patient outcomes and research-based nursing practice. These include the following:

- Development of nursing interventions directed at high-risk, complex patients and/or

those experiencing depression and perceiving their illness as a major harm, threat, or loss
- Implementation of care delivery models that support continuity of care for patients across the continuum
- Expanded development of interdisciplinary collaborative practice models for patient care
- Focused effort to improve analysis capability for evaluating quality-cost benefit of CCM interventions and patient outcomes for functional status, satisfaction, and cost

Nursing research is needed on the relationship between specific nursing interventions and patient outcomes. This will be extremely valuable for the future of quality, cost-effective professional nursing practice. Outcomes-research foci of interest include functional and social status, patient and family satisfaction, care provider satisfaction, and financial outcomes. The potential for this model is unlimited, the outcomes noted are possible, and the model is successful because of the breadth and depth of expertise the CNS brings to the model as case manager.

References

Aguilera D, Messick J: *Crisis intervention: theory and methodology*, ed 6, St Louis, 1990, Mosby.

American Nurses' Association: *Scope and standards of advanced practice registered nursing*, Washington, DC, 1996, American Nurses' Publishing.

Frost M et al: An analysis of factors influencing psychosocial adjustment to cardiomyopathy, *Cardiovascular Nursing* 30(1):1-7, 1994.

Johnson M, Maas M, eds: *Nursing outcomes classification (NOC)*, St Louis, 1997, Mosby.

Lazarus RS, Folkman S: *Stress, appraisal and coping*, New York, 1984, Springer Publishing.

McCloskey J, Bulechek G, eds: *Nursing interventions classification (NIC)*, ed 2, St Louis, 1996, Mosby.

NANDA nursing diagnoses: definitions and classification 1995-1996, Philadelphia, 1994, North American Nursing Diagnosis Association.

Rich M et al: *Journal of General Internal Medicine* 8:585-590, 1995.

Valentine KL, Stiles MK, Mangan DB: Values, vision and action: creating a care-focused nursing practice environment. In *Power, politics, and public policy: a matter of caring*, National League of Nursing Press. New York, NY, 1995.

Ware JE: SF-36 *Health survey manual and interpretation guide*, The Health Institute, New England Medical Center, Boston, 1993.

Deborah Mangan and Jan Stone wish to dedicate this chapter to the memory of Bonnie Closson, a professional nursing colleague and friend, for her dedication and contribution in the development of Clinical Case Management.

CHAPTER 13

Mental Health Nursing and Case Management in Great Britain

BEN THOMAS, MSc, RMN, RGN, Dip N, RNT, FRCN
KARINA LOVELL, BA, MSc, PhD, RMN, ENB650, DpEd

OVERVIEW

Mental health nurses are well positioned to take on the role of case managers for the seriously mentally ill. In order to do so they require adequate training, management support, and an ability to articulate client outcomes resulting from case management.

Mental health services in the United Kingdom are going through major reform. The advent of community care has enabled nurses to reappraise their role in providing comprehensive mental health service and to think beyond existing structures. Case management has been well received as an innovative service model by clients and professionals alike. There is a growing body of research studies investigating the efficacy of case management. Many of the studies are concerned with the success of case management in reducing hospital admissions. However, it may be more helpful to examine how successful case management is in determining the appropriateness of hospital admissions. Training in case management has been slow to materialise. However, one training programme is an exception. The Thorn training programme has been running for five years and has produced 260 graduates. Recommendations are made for more training of a similar type, based on the latest effective treatments and advances in community health care provision such as case management. Despite these initiatives problems still remain for nurses to work across boundaries and to articulate their worth. Nevertheless, mental health nurses are well positioned to take up the role of case managers and to demonstrate the model's effectiveness on client outcomes. ▲

For the last two decades there has been an increasing move from institutional or hospital care to community-based mental health services. Case management has been gradually introduced along with this movement. The origins of case management derived from North American community care development in the late 1960s and early 1970s. British mental health policy documents from the 1970s, including the 1975 White Paper *Better Services for the Mentally Ill,* highlighted the need for such community-based services. The White Papers *Caring for People* (Department of Health, 1989a) and *Working for Patients* (Department of Health, 1989b), which were based on the recommendations of *Community Care Agenda for Action* (Griffiths, 1988), put forward the case for care management for clients with long-term mental health problems.

Despite these policies, the transition from hospital-based care to community care for the mentally ill remains problematic. Much concern is continually expressed about the so-called failure of community care as a result of insufficient resource allocation and patchy, inadequate, and uncoordinated services. Ryan et al (1991) cite the Audit Commission's finding of 1986 that inadequate community services had been developed and identified five major problems (Box 13-1).

In 1990 the NHS and Community Care Act stated that care plans were to be developed for people with complex social needs that were the responsibility of the local authority. In a similar vein the Department of Health (1990) in HC(90)23 required all people accepted by secondary mental health services, including inpatients, to have a designated keyworker to arrange and coordinate care in the community. Following this the Care Programme Approach (CPA) was introduced in 1991. The CPA requires specialist mental health services to ensure that adequate care plans are agreed to meet the health and related social care needs to provide a framework for the care of the seriously mentally ill living in the community. The *Building Bridges* document (Department of Health, 1995) outlines four main elements to the Care Programme Approach (Box 13-2).

The Community Care Act (1994) identified the need for the role of the "care manager" and described the role as assessing clients' individual needs and coordinating and monitoring services to these clients in response to these needs. More recently the Government Green Paper on developing partnerships in mental health (Department of Health, 1997), outlines four options for structural change, each of which would adjust the current

---

BOX 13-1
Problems With Inadequate Community Services Identified by the Audit Commission, 1986

1. A mismatch of resources to meet the requirements of community policies
2. The lack of short-term bridging finance to further allow a transition to community care
3. Social security policies that provided a perverse incentive for residential as opposed to domiciliary care
4. Inadequate arrangements for training and the provision of opportunities in community services for existing staff in long-stay hospitals, and for training sufficient numbers of community-based staff
5. Fragmented organisation in, and lack of effective joint working and planning among, the different agencies involved in the provision of services

---

BOX 13-2
Main Elements of CPA

1. Systematic arrangements for assessing the health and social needs of people accepted by specialist psychiatric services
2. The formulation of a care plan that addresses the identified health and social care needs
3. The appointment of a keyworker to keep in close contact with the patient and monitor care
4. Regular reviews and, if need be, agreed changes to the care plan

From Department of Health: *Building bridges: a guide for interagency working for the care and protection of severely mentally ill people,* London, 1996. Crown copyright is reproduced with the permission of the Controller of Her Majesty's Stationery Office.

boundaries between health and social care for people with serious mental illness. *London's Mental Health: The Report to the King's Fund London Commission* (Johnson et al, 1997) examined service provision in London and proposed strategies for tackling the gaps between need and provision.

It has been argued that uncoordinated and fragmented services for the seriously mentally ill have three main consequences: first, they lead to an increase in hospital admission rates; second, a high proportion of those individuals with a serious mental illness lose contact with mental health services; third, some individuals with serious mental illness deteriorate as a result of a failure of the services to offer appropriate care (Marshall et al, 1996). Individuals with serious mental illness have many health and social needs, and require help from a number of sources. If such needs are to be met, a coordinated service is clearly necessary. Case management is proposed as a solution to overcome the difficulties of fragmented services and their lack of planning, and is meant to develop more effective working relationships between agencies.

Definitions of Case Management

Case management is described as "the cornerstone of community care" (Shepherd, 1990). A plethora of definitions of case management are identified. Ryan et al (1991) succinctly define case management as "a system of service delivery designed to provide care and support for people with severe and long term mental health problems who would otherwise be at risk of losing contact with services. Case management recognises that these people risk being unable to cope with personal, social, financial and other difficulties which arise either as a result of their mental health problems (or the treatment for them), or the unemployment, poverty and stigma attached to mental health problems." Intagliata (1982) states, "Case management involves having a single person responsible for maintaining a long-term supportive relationship with the client, regardless of where the client is and regardless of the number of agencies involved. The case manager is a helper, service broker, and advocate for the client. . . . "

Reviews have identified four main categories of case management models (Holloway et al, 1995;

Solomon, 1992; Oynett, 1992). The four main models identified include the following:

1. Assertive Community Treatment (ACT), developed by Stein and Test (1980), which emphasizes assertive outreach
2. Personal Strengths Model, developed by Modrcin et al (1988), which stresses the development of an individual's strengths rather than concentrating on his or her deficits
3. Psychosocial Rehabilitation Model (Goering et al, 1988), which focuses on rehabilitation—in particular, medication management and social skills
4. Brokerage Model (Kanter, 1989) which emphasises the coordination and organisation of services for clients.

Much of the British literature is fraught with confusion regarding the terms "case" and "care" management. However, the main distinction is that care management focuses on coordination and purchasing responsibilities, whereas case management stresses the provision of direct care to clients with serious mental illness in the community (Armstrong, Ward, 1996; Clifford, Craig, 1988; Ford et al, 1995).

Burns (1997) distinguishes clearly between case management, care management, and care programming. He argues that clinical case management follows an ACT model as described earlier, whereas care management is the term used by British Social Services to describe their approach to case management and describes the brokerage model.

Ford and Ryan (1997) argue: "Care management and Care Programme Approach (CPA) have primarily led to bureaucratic changes in the system of care delivery, and there is no evidence of their effectiveness. Indeed, there is clear evidence of their ineffectiveness. Mounting evidence shows that case management programmes such as the Daily Living Programme, which are clinically driven, incorporating low case-loads and assertive outreach, can be effective." Thus, as will be detailed later, there is more evidence of clinical case management models being effective than the brokerage type of model.

In a recent review of case management (Marshall et al, 1996), the ACT model described above was the only model to have been used as an alternative to acute admissions to a psychiatric hospital. Moreover, the ACT model (unlike other models) was able to demonstrate four principal elements of clinical practice: case management teams were multidisciplinary, they provided interventions in the community as well as in the client's own home, case loads were kept between 10 and 15 clients, and ACT case management teams tried to provide all or most of the interventions as opposed to referring them to other services and agencies.

Most United Kingdom case management services do not tend to adhere strictly to any of the particular models identified above. There is an overlap of certain aspects in all these models; however, the critical and most effective elements of case management are still to be determined (Gourney, 1995). Although a number of models of case management exist, there is a wide consensus that they should include "assertive outreach." Assertive outreach involves the case manager in long-term persistent efforts to keep in contact with the client (Ford et al, 1995). The very clients whom case managers deliver services to are those with difficulties with compliance and those who persistently lose contact with the mental health services. This aspect of the work would seem to be an essential feature of case management. Moreover, assertive outreach attempts to ensure that those clients not compliant with treatment are actively engaged in services. Maurin (1990) contends that assertive outreach helps clients to achieve maximum levels of functioning in the least restrictive settings.

A whole array of aims of case management can be found in the literature. Primary aims include improving social functioning rather than achieving "cure" of mental disorder, reducing hospital admissions, improving clinical outcome, and maintaining contact with clients (Marshall et al, 1996). The basic principles of case management are that a case manager takes responsibility for a particular client or clients, arranges an assessment of need, develops a comprehensive service plan, organises delivery of suitable services, and monitors and reviews the effectiveness of the services delivered (Box 13-3).

Clifford and Craig (1988) also argue that the goals of case management should be to:

- Provide a focus for establishment of satisfactory working arrangements among health, local authority, and the voluntary and private sectors

---

BOX 13-3
Functions of a Case Manager

1. Identifying clients who need and desire case management services
2. Working with the client to develop a comprehensive service plan based on the client's needs and goals
3. Providing information to help the client make an informed choice about opportunities and services
4. Assisting the client to obtain needed services, supports, and entitlements
5. Being available and accessible during and after regular working hours
6. Advocating at the systems level for needed systems improvements

From Clifford P, Craig T: Case management systems for the long-term mentally ill: a proposed system inter-agency initiative, London, 1988, Sainbury Centre for Mental Health.

- Improve the coordination and continuity of care given to the individual client
- Facilitate rational planning and resource allocation by improving feedback to manager and care staff
- Increase the accessibility and accountability of services to clients and their relatives

It is important to reiterate that case management is primarily a vehicle by which health care and related interventions are delivered. Those might include medication management and compliance, assertive outreach, the use of negotiation skills, services for dual diagnosis, psychological interventions in the management of symptoms in schizophrenia, family work, and so on. Many sufferers of severe mental illness require support and assistance in successfully accessing adequate housing, employment, and general medication and dental services.

Appropriate models of day care and vocational services can prove invaluable in providing appropriate daytime structure and moving beyond the experience of illness and the identity as a "sick" person. Service models that offer opportunities for service users to make meaningful contributions to and allow opportunities for personal, vocational, and social development are increasingly seen as part of the necessary and comprehensive range of services to be offered to persons with major mental illness.

Two such services are "Clubhouse" and "Feathers." The "Clubhouse" offers the opportunity to be a fully participative member of a club offering a range of material, social, leisure, and vocational opportunities within a community supportive of people with major mental illness. This model, originating in the United States in 1952, now has in excess of 400 clubs worldwide and is the fastest growing model of social rehabilitation in the United Kingdom. "Feathers," developed in London in 1988, offers a range of "real life" work opportunities in an empowering and nonstigmatising way. These include salaried positions within the service, which demonstrate the potential value of each member of the "work force" within a model based on human and worker rights. A number of replicated services have been developed under the auspices of "The First Step Trust," a charitable body. Neither model offers "medical" or "therapy" services, but rather seeks to emphasize the person rather than the patient.

There is a wide variety of case management teams, practice, organisation, and makeup in the United Kingdom, as there is elsewhere. Some case management teams in the United Kingdom work from mental health services. Others are jointly managed by social services and mental health services, and some work from social services alone. In addition, case managers can work as independent agents or as part of a team of case managers (Armstrong, Ward, 1996).

A central consideration in the development of case management teams is the selection of clients who will receive case management. Given current resources, it is evident that not all seriously mentally ill clients will receive case management. Onyett (1992) argues that much British case management has concentrated on the "long-stay" patients as they leave hospital. However, as he correctly argues, "Diagnosis and clinical factors are often used to differentiate groups of users for the purposes of service provision. However, social factors are far superior in predicting the onset, course and out-come of mental distress and the ways people make use of services."

Much of the research literature regarding case management focuses on seriously mentally ill clients with long histories of schizophrenia and repeated admissions to hospital. It is rare that individuals with newly diagnosed serious mental illness are offered the benefits of a case management approach. However, it may be this very group who would significantly benefit from such an approach. Given the importance of social factors in determining the impact and course of a severe mental health disorder, it may be appropriate to target case management interventions to individuals who are judged likely to successfully engage in services that would improve their accessing and maintaining adequate housing, employment, educational, and leisure opportunities, as well as effective clinical alliances.

In the United Kingdom, case management teams are generally said to be multidisciplinary (Ford et al, 1993); however, the reality seems to be that for the most part they are made up of more nurses than members of other professions. Some authors suggest that support workers (unqualified mental health workers) can act as effective case managers as part of a case management team (Ford et al, 1995; Hatfield, 1996). Others suggest that the way forward is for users themselves to become part of the case management teams. Although this suggestion has only a very recent history in Britain, it has been well tested in the United States. Twenty mental health users were trained and employed to act as case managers (Sherman, Porter, 1991). At two-year follow-up 15 of the trainees remained employed as case managers and had required a total of only two bed days of psychiatric hospitalisation.

There is a general consensus in the literature that case loads of case managed clients should be small in order that clients' needs can be met. Gourney (1995) argues that case loads should be between 6 and 8, whereas others argue that between 10 and 25 is a more reasonable number (Craig, Pathare, 1996).

A whole number of organisational issues are evident in case management (Oynett, 1992), and many problems can arise. McNamee (1993) gives an eloquent account of many of the inherent difficulties in establishing an effective case management team.

Efficacy of Case Management

In the last decade there have been attempts to determine the efficacy of case management across a number of variables. However, much of the research conducted is typified by small patient numbers and methodological problems. Therefore research in this area is thought to be in its infancy.

There is mounting evidence that clinical case management models have demonstrated some efficacy, although, in contrast, little efficacy has been found with brokerage models of case management (Holloway et al, 1996; Burns, Santos, 1995). A recent review of the effectiveness of case management by Holloway et al (1995) examined outcome studies of case management and community treatment of psychiatric illness between 1987 and 1993 in Australia, the United States, Canada, and the United Kingdom. Of the 23 outcome studies, most are from the United States and only three are from the United Kingdom.

The authors break down the studies into the type of case management used. Most of the studies were based on the clinical case management (nine of which were based on ACT) and two studies were based on the brokerage model of case management.

With regard to outcome, the most frequently reported variable is hospital utilisation. Other variables are cost analysis, compliance with medication, symptomology, client satisfaction, social functioning, and the effect of case management on clients' social networks and relationships. The results vary from study to study; some show favourable results when compared with a control group, whilst others show no difference between case management and a control group. Cross-study comparisons in any research are difficult because of differences in client groups, methodology, case loads, case management models, assessment tools, and periods of follow-up. Because of such differences it is difficult to make conclusions.

The overall results of the review indicate that case management is generally successful in reducing the number and duration of hospital admissions. However, using hospitalisation as an outcome measure has its criticisms (Bachrach, 1982). Other variables, such as economic analysis, symptom reduction, quality-of-life measures, social and global functioning, family burden, and social network and relationships, are equivocal and vary

from study to study. The authors highlight the inherent difficulties in cross-study comparisons, but suggest that research into case management should now be directed at comparing elements of case management and different models of case management to identify the necessary effective and essential components. They also highlight an important point—that there is some evidence in the literature that gains from case management do not become apparent until after the first 18 months.

In mental health one of the largest studies to be conducted is that by the Sainsbury Centre for Mental Health (Ford et al, 1995). In four sites across the United Kingdom, leaders and their teams (across a range of professionals) were trained in case management. Their model of case management focused on assertive outreach and developing a long-term supportive relationship. In three of the sites an open trial was conducted, and in one site clients were randomised to either case management or standard psychiatric care over an 18-month period.

In the site where clients were randomised, 39 clients received case management. These clients were deemed to have a serious mental illness; 77% had a diagnosis of schizophrenia, 40% had some difficulty in complying with medication, none were employed, and 63% had had an admission to a psychiatric hospital in the previous two years. The experimental group and the control group did not differ significantly in terms of these variables. At 18 months only one client (3%) in the case management group had lost contact with the service, compared with nine clients (24%) of the control group. Furthermore, clients in the case-managed group had significantly more contact with psychiatric care than those in the control group. In the other three sites a similar picture was found, with low levels of lost contact. In contrast to some other outcome studies, costs in case-managed groups were significantly higher than in the control or matched groups.

A study by Marks et al (1994) randomised 92 clients with serious mental illness to the Daily Living Programme (DLP) and 97 clients to standard inpatient care followed by outpatient care. In brief, the DLP offered 24-hour care, treatment at the site of breakdown, case management, problem-oriented care, help to acquire and maintain daily living skills, support and education of people important in daily life, and advocacy.

This study found that over 20 months, those receiving DLP improved in symptoms and social adjustment slightly more than the control group, and the duration (but not the number) of crisis-based admissions was reduced by 80%. Consumer and relative satisfaction was significantly higher in the DLP group than the control group. A later paper (Knapp et al, 1994) found that the DLP was significantly less costly than the control treatment.

A further study (Audini et al, 1994) followed up patients who had received DLP care at 30, 34, and 45 months and found that many of the gains made during the first phase of the study had been lost in the second stage of the study. The authors suggest that the loss of gains may have been due to "attenuation of home-based care quality and to benefits of Phase I home-based care lingering into Phase II in DLP controls." They also state that the home-based care team were suffering low morale (because of policy and personnel changes).

A number of studies have investigated the level of client satisfaction with case management compared with standard services. In a randomised controlled study (Cullen et al, 1997), 70 clients with serious mental illnesses were allocated to either case management or a control group. Clients were assessed at baseline and at 9 and 18 months later. The four main elements of the case management teams' functioning included engagement and assessment, direct "clinical work," "social care," and brokerage or advocacy. Results showed that there was a significantly higher level of satisfaction in the case management group than the control group at 9 months but not at 18 months.

A recent study has looked at user evaluation of case management (Beeforth et al, 1994). This was a user-led project. The methodology included individual interviews and questionnaires with users of mental health services receiving case management. Mental health users were also the researchers. Although numbers were small, with 23 users interviewed, overall the respondents were positive about their experience of case management. The interviews showed that most users were satisfied with the accessibility of their case managers, and most of the users felt that they had a major input into discussions and decisions regarding their treatment; most had set goals with their case managers. Of importance is that users felt that they had some control about what happens to them and that they are involved in decision making. The three main areas of dissatisfaction amongst users were daytime activities, hospital admission, and medication.

A randomised controlled study (Muijen et al, 1994) compared community psychiatric nurses giving either intensive support (case management) or generic care to 82 clients with serious mental illness. Clients were assessed at baseline, and again at 6, 12, and 18 months. Despite case-managed clients having a much higher proportion of nurse contacts and more interventions, the study found no significant differences between groups in terms of psychopathology, social functioning, number or duration of hospital admissions, or patient and relative satisfaction.

The authors give some potential explanations for this negative result (e.g., lack of staff training). This study was also subject to a costing analysis (McCrone et al, 1994), which found that the service was more expensive in the short term for the control group; however, no significant differences were found at 12- and 18-month follow-up.

One of the striking issues about all these outcome studies is that whilst scientific rigour has been adhered to, with the studies having been well designed, there has been a general lack of training in case management and relevant interventions. A number of studies have argued that this may have been the reason for negative results (Muijen et al, 1994) or that there was a trend for benefits later as the teams developed (Ford, Ryan, 1997).

Future Developments

Most people with mental health problems live in the community, including those with serious mental illnesses. The Mental Health Nursing Review (Department of Health, 1994) recommends that the essential focus of mental health nurses should be on working with clients with serious mental illness. It is clear that mental health nurses need to respond to the challenges of the serious mentally ill and the wealth of interventions that have been developed. Despite the inconclusiveness of the research studies into case management so far, it does appear to have much to offer the seriously mentally ill. Case management can provide an alternative to hospital admission, continuity of care, coordination of services, and, importantly, the ability to keep clients in contact with mental health services.

Unfortunately, despite the increasing literature about case management, there is a paucity of research about the makings of a good care manager and the skills required. One recent paper (Sherlock-Storey, Milne, 1995) examines this issue and uses a variety of sources to identify some of the skills necessary for care managers in mental health settings.

Clifford and Craig (1988) report that existing professional training does not provide the necessary skills for case management. The multiskilled work necessary for nurses and other professionals to act as case managers requires a diversity of skills; for the most part these are sadly lacking in professional training. This situation has to be rectified without delay if we are going to provide comprehensive mental health services capable of responding to a wide spectrum of need. An exciting development in Britain is the Thorn Initiative. The initiative was named after the Sir Jules Thorn Charitable Trust, which initially funded the project. The course was developed in 1992 to provide training for the mental health nurse (but more recently has been extended to other mental health professionals). Essentially it focuses on high-quality case management for clients with serious mental illness (Gamble, 1991). Three core modules are taught: an introduction to schizophrenia and case management, behavioural family interventions, and psychological management of psychotic symptoms. The interventions taught are those with a proven track record of reducing relapse and readmissions to hospital. Final results of outcomes from this training have not yet emerged. However, preliminary outcome data (Lancashire et al, 1997) show that clients receiving care from nurses who had been trained showed improvement in positive and affective symptoms, although no change occurred in their negative symptoms.

However, skills-based training is not enough to bring about the successful implementation of case management. In addition, there have to be changes in attitude and service models. For example, managers and members of the multidisciplinary team must be willing to support colleagues who have undertaken research-based training and who want to implement these new approaches. Those involved in implementing case management must realise the importance of working across boundaries.

The boundaries may be structural, professional, or organisational. For example, it is generally accepted that it is not possible to do without hospital care altogether for people with severe mental illnesses; however, when people are rehospitalised, case managers often have no further contact with the clients until discharge. Such disjointed working between inpatient nurses and case managers is not only detrimental to the client but also inefficient, with duplication and repetition of assessments and care planning. Case managers must be able to work across all settings and with all agencies. Unfortunately, although this is accepted in principle, in reality we still have a long way to go to ensure proper integration and collaboration.

The role of the case manager is developing fairly rapidly in mental health services. Mental health nurses are well placed to take on this new and challenging role. Nurses must seize this opportunity, since the role of the case manager lies at the heart of providing a comprehensive and effective mental health service. Training based on interventions that have been shown to be effective has already commenced, albeit in a small way. In addition, we now need more integrated research that assesses the outcomes produced by these nursing interventions and their delivery through case management. In this way we will be able to more clearly articulate the best way of caring for people with a serious mental illness.

References

Armstrong C, Ward M: Case management: an audit of the training, skills and caseloads of community mental health support workers involved in case management. The National Institute for Nursing Interim report (report no. 12), National Institute for Nursing, Centre of Practice Development and Research, Radcliffe Infirmary, Woodstock Road, Oxford, England, 1996.

Audini B, Marks IM, Lawrence RE, Connolly J, Watts V: Home-based versus outpatient/inpatient care for people with serious mental illness: phase II of a controlled study, *British Journal of Psychiatry* 164:204-210, 1994.

Bachrach L: Assessments of outcomes in community support systems: results, problems and limitations, *Schizophrenia Bulletin*, 8(1):833-834, 1992.

Beeforth M, Conlan E, Graley R: *Have we got views for you: user evaluation of case management*, London, 1994, Sainsbury Centre for Mental Health.

Burns BJ, Santos AB: Assertive community treatment: an update of randomised trials, *Psychiatric Services* 46:669-675, 1995.

Burns T: Case management, care management and care programming, *British Journal of Psychiatry* 170:393-395, 1997.

Clifford P, Craig T: *Case management systems for the long-term mentally ill: a proposed system inter-agency initiative,* London, 1988, Sainsbury Centre for Mental Health.

Craig TKJ, Pathare S: Continuing care: theory and practice, *British Journal of Hospital Medicine* 56:(9),461-464, 1996.

Cullen D, Waite A, Oliver N, Carson J, Holloway F: Case management for the mentally ill: a comparative evaluation of client satisfaction, *Health and Social Care in the Community* 5(2):106-115, 1997.

Davies B, Challis D: *Matching resources to needs in community care,* Aldershot, England, 1986, Gower.

Department of Health and Social Security: *Better services for the mentally ill,* London, 1975, HMSO.

Department of Health: *Caring for people,* London, 1989a, HMSO.

Department of Health: *Working for patients,* London, 1989b, HMSO.

Department of Health: *Care programme for people with a mental illness referred to the specialist psychiatric services,* HC(90)23/LASSI (90)11, London, 1990, HMSO.

Department of Health: *Working in partnership: a collaborative approach to care*—report of the Mental Health Nursing Review Team, London, 1994, HMSO.

Department of Health: *Building bridges: a guide for inter-agency working for the care and protection of severely mentally ill people,* London, 1995, HMSO.

Department of Health: *Developing partnerships in mental health,* London, 1997, HMSO.

Ford R, Beadsmoore A, Ryan P, Repper J, Craig T, Muijen M: Providing the safety net: case management for people with serious mental illness, *Journal of Mental Health* 1:91-97, 1995.

Ford R, Repper J, Cooke A, Norton P, Beadsmore A, Clark C: *Implementing case management* London, 1993, Research and Development for Psychiatry.

Ford R, Ryan P: Labour intensive: how effective is intensive community support for people with long-standing mental illness? *Health Service Journal,* pp 26-29, 1997.

Gamble C. The Thorn nurse initiative, *Nursing Standard* 9(15):31-33, 1995.

Goering PN, Wasylenki DA, Farkas M, Lancee WJ, & Ballantyne R: What difference does case management make? *Hospital and Community Psychiatry* 39(3):272-276, 1988.

Gournay K: Changing patterns in mental health care: implications for evaluation and training, *Psychiatric Care* 2(3):93-95, 1995.

Griffiths R: *Community care: agenda for action.* London, 1988, HMSO.

Hatfield B: Case management in mental health services: the role of community mental health support teams, *Health and Social Care in the Community* 4(4):215-225, 1996.

Holloway F: Case management for the mentally ill: looking at the evidence, *International Journal of Social Psychiatry* 27(1):2-13, 1991.

Holloway F, Oliver N, Collins E, Carson J: Case management: a critical review of the outcome literature, *European Psychiatry* 10:113-128, 1995.

Holloway F, Murry M, Squire C, Carson J: Intensive case management: putting it into practice, *Psychiatric Bulletin* 20:395-397, 1996.

Intagliata J: Improving the quality of life for the chronically mentally disabled: the role of case management, *Schizophrenia Bulletin* 8(4):655-674, 1982.

Johnson S, Ramsay R, Thornicroft G, et al: *London's mental health,* London, 1997, Kings Fund.

Kanter J: Clinical case management: definition, principles, components, *Hospital and Community Psychiatry* 40(4):361-368, 1989.

Knapp M, Beecham J, Koutsogeorgopoulou A, Hallam, Fenyo A, Marks IM, Connolly J, Audini B, Muijen M: Service use and costs of home-based versus hospital based care for people with serious mental illness, *British Journal of Psychiatry* 165:195-203, 1994.

Lancashire S, Haddock G, Tarrier N, Baguley I, Butterworth A, Brooker C: Effects of training in psychosocial interventions for community psychiatric nurses in England, *Psychiatric Services* 48(1):39-41, 1997.

Marks IM, Connolly J, Muijen M, Audini B, McNamee G, Lawrence RE: Home-based versus hospital-based care for people with serious mental illness, *The British Journal of Psychiatry* 165(2):179-194, 1994.

Marshall M, Lockwood A, Gath D: Social services case-management for long-term mental disorders: a randomised controlled trial, *The Lancet* 345:409-412, 1995.

Marshall M, Gray A, Lockwood A, Green R: Case management for people with severe mental disorders, *The Cochrane Library* 3:1-25, 1996.

Maurin J: Case management: caring for psychiatric clients, *Journal of Psychosocial Nursing* 28:8-12, 1990.

McCrone P, Beecham J, Knapp M: Community psychiatric nurse teams: cost-effectiveness of intensive support versus generic care, *British Journal of Psychiatry* 165:218-221, 1994.

McNamee G: A changing profession: the role of nursing in home care. In Weller MPI, Muijen M, eds: *Dimensions of community mental health care,* London, 1993, Saunders.

Modrcin M, Rapp CA, Poertner J: The evaluation of case management services for the chronically mentally ill, *Evaluation and Programme Planning* 11(4):307-314, 1988.

Muijen M, Cooney M, Strathdee G, Bell R, Hudson A: Community psychiatric nurse teams: intensive support versus generic care, *British Journal of Psychiatry*, 165, 211-217, 1992.

Oynett S: *Case management in mental health,* London, 1992, Chapman Hall.

Pierides M, Roy D, Craig T: The care programme approach: preliminary results one year after implementation in an inner city, *Psychiatric Bulletin* 18:249-257, 1994.

Ryan P, Ford R, Clifford P: *Case management and community care,* London, 1991, Research and Development for Psychiatry.

Shepherd G: Case management, *Health Trends* 22:59-61, 1990.

Sherlock-Storey M, Milne D: What makes a good care manager? An analysis of care management skills in the mental health services, *Health and Social Care in the Community* 3:53-64, 1995.

Sherman PS, Porter R: Mental health consumers as case management aides, *Hospital and Community Psychiatry* 42(5):494-498, 1991.

Solomon P: The efficacy of case management, *Community Mental Health Journal* 28(3):163-179, 1992.

Stein LI, Test MA: Alternative to mental hospital treatment, *Archives of General Psychiatry* 37:392-397, 1980.

CHAPTER 14

The Broker Model of Case Management

ROBERTA M. CONTI, RN, PhD

OVERVIEW

The broker model affords case managers the greatest leverage of responsibility for identifying the client's needs, matching appropriate health and community resources in a timely, cost-effective fashion, and monitoring the results of the match between the client's needs and the provided services.

This chapter describes models of case management, with specific discussion of the broker model. Content on specific operational aspects of case manager practice within this model is presented, along with three exemplar case studies illustrating these practice attributes. The chapter concludes with a literature-based discussion of case manager roles in general and those found in the broker model in particular. ▲

The high cost of health care is a major problem for all. Although cost escalation has many causes, research shows that patients receive much care that is inappropriate for their conditions, not beneficial, sometimes harmful, and more intense and expensive than necessary. Consequently many stakeholders, but especially the payers of health care, are demanding more accountability and better performance from those who are making health care decisions, in order to ensure that patients receive valued care for the money spent. Case management is the recognized primary mechanism for achieving efficient, cost-effective, and quality care through its strategic approach to health care delivery.

Case management's core concepts are that it is a *process,* that there is *integration* and *coordination of services* within a *service network,* and that its purpose is to meet client needs effectively and efficiently. Case management is defined as a purposeful interaction coordinated among multiple providers and vendors with the intention of meeting the client's needs effectively and efficiently, and with cost effectiveness (Weil, Karls, 1985).

Models of Case Management

A plethora of case management models are described in the social services, health care, and nursing literatures (Brault, Kissinger, 1991; Desimone, 1988; Papenhausen, 1990; Weil, Karls, 1985). These models exist because case management is recognized as a system, not simply a service, with roots in general systems theory.

Conceptual models or frameworks provide a way to depict the key concepts and the relationships among them for a particular phenomenon. Thus, a conceptual model or framework of case management would propose ways to define and describe the phenomenon called case management by focusing on the models associated with it. The following presents my conceptualization of one such framework. This classification organizes case management models as grand, middle-range, and practice-based models, terms consistent with the stratification of nursing theory. In this proposed framework, *grand* models of case management would include general systems–based ones, such as discussed by Zander (1988a, b, c) and Ballew and Mink (1986), consisting of core behaviors of coordinating and integrating, and targeting these behaviors to services, resources, communications, and expectations. Patients, families, treatment team members, and payers are the recipients of these coordinating and integrating actions. While they are conceptually interesting, I do not believe that *grand* models of case management lend themselves easily to application and/or testing. *Middle-range* models are divided into purchaser-based and provider-based. Purchaser-based models can be further divided into public and private purchasers, with the former including health departments, public hospitals, home health care agencies, and the Medicare and Medicaid programs, and the latter consisting of HMOs, PPOs, insurance companies, self-insured employers, and private individual purchasers. Flarey and Blancett (1996) discuss purchaser-based middle-range models as examples of private, social/community-based, and vendor/gatekeeper case management models. Provider-based models in this group include acute care case management and primary care case management. Of these two, models of primary care case management are continuing to evolve, with many extending the delivery of services into the community and maintaining case management arrangements with some clients for months and years. *Practice-based* models, the last level in this framework, include ones tailored to specific client populations. Examples include the model of case management services delivered by the New Jersey Department of Health's Perinatal AIDS Prevention Project, head injury rehabilitation programs, and geriatric case management systems (Bower, 1992). Within the conceptualization of case management models, the *broker model* represents a purchaser-based middle-range model that can be implemented by either public or private purchasers.

The Broker Model of Case Management

One rationale for case management is based on the notion that often clients in need of health care are individuals who have multiple and complex needs as a result of a catastrophic incident, a long-term-care illness, a complex disability, and so on. The emphasis is on managing the complexity of the medical and social care necessary with such vulnerable populations in order to prevent additional problems and to establish equilibrium and cost effectiveness (Brault, Kissinger, 1991; Netting, 1992).

Often, because of inadequate knowledge and information, clients have significant limitations in maneuvering in the health care services arena, reducing their capacities to locate appropriate assistance on their own, bring combinations of service together that are compatible and coherent, and negotiate with multiple providers for service provision. Through enactment of the brokering function, case managers in the broker model provide clients with unbiased, comparative information that otherwise is not easily available to them.

Moxley (1989) defines brokering as an indirect service strategy requiring knowledge that includes:

1. Available, adequate, appropriate, acceptable, and accessible services
2. Provision of services according to need-, diagnostic-, or means-based eligibility criteria
3. Quality of past services, client feedback, and accreditation status
4. Service provider competence
5. Agency reputation
6. Service domain of the agency

Within a context of a broker model of case management, case managers assist clients, families, providers, and payers through these tasks by assessing the client's needs, identifying efficient and effective resources, advocating for the client, the payer, and the case management program, and monitoring the delivery of services.

CASE MANAGER PRACTICE WITHIN THE BROKER MODEL

Case manager practice within the broker model is dynamic from the time a case is opened until it is closed. In my experience with the broker model, upon receiving a case, the case manager calls the client and/or family to gain receptivity to the offer for case management. Once the client and/or family have agreed to see the case manager, an appointment is made to meet the client either in the hospital, another health care facility, or his or her home. The purpose of this initial visit is to achieve a holistic assessment of the client, his or her health status, and the medical management necessary for the present, and to consider needs for the future—in most cases to support quality of life and/or gainful employment.

During the assessment process, the case manager elicits historical information on the client's health status and the precipitating data to warrant case management, and gain insight into the psychological, educational, family, and cultural dimensions of the client and other issues significant to the client. Based on the assessment, a hierarchy of needs or problems is identified, with concurrent, measurable goals aimed at problem resolution. The case manager then discusses with the client and family the potential aspects of an initial program plan and assists with the development of a vision for the future in order to get the client to a point of having positive quality of life or back in employment realistic to the client's disability. This process requires the case manager to be both clinically and managerially knowledgeable about public and private community resources, including providers and vendors of services and material resources.

Once the problem list is established, the case manager ascertains what specific services, resources, and/or providers are needed to initiate resolution of the problem. As the case manager reviews and periodically reevaluates the problem list, there might be multiple elements that could be undertaken by a provider (e.g., providing both a hospital bed and a commode chair), or specialty services (speech, occupational, or physical therapy) may be needed.

At all times, it is important, to whatever degree possible, for the client to be mentally and physically in balance and participating in the development of the case management plan. The case manager has a responsibility to the client and family to provide information about options that are available under particular insurance coverage and, at the same time, to keep the payer involved and knowledgeable about the differences and potential options. The client's primary care provider is always included in the planning process, but often the client's needs are beyond the scope of that provider's practice and experience. The case manager creates the linkages with necessary service providers and vendors and specifically determines with them the goals to be achieved within specific periods of time, and then continuously monitors the situation to see that whatever expected outcomes were established are achieved. This requires the case manager to follow up with client and family, as well as with provider and vendors. If a discrepancy occurs, the case manager can ensure that services remain coordinated and are efficient and effective for the client and the payer. The continuum of practice requires dissemination of information and collaboration among the client, providers, and the payer to maintain as aggressive a coordinated plan as is possible. The client situation requires constant reevaluation over time. Most often, the medical status determines the frequency of oversight and reevaluation; that is, a person whose physiological status is in imbalance may require more frequent case manager interaction in order to determine what is happening with medical treatment, what is not happening, and what is needed.

Because many of these clients end up in their own home environments, the case manager must work cooperatively with family members, service providers, and vendors to make sure that the services provided are efficiently and effectively coordinated. Often groups of providers in a case have not worked together in the past. Thus, the case manager must identify and clarify among them who has the lead role in service provision and what monitoring of each provider's action will be necessary. A good example is a client discharged to home who needs hyperalimentation, abdominal wound dressings, and relatively frequent physiological assessment. The broker model case manager must be precise in laying out and activating a plan for implementation and evaluation of needed services. To achieve this, the case manager communicates with the providers, as well as with the management component of the organizations for whom they work. Similarly, the case manager must know and ensure provision of adequate expendable supplies to support the hyperalimentation therapy, wound care, and so on. Someone must be given responsibility and held accountable so that the client is not jeopardized. At the same time, the appropriate provider must be held accountable to do routine physiological assessments.

One major characteristic of practice under the broker model is that the case manager researches the options appropriate to assist in resolution of one or more of the client's problems or needs. The identity of options includes the names, addresses, and phone numbers of providers and the costs of their services for this specific case. This information is shared with the payer before options are presented to the client and family, to ensure that the

payer is willing to pay for these options and/or to go outside the plan if appropriate. Critical to the case manager role is that the case manager delineate very specifically the differences among the options in terms of descriptions of services and costs. The case manager also is responsible for identifying and obtaining cost discounts. Clinical and cost information provided to payers can allow for an option to be chosen that over time will prove to be more cost effective than others of initially lower costs.

Once the case manager presents to both the payer and the client and family what options may be considered for required services, both the payer and the client retain elements of choice. The client has choice in selecting across comparable services, based on location, while knowing significant elements of differences among them.

The case manager in the broker model can serve a wide range of client populations. As a generalist, the case manager often will obtain assistance from clinical specialty subject matter experts. Success here requires establishment of a broad network of colleagues, service providers, and vendors based on establishing and nurturing positive relationships over time.

Broker-model case managers interact primarily with industry payers who contact them to arrange for provision of services. These contractual arrangements require timely reporting of exactly what is happening with each case in terms of problems, needs, and outcomes. Written reports include discussions of the plan of management agreed to by the payer and client, usually for 30-day periods of time.

The broker model affords case managers the greatest leverage of responsibility for identifying the client's needs, matching appropriate health and community resources in a timely, cost-effective fashion, and monitoring the results of the match between the client's needs and the provided services. Research indicates that nurses practicing in the broker model demonstrate a wide range of role behaviors (Conti, 1996).

EXEMPLAR CASE STUDIES

The following are summaries of actual case studies with related discussion. They illustrate enactment of the broker model of case management and the specific case outcomes associated with the model.

In addition, these cases provide a glimpse into the complexity, diversity, and clinical and managerial knowledge necessary to enact the practice of case management under the broker model.

Case Study 1: Mrs. S. Mrs. S was a 34-year-old, divorced, white woman, with two teenage children, who was diagnosed with chronic fatigue syndrome. She had not worked in her job as a nurse in the ambulatory operating room of the local hospital since the symptoms of her diagnosis worsened to the extent that she could not cognitively handle multiple stimuli. Mrs. S felt that she had never recovered her stamina after an episode of severe chickenpox 5 years earlier. Her current symptoms included significant arthralgias, severe fatigue, pharyngitis, irritable bowel syndrome, subnormal temperatures, lymphadenopathy, and severe headaches. In addition, she suffered from sleep disturbance, neurocognitive symptoms (e.g., photophobia, forgetfulness, short-term memory loss), and emotional lability. Also, the laboratory findings and her history, which strongly supported the diagnosis, fit the Centers for Disease Control, Chronic Fatigue Disease Syndrome case definition criteria.

Mrs. S stated that she had been under the care of several local physicians, who she felt heard her complaints but did not take them seriously. She discovered a physician expert in her diagnosis in another state and decided to seek him out for evaluation and treatment. Her employer, however, questioned the necessity for this action, and, together with the payer, decided to use case management (i.e., broker model) to work with this client. From the perspective of the employer and the payer, this was an unbelievable diagnosis, virtually unknown outside of medical center communities.

The payer requested case management to determine the medical rationale for coverage and to develop an appropriate and comprehensive plan of treatment and care. Mrs. S agreed with this request and authorized release of her medical records to the case manager. The case manager visited Mrs. S in her home and conducted an initial, comprehensive assessment of her medical and psychosocial status.

Next, the payer asked the case manager to obtain, in any way possible, comprehensive, definitive information regarding this unusual diagnosis. The case manager researched the diagnosis by contacting the then-current treating physician and

other physicians and nurse experts located at premier medical centers across the country, and did a thorough medical literature review. The findings from this process were summarized and provided as a written report to the payer and the employer. The case manager also used the information to write a letter to the treating physician requesting the following:

1. Information on all potential diseases or illnesses that had been ruled out, including all supporting data
2. Information about the current diagnosis, including all supporting data
3. Current treatment plan
4. Academic and research data supporting the treatment plan
5. Anticipated time frame for Mrs. S's recovery and return to work

In addition, the case manager negotiated a fee with the physician for the collection and provision of this information.

The case manager systematically reviewed all of the data and findings regarding this client and provided the employer and the payer with the following initial recommendations:

1. Have Dr. K at the out-of-state CFIDS specialty clinic manage Mrs. S's medical treatment plan for 6 months. This would be the most comprehensive and cost-effective approach to this client's treatment. Medical management would consist of visits to the clinic every 3 to 4 months and monthly phone consultations. This arrangement also ensured that the client maintained access to a new immune modulator drug.
2. Have Dr. K prepare the explanatory letter and provide it to the payer. The letter would serve as documentation of the review and analysis of the case and provide the payer with substantive reasons for action, in the event of approval of continuing care as recommended.
3. Provide monetary support for housekeeping services twice weekly for 3 months. Housekeeping services would help the client to conserve limited energy for performance of more necessary daily activities.

The broker model case manager interventions related to the following needs:

- Resolving the dilemma as to who would be the treating physician

- Obtaining sufficient authoritative medical research to validate the uncertainty and complexity of this diagnosis
- Validating medical information, the determining client's crisis level of fatigue, and determining options for assistance

Using the broker model, the following two options were devised:

	OPTION A	OPTION B
Medical coverage	Monthly visits to multiple physicians (e.g., internists, neurologists); $100/visit; 3 to 4 visits/month; 3 months = $1200	Visit to CFIDS specialist every 3 months; $300/visit; $150/hr monthly phone consultation; 3 months = $750
Specialty physician letter	Not applicable	$120
Housekeeping services	Company A: 2 times/month; $100/month	Company B: 2 times/month; $70/month
TOTAL COSTS	$1300	$890

After discussion with the family, client, employer, and payer, option B was selected, with a cost savings of $410.

On the basis of the employer and payer's request for services, the case manager achieved the following outcomes:

1. A comprehensive medical treatment plan for 6 months with the CFIDS medical specialist that would be consistently monitored by the case manager
2. Documentation and coordination of dissemination of CFIDS diagnosis relative to national medical research, expert opinions, and the client's medical record
3. Acceptance by the employer and payer for the client to have 3 months of housekeeping services and then review this for necessity of renewal based on the client's well-being
4. Elimination of the perceived animosity between the client and the employer and payer by identifying the available medical knowledge and facts, in addition to precipitating development of a comprehensive medical plan

for several months that provided role and outcome expectations for client, medical specialty physician, and employer and payer.

Case Study 2: Mr. S. Mr. S is a 22-year-old, single male who sustained massive traumatic brain injury in a motorcycle accident. This brain injury occurred because he was riding without a helmet when his motorcycle struck a telephone pole. The injuries sustained in this accident included a depressed right frontal skull fracture; left epidural hematoma, requiring emergency craniotomy; left temporal lobe contusion with ligation of the left common carotid artery; left basilar skull fracture; right tripod facial fracture; right superior pubic fracture; right orbital fracture; left trochanteric fracture; left clavicular fracture; and pulmonary contusions. Mr. S remained in a coma for a number of weeks. After numerous weeks of acute hospital care and rehabilitation, Mr. S was referred to a case manager.

At the time of referral, Mr. S was cortically blind bilaterally and deaf in his right ear. He also had expressive aphasia and ambulated with difficulty because of weakness to his right lower leg and ankle. He also demonstrated impaired ability to locate items in his environment. His reduced mental endurance resulted in an inability to participate in daily, scheduled activities without experiencing extreme fatigue and needing rest periods.

Mr. S also had impaired auditory short-term memory, suggesting significant difficulties in attending to and concentrating on verbally provided information. He had severe problems focusing on instructions and was easily distracted by external environmental stimuli, as well as by his own internal thoughts.

His aphasic disturbance undermined his ability to process auditory-verbal information with a realistic degree of accuracy. At times, he was able to comprehend only rudimentary verbal instructions and became confused when presented with verbal information of moderate abstraction and complexity. He was unable to comprehend and follow multiple-step verbal instructions and was very slow to respond to environmental information.

Mr. S demonstrated impaired ability for abstract reasoning, deficiencies in verbal judgment, and inappropriate thematic content. Behaviorally, he frequently displayed inappropriate social behavior, including raising his voice, being sexually inappropriate, being aggressive, and using profanity.

The following are the related broker-model case manager interventions:

- Independence in self-care (e.g., bathing, dressing, personal hygiene, feeding)
- Ability to function in a risk-familiar environment safely and with some assistance in a new environment
- Assist father and his new bride in potential options for client's care at home
- Establish expectations and direction for vocational rehabilitation

Using the broker model, the following two options were devised:

	OPTION A	OPTION B
Independence in ADL	Comprehensive home health care (e.g., PT, OT, speech)	Admit to a neurological rehabilitation program (e.g., PT, OT, speech, cognitive therapy, family counseling, risk environment vocational rehabilitation)
Costs	Three professionals 3 times/week at $110/visit = $990	$503.50/day for 5 days/week = $2517.50
Function in risk environment	Not provided	Included in program
Family counseling	Not provided	Included in program
Plan and direction for vocational rehabilitation	Not provided	Included in program
TOTAL COSTS	$14,880 for 4 months	$40,280 for 4 months

The significantly lower costs in option A were the result of nonprovision of services related to three of four identified client needs, thereby making this option unacceptable. After discussion of the options with family, client, and payer, option B was

selected as the best value both economically and in terms of the client's long-term health and quality of life, as well as being a productive member of society.

Based on these findings, the case manager's plan of care achieved the following outcomes:

1. Self-care: Independent with basic self-care; able to perform advanced levels of tasks with supervision
2. Self-protection: Able to function with minimal assistance in a familiar environment with supervision; able to recognize and problem solve environmental hazards; able to function in new environments with direct supervision
3. Domestic outcome: Members of the family will redistribute their roles and responsibilities and will be able to identify and use outside assistance to manage their affairs
4. Work/educational outcome: Able to participate in a structured, productive, hands-on activity for up to 2 hours with supervision

Case Study 3: Ms. R. This client was a 21-year-old, single female with a C7 complete spinal cord injury from an all-terrain-vehicle accident. She was a high school graduate and had been working as a waitress at the time of the accident. Initially, she had surgery for decompression and corpectomy of C7 and anterior stabilization with left iliac crest bone graft. Her acute care stay was compromised by the development of right lower lobe pneumonia with right lung atelectasis requiring bronchoscopy and tracheostomy. After 47 days of acute care, at a cost of $104,467, the client was transferred to a specialty acute rehabilitation facility 100 miles away from her parents' home, where she had lived at the time of the accident.

On receiving this case, the case manager's assessment of the client's medical status revealed the following:

1. Quadriplegia, C7 level
2. Neurogenic bowel and bladder
3. Total dependence for all activities of daily living
4. Intermittent orthostatic hypotension (sitting)
5. Healing tracheostomy stoma
6. Depression
7. Tolerance to sit/wear shoes for 1 hour
8. Tolerance to propel her wheelchair 100 feet across a level surface

Broker-model case manager interventions related to the following need:

- The client needed acute rehabilitation as an inpatient. The options included a choice between two institutions that were 75 miles apart and of like rehabilitation programs. Using the broker model, the following two options were devised:

	OPTION A	OPTION B
Inpatient rehabilitation	Average daily cost = $750; cost for 8 weeks = $42,000	Average daily cost = $1200; cost for 8 weeks = $67,200
TOTAL COST	$42,000	$67,200

After discussion of the options with family, client, and payer, the facility in option A was selected, with a cost savings to the payer of $25,200.

The case manager then researched other options for care after the acute rehabilitation phase. Taking into account the client's educational status and the need for maximum independence, choices focused on organizations providing both physical and vocational rehabilitation services. Fortunately, the state of residence had a state facility that offered both programs and was the location of choice in terms of quality and cost.

The case manager's responsibilities included monitoring the client's progress over time while the client was at the option A facility and working through necessary details with client, providers, family, and payers to move the client into the comprehensive rehabilitation program as soon as possible.

The outcomes achieved included the following:

1. Increased knowledge of spinal cord injury and potential complications
2. Ability to verbally direct any remaining dependent care
3. Adjustment to disability
4. Independence in bathing with appropriate equipment
5. Minimal assistance in transferring despite 6-inch height difference and 4-inch gaps
6. Minimal assistance for lower extremity dressing
7. Independence in upper extremity dressing
8. Independent wheelchair propulsion across level surface and some rough terrain
9. Independence in wheelchair setup
10. Independence in routine transfers
11. Independence in bowel and bladder program
12. Independence in feeding self
13. Independence in personal hygiene
14. Completion of driver evaluation and training

Case Manager Roles

Role theory is concerned with an important feature of social life, that of characteristic behavior patterns or roles. Roles are explained by the presumption that persons are members of social positions and hold expectations for their own behaviors and those of other persons (Biddle, 1986). A role is both the expected and the actual behaviors that are associated with a position (Biddle, 1979; Hardy, Conway, 1978). Role behaviors can be defined as anticipated behaviors to be performed by individuals who are engaged in certain roles within society. These anticipated behaviors can be influenced by learning and socialization and are known as role expectations (Biddle, 1985; Hardy, Conway, 1978).

Establishing role clarity for case managers is critical for the effectiveness of any program of case management. In every case management system, there needs to be a clear understanding across the organization as to the role set required to achieve desired client and program outcomes. That same understanding must be conveyed to all agencies participating in the case management program. The effectiveness and efficiency of case manager practice are dependent upon attainment of role clarity.

The selected set of roles taken on by a case manager determines the emphasis on service integration and coordination. The health care and social services literatures attribute a variety of roles to case managers, including problem solver, advocate, broker, planner, community organizer, boundary spanner, service monitor, record keeper, evaluator, consultant, collaborator, coordinator, counselor, and expediter (Brault, Kissinger, 1991; Burdett, 1960; Kemp, 1981; Redford, 1992; Weil, Karls, 1985). Many of these roles are enacted in the context of interaction with the clients, the service network, and the case management system (Weil, Karls, 1985).

The nursing literature generally does not stipulate roles or practice behaviors as being unique to case managers. Instead, it reports on convergence of them into other roles, or posits that existing advanced practice roles adequately incorporate and implement the majority of identified case manager roles. Discussions of convergence include that of the nurse case manager and clinical nurse specialists/advanced practice nurses (Glettler, Leen, 1996; Norris, Hill, 1991; Nugent, 1992; Schroer, 1991; Wells, Erickson, Spinella, 1996), case manager/nurse practitioner (Schroer, 1991), case manager/rehabilitation nurse (Mound et al, 1991), and case manager/trauma/critical care (Simmons, 1992; Tidwell, 1995). This literature indicates that the practice of nursing case management is discipline-specific and that nurse case manager role behaviors do not differ significantly from already existing nursing roles. Nugent (1992) described the case manager roles of the clinical nurse specialist as coordinator, monitor, evaluator, and director of the care of a patient through the patient's illness. Schroer (1991) discussed the three converging roles of the case manager/clinical nurse specialist/nurse practitioner. The foundation of the convergence is the case manager role with espoused behaviors of overseeing patient care, providing monitoring and assessment of the patient's health care status, and providing the communication medium for coordination of care among disciplines. Mound et al (1991) described the expanded role activities of the rehabilitative nurse/case manager as including family counseling, public education, advocacy, community involvement, and research. Simmons (1992) described the trauma nurse/case manager roles to be expert clinician, manager, consultant, educator, and researcher. I believe that authors demonstrate a lack of consensus regarding nurse case manager role behaviors. Of the identified behaviors, none were examined within the framework of a specific practice model or conceptual framework.

A review of the social services, health care, and nursing literature on case management revealed few articles discussing case manager roles. Articles began to appear in the early 1980s, specifically in the social services literature (Austin, 1983; Kemp, 1981; Billig, Levinson, 1987; Rapp, Chamberlain, 1985; Wagner, 1987). Collectively, they describe the roles as practiced in social services, mental health, geriatrics, and rehabilitation.

A search of the nursing, health care, and social services periodical literature from 1985 through 1997 identified three studies reporting on case manager roles (Middleton, 1985; Rothman, 1991; Zimmerman, 1987). First, Rothman (1991) identified 14 functions of case management derived from a field survey of 48 case managers and an applied field study. The functions, or role behaviors, identified were as follows: accessing an agency, intake, assessment, goal setting, intervention planning, resource identification, linking clients, monitoring, reassessment, outcome evaluation, interagency coordination, counseling, therapy, and advocacy. In the second study, Zimmerman (1987) gathered data from case records, agency personnel, and the clients themselves in a program to provide integrated case management services for multiproblem children. The roles most frequently identified by case managers in face-to-face contact with clients were discussion of client concerns, explanation of agency services, and counseling. In the third study, Middleton (1985) determined that the majority of case managers were involved in the tasks of service plan development, making agency contacts, recording and reporting, and evaluation of community services. These findings attest to the diversity across disciplines in case manager roles.

Broker Model of Case Manager Roles

Recent research on the broker model of case management is contributing to further clarifying attendant roles and competencies (Conti, 1996; Yeager, 1997). Studies are emerging that identify and describe the role behaviors of nurses practicing in the broker model of case management. Conti (1993; 1996) examined the role behaviors of nurse case managers practicing under the broker model while they were employed by a large health care insurance company. Qualitative field work and survey methods were used to identify the role behaviors, attendant roles, and sources of learning of these nurse case managers. The study identified the sixteen distinct roles of public relator, educator, expeditor, monitor, problem solver, explainer, negotiator, planner, communicator, contactor, recommender, broker, researcher, assessor, documentor, and coordinator. Additional research is necessary to determine the interdisciplinary applicability of these findings.

Conclusion

Broker-model case managers need to be critical thinkers, able to make decisions and recommendations that acknowledge and balance the needs and requirements of client, family, treatment team, and payer. They need to know all about a broad base of community resources, and to be able to differentiate among providers and vendors of the same services, sort out the unrevealed aspects, and make clinically credible conclusions, decisions, and recommendations. Finally, they need to be astute in bargaining to obtain the most cost-effective services on behalf of the client and the payer.

References

Austin C: Case management in long term care: options and opportunities, *Health and Social Work,* pp 16-30, 1983.

Biddle BJ: Recent developments in role theory, *Annual Review of Sociology* p 12, 1986.

Biddle BJ: *Role theory: expectations, identities, and behaviors.* New York, 1979, Academic Press.

Biddle BJ: *Role theory: expectations, identities, and behaviors,* New York, 1985, Academic Press.

Billig N, Levinson C: Homelessness and case management in Montgomery County, Maryland: a focus on chronic mental illness, *Psychosocial Rehabilitation Journal* 11:1, 1987.

Bower KA: *Case management by nurses,* Washington, DC 1992, American Nurses' Association.

Brault GI, Kissinger LD: Case management: ambitious at best, *Journal of Pediatric Health* 5:4, 1991.

Burdett AD: Pinpointing the counselor's role in rehabilitation, *Journal of Rehabilitation* 26:9-12, 1960.

Conti RM: *Role behaviors of nurse case managers* (doctoral dissertation, George Mason University, 1993), *UMI Dissertation Service* 9316549.

Conti RM: Nurse case manager roles: implications for practice and education, *Nursing Administration Quarterly* 21:67-80, 1996.

Desimone BS: The case for case management, *Continuing Care,* July 1988.

Flarey DL, Blancett SS: *Handbook of nursing case management,* Gaithersburg, Md, 1996, Aspen.

Glettler E, Leen MG: The advanced practice nurse as case manager, *Journal of Case Management* 5(3):121-126, 1996.

Hardy M, Conway M: *Role theory: perspectives for health professionals,* Norwalk, Conn, 1978, Appleton-Century-Crofts.

Kemp R: The case management model of human service delivery, *Annual Review of Rehabilitation* p 2, 1981.

Middleton J: Case management in mental retardation service delivery systems: a view from the field (doctoral dissertation, University of Pennsylvania, 1985).

Mound B, Gyulaz R, Kahn P, Goering P: The expanded role of nurse case managers, *Journal of Psychosocial Nursing* 29:6, 1991.

Moxley DP: *The practice of case management,* Human Services Guide 58, Thousand Oaks, Calif, 1989, Sage.

Netting FE: Case management: service or symptom? *Social Work* 37:2, 1992.

Norris M, Hill C: The clinical specialist: developing the case manager role, *Dimensions in Critical Care* 10:6, 1991.

Nugent K: The clinical nurse specialist as case manager in a collaborative practice model: bridging the gap between quality and cost of care, *Clinical Nurse Specialist* 6:2, 1992.

Papenhausen J: Case management: a model of advanced practice? *Clinical Nurse Specialist* 4:4, 1990.

Rapp CA, Chamberlain R: Case management services for the chronically mentally ill, *Social Work* 30:417-422, 1985.

Redford LJ: Case management, *Journal of Case Management* 1:1, 1992.

Rothman J: A model of case management: toward empirically based practice, *Social Work* 36(6):522-527, 1991.

Schroer K: Case management: clinical nurse specialist and nurse practitioner: converging notes, *Clinical Nurse Specialist* 3:4, 1991.

Simmons F: Developing the trauma nurse case manager role, *Dimensions in Critical Care* 11:3, 1992.

Tidwell SL: The role of the critical care CNS in case management, *American Journal of Nursing* 95:16E-16F, 1995.

Wagner DM: Client case management: a systems development process. *Caring,* December 1987.

Weil M, Karls J: *Case management in human service practice,* San Francisco, 1985, Jossey-Bass.

Wells N, Erickson S, Spinella J: Role transition: from clinical nurse specialist to clinical nurse specialist/case manager, *Journal of Nursing Administration* 26(11):23-28, 1996.

Yeager MA: *Role behaviors in nurse case management.* Unpublished manuscript. Columbia Union College, Virginia, 1997.

Zander K: Nursing case management: strategic management of cost and quality outcomes, *Journal of Nursing Administration* 18(5):23-30, 1988.

Zimmerman JH: Negotiating the system: clients make a case for case management, *Public Welfare* 45:2, 1987.

CHAPTER 15

Carondelet/Santa Cruz Parish Nurse Program

The Church as a Place of Healing

BELINDA J. ACOSTA, RN, BSN, **DELMA B. HUGGINS**, RN, MS, FNP, **ISELA LUNA**, RN, PhD, and **CATHERINE MICHAELS**, RN, PhD, FAAN

OVERVIEW

Our efforts have been successful not only because the services are culturally competent, but because the outcomes that we search for lie within the context of the lived experience of the people we serve and our relationships with them.

The Carondelet/Santa Cruz Parish Nurse Program is a joint effort of the Santa Cruz parish and Carondelet Health Network. The Catholic parish is mostly Mexican-American. Bilingual, bicultural Mexican-American nurses provide culturally competent health care services to individuals and groups within a spiritual context. The recipients are members of the parish and others who live within the parish. Health issues range from teenage pregnancy and violence to diabetes and heart disease. Working from the philosophy that individuals are connected to their community as a living system and that change in any part of the system affects the whole, the parish nurses serve individuals, families, and communities to improve health and well-being. ▲

"And these signs shall follow all who believe, they shall lay their hands upon the sick, who will recover."
(Mark 16:17)

The Carondelet Parish Nurse Program supports the Santa Cruz Catholic parish, providing services to an underserved, impoverished, and primarily Mexican-American community known as South Tucson. South Tucson is known as a high-crime area, with the main street dissecting the city and passing in front of the main church being regarded as the most violent in the larger Tucson community. Besieged by years of crime and gang violence, drug dealing, drug use, and prostitution, the people who live in South Tucson have many health issues that have been associated with poverty. Poverty is also linked to teenage pregnancy, mental health problems, and many chronic diseases such as heart disease, cancer, chronic lung disease, cirrhosis, and diabetes. It is believed that given meaningful access in terms of time, proximity, culture, and language, risk factors for these health problems can be modified. The Carondelet/Santa Cruz Parish Nurse Program has as a goal to meet this challenge. The Carondelet/Santa Cruz Parish Nurse Program is providing accessible, bilingual, bicultural primary care, health screening, monitoring, and education interspersed with prayer and healing. The parish nurses offer opportunities for improved health and well-being and, in that regard, depart from the model in which the parish nurse offers education and counseling only from a church site.

Carondelet Community Nursing has traditionally designed services to meet the needs of the people in a co-creative process. Following suit, the parish nurses partnered with members of the Santa Cruz parish to form the *Consilio de Salud* (Health Cabinet) to develop programs to help meet the health care needs of the community. The outcome was to transform the program in one community health center into three parish nurse health centers, providing primary care services and organizing community events. In less than two years, the Carondelet/Santa Cruz Parish Nurse Program has become an accessible provider for people who are undocumented, a bridge for others who have a medical home but do not know how to use it for either primary, secondary, or tertiary prevention, a primary provider of sports physicals, a school health service, an organizer of health events, and the leader of an annual Walk 4 Peace.

Why the early success? The foundation for the Parish Nurse Program is partnership. Lisbeth Schorr, author of *Common Purpose: Strengthening Families and Neighborhoods to Rebuild America*, described relationships in this way:

I have concluded that I have been observing the evolution of a new form of professional practice, often at odds with more conventional ways of working. The new Practice has emerged, more pragmatically than ideologically, from many disciplinary origins, often in opposition to professional traditions. The touchstones of the new practice are a new mind-set about what it means to be a professional . . . the new professional aim, quite consciously, to strengthen the ability of clients, students, young people and families to make their journey toward independence and to take greater control over their own and their children's lives. To this end, practitioners elicit client strengths and assets rather then pathology (pp 12-13, 1997).

With this kind of professional nursing practice as the foundation, the Carondelet/Santa Cruz Parish Nurse Program is unfolding as a strong contributor to the health and well-being of individuals, families, and the South Tucson community. The mission being realized, just as what started as a dream grounds itself into the reality of daily life in the Santa Cruz parish and the city of South Tucson.

Mission Statement

We, the Nurses of the Carondelet/Santa Cruz Parish Nurse Program (Parish Nurse Program) have as our mission to serve physically, mentally, and spiritually, any individuals in need, regardless of ethnic group, color, or religion, in a spirit of partnership. We provide a safe compassionate environment to offer health care services, facilitating medical care, health education, social services and spiritual support, through culturally sensitive, compassionate, focused nursing practice that facilitates the health and well-being of people and communities.

The Dream

The Parish Nurse Program began as a dream. For years, we, the founders, shared a dream of helping their community, and the Mexican-Americans, in particular. As Mexican-Americans ourselves, we were drawn by the unmet needs of our people, especially in the city of South Tucson, a one-square-mile town located south and central of Tucson, Arizona. We could imagine ourselves serving this small and poor Mexican-American community that lacked the level of health care services to prevent disease and disability. But we did not know where and how to begin such an endeavor.

Years later, having increased our education and experience as baccalaureate-prepared professional nurse case managers, we continued our dreaming. Our employer, Carondelet Health Network, had implemented several Community Health Centers to serve seniors. Yet none of these centers was located in South Tucson, where we continued to see the greatest need for Mexican-Americans. In a professional nurse case management meeting, we told Phyllis Ethridge, our Vice President of Patient Services, that the one-to-one approach of case management was not reaching the family-oriented Mexican-Americans. Phyllis said, "Then do what you need to do to reach them." With the Community Health Center as our model, we seized this opportunity to translate our dream into reality. We proposed a health clinic in South Tucson, the community we had talked about serving so many years ago. This was our first step in fulfilling the dream. We contacted the city of South Tucson for assistance in locating a site. After several months without any response from the community authorities, we thought of an alternative. There were several chapels in the area, but one stood out, a small Catholic chapel in a Mexican-American neighborhood. The limited medical services available in the community made the chapel an ideal location for our work. The next step was to contact the pastor and obtain consent for its use. The pastor gave his blessing for the chapel's use as a screening clinic. The chapel was one of two satellite missions administered by Santa Cruz Catholic Church parish in the Diocese of Tucson. The parish is located in an area of Tucson made up mostly of Mexican nationals and Mexican-Americans who for the most part are monolingual, Spanish-speaking. This was the ideal site for two Mexican-American nurses who were bilingual and bicultural to work with their people. In April of 1991, Our Lady of Guadalupe Chapel became the Health Screening Clinic site.

Reaching Out to People Where They Pray

The people seemed open to having us at the church at first. The issue of accepted uses for the church building came into play. The traditional belief that a church was for worship, not for other uses, was voiced by people in the neighborhood. In time, the nursing team was able to help individuals get beyond this issue. People began to understand that, yes, a church is a place for worship, and, because the people are the Church, and because Jesus offered many self-care teachings for improving health and well-being, both worship and health services can take place in the same building. The people grew to accept us and the work that we were doing in the church as help from God and His Mother, Our Lady of Guadalupe. By then, we had joined the parish and had become active members of the parish community.

We were functioning in the roles of: educator, counselor, and service coordinator at the clinic. Our peers and our clients provided us with positive feedback on the work we were doing. Our work was seen as making a difference in people's lives. Because of the location of our work, the church, it was seen as a ministry connected to God; there was a natural relationship of spirituality and health. The clients came to realize this relationship, and they facilitated the process. A people devoted to prayer, they began to request our prayers and asked us to join in their prayers. We had become healers through the word. It was as if we had become one of their traditional healers, *curanderos/curanderas*, who heal through prayer, herbs, and healing touch.

Partnering With People

We discussed our work with our parish pastor; he was supportive of what we were doing. He also encouraged us to grow in other directions. He saw the need for nursing care, "hands-on" care, as we did. We saw the need to involve others in providing the care that was needed. When we presented the idea of bringing other health care professionals and services to the clinic, at first the clients refused, with a resounding, "NO, we don't want others who don't understand us." Our clients had developed a trusting relationship with us as the providers and as church members. They did not want to accept other providers, especially those outside the faith and culture. They were afraid we would leave if others came. They were at ease with us. Finally, they agreed we could bring others in to help and observe, but identified us as the providers. We treated them in a culturally sensitive manner and gave them the care they felt they needed. We had become their nurses, "the parish nurses, at Santa Cruz Catholic Church parish." Thus, the Carondelet approach to parish nursing had evolved. We all now shared the dream, and partnering our work with what the people wanted has become the framework for parish nursing.

The Program Grows

Shortly after the screening clinic was established, we read about parish nursing and how popular it was becoming. We started to explore the concept, and thought about how it might apply to the population and work we were already doing. We were not only serving a church congregation. We were serving a population residing within a delineated diocesan parish boundary, and a community. We were functioning in roles such as those described in parish nursing literature: educators, counselors, spiritual supporters, service coordinators, and nursing care providers. We were recognized by our pastor as the "parish nurses"; he referred all health care matters to the parish nurses.

In 1995, with the support of our employer, two additional sites were opened to provide screening services. A site at the primary church, Santa Cruz Catholic Church, and another at the San Antonio Chapel, the other satellite chapel, were established. The three sites are logistically separated by main streets creating individual neighborhoods. Each neighborhood has its own individual characteristics, but with similar needs. With the addition of the Santa Cruz site, we also became the school nurse on the day of clinic. The work continued to evolve, and the program was designated a parish nurse program in 1995.

The Carondelet/Santa Cruz Parish Nurse Program (Parish Nurse Program) became official in August 1996 with incorporation of primary care services. This was facilitated by the financial support of the Carondelet Community Trust, Hughes Missile Systems, and the Marshall Foundation. Because of these benefactors, the Parish Nurse Program was able to improve its resources and provide additional services as the client numbers continued to grow at all the sites and the need for new services continued to be identified.

The responsibilities of the parish nurse have increased with addition of new services. With availability of a family nurse practitioner to provide primary care, the parish nurse has taken on a "hands-on" role in the practice. The parish nurse now carries out orders of the nurse practitioner, as well as from collaborating or referring physicians. Community outreach and intervention responsibilities have been added to the parish nurse role as we reach beyond the health care system to work with communities on health issues of their concern. The added responsibilities have taken the parish nurse beyond the traditionally described role of parish nursing. The providing of nursing care and social responsibilities differentiate the Carondelet approach to parish nursing from other programs.

The program incorporates volunteers to assist in providing service and care. For the most part the volunteers are bilingual; however, being bilingual is not a requirement. The volunteers are housewives, nursing students, nurses, nuns, and parents of the schoolchildren. Some volunteers are parish members. Others come from the community at large. Their contributions to the program range from assisting with patient care to performing clerical duties that maintain the efficiency at the different sites. Volunteers are a valuable part of the program, because of the time they give and share with staff and patients.

Honoring the Culture

Our working philosophy in the practice of the parish nursing is to develop a working relationship with the clients. Respect for client choice is the key that facilitates the work of the parish nurse and relationship building. Everything revolves around practicing respect for the client as a person and respect for the choices that the clients make in all aspects of their lives. We practice respect for client healing practices, faith beliefs, traditions, and culture orientation; in turn the respect is allotted to us.

Acceptance of these practices was facilitated for us because of our Mexican-American descent.

Because of nurse case management experience, we also look at client patterns of choice making. As nurses we provide the client with information; the client makes the choice about what to do with the information. Social and health care choices become patterns practiced by the client. At times choices become a series of trials and errors, until the client comes to realize that he or she is going around in circles and may be open to a different choice. At this point as case managers, we assist with new choice outcomes.

The use of herbs for healing is a health practice of Mexican-American families. Herbs are traditional medicines passed down from one generation to the next and shared between families and friends. It seems that everyone has an herbal remedy for any complaint or problem. The remedies are shared openly among clients. Sharing of remedies is the client's way of helping others. Accepting the use of herbs and allowing the sharing by us is a show of respect. The client becomes more open to listening to our information as he or she accords us mutual respect. This allows the relationship to blossom and grow with mutual respect through sharing of knowledge, and allows the introduction of Western Medicine ideas, therapies, and treatments for consideration.

An example of alternative choices used by the clients is the use of herbs to control blood sugar levels in treatment of diabetes. There are different teas, pills, herbs, and even cactus plants that are used in an attempt to lower blood sugar levels. Some of these treatments are perceived as healing, others not. With time the choice made by the client may lead to positive outcomes, or it may not be beneficial for the client. Allowing clients to try the herbs and other alternatives is evidence of respect and is important to the relationship building between client and nurse.

Respect for religious practices is an example of our acceptance of the clients' beliefs. In the Mexican-American culture religious faith plays an important role in everyday life. Faith in prayer that heals, protects, and directs one's life is the essence of daily life. Along with prayer is penance, promises to a saint, God, or His Mother, to do something in return for an answered prayer. Prayer to the Blessed Mother, in whatever apparition that the person believes in, is seen as paramount. The Blessed Mother is seen as God-like in nature, able to grant every prayer through her intercession. For this parish as with most Mexican-American and Latin American cultures, Our Lady of Guadalupe, the mother of the Americas, is the revered representation of the Blessed Mother. Penitent prayer to other statues of saints is also practiced. Offering of penance and *milagros* (metal images of body parts) in request for healing or as payment for an answered prayer is also integrated into the faith practices of the culture.

Another accepted healing practice that combines prayer, herbs, and healing touch is the use of healers (*curanderos* or *curanderas*). It is believed that healers have a healing power given them by God. Healers use prayer as an intercession to God to heal through them. Herbs are their medicines, and touch as massage conveys the healing to the patient. Healers are sought out by Mexican-American culture for many health concerns. Among these concerns are stomach aliments, sleeplessness, and assorted pains and diseases. It is further believed that the power of the healer can ward off evil and prevent illness. Many times this population does not seek health care from Western Medicine providers until they have exhausted their traditional practices.

Maintaining confidentiality is an example of respect as well as key to the work of health care. We strive for confidentiality, in the process of providing service to our clients. However, confidentiality takes a backseat at times, as is evident when clients share with each other their beliefs, problems, and concerns. When confidentiality is an issue, clients respect each other's privacy. As health care providers, we provide the necessary environment to maintain confidentiality when necessary.

Our Services and Staff

When we opened, the first clinic clients came either out of curiosity or because they had a health care issue that needed to be addressed. Others came for socialization. The lack of health care services for the Mexican national, Mexican-American population on the south side of Tucson brought us to the neighborhood. What we found was a high incidence of hypertension, heart disease, diabetes mellitus, obesity, and some autoimmune diseases. In most cases, the patients were not even aware of having a problem with their health. Many had never been to a physician except in a time of need, such as childbirth.

We also found that there were social issues that were not being recognized and that people were not being assisted. Other issues that evolved were legal residency status, illiteracy, lack of finances, inappropriate or absent nutrition, deplorable housing, and lack of transportation. People with small children or frail elderly with disabilities have great difficulty with public buses, as there are long waits, and often long walks between bus stops. This gave the nurse team an opportunity to facilitate the creation of social networks for individuals to help each other out with shopping needs, child care, and the development of volunteer networks. Soon, families were helping families, and friends and neighbors were coming together to help each other out with transportation as well as other needs. Through our work, processes were developed to facilitate and assist individuals to assume responsibility for their health, and sometimes assist with the health of others.

At the beginning we had elected to work with an elderly high- to moderate-risk population. Within a short time, however, it became evident that the elderly in this community were not the only ones lacking in health care services. Our clients started to bring younger family members with them, and over time we found ourselves serving many generations of the same family with various service and health care needs. The Parish Nurse Program now serves all age groups.

The Parish Nurse Program now provides services that include nursing care, primary care services, advocacy, facilitation, coordination, support, counseling, spiritual nurturing, and referrals to a variety of community and health services. We are also involved in providing community outreach (support groups, family retreats) and participating in community-level interventions (Walk 4 Peace, anti-violence). Our model of care was based on a wellness model of service, which provided health promotion, illness prevention, and disease management through education, monitoring, and screening.

Because of our familiarity with community agencies, we were able to refer clients into systems for medical, legal residency status, and, in some cases, better housing situations. We are looking at the needs and concerns of the Mexican-American people and try provide the necessary information, support, and guidance in a gentle, respectful, and nonjudgmental way in the hope of helping the community and the people.

The Health Screening Clinic at Our Lady of Guadalupe was originally staffed by two dreamers and a licensed practical nurse. We were all bilingual and bicultural Mexican-American nurses. Now the Parish Nurse Program is staffed by three registered nurses and several volunteers. Together, three nurses serve as parish nurses as well as fulfill other roles in the program. The primary parish nurse staffs all three sites. She is a baccalaureate-prepared nurse who provides nurse case management services, skilled nursing care, school nurse services, service coordination, and the clinic coordination. Primary care is provided by a master's-prepared family nurse practitioner with case management and parish nurse experience. A third, part-time registered nurse supports the parish nurse centers, freeing the nurse practitioner for primary care and the primary parish nurse for counseling and education related to complex chronic and behavior health issues. The Parish Nurse Specialist, a doctorally prepared nurse, assists with community-based interventions, program development, and program evaluation. The Parish Nurse Specialist also serves as a liaison to the Carondelet Foundation and other Parish Nurse Program funders. All the parish nurse staff oversee finances and program development, in collaboration with the Health Cabinet.

Specific Health Services

HEALTH PROMOTION

We have identified that hypertension, diabetes, cardiac diseases, and obesity are prevalent in the Mexican-American culture in our area of the country. We have also noted that there is a significant lack of knowledge of prevention or treatment of the problems. Many are on medications, but have no knowledge of why they are taking the medicine, what it is for, how long to take it, or what the medicine is. This knowledge deficit has created a need for the staff of the Parish Nurse Program to prioritize our work in educating the clients: disease processes, prevention of complications, managing disease, and maintaining the maximum level of wellness within the mental, intellectual, and physical capabilities of the clients.

HEALTH SCREENING AND MONITORING

Health screening is the first step in health promotion and illness prevention education, and is the most important of the services provided at the parish nurse sites. Many clients arrive at the clinic feeling confident, believing themselves to be free of diabetes or hypertension. Some will say, "I used to be a diabetic" or "I used to have high blood pressure . . . but the doctor gave me some pills five years ago and I was cured." Others come because a relative (including in-laws) has had some complications from being diabetic and they "don't want to get it." Often we have clients who state that their doctors have told them they are "borderline" diabetics, present with a blood glucose of 300 mg/dl, and are not symptomatic. Through screening interventions, we are given opportunities to begin the clients' education process on disease identification, management, facilitation of lifestyle change, and/or medication compliance.

Regular visits to the sites for monitoring of weight, blood pressure, and blood sugar levels are a mainstay of the clinics. Providing glucose monitors to clients for the purpose of self-monitoring has brought about changes in eating patterns and control of blood sugar levels and given the staff an opportunity to become cheerleaders in support of the clients' success. Blood pressure monitoring by staff at each visit provides client feedback on status and also affords a teaching opportunity for the staff. Weight management, because of our clients' predisposition to obesity, was incorporated as part of the screening process. Disease management through nutrition is automatically included in our clients' education plans. Most of the clients seen at the parish nurse sites are dealing with two if not all three problems.

PRIMARY CARE

Services at the parish nurse sites have become family oriented, as previously noted. With the addition of primary care services, the focus of service has become more family oriented; services are provided to all age groups. This has occurred for two primary reasons. One reason is that the primary care site is located on the same campus as the church and school, and the other is the circumstances that identify this community as high risk: the lack of health services in the neighborhood, low-income status of families, and lack of or insufficient insurance coverage. Primary care services provided include wellness checks for all age groups, physical exams for adults who do not have health care providers, children's sports physicals, preschool physicals, and episodic illness visits for assessment, problem identification, treatment, and follow-up. Services are provided by a family nurse practitioner (FNP) on the site. The FNP is on call for the other sites as needed. There are limits to the services that the nurse practitioner can provide. For example, complicated medical problems or clients with multiple medical problems that are out of control or require in-depth evaluation are referred to health care services that can provide needed evaluation. The nature of the population that is seen in the Parish Nurse Program has provided a challenge to the staff. Contacts with providers that are responsive to the economic and health status of the clients have been difficult to find. With persistence, collaborative relationships have been established that provide clients with affordable and quality health care services.

SUPPORT PROGRAMS

Weekly visits to the clinics have led to the development of client-nurse relationships, but also client-client relationships. The clients look to us to provide information about their status. We also provide them with positive support for progress or maintenance in meeting their goals. The clients lend support to one another when one of them does not meet a goal for the week. The clients have established informal support groups and cheer each other when blood sugars, blood pressures, or weights are down. They form friendships, walk to clinic together as a form of exercise, and wait for one another to share results. They share the successful attempts to lower blood pressure or blood sugar, but also the experience of what they are doing to achieve that lower value. The need for client support from not only the nurses and clergy but other persons who have similar problems or concerns has led to the development of support groups. Some of these groups are informal; others are led by the staff. The support groups are specific to the site. The groups spend time socializing, comparing outcomes, and giving each other moral support as well as suggestions on what to do about the medical as well as family problems. Structured support groups for grieving and coping have been provided to a small number of clients. Formal support programs are facilitated as needs are identified.

COUNSELING

A counseling program using a nursing and spiritual perspective has been developed and implemented to serve the concerns of the clients. The counseling is generally one-to-one with client, caregiver, or family. The focus is usually on self-care, health care issues, or coping strategies.

SPIRITUAL SUPPORT

The spiritual component of the counseling is in the realm of spiritual nurturance, which takes on a life of its own. Some spiritual issues addressed by our team include healing through forgiveness, "letting go" in order to move on with life, and acceptance (unconditional love for others and for self). Often, we remind the clients of Jesus' great and unconditional love for each of His children, His forgiveness, and the need to ask for help. We bring to clients' attention their need to be participants in the health process in order to obtain better results. This created a need for increased involvement in the parish community as well as working more closely with the parish clergy. Two of our nurses participate as readers and Eucharistic Ministers in the Parish. Our participation has brought together the physical as well as the spiritual role of a healer for the people of the parish. This has facilitated the collaboration between the clergy and the nurses in working on spiritual issues and family concerns of clients. We have established a referral process for spiritual issues. At times, more deeply rooted needs for spiritual guidance are identified; these are referred to the parish clergy.

Nurse-client joint prayer, group prayer, or just wishing clients Godspeed as they leave the clinic assists in meeting spiritual needs. The faith component of nursing service evolves from the interaction between nurse and client. The nurses need to be open to listening to key words that warn of spiritual distress or dependence of the client on healing by faith. Clients have also formed prayer groups, spending time in prayer before leaving the clinic setting, especially at the clinic in the church. At one clinic, clients routinely spend time in prayer as they await their turn to be seen by the nurse or before they leave.

HEALTH MINISTRY TO YOUTH AND ADOLESCENTS

The issues identified by the *Consilio* were brought to the *Consilio de Ninos* (Health Cabinet of Children). This *Consilio* is a group of seven children from 7 to 12 years old, who are representatives of their school classes at the Santa Cruz Parish School. Each member brings to the group the health concerns of his or her class. This group, in turn, develops teaching strategies to address those concerns, and identifies one member of the group to be the expert and spokesperson on the issue for that community. Violence, especially in the streets, was the number one concern of the youth and adults whom we work with. The health cabinets, the Parish Nurse Program, and numerous community agencies, church groups, churches, and interested individuals formed a partnership in an effort to begin to address this issue.

Funding from the Flinn Foundation, an Arizona-based funder, has allowed us to reach out to adolescents in regard to sexual abstinence. We implemented a sexual abstinence program that is grounded in sex education, ethnic identity issues, career planning, and spiritual issues. We have educated a group of teens on these issues. They, in turn, educate others. Teen members belong to the parish and the surrounding community.

Evaluation of Outcomes

Evaluating the outcomes of the Parish Nurse Program consists of several components. Components evaluated include the number of church center visits as a measure for seeking health services, self-care management, and community-based interventions. We believe that relationship is the mediator for these and other measurable outcomes. Our work with the Mexican-American population, especially that of lower socioeconomic levels, has taught us that providing a supportive environment and giving permission to express one's cultural practices of healing in a respectful manner allow for the building of relationships and partnerships. For our work, we have identified several signs to indicate that a relationship has been formed. These signs are:

Asking for a specific parish nurse

Knowing the parish nurse's first name

Being familiar with the parish nurse's family situation

Offering personal invitations to their homes

Giving personal gifts, including food and items of personal value, to the parish nurse

Sharing spiritual practices, prayer, and special devotions to *santos* (religious saints)

Acknowledging use of nontraditional health practices such as *hierbas* (herbs) and other nontraditional *remedios* (remedies), such as *limpias* (spiritual cleansings)

Once we see these signs, we believe we have achieved a partnership that can be used as a springboard to negotiate changes in health behavior.

Evaluation of Health-Seeking Behavior Through Church Center Visits

The number of church center visits varies in each of the churches where we practice, reflecting the slight differences in client population (Figure 15-1). At Our Lady of Guadalupe Chapel, a site that is visited mostly by elderly women (although we are beginning to see men and younger women with children visit the site), we saw a 91% increase in the number of church center visits in the last fiscal year. At the Santa Cruz Church site, where we offer the most comprehensive services, like health fairs, sports physicals, school screening, primary care, and

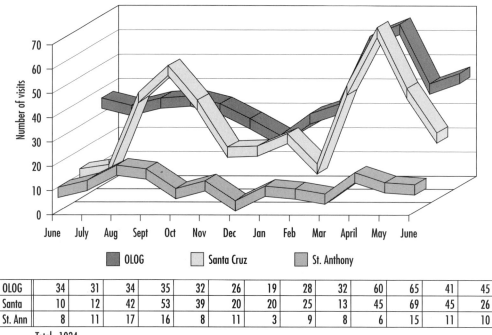

June 1996 to June 1997

	June	July	Aug	Sept	Oct	Nov	Dec	Jan	Feb	Mar	April	May	June
OLOG	34	31	34	35	32	26	19	28	32	60	65	41	45
Santa	10	12	42	53	39	20	20	25	13	45	69	45	26
St. Ann	8	11	17	16	8	11	3	9	8	6	15	11	10

Total = 1034

FIGURE 15-1 Church center visits by month and site.

health monitoring and screening, to the most age-diverse population, infants to elderly, the number of visits increased 590% in this fiscal year. At the third site, San Antonio Chapel, visited mostly by elderly women, we saw an increase of 87% in church center visits in the last fiscal year. Church center visits, and/or use of the services available to the community, have been one way in which we have measured the success of the Parish Nurse Program and the building of relationships in the community.

Evaluation of Self-Care Management

Self-care management is a valuable component to us, since it reflects client strengths and assets. In evaluating this effort, we have focused our clinical outcomes on self-care management of diabetes and hypertension. We used the Omaha Classification System to document the self-care management outcome of our interventions. The Omaha Classification System uses an evaluation approach based on a five-point Likert-type scale for measurement of client knowledge, behavior, and health status. For knowledge, the scale ranges from minimal knowledge (score 1) to superior knowledge (score 5). Behavior and status have similar ratings, with a score

of 5 indicative of optimum health behavior and health status.

In the analysis of early data, we found the ratings for measuring knowledge, behavior, and health status (KBS) inadequate for our evaluation. Therefore, we developed a comprehensive and culturally appropriate diabetic and hypertension protocol aligned with the American Heart Association and the American Diabetes Association, to augment the Omaha KBS. The diabetes and hypertension protocol was implemented with 100% of our clients who met the eligibility criteria (that is, having hypertension and diabetes), and data were collected on 15 clients twice, when the protocol was initiated and three months later.

We found that the mean knowledge (time 1, mean = 2.4; time 2, mean = 3.3) and behavior (time 1, mean = 2.7; time 2, mean = 2.9) of the clients increased over a three-month period (Figure 15-2). This was interpreted as a positive indicator of clients' increase in knowledge and incorporation of positive health behaviors. The health status rating consisted of a combination of subjective and objective ratings of symptoms present. We found a slight decrease in the mean health status, indicating a decline in status over a three-month period (time 1, mean = 2.8; time 2, mean = 2.5). We have several possible explanations for this finding. One explanation relates to instrumentation problems that we encountered, and the other possibility is our observation that as our clients began to learn more about their disease processes, often their perception of their health status decreased. How the perception of health changes over time with increased knowledge and behavior is an interesting question to explore in a long-term study. We concluded that we must continue to explore effective and reliable ways to measure culturally appropriate clinical outcomes, incorporating subjective and objective ratings such as those used in Omaha.

Evaluation of Community-Based Interventions

A third important outcome of our work has included population-based interventions. In 1996, a *Consilio de Salud* (Health Cabinet) was formed to steer the efforts of the Parish Nurse Program, with the philosophy that the members of the community

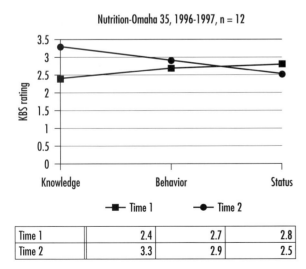

Nutrition-Omaha 35, 1996-1997, n = 12

	Knowledge	Behavior	Status
Time 1	2.4	2.7	2.8
Time 2	3.3	2.9	2.5

FIGURE 15-2 KBS before and after means of hypertension/diabetes study.

itself know best what the needs of the community are. This cabinet is composed of representatives of the parish, people who live in the surrounding community, and other community leaders who are nonprofessional. Together with the Parish Nurse Program team, the areas of health of priority were identified. These include violence (mental health issues, domestic violence, gang activity, substance abuses), teenage pregnancy, diabetes prevention, and cancer screening. Our efforts in the past year have concentrated largely on these issues.

One of the areas of great concern to our community has been the increase in violence over the last few years. This was initially brought to our attention by the *Consilio de Salud* that steers the community-based programs. Violence, especially in the streets, was the number one concern to the youth and adults whom we work with. The health cabinets, the Parish Nurse Program, and numerous community agencies, church groups, churches, and interested individuals formed a partnership in an effort to begin to address this issue. With the leadership of the parish nurses a 1.3 mile Walk 4 Peace (*Caminata por la Paz*) was organized along a street often labeled by the police as the deadliest in town, according to newspaper accounts: "Police say, shots are fired on this stretch of South Sixth Avenue nightly" (Tucson *Citizen*, December 2, 1996). More than 500 people took a stand against violence in their neighborhood on December 6, 1996, a Friday night. The crowd of marchers, many of them children, gathered at a shopping center with banners, signs, and photos of loved ones lost to violence. The event concluded at Santa Cruz Church, one of the Parish Nurse Program sites, with an ecumenical prayer service and a pledge for peace developed by the *Consilio de Salud de Ninos* (Box 15-1). For many participants, this was a beginning effort to integrate the loss of a loved one.

BOX 15-1
Dreams of Peace

I promise to increase the peace and erase the hate, and stand united against violence, by accepting differences in others, and by showing the universal love of my Creator.

Conclusion

The Parish Nurse Program provides bilingual, bicultural, and spiritually based services to a Mexican-American population. Our efforts have been successful not only because the services are culturally competent, but because the outcomes that we search for lie within the context of the lived experience of the people we serve and our relationships with them. This is often manifested in the hugs that we share with our clients as they leave or arrive at our church centers. The changes that take place within the format of the relationship building have transformed not only our clients, but ourselves and our practice. The most important collaborative effort that we engage in, as parish nurses, is our own desire to serve God in whatever way we are guided, knowing that we are only vehicles for continuing God's work.

References

Schorr LB: *Common purpose: strengthening families and neighborhoods to rebuild America*, New York, 1997, Doubleday.

CHAPTER 16

New Roles in Building Healthier Communities

Relationship-Centered Care

ELAINE R. COLVIN, RN, BSN, MEPD, RANDI FRIEDL, RN, MPH, and JULIE MacDONALD, RN, MS

OVERVIEW

The concepts of health, community, and consumer-driven care have roots that are common. Each calls for active participation and partnerships from a deeper knowing, understanding, and acceptance of those being served.

The traditional mode of patient and provider interaction and relationship is insufficient in a reforming health care system that is moving from institutions to communities and is more reliant on the health and active involvement of those being served. A transformation of both the role of patient and the role of provider is necessary. This chapter explores the framework of relationship-centered care as the vehicle for this transformation and examines Gundersen Lutheran's involvement and outcomes in two community partnerships, end-of-life planning and parish nursing. ▲

The pace and amount of change that is occurring within health care itself, the organizations that provide the care, and the systems that fund it are cataclysmic. Moreover, despite the fact that health care system reform and the chaos it has produced in the industry are not new, there is not a single structure that is emerging or a predictable pattern of change for others to emulate. However, multiple factors are beginning to converge that are creating a demand for a more integrated approach to care. This approach takes into account the many factors that interact to promote health or that cause illness and that request individual responsibility for one's own health as well as a collective responsibility for the health of the population at large (Tresolini, Pew-Fetzer Task Force, 1994). At the same time, clear themes are emerging from stories in communities across the country that offer a direction and a challenge for both providers and consumers. These themes are simply that health care is becoming more of a genuine balance of health and illness care, with more solutions being generated out of local community efforts and with more consumers of health care shifting into the driving seat (AONE, 1997; DeBack, Cohen, 1996; Quill, Brody, 1996).

The concepts of health, community, and consumer-driven care have roots that are common. Each calls for active participation and partnerships that result from a deeper knowing, understanding, and acceptance of those being served.

As the industry begins to reframe what health is, we are coming to understand health not as the absence of disease, but rather as the process by which individuals maintain their sense of coherence (i.e., a sense that their lives are comprehensible, manageable, and meaningful) and are able to function in the face of the changes in themselves and their relationships within their environments. Health is not given to people, but it is generated by them (Tresolini, Pew-Fetzer Task Force, 1994).

Role Reform

In discussion of efforts to move toward community-based care, Carole Schroeder emphasizes increased community participation and responsibility in health, but identifies problems in imposing the medical model of care within community partnerships. "Approaching communities as partners," writes Schroeder (1994), "will require a profound shift in professional values and beliefs, for most professionals are accustomed to medically designated models of health. Partnerships mandate relationships based on mutual respect, expertise, knowledge and authority."

An imbalance of power exists when communities are seen and patronized as simply the clients of health care professionals. Moreover, identifying the community as client connotes an image of the community as passive and needy and the professional as expert, authority, and normalizer (Schroeder, 1994). Professionals can no longer act unilaterally in attempting to solve problems for people; people must be actively involved and invested in discovering their own solutions.

As the health care industry begins to rely more on each individual's health and on communities as core solutions to many of its ailments, new roles for both consumers and professionals must be actively pursued. These role changes call for a transformation of the professional role into that of facilitator and enabler of self-care and empowerment for individuals, families, and communities as necessary (Courtney, 1995).

Courtney et al (1996) use an illustration of the partnership model (Table 16-1) to demonstrate the dimensions of the role changes necessary. The expected outcome with the role shift is enhanced knowledge, skill, and capacities of individual, family, and community partners to act more effectively on their own behalf. "It is only through partnerships that individuals, families, and communities can realize the power of their own contribution to improving their health and well-being" (Courtney et al, 1996). To continue to determine another's needs and to plan unilaterally for them results in continued dependence on professionals.

Patient as Partner: The Cornerstone of Community Health Improvement (AONE, 1997) explores the processes involved in these role changes. Despite the policy and economic issues surrounding health care today, old boundaries for roles are actually being dismantled and new partnerships between patient and provider are evolving. These new partnerships are not seen as transitional strategies, but rather as the cornerstone of a new health care delivery system.

TABLE 16-1
Comparison of Professional Model With Partnership Model

PROFESSIONAL MODEL	PARTNERSHIP MODEL
Focus	
The problem or the diagnosis	Fostering the skills and capacity of the partner as a primary focus in the process of improving health and well-being (the initial stimulus may be a problem, but the primary focus will be strengthening/facilitating empowerment of the partner)
Health Professional's Role	
Expert who does "to" or "for," not "with"; the professional serves as decision maker and problem solver	Professional working "with," not "doing to"; facilitator, enabler, resource person who shares leadership and power with partner; services are provided in nonjudgmental, noncontrolling manner
Partner's Role	
Often passive recipient of "service" that is defined by professional	Active and willing participant in self-determination of strengths, problems, and solutions
Nature of Relationship	
Professional is director of the process, instructing or "telling" other what to do; interventions tend to be standardized and are seldom tailored to individual or cultural needs; interventions tend to focus on the problem, not the person	Professional actively facilitates the partner's participation in the relationship; requires ongoing negotiation of goals, roles, and responsibilities; respects individual and cultural differences
Goal/Plan	
Determined by the professional; focused totally on the problem, not the person	Mutual goal setting; plan of action developed with partner who is involved as active participant
Activity/Service	
Unilateral action by the professional to diagnose problem, establish intervention, assess progress, and revise intervention as needed	Joint action and assessment of progress that includes ongoing negotiation of roles and responsibilities; implements the partnership process; emphasizes involving natural helpers, families, groups, and/or coalitions as resources
Expected Outcome	
The problem is solved or corrected or the patient is considered noncompliant	The partner's capacity to act more effectively on his/her own behalf is strengthened (i.e., more empowered); the "problem" may or may not be solved, but the partner's capacity is enhanced to prevent future problems or to address them more effectively

From Courtney R et al: The partnership model: working with individuals, families and communities toward a new vision of health, *Public Health Nursing* 13(3):177-186, June 1996.

Gundersen Lutheran and Relationship-Centered Care

Relationships serve as the basis and vehicle for partnerships. Although relationships seemingly have always been central to health care, relationships that practitioners form with patients, communities, and other practitioners have not generally been explored or taught explicitly. In the report of the Pew-Fetzer Task Force on Health Professions Education and Relationship-Centered Care (1994), areas of knowledge, skills, and values that allow practitioners to work more competently within relationships with their patients, their patients' communities, and each other are identified. These relationships are identified as the vehicle for putting into action a paradigm of health that integrates caring, healing, and community.

As Gundersen Lutheran began its work in 1995 as a newly formed integrated delivery system, the need to commit in a meaningful way to the health of the communities it serves emerged. The concept of community partnerships was designed into a freshly chartered mission statement. There was not, however, a clear strategy for moving it forward. Moreover, the concept of community partnerships and how these partnerships related to the care that traditionally went on within the walls of the institution were yet to be discovered.

Moving resources and key aspects of the work of Gundersen Lutheran into the community settings at a time when we were actually novices in these settings called for a new table to be set where relationships were the focus. Practitioners needed to step back and examine their own values and capacities before they could successfully do the work at hand. Accepting and relying on our community residents as the experts resulted in a profound role and power shift. Gundersen Lutheran discovered that moving from the walls of our institutions into the cultural context in which our people live and make decisions may be the best environment for new roles to evolve and partnerships to emerge.

Two programs that illustrate this shift to our communities and learning about relationship-centered care are end-of-life planning and parish nursing.

END-OF-LIFE PLANNING PARTNERSHIPS

In 1991 four major health care organizations in La Crosse, Wisconsin, recognized the need to form a partnership and to address a growing health concern for both patients and health care providers in regard to end-of-life planning. The task force formed by these health care organizations in La Crosse was asked to develop a common advance-directive educational program that would have broad community support and would ultimately result in at least half of the adults in the community having done end-of-life planning in advance (Hammes, in press).

An interdisciplinary group of health professionals, including nurses, administrators, social workers, a health educator, a clinical ethicist, and a community church pastor, constituted the task force. The members represented hospitals, ambulatory care facilities, and nursing homes. The task force worked with and was accountable to the four administrative presidents and the physician leadership in the organizations.

The task force recognized that as health care providers form partnerships with patients, they need to promote patient autonomy and self-determination when patients are making health care decisions. However, if patients are to act autonomously, they need to be informed about the decisions they need to make, and they need the knowledge that is necessary to make those decisions.

Health care providers need to be aware of patients' values and beliefs and understand the patients' goals for their health care in order to assist them in making health care decisions (Colvin et al, 1993). The use of an advance directive is one way to promote patient autonomy and to involve patients' values and beliefs in health care decision making when patients cannot speak for themselves. An advance directive could be something as simple as a verbal discussion with family members or with health care providers in regard to end-of-life care. It could also mean a written expression by the patient, which may or may not be documented on a statutory form such as a Power of Attorney for Health Care or a Living Will (Miles, Koepp, Weber, 1996).

These oral or written expressions about future health care decisions provide patients with the opportunity to maintain their autonomy and to exercise their self-determination even if they are unable to speak for themselves. The need to educate people about their choices on end-of-life decisions is a serious national health care issue and is also important when practitioners are forming relationships with patients.

The first strategy as the task force began its work was to conduct a literature review of advance-directive education programs (Hammes, in press). Second, the experiences from an advance-directive educational program that had been developed in the dialysis unit at Gundersen Lutheran in 1986 were discussed. The development, implementation, and history of this program, called "If I Only Knew" (Colvin, Hammes, 1991), provided a base for development of the community-based program. Last, the task force did a study to determine the "knowledge, attitudes, and needs of the area adults" in regard to advance directives (Hammes, Rooney, Bendiksen, 1991).

This study, which was done in March of 1991, included a random phone survey of 304 adults (Hammes, in press). The demographic makeup of the community was represented in the adults who were surveyed. The survey results indicated that 47% of the adults were having discussions with their families about end-of-life care, but only about one third of those adults had actually completed written advance-directive documents. The survey also revealed that the two most important needs of these adults were the need to have some assistance in "how to talk with my family" and the need to know "how to talk with my physician." People also requested information about medical treatments and legal issues in regard to advance directives.

A structure for the advance-directive program was agreed upon as a result of the information the task force had gathered. The strategies the task force agreed to use were:

1. Promote an adult educational model
2. Use stories as teaching tools
3. Develop a common image for the program
4. Make the materials readily available to the people in the community
5. Educate staff so they could provide assistance to patients and families
6. Develop common policies and procedures so all the health care organizations in the system

could follow the program (Hammes, in press).

The task force also agreed that the primary aims of the educational program, which was called "Respecting Your Choices," would be to "increase understanding of end-of-life decisions, assist in personal reflection about end-of-life decisions, and to promote discussion and communication of these decisions among loved ones and between patients and physicians" (Hammes, in press). A secondary goal was to create more advance-directive documents.

Community education programs, written materials, and a video were designed by the task force members to be used in this educational process by healthy adults as well as those facing a medical crisis. The educational materials could be used in a variety of settings, with different people at different levels of understanding, in regard to advance directives.

A training program for advance-directive educators also was a result of the task force's efforts. Currently over 400 individuals have completed this training in a nineteen-county area. These counselors are predominantly social workers, nurses, and chaplains. Volunteers are also participating in patient and staff education in some of the health care organizations. The public libraries have educational materials available as well.

Not only were the materials and the training program developed and implemented, but efforts are continually being made to improve how patients are asked about advance directives in the health care organizations. As part of a quality improvement effort at Gundersen Lutheran, nursing staff were surveyed to identify ways in which nurses could more effectively interact with patients about advance directives. As a result, a script was developed to assist nurses when they had conversations with patients on admission about advance directives. The survey also helped to identify ways in which documentation and communication could be improved between health care providers.

From April of 1995 until March of 1996, an extensive, community-wide retrospective study was done to look at end-of-life planning and end-of-life decisions in all health care organizations in the La Crosse community (Hammes, Rooney, 1997). The study revealed that of the 540 deaths reviewed, 85%

of adults had written advance directives and 81% had these documents in their health records (Hammes, 1998). The study also showed that families and physicians were aware of treatment preferences expressed in the advance directives and that these preferences were typically followed.

The results of the study indicate that the educational program, "Respecting Your Choices," developed from the partnership in the community of La Crosse, has had an impact on end-of-life planning. A significant number of advance-directive documents have been completed with patients. These documents could be found in the patients' medical records in the various health care organizations, and the decisions that were made at the end of life were consistent with the patients' wishes (Hammes, 1998). More important, partnerships developed and relationships were strengthened between providers and between providers and community as this community-wide program was developed and continues to be developed.

Discussions with patients about their preferences at the end of life are certainly not easy. However, not only do patients welcome these conversations, but they expect health care providers to initiate them (Towers, 1992).

These important end-of-life discussions with patients will further support the role shift that is needed, in which consumers of health care are acting more effectively on their own behalf by making choices based on *their* beliefs and values and exercising their self-determination. As patients become more involved, the relationship between the patient and the provider will take on a deeper meaning, and a true partnership will form.

HEALTHY LIVING PARTNERSHIPS THROUGH COMMUNITY-BASED PARISH NURSING

Parish nursing is one community-based application of nursing that is currently being initiated on a grass-roots level nationwide. The concept was introduced by Reverend Granger Westberg in 1984. Parish nurses are not direct service providers; rather they are stewards of the congregation's health. They encourage communities to assess their own health needs and develop their own solutions, while drawing on the resources of the health care partners. Parish nursing is a unique practice in that

it combines theology and nursing, focusing on the whole person and encouraging individuals to define their own quality of life. One of the primary functions of theology, says Engebretson (1996), is to provide explanatory models of life's purpose and meaning. Thus, experiencing a physical crisis can be looked upon as a learning experience about oneself, and rather than being paralyzed by the health crisis, one can be able to grow and move on.

When parish nurses are prepared and utilized, the community addresses not only the physical needs but also the spiritual needs of the population it serves. This link returns the church to its central place in the community as healer of body, mind, and spirit. The community-based parish nurse program encourages churches to participate in the program and help communities to become healthier.

The role of the parish nurse in the community is one of health educator, counselor, community resource liaison, facilitator of volunteers, and interpreter between faith and health (Westberg, 1990). Parish nurses also act as advocates to assist the congregation members in finding their way through health systems. They can make formal or informal referrals within the congregation to community services or to health services. Parish nurses serve as members of the church staff and become a link between the assessed needs of individuals and congregations and the health delivery systems in the community.

As Gundersen Lutheran stepped beyond its traditional institutional walls and into the communities it serves, the primary goal of the Parish Nursing Program was to prepare nurses for their new role in their congregations. The projected outcome of the program is for parish nurses (and thus churches) to be aware of and knowledgeable about the community and health resources and assist their church families in accessing them. The parish nurse is taught to walk with the individual, not do for the individual (Courtney et al, 1996).

Within the first two years, 55 nurses have gone through the Gundersen Lutheran parish nursing preparation course. The majority of these nurses are currently functioning in a nonpaid staff capacity within their churches. Two of these nurses have replicated Gundersen Lutheran's community-based program in their own communities and have trained an additional 53 nurses.

Parish nurses realize that people must be actively involved and invested in discovering their own solutions. With a clearer understanding of human existence and a view of life as a process, nurses are able to be with people in ways that respect and inspire them as they make personal choices. It is in this experience that deeper knowing, understanding, and acceptance occur, not only individually for the patient and the practitioners, but also globally in and for the community in which they live (Courtney et al, 1996).

Parish nurses have both a scientific and a spiritual background; thus they can establish a unique relationship with the people they come into contact with. This has been described as having "presence with another human being." Borysenko (1987) described presence as "holy moments" in which the professional boundaries shift from doing to patients, to working and being with other humans, traveling with them on their journey, respecting them and not judging, and loving and appreciating them for where they have been and who they are at this moment. The parish nurse practice environment sets the stage for this by allowing the nurse to go where those whom he or she serves live. This one act, in and of itself, demonstrates acceptance of another and allows the individual experiencing a health care crisis to be in his or her "safe environment." Parish nurses then are really seen as a caring partner, which allows the relationship to anchor this partnership model. When the relationship leads, the patient's capacity to act more effectively on his or her own behalf is strengthened; the "problem" may or may not be solved, but the patient's capacity to act is enhanced, which allows problems to be better handled in the future (Courtney et al, 1996). This "capacity to act" is perhaps the most significant outcome reported by parish nurses who are serving in community ministry from Gundersen Lutheran's parish nursing program.

Rydholm (1997) documented practitioners' outcomes from research he has done with parish nurses. In the 1800 stories of record, half the concerns that parish nurses address with patients are related to spiritual-psychosocial concerns such as unresolved feelings, transitions, caregiver stresses, and isolation. The other issues are related to physical concerns such as symptom disregard and struggles pertaining to functional safety or in-

dependence. Rydholm's documentation reveals that when parish nurses intervene, outcomes are favorable.

To illustrate this point, two stories from this parish nurse's experiences will be presented. The first describes the debilitating effect of isolation and the second of symptom disregard.

Story One. An 82-year-old man had not been to church for 18 years. On my first two attempts to visit him at his home, I was not permitted to enter. When I finally obtained permission to enter the kitchen on my third try, I noticed a deck of cards on the table. I asked if he played cards. The answer was a resounding yes. For the next two hours we played cards. Not much dialogue was shared. I asked if I might return again the same time next week. A positive response was given. After three weeks of card playing, the man began to tell his story of life. The man had lost his wife to cancer 18 years ago and had been left with an 11-year-old daughter to raise. He was the postmaster of a small town, and the mail had to continue being delivered. Through his own reflection and discovery, he realized he had never cried. He was able to do so with me and thus began the grieving process. He realized that he had become paralyzed with fear and that in his living he was just trying to survive. Through our discussions he was able to accept a referral to a physician for treatment of depression.

After two months he began to come to church for the potlucks. He was welcomed back enthusiastically and rekindled two old friendships. After four months of telling his story, he was volunteering and coordinating the mailing of the church's newsletter. He also was coordinating a team of three other volunteers who were assisting him. As a parish nurse, I was able to be with this individual in his journey and was able to allow him to rediscover who he was and where he had been. This ultimately helped him to reclaim life with a quality he desired.

This example clearly shows what can happen when the practitioner utilizes the knowledge, skills, and values of an individual. It was through the values of self-awareness, appreciation of the patient's whole person, respect for the mind/body/spirit unity, and the importance of being open and non-judgmental that I was able to establish a relationship that allowed the individual to rediscover who he was and become a functioning human being and a contributing member of a community.

Story Two. I was called by my minister to visit a 68-year-old woman. The minister stated that he had gone to visit the parish member, who had not been out of her house for one year. He stated that at this time she was only able to get to the bathroom by crawling, and he was unable to get her permission to seek medical assistance. I arrived to help the minister evaluate the situation. The parishioner was crying when I entered the home with the minister. I began to experience the home. I noticed the home was dark, unkempt, and smelling of urine. The parishioner was the same. I noticed pictures of family and of a farm. I had grown up on a farm and began talking about farming. After a few moments the patient stopped crying and engaged in a 45-minute conversation on farming and hauling manure. We shared much in common. I then came to hear her story. She had had severe degenerative arthritis for the past eight years and was on no medication. She felt that this was her burden in life and did not want to bother the doctor. Her mother had had this same condition, and nothing could be done for her forty years ago. She had learned just to accept and bear the pain and not be a "bother" to her scant family or society. I had happened to make this visit in my truck. I taught the minister how to do a two-man lift and took her to the emergency room, bundling her up in afghans from her home.

With support from social services and the Rheumatology Service, the patient was able to walk with a walker and went home three weeks later on steroids and pain medication. Public health nurses were involved to assist with her needs. After one week of being at home, the patient called me at my home to say that she was unable to get out of bed. I went to her home and called an ambulance. The patient was readmitted to the hospital and after one week discharged to a nursing home. The patient is currently in a wheelchair, able to move herself throughout the nursing home. She has told me how "bad off" these "poor" folks are and is now making visits to the other residents. She is coordinating the folding of linen for the nursing home, but still misses her home a lot. At the same time, the patient has rediscovered how much she missed being with others, and she enjoys being able to "help" these

people by visiting with them. She continues to feel that she is not a burden to her family or society.

This patient clearly had a stoic independence, a reluctance to burden physicians, and a knowledge deficit regarding current available treatment. Through the establishment of trust and a reframing of how intervention can facilitate greater independence and health, she was able to improve her quality of life, maximize her self-care capacities, and increase her socialization.

According to Rydholm (1997) few systems are able to troubleshoot patients' reluctance to seek health care as easily as parish nurses can. She believes parish nurses can do this because of the relationships they have developed with patients. Rydholm refers to parish nurses as "insider experts." These nurses use their relational understanding to teach empowering self-care according to their patients' own agendas. Honoring the patients' values and understanding their stories of life are key capacities of the parish nurse, which foster the patients' capacity to act more effectively on their own behalf.

Bringing the Learning Back to Health Care Institutions

You cannot change one aspect of care delivery in an integrated delivery system without it affecting all others. The work by health care practitioners in the homes and communities of the patients we serve is beginning to have implications for providers in Gundersen Lutheran's acute hospital and ambulatory clinics. These implications center around patients who are clearer and more articulate in discussing their values and their needs. Moreover, these patients understand what quality of life means to them. They expect to participate in care that is given and in decisions made about that care.

This evolving role for our patients is exactly what is needed as health care reforms itself. The expectation by patients that providers along the entire health care continuum will foster development of this role is one way of building consistency and accountability by all caregivers. Our struggles as a large organization remain in the consistency of this approach across the entire system. To assist in strengthening our accountability as providers in meeting patients' new expectations, a Patient

Health and Resource Center is being constructed on the main campus of Gundersen Lutheran. The purpose of the center is to foster the development of knowledgeable and confident patients as they address their health care issues and decision making. The learning resulting from the work in our communities with advance-directive and parish nursing programs has informed us and provided the cornerstone for the center's work and approach to relationships with those we serve. The opportunities for change within our system and the real reform necessary in health care delivery relate to *fully maximizing the contributions of our new partners* and learning more from them about health as it is being generated.

References

American Organization of Nurse Executives: *Patient as partner: the cornerstone of community health improvement,* Chicago, 1997, American Hospital Publishing, Inc.

Borysenko J: *Minding the body, mending the mind,* Reading, Mass, 1987, Addison-Wesley Publishing Co.

Colvin ER, Hammes BJ: If I only knew: a patient education program on advance directives, *ANNA Journal* 18:557-560, December 1991.

Colvin E, Myhre M, Welch J, Hammes B: Moving beyond the patient self-determination act: how do we educate patients to be autonomous? *American Nephrology Nurses Association Journal* 20:564-568, October 1993.

Courtney R: Community partnership primary care: a new paradigm for primary care, *Public Health Nursing* 12(6):366-373, December 1995.

Courtney R, Ballard E, Fauver S, Gariota M, Holland L: The partnership model: working with individuals, families and communities toward a new vision of health, *Public Health Nursing* 13(3):177-186, June 1996.

DeBack V, Cohen EL: The new practice environment. In Cohen EL, ed: *Nursing case management in the 21st century,* St Louis, 1996, Mosby, pp 3-9.

Engebretson J: Considerations in diagnosing in the spiritual domain, *Nursing Diagnosis* 7(3):100-107, 1996.

Hammes, BJ. Respecting your choices: one community's successful advance directives program. In: Miles S, Faber-Langendoen K, eds. *Improved End-of-Life Care: The HMO Challenge.* Frederick, Md: University Publishing Group. In press.

Hammes BJ, Rooney BL: Death and end-of-life planning in one midwestern community, *Arch Inter Med* 158: 383-390, 1998.

Hammes BJ, Rooney BL, Bendiksen BA: Advance directive survey of adults before the patient self-determination act. Unpublished report, Gundersen Medical Foundation, La Crosse, Wis, 1991.

Miles SH, Koepp R, Weber E: Advance end-of-life treatment planning, *Archives of Internal Medicine* 156:1062-1068, 1996.

Quill TE, Brody H: Physician recommendations and patient autonomy: finding a balance between physician power and patient choice, *Annals of Internal Medicine* 125(9):763-768, November 1996.

Rydholm L: Patient-focused care in parish nursing, *Holistic Nursing Practice* 11(3):47-60, 1997.

Schroeder C: Community partnerships and medical models of health? I don't think so . . . *Public Health Nursing* 11(5):283-284, 1994.

Towers J: Advance care directives: counseling the patient and family in the primary care setting, *Nurse Practitioner Forum* 3(1):25-27, 1992.

Tresolini CP, Pew-Fetzer Task Force: *Health professions education and relationship-centered care,* San Francisco, 1994, Pew Health Professions Commission.

Westberg GE: *The parish nurse,* Minneapolis, 1990, Augsburg Fortress.

CHAPTER 17

Longitudinal Profiling

A Differentiated Community Nursing Model

GWENNETH A. JENSEN, RN, MN, CNS, **and JoELLEN GOERTZ KOERNER,** RN, PhD, FAAN

OVERVIEW

Interdisciplinary collaborative management of increasingly complex patients replaced the old paradigm of care planning and task completion, while broadening the accountability for outcomes care.

This emerging community model integrates the following elements: theory-based practice with respect for the client's lived experience of health, personal definition of health care value, and right to informed choices for health care; an evidence-based search for the irreducible minimum in quality patient management through differentiated case/population management, risk appraisal, risk analysis, and stratification; and a commitment to integration of clinical and financial outcomes measurement. This model is applied in a differentiated group practice, led by advanced practice registered nurses (APRN) who embrace core principles of first-party dialog, mutual valuing, collaboration, and co-consulting. The model is based on a belief that nursing is inherently relational, cognitive, and active-collaborative, as opposed to technical, passive, and delegated. It recognizes the contextual imperatives of corporate constraint and financial necessity, but harbors the professional courage to innovate, advocate, and negotiate for consumer-centered health programs. ▲

In a rapidly changing health care world, connected by information systems, driven by sociopolitical and corporate ideology, the relational essence of health care delivery and the mindset of its practitioners are being challenged. The relationship between quality, consumer value, and measurable outcomes of care must be explored and *co*-analyzed by teams of administrative and clinical experts, acting in concert to invite change in a budget-neutral, cost-reducing manner. This requires *new ways of thinking* about health care delivery, *new ways of being* with health consumers, and *new ways of doing* hands-on care.

Reengineering of health care systems is bringing redefinition of provider roles and work space in community settings. Institution-based episode of illness is shifting to continuum-based health that focuses on patient flow across the system. Health, self-care, and life-management skills are taking the place of illness-focused, provider-stipulated care (Porter-O'Grady, 1997). Successful health plans are offering portable services in various community settings for convenience, easy access, and "health appeal" to busy subscribers. In concert, the role of the RN shifts to primary provider, case manager, service broker, health partner, teacher, and coach. The RN expands from the traditional "bedside" role to "clientside," moving with the client through the system continuum.

The most successful portable services are flexible, user friendly, low cost, mobile, and computerized. The accompanying information system infrastructure needs the capacity and flexibility to build and network common and special databases. Episodic and longitudinal clinical and financial outcomes must be tracked for patterns and relationships over time. Trackable indicators sensitive to the effects of nursing and interdisciplinary clinical interventions must be created, researched, and embedded in emerging systems. National standards, guidelines, protocols, and benchmark data from comparable health systems are already in use to reduce variation in practice. Standardized, but customizable, methodologies are being created, such as integrated clinical pathways that guide interdisciplinary providers with the health system continuum.

Mass Customization

Mass customization concepts applied in manufacturing can be adapted and applied to health care to create customer-unique value (Gilmore, Pine, 1997) (Box 17-1). We are challenged with the paradoxical thinking of simultaneously standardizing and customizing care. As in business, health providers must be sensitive to consumer sociocultural characteristics, perceived health needs and desires, and the demand patterns of targeted populations. These softer social and behavioral elements are being integrated with the most up-to-date scientific clinical evidence to create a case/population management approach with personal "fit." For instance, Mrs. Jones, a recently retired widow with three chronic conditions, who screens positive for depression, may be less interested in trying a costly new medication than in finding an apartment before winter that will fit within her current budget. A housing authority or social services referral may be prerequisite to other health interventions. A standardized health appraisal with customized or population-specific risk "triggers" may red flag such issues for quick review and dialogue between the consumer/subscriber and the provider, thus preventing an unnecessary decline into illness and costly hospitalization.

Standardization of risk assessment and intervention strategies is informed by such bodies as the Joint Commission on Accreditation of Healthcare Organizations (JCAHO) and the National Committee for Quality Assurance (NCQA). These agencies have introduced sets of standardized clinical and utilization indicators for outcome measurement and monitoring for health systems.

Differentiating Outside the Walls

Nursing case management has been in existence in our 400-bed hospital since the practice differentiated in 1989 (Koerner, Karpiuk, 1994). That model was founded on principles of the original primary nursing concepts of the 1970s and 1980s: consistent caregivers; holistic, patient-centered planning; and coordinated care and services within a hospital setting. The primary nurse, or case manager, had the authority and autonomy for care decisions and was accountable to guide care delivery toward financially sound goals. Early outcomes of primary nursing models included reduced hospital length of

BOX 17-1
A Health Care Application of Mass Customization

Standardized

Evidence-driven practice

Core appraisal and care process

Structured care methodologies to reduce and track practice variation (e.g., pathways, guidelines)

Customized

Consumer-responsive; service-oriented

Identifiable risk triggers; timely referral, follow-up

Critical thinking

Collaborative, interdisciplinary care

Consumer Driven

Relational, interactive dialogue

Consumer-provider partnerships

Care delivery models that support shared decision making and informed consumer choice

Packaged and Convenient

Accessible, timely, portable

Knowledgeable, approachable, low-cost providers

Coordinated, one-stop service brokerage

Informed and Networked

Common languaging to organize data, foster meaningful analysis, and communicate across public and private systems

Research and Development

Feedback and feedforward mechanisms

Real-time outcomes analysis

Valid consumer satisfaction measures

Partnerships with higher education, public and private agencies, and community groups

---

stay (LOS) and cost of care, reduced recidivism, and increased patient satisfaction. However, this early single-case or unit-based approach to care delivery in the hospital setting lacked aggregate analysis of populations and did not extend across the continuum. It also lacked measures related to physiologic outcomes, quality of life, functional status, and identification of high-risk subgroups within populations.

In the first generation of an Advanced Practice RN case management model, focus was on the one-to-one relationship of an APRN and single high-resource-user cases, or HULAS (*h*eavy *u*sers, *l*osers, and *a*busers). This model was usually initiated after an inpatient acute care stay and extended into the patient's home setting after discharge. Case finding was based on case complexity, recidivism, or other pattern of unusual utilization or high cost. This method of case finding during or after crisis and in the midst of intensive resource use is a high-cost method for subscriber systems. As the concept of outcomes management developed in the literature, the one-to-one nursing case management model within its differentiated practice context began to shift. Episodic care gave way to longitudinal management of whole populations of patients. Risk as-

sessment of managed subscribers increased. Evidence-based care practices and evolving national guidelines mandated continuous scrutiny of local practice patterns, care methodologies, and outcomes of care. Interdisciplinary *collaborative management* of increasingly complex patients replaced the old paradigm of care planning and task completion, while broadening the accountability for outcomes of care.

The advent of integrated clinical pathways (ICPs), reflective of "re-modeling" in the next generation, provided a collaborative, multidisciplinary foundation for care delivery coordination, and, later, for outcomes management. Clinical pathways are evolving to facilitate coordination of complex, longitudinal care driven by evidence-based care methodologies. They assist in targeting, documenting, and tracking abstractable outcomes reflecting physiological, functional, utilization, and cost outcomes. As hospital-based care moves into the community, longitudinal clinical pathways, with greater emphasis on health maintenance and self-care of chronic disease, help to focus attention on longitudinal outcomes. In the future, visual trajectories from these outcomes may be consumer-friendly tools to help client-provider partnerships

BOX 17-2
Outcomes: Measuring, Monitoring, or Managing?

Ellwood defined outcomes management as a "technology of patient experience designed to help patients, payors and providers make rational medical care-related choices based on insight into the effect of these choices on the patient's life" (Ellwood, 1988). According to Ellwood, outcomes management programs should include:

- An emphasis on standards to help guide interventions
- Measurement of functioning, well-being, and disease-specific clinical outcomes
- Large-scale, aggregate pooling of outcomes data
- Analysis and dissemination of the database to appropriate decision makers.

Definitions of Outcomes Measurement, Monitoring, and Management

Outcomes measurement is the systematic, quantitative observation, at a point in time, of outcome indicators.

Example A: In the initial data set, 50% of patients with a secondary diagnosis of DM had Hgb A1C's and foot evaluations performed in the previous 6 months.

Outcomes monitoring is the repeated measures over time of outcome indicators in a manner that permits causal inferences about what produced the observed patient outcomes.

Example B: After repeated measures on all DM patients in the clinic, Hgb A1C's were obtained twice yearly on 80% of those attending an education session and receiving newsletter updates; 90% of all member diabetics had been seen in the health maintenance clinic for foot evaluations within the past 3 months.

Outcomes management is the use of information and knowledge gained from outcomes monitoring to achieve optimal patient outcomes through improved clinical decision-making and service delivery.

Example C: A longitudinal clinical pathway for DM was amended to include twice-yearly Hgb A1C draws and quarterly foot clinic checkups, with referral to podiatric services as needed.

to understand and manage self-care and health maintenance (Box 17-2).

Longitudinal Profiling: The CareSpan™ Community Project

A pilot template for interdisciplinary population management was developed for a community outreach project (Figure 17-1). The project is based on a model of care delivery called "longitudinal profiling" and is targeted to the longitudinal management of persons with chronic disease.

The shared vision for the CareSpan project was created after months of dialogue by advanced practice nurses who sought a new approach to case management of populations within the context of differentiated practice. Guiding principles for the APRN practice group are listed in Box 17-3.

Longitudinal profiling is defined as a process of health management involving a longitudinal thera-

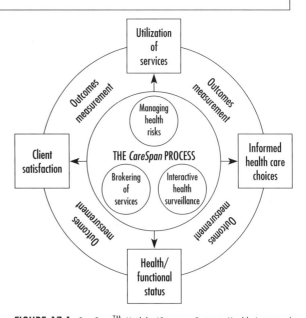

FIGURE 17-1 CareSpan™ Model. (Courtesy Geriatric Health Institute/ Sioux Valley Hospital.)

BOX 17-3

Advanced Practice Registered Nurse Guiding Principles

True presence
Authenticity
Expert knowledge
Theory-based practice
Evidence-based practice
Outcomes measurement
Collaboration
Co-consulting
Co-creating

---

peutic alliance with a client or client group that involves:

- Advanced application of a clinical reasoning process
- Brokering of identified resources/service needs
- Interactive surveillance of clinical status, utilization, health behaviors, and quality of life
- Outcomes tracking, including longitudinal clinical and functional trajectory, perceived satisfaction with the mutually determined health plan, and utilization of services and cost

The CareSpan model targets more homogeneous groups of non-acutely ill clients across the life span and takes the service "client-side," outside the institution to wherever the client resides. It incorporates concepts of mass customization through targeted, core risk appraisal and screening, followed by individualized risk analysis and prescription within the client's lived experience of health and personal health choices. Within this model, the client is considered expert in his or her own health (Parse, 1995). The client, not the provider, drives health management strategies in partnership with the RN as coach and broker. The provider's menu of services along with community resources provides the RN and client an array of choices to "fit" both client and system goals. Foci of the model include risk reduction, measurement, functional health maintenance or improvement, and perceived quality of life within the client's definition and experience of health.

This project targets older adults, the fastest-growing segment of the United States population. Technology, better public health practices, and lifestyle modifications are increasing longevity. This, in turn, creates a strategic need for longitudinal management of costly chronic illnesses, an ideal venue for APRN interventions. Unfortunately, timely opportunities for potent low-tech interventions are often missed in community-dwelling populations of older adults.

The Role of the Advanced Practice RN: Risk Reduction and Population Management

The clinical reasoning process begins with assessment of the client's current and potential problems. Advanced practice RNs (APRNs) possess "a high level of expertise in the assessment, diagnosis, and treatment of the complex responses of individuals, families, or communities to actual or potential health problems, prevention of illness and injury, maintenance of wellness, and provision of comfort" (ANA, 1996). According to Harris (1997), APRNs not only recognize and treat complex responses related to health and illness but also demonstrate expertise in reducing the risks of complex responses. This dimension of advanced practice, according to Harris, focuses on the "integration of clients within complex health care systems and environments, and on the complex trajectories of cascading events that can result in complex responses."

These complex responses often result from multiple interacting factors and can result in exacerbations of chronic conditions, critical events, increased use of health services, and deteriorating quality of life. Harris suggests that reducing the risk of complex responses is an unrecognized outcome of advanced practice nursing, related to risk assessment and risk management.

Risk appraisal is a survey for the presence of, or exposure to, factors known or suspected to be associated with adverse consumer or provider outcomes, including clinical, functional, satisfaction, and financial outcomes. Risk analysis assists decision making and stratification of the degree of risk for adverse outcomes. Risk management seeks to control or ameliorate internal and external conditions leading to greater risk of adverse outcomes for targeted groups or populations.

Coordination of collaborative interdisciplinary risk appraisal, analysis, and clinical management has become part of the expanding role of the APRN in health systems. In addition to expert clinical knowledge and process consulting, the APRN brings expertise in communication and group leadership (Grady, Wojner, 1996). By using these skills in an on-site interdisciplinary group practice, or virtual group practice, he or she is also in the unique position to help frame and integrate clinical and financial outcomes measurement and management. By analyzing clinical iterations of health maintenance intervention strategies combined with financial and utilization outcome measurements, the APRN can lead the effort toward "best practice" for patient populations in community.

Risk Appraisal

Risk appraisal has become the cornerstone of managed care plans. A variety of instruments have been developed in an effort to target subscribers and conditions most amenable to early intervention. Few evidence-based instruments, however, have been developed specifically for the needs of older adults. Such an assessment should target high-risk health behaviors, preexisting chronic conditions and current treatments, and functional and cognitive deficits as measures of impairment and unique risk. To date, the relationships between functional health status, health perception, health behaviors, preexisting conditions, and utilization of services by older adults are unclear.

A rather extensive evidence-based, risk appraisal process was developed for this demonstration. A more concise, "drilled down," process is expected and would be recommended for implementation in a full-scale program.

The appraisals were carried out at four sites, three of which were independent community residential complexes, within an upper-midwestern city of approximately 120,000 people. The purpose of this front-end comprehensive assessment process was to thoroughly describe client health status, health behaviors, functional performance, and utilization patterns. Abstractable and reproducible data sets were developed for each client as well as for the aggregate population. Evidence-based mea-

sures were abstracted from the risk-appraisal compendium, resulting in individual, confidential health profiles. Domains of measurement included prevention and wellness practices, self-care function, mobility, nutrition, cognition, affect, social integration, physiological stability, and sensory status. Proxy indicators for measurement were guided by current literature, Health Employee Data Information Set 3.0 (HEDIS 3.0) guidelines for measurement and reporting, Healthy People 2000 recommendations and targets, and a select battery of instruments and performance tools derived from the literature for this population.

In the CareSpan project, the first contact comprehensive assessment required anywhere from 20 to 90 minutes of RN time, depending on the self-report ability and desires of the clients in the demonstration project. Some clients preferred interview to self-report because of sensory problems or other issues that make paper-and-pencil self-appraisal difficult. For those who chose the self-report method, RN contact was limited to a brief functional performance measure and APRN review of the paper-and-pencil data. This review gave the APRN an early "gestalt" of risk level and was enhanced by real-time review of the SF-36 Health Status Profile, generated on-site by computer printout. Direct health counseling by the RN for low-risk clients may begin and end with this review, although indirect health education is continuous via other accessible programs within CareSpan.

The flexibility of the data collection methodology/appraisal process has enhanced recruitment for this stage of the project. The current appraisal process is expected to be significantly reduced when only known potent variables are assessed.

Using statistical analysis of this broad data set, the search for patterns and relationships begins, leading to application of appropriate meaning. A by-product of this risk assessment and analysis process is the continued search for the "irreducible minimum," that is, the most meaningful, yet succinct, assessment data set for a given population.

After risk analysis and client consultation, management strategies based on risk level, client readiness, and informed choice are developed. These strategies are developed to reduce risk, decrease critical events resulting in high-cost hospitalizations, stabilize the trajectory of chronic decline while improving quality of life, and reduce overall cost of care.

Program Implementation

Embedded within the framework of differentiated practice, implementation of this model partners an APRN and a Primary Nurse (PN) with a client group (Box 17-4). Within the model, the relational aspects of trust and accessibility, so important to clients with chronic disease and considerable risk, are largely accomplished through a lower-cost, on-site PN who staffs a tri-weekly nursing clinic, brokers services, and manages episodic health concerns in collaboration with the APRN. Profiles of each client are reviewed for risk stratification and categorization, and succinct plans of interactive surveillance and monitoring are developed with at-risk clients. Low-risk clients generally have minimal contacts and interventions compared with high-risk clients. A second-level focused assessment results for moderate and high-risk clients, with possible referral to other appropriate disciplines involved in the management of complex, high-risk populations. For instance, first-level screening for fall risk includes three simple measures and history of a fall within the past year. A second-level assessment includes a gait and balance screen and possible referral to a sister program called *On Your Feet,* a no-cost fall prevention program staffed by a physical therapist

---

BOX 17-4
A Differentiated Practice Community Model

Risk appraisal by APRN and PN
Risk analysis by APRN
Client-driven goal setting
Collaborative planning with client, PN, and APRN
Portability: client-side in community
Interactive surveillance and on-site clinics by PN
Telephone consultation and periodic on-site visits by APRN
Data tracking by APRN and PN
Data analysis by APRN and PhD

---

and an APRN and sponsored by a partnering program.

Higher-risk CareSpan enrollees may meet with the RN/APRN in tri-weekly on-site health maintenance clinics within their residential living centers to discuss the clients' health goals. Intervention strategies are mutually determined in partnership with the RN coach, based on the client's preferences and lived experience of health. Health education, ongoing monitoring of chronic health issues, and evaluation of acute episodes or critical events are also conducted in clinic.

The client's priorities for health and lifestyle options are considered within the risk assessment and analysis process. By ongoing partnering and co-consulting, the APRN collaborates with the client, the PN, and a customized network of care providers to create an efficient intervention and surveillance plan driven by the client's informed choices. In addition, health education programs and screenings are held for the target population each month, teaching clients primary, secondary, and tertiary prevention strategies and self-management skills for existing chronic problems.

Early Programming

In addition to the health maintenance clinics and the health education and screenings cited above, special programs are being developed in concert with the older adults, based on needs identified in the profile process.

Of these emerging programs, some of the greatest "satisfiers" have been group activities and a brief, bimonthly newsletter.

The newsletter captures activities and health topics that are relevant to the expressed interests and needs of the older adults in the CareSpan project. Participants comment frequently about information they have read and ask for clarification in applying it to their own health care situations and needs. Clients have been empowered to dialogue with physician-providers about medications and symptom management, as well as to take charge of self-care decisions and lifestyle adjustments for health promotion and maintenance of chronic conditions.

Group health promotion activities are also popular for their health impact and socialization opportunities. For instance, a low-impact-exercise group now meets regularly for those older adults with arthritis or other painful physical ailments who did not attend a preexisting exercise group. Led by a PN, the class started after a kickoff education session by a physical therapist. The group now "swings" to classic oldies music and special chair sitting exercises, augmented by stretchable bands and soup cans, to improve flexibility and strength for upper and lower extremities. Socialization and peer support have attracted new membership to the group and to the CareSpan membership project.

Inside walking clubs are also starting in residential complexes, with modest incentives built in to motivate participation and track progress. Plans are underway for other groups or clubs, such as Tai Chi and a "mental gymnastics club" with an array of puzzles, games, and mind teasers of varying difficulty to maintain mental fitness.

Outcomes

Clinical and utilization outcome indicators for the CareSpan project reflect measures of primary, secondary, and tertiary prevention and health maintenance behaviors, some of which are listed in Box 17-5. The Consumer Assessment of Health Plans Survey (CAHPS) from the Medical Outcomes Study served as a template from which a consumer satisfaction survey was adapted.

Prior health service utilization patterns were assessed by self-report for a period prior to the health appraisal. Following the appraisal survey, utilization is being tracked each month for each participant. Utilization indicators include: inpatient and outpatient visits, such as clinic visits or overnight hospitalizations or nursing home stays; LOS and recidivism; other resource consumption, such as x-rays and medications; descriptions of usual providers in the last year, such as primary and specialty physicians, nurse practitioners, and physician assistants, and duration of time with the primary provider.

Nursing activities and costs within the clinic are also being tracked. Clinic visits are counted, timed, and catalogued by reason for visit. Clients receive recommendations on a CareSpan Health Maintenance Rx slip, which also serves to track client needs and provider interventions and can be added to the clinic chart for ease of documentation and follow-up. In the initial 2 months of the demonstra-

---

BOX 17-5
Clinical Indicator Categories

Primary Prevention

Definition
Health promotion, education, immunizations, risk reduction

Indicators
Age-appropriate immunizations
Medications
Attendance at health education programs
Self-perception of health

Secondary Prevention

Definition
Screening, early detection, and containment to arrest or slow progression of of illness after presymptomatic diagnosis

Indicators
Mammography
Prostate screens
BP screens
Stroke screens
Fall risk assessment

Tertiary Prevention

Definition
Chronic disease symptom management to mitigate debilitation and minimize acute exacerbations

Indicators
Select measures of functional performance (e.g., SF-36)
Physiological indicators of disease management (e.g., diabetes mellitus, chronic lung disease, congestive heart failure)
Tracking of critical events and complications of illness

---

tion project, walk-in visits have increased to about 40 to 50 per week at two clinic sites. The interactive surveillance model includes not only client-initiated contacts but also some nurse-initiated telephone follow-up and an occasional home visit.

The most common referrals are collaborative-care calls to physicians' offices for medication adjustments or new complaints (some of which have resulted in new diagnoses) or to report on monitoring activities, such as blood pressure regulation. Because the project is only in its second month of full implementation, nursing utilization data are in the very early stages of collection and analysis.

The clinics have been a real satisfier for the populations served. Initial client satisfaction survey results indicated overwhelming support for easily accessed on-site health maintenance clinics and the security of knowing someone was available to help with health issues. The trust relationship between the PNs and the clients is a major satisfier for both. The relationship with the private agency has also client satisfaction and increased marketing potential for the private agency. An overview of outcomes and facility benefits is presented in Box 17-6.

Demonstration project data analysis is underway at this writing. Profile data for the current demonstration have been collected on nearly 150 older adults; about 85 of these will have access to the population/case management program. A second appraisal will be conducted at the end of the demonstration, comparing the case-managed group with a control group.

The initial pilot project, prior to the current demonstration, operated by contracts with private

agencies serving older adult populations in the community. The current demonstration is partially grant funded, with in-kind support from the agencies and our health system.

During the previous pilot project, start-up profiling, risk analysis, and mutual planning with each client required an average of 1.5 hours of APN time and 0.75 hour of Primary Nurse time. That time requirement has already been reduced in this revised demonstration, partially by the self-report option for the health profile. The maintenance cost of the program is primarily personnel time, with minimal overhead costs for the clinic. Rental expense for clinic space on site was bartered back for partial payment of contracted services. The PN spends 6 hours per week in each clinic and 1 to 3 hours per week in follow-up and brokering of services for at-risk clients. Utilization of the walk-in clinic by clients is related to their risk index and the need for ongoing monitoring and periodic intervention and follow-up for illness episodes and clinical monitoring.

In a future subscriber-enrollment model, the profile data could be updated at intervals to create a longitudinal database and "longitudinal profile" of client progress through the later years. These data would also invite ongoing intervention and program evaluations, building future community "best practice" models.

Conclusion

In this age of exploding information, rapid change, and paradoxical downsizing for more efficient health care delivery, providers struggle with sustaining quality of care in efficient patient-management systems. Foundational to development of successful management systems that can demonstrate cost-effective and consumer-satisfying outcomes is a dynamic set of tools and processes that can be applied to an aggregate population or an individual in a relevant, timely fashion. As clinicians increasingly adopt skills that include population-based thinking and methods, evidence-based management, quality improvement, and consumer empowerment, the health of society will be enhanced. Improved quality of life for the person and the family also increases professional satisfaction of the clinician privileged to provide services. This increases the quality and productivity of the

---

BOX 17-6
Overview of Outcomes From Initial CareSpan Pilot

- 100% influenza immunizations
- Increase in healthy behaviors (e.g., diet modification, exercise)
- Decrease in falls and fallers
- Increase in participation in health screenings
- Increase in participation in health education
- Increase in health monitoring for high-risk residents
- Decrease in medication use and cost
- Zero deficiencies in facility regulatory survey
- High consumer satisfaction with on-site services
- Coordination of other brokered services

health system serving communities, enhancing the well-being of humanity. In interdependent fashion, we are moving closer to whole-earth health.

References

American Nurses' Association: *Scope and standards of advanced practice registered nursing*, Washington, DC, 1996, The Association.

Ellwood PM: Outcomes management: a technology of patient experience, *New England Journal of Medicine* 318:1549-1556, 1988.

Forkner DJ: Clinical pathways: benefits and liabilities, *Nursing Management* 27(11):35-38, 1996.

Gibson SJ: Differentiated practice within and beyond the hospital walls. In Cohen EC, ed: *Nurse case management in the 21st century*, St Louis, 1996, Mosby, pp 222-244.

Gilmore JH, Pine BJ: The four faces of mass customization, *Harvard Business Review,* pp 91-101, January-February 1997.

Grady GF, Wojner AW: Collaborative practice teams: the infrastructure of outcomes management, *AACN Clinical Issues* 7(1):153-158, 1996.

Harris M: Reduced risk of complex response: an invisible outcome, *Nursing Administration Quarterly* 21(4):25-31, 1997.

Koerner JG: Differentiated practice: the evolution of professional nursing, *Journal of Professional Nursing* 8(6):335-341, 1992.

Koerner JG, Karpiuk KL: *Implementing differentiated nursing practice: transformation by design,* Gaithersburg, Md, 1994, Aspen Publishers, Inc.

Parse R: The human becoming theory. In Parse RR, ed: *Illuminations: the human becoming theory in practice and research,* New York, 1995, National League for Nursing.

Porter-O'Grady T: Over the horizon: the future and the advanced practice nurse, *Nursing Administration Quarterly* 21(4):1-11, 1997.

CHAPTER 18

The Changing Environment for Outcomes Management

Which Way to Go

MARITA MacKINNON SCHIFALACQUA, RN, MSN, **and VICKI M. GEORGE**, RN, PhD(c)

OVERVIEW

There are always benefits and losses to every management approach. The key is to have the outcome drive the structure and not the structure drive the outcome.

The journey of change began with the assessment of the hospital and community environment and continued with the adaptation and development of a specific plan for that environment. The implementation and evaluation of the innovation are the cornerstones for any change. The following is a description of the outcomes management journey of St. Luke's Medical Center, Milwaukee, Wisconsin. The multidisciplinary outcome facilitation team structure was developed into a two-level model. The levels consisted of both an aggregate and an individual patient focus. The structure and processes were based in theory and principles of systems thinking, case management, and decision making. The evaluation reflects increases in patient satisfaction and overall decreases in unit length of stay. ▲

"It is all around people—in the seasons, in their social environment, and in their own biological processes. Beginning with the first few moments of life, a person learns to meet change by being adaptive" (Davis, Newstrom, 1989). This quotation implies that change has been with every person since the beginning of time. In health care organizations the acceleration and the amount of change are on an upward trajectory. Many of the driving forces for change are being exerted from external influences, including government policies, accrediting bodies, reimbursement, and technology. Some of the internal forces of change include the quality-improvement momentum, the focus on outcome-based care, the access to care, and the necessity to have a financially solvent health care delivery system.

The need for change was recognized at St. Luke's Medical Center (SLMC), but identifying the nature and scope of that change was a bit more challenging. SLMC is a 700-bed tertiary, not-for-profit, community hospital located on the south side of Milwaukee, Wisconsin. SLMC is recognized nationally and internationally for its clinical excellence in cancer and heart care. It is a part of Aurora Health Care, the leading provider of health care services in eastern Wisconsin, which is dedicated to personalized, high-quality, cost-effective care.

Environmental Assessment

The assessment of SLMC's environment revealed that the market demands for high quality and reasonable costs were the same forces that were driving the evolution of health services in the United States in general. These forces are rapidly giving way to consolidation of providers, standardization of health care processes, and mass marketing to improve market share through increased levels of patient satisfaction.

The administrative staff attributed much of the financial and customer-satisfaction success at SLMC to the organizational structure of product/service line management that was adopted in the early 1980s. A key issue in patient care was viewing the nature of health care services as a delivered product or service. Unlike raw materials and manufactured goods, services are not highly tangible. Services are more or less spontaneous, and the customer is an active participant in the delivery process.

The health care customer interfaces most frequently with the point-of-service provider. For providers to perform their jobs well, they must be able to assess services and to personalize them according to the needs of its customers. The SLMC management philosophy was to create the climate to empower the staff to make the outcomes happen successfully, both to be satisfying to the customer and to be fiscally responsible to the organization. A bond develops between the staff and the customer that must be reconciled between the staff and the organizational goals. The SLMC unit-based manager has the accountability on a daily basis to help manage the system. The staff needs to be able to balance the customer needs and to be fiscally proactive by aligning all the interested parties (Porter-O'Grady, 1997).

The nursing shared governance model at SLMC's integrated nursing across the product/service lines. The shared governance model has been in place at SLMC since the early 1980s. In 1990, the model focused on the need for the structure to foster an accountability-based system. The staff nurse's councils (Figure 18-1) were charged with decision making and futures planning. The nurses and the council infrastructure were well accepted by members of the multidisciplinary team. For example, a registered nurse leader of the hospital-wide quality council and the chair of the practice are members of the Medical Executive Committee and the Patient Care Council.

In the early 1990s the nursing division adapted the following two influential processes:

1. The transition from a clinical ladder to a clinical practice development model based on Benners' (1984) novice-to-expert framework. The novice-to-expert developmental model had produced the structure that allowed SLMC the ability to measure the level of expertise of the clinical staff nurse. All 1200 SLMC registered nurses were staged along that continuum, with 75% of the RNs being assessed at the proficient or expert status. These results indicated that the nurses at the bedside had strength in practice for care coordination, which is a behavior associated with the proficient or expert nurse.

2. The redesigning of the nursing shared governance council (see Figure 18-1). The nursing practice council makes decisions regarding professional nursing practice. The new practice council determined that the staff nurse was the coordinator of patient care delivery.

The structure and accountabilities depicted the importance of the nursing practice for decision making and the strengths of the nurses themselves. The staff nurse is the single most important variable in assessing the environment for a practice change.

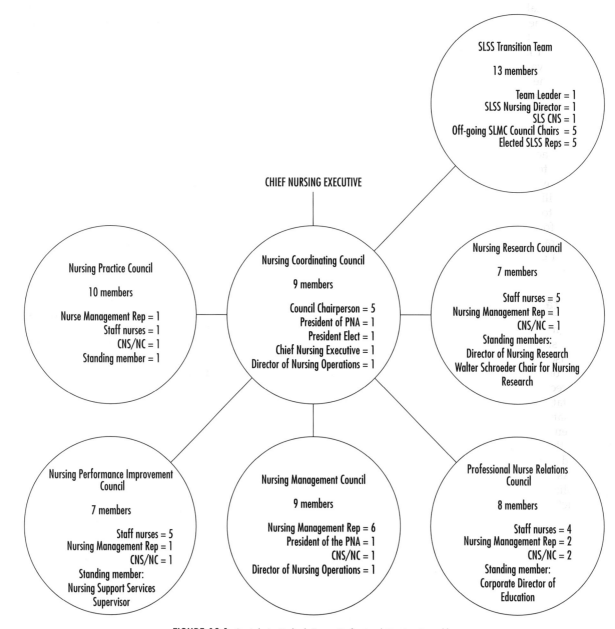

FIGURE 18-1 St. Luke's Medical Center Professional Nursing Assembly.

The challenge of the leadership was to design a unit-based infrastructure to enhance care coordination. The care coordination function of the bedside practitioner needed to be supported through many avenues. Examples of support included but were not limited to having the appropriate staffing resources and the mentorship of a clinical nurse specialist (CNS) to grow the staff nurse's practice. The service standards of SLMC defined stated that the care coordination needs of the patient and family need to be individually identified and evaluated.

After the assessment of the environment, the new structure needed to bring together identified major strategic elements, including the product/service line management successes and staff nurse autonomy. The high level of recognized professional practice allowed for the point-of-service provider to be the key decision maker for overall improvement in service delivery to patients and families. A new collaborative structure was needed to determine an integrative, consistent process for the service line delivery and professional practice. The outcomes needed to be realized in a comprehensive, timely, and cost-efficient manner.

Adaptation to the Environment

A design team was initiated for the purpose of creating a structure and process that would support multidisciplinary planning and accomplishment of patient outcomes. The team consisted of the service line directors, the vice president/chief nurse executive, staff nurses, and the project coordinator for case management.

Essential to success was designing care outcomes through a multidisciplinary structure, which needed the full support of the product line directors. As major stakeholders, the directors needed to realize how a new process could benefit the product/service line goals and products. These directors needed to become the leadership for the structure change, as they would be supporting the implementation.

Many motivating forces brought the design team to the table. One of the external forces was the new emphasis of the JCAHO survey on the multidisciplinary focus of patient care design. An internal force was the opportunity to strengthen the product/service line efficiencies and effect

quality patient outcomes measures. Each product/service line team leader was charged in his/her goals to develop measures that would reflect that the care delivered fell into the 75 percent of quality and the bottom one third of cost as benchmark to other competitive and perceived equality products.

There are always benefits and losses to every management approach. The key is to have the outcome drive the structure and not the structure drive the outcome. The process needs to be fluid enough to embrace diversity of interventions, and that will improve the defined outcome and product.

The design team agreed to integrate the principles of case management into the product line structure. This structure would meet the JCAHO requirements for multidisciplinary team involvement in patient care delivery. The design team agreed that the outcomes would be data driven in the following categories: clinical quality; service/satisfaction; process; and financial.

The essence of that coordination lay in the principles of case management, which is defined as the organization and sequencing of services to respond to an individual's health care problems and to plan, coordinate, and provide care to meet those needs (Merrill, 1985). The elements of case management were integrated into the framework: health assessment, planning, procurement, delivery, and coordination of services; monitoring the multiple service needs of the client (ANA, 1988). The goals of case management are to provide quality health care along the continuum, decrease fragmentation of care across many settings, enhance the client's quality of care, and contain costs (ANA, 1988).

The Outcome Facilitation Teams were created at two levels—the Aggregate Outcome Facilitation Teams (A: OFT) and the Unit-Based Outcome Facilitation Teams (UB: OFT). Each team had a different makeup in structure but was similar in purpose, the global purposes being to focus on the patient, to determine quality and cost-effectiveness benchmarks, to promote a seamless care experience, and to support the philosophy of service management.

Several theories formed a basis for this design. For example, general systems theory views the holism and synergism of the system as a whole, and not just a sum of its parts (Kast, Rosenzweig, 1981). A system is defined as a composition of interrelated parts or elements. If one part succeeds and another does not, the whole will not be accomplished to the fullest. Systems have a hierarchy of relationships with subsystems: one part of the system will affect another part of the system (Kast, Rosensweig, 1981; Senge, 1990).

The Outcome Facilitation Team (OFT) process was developed to be an open system that would exchange information. A strength of this model is the focus on the system rather than on individual behavior. The integration of understanding the dynamic of the whole and the value of looking at trends over time instead of at one-time occurrences are other strengths of the systems thinking approach (Gardner, Demello, 1993; Miller, Winstead-Fry, 1992).

The OFT structure and process are based on some basic assumptions. Assumptions are the statements that connect concepts; assumptions are the thread that holds the fabric of knowledge within a theory together (Meleis, 1991). The OFT process is based on the following assumptions:

1. The nurse-patient relationship is a dynamic relationship.
2. The interpersonal commitment of the professional nurse gives direction to the care provided (Arnold, Boggs, 1989).
3. The multidisciplinary team will determine the case management actions needed to address the complexities of the patient's needs.
4. The coordination of the patient's services will decrease fragmentation and increase efficiencies of that care.
5. The coordination and achievement of the outcomes will decrease the cost of care.

AGGREGATE OUTCOME FACILITATION TEAM

Seven different A:OFTs were structured around the service lines: Cardiac, Orthopedics, Oncology, Women's Health, Emergency, Rehabilitation, and Primary Care. The aggregate structure, purpose, process, and initiatives are as follows:

Structure
- Service line director or designee
- Physician representation
- Representation from unit-based OFTs from that service line
- Disciplines as appropriate per service line

Purpose
- Aggregate patient focused
- Service line system focused
- Develop quality and cost-effective benchmarks
- Promote seamless care experience
- Support service management philosophy

The aggregate team defined the processes of care delivery and invited appropriate team physician members to the planning table. The team would determine the initiatives for development and implementation.

Process
- Define priorities: service line
- OFT and disciplines set direction for initiative (e.g., stakeholders, baseline data)
- Plan for evaluation (e.g., clinical quality, service, functional, fiscal)
- Develop timeline and communication plan

Multidisciplinary Initiatives
- Identify patient population needs (e.g., patient pathway)
- Collaborate to support the goals of the service line
- Care continuum evaluation (e.g., pre-admission through discharge)
- Disseminate learning and successes (e.g., service line, Aurora)

• • •

An example of an aggregate initiative was that the primary care team received data on the high-volume casetypes of patients who were cared for on the primary care units. The data revealed that the majority of the patients had a chronic illness with underlying co-morbid conditions. The team decided to format a pathway template that other teams could use in addressing the multitude of chronic illnesses specific to the patient population of each primary care unit. This work decreased the variation in defining the outcomes and processes for this patient population. This enhanced the speed of developing other specific chronic illness pathways.

UNIT-BASED OUTCOME FACILITATION TEAM

The UB:OFT was designed to meet the need for consistency in service delivery and evaluation of the outcomes. The design team reviewed the literature on case management models and recognized that this consistency is often managed by the role of a case manager. St. Luke's Medical Center's nursing practice council decided that the staff nurse is the designated coordinator of patient care. The specific role of a case manager was not acceptable or needed.

Considering that SLMC's 700 beds were spread over 40 units, developing an infrastructure for an effective unit-based design was essential. The unit-based structure needed to be grounded in the principles of case management, in which the nurse is the designated coordinator of patient care and collaborates with the members of the health care team to efficiently accomplish patient outcomes. For unit-based implementation, there were three guiding principles:

1. Staff RNs are the care coordinators.
2. The manager would be the systems linker.
3. The CNS would serve as facilitator and role model for those staff nurses needing mentoring in critical thinking skills.

These three individuals would be accountable to the unit-based patient populations and would be core members of the unit-based OFT. It is the unit-based OFT's role to ask daily, "What is keeping the patient here today?" and "What are we doing to meet patient outcomes?"

Structure

- Physician
- Social worker
- Patient care manager
- Clinical nurse specialist
- Staff nurse
- Disciplines as appropriate per patient population
- Collaboration and communication to the service line directors

Purpose

- Individual patient focused
- Unit system focused
- Implement and monitor quality and cost-effective care delivery
- Implement initiatives from A:OFT
- Promote seamless care experience
- Support service management philosophy

Process

- Define priorities: per patient and per unit
- Implement initiatives from A:OFT
- UB:OFT and disciplines set direction for the collaboration process
- Plan for evaluation . . . service, fiscal, quality, functional, process, etc.
- Timeline and communication plan

Multidisciplinary Initiatives

- Identify unit-specific patient population needs
- Collaborate daily to coordinate the individual plan of care

• • •

An example of a unit-based team for a medical unit consisted of the core team as the manager, CNS, social worker, dietitian, pharmacist, home care, and the chaplain. The team meets five days a week to address individual patient needs. An OFT note is written in the chart describing the planned interventions of the specific discipline.

Medical staff involvement at the unit level became critical. One unit that admitted primarily medical/chronic illness patients began a process on admission of setting goals with the physician in terms of what he or she wanted to get accomplished for the patient this admission. One group of physicians would call the day ahead of the patient's nonurgent admission and have the plan of care ready to dictate. The physician would speak with the CNS as the entry point of service provision, and the CNS would collaborate with the staff nurse on the day of admission.

The physician and nurse collaboration were increased as a measure of success. Physicians could round with knowledgeable care coordinators or attend OFT rounds on their patients. A particular unit was asked by medical staff leadership to help monitor a specific physician's practice pattern of overutilization and get him back into credentialling compliance.

The principles of group process are key for the OFTs to be effective. The elements of group process include problem solving, conflict management, communication, and boundary management (Wheeler, Chin, 1991). The interventions of OFTs were based on the development of a communication structure and process to promote consistent collaboration of multidisciplinary health care professionals, with the focus on identifying and achieving patient outcomes.

The roles of the manager and the CNS are consistent with the characteristics of coach and facilitator for the UB:OFTs. These unit-based leaders are to inspire a shared vision with the staff. Scholtes (1990) states that managers must lead the transformation effort to foster long-lasting success. The manager and the CNS needed to focus on preventing and eliminating problems related to the systems of patient care.

Outcome Evaluation

The evaluation of the outcome facilitation teams was based on patient satisfaction data, average unit length of stay data, and multidisciplinary provider satisfaction data. The implementation of the outcome facilitation teams was completed by the end of 1996. Thus the benchmark data represent all four quarters of 1996. The satisfaction and fiscal data of 1996 were compared to those for the first two quarters of 1997.

The patient satisfaction data were compiled from the standardized survey sent to all patients after discharge. Two survey indicators were part of the evaluation: "The nurses were sensitive to your condition and needs" and "The nurses provided adequate information on discharge and follow-up care." This information is based on the patient's personal experience. Patients were ask to use these indicators to rate nurses on a Likert scale of 1 to 7, 1 being "did not meet expectations" and 7 being

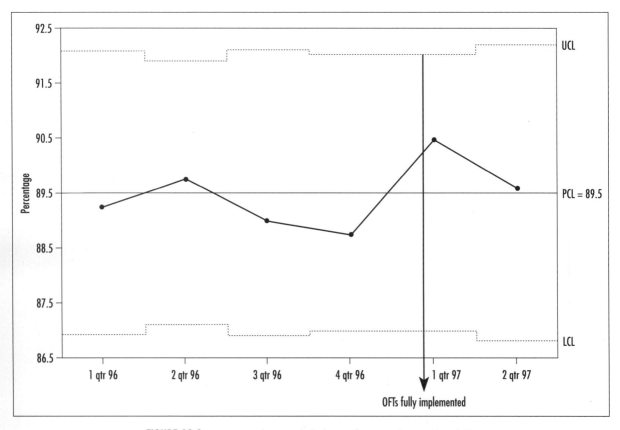

FIGURE 18-2 Inpatient satisfaction with discharge information: Percent 6's and 7's.

"extremely satisfied." The benchmark satisfaction data show an increase in the number of patients scoring nurses as a 6 or 7 in the first two quarters of 1997 (Figures 18-2 and 18-3).

The average unit length of stay data showed that 91% of the fourteen inpatient medical-surgical units had a decrease in length of stay, within a 3% margin. The data for the five intensive care areas indicated that 60% of the units showed a decrease in unit length of stay, within a 3% margin. The obstetric data did not show a change in average unit length of stay.

The provider satisfaction data are qualitative in nature. They were collected by interviews with various outcome facilitation teams. The data indicated an overall satisfaction with the innovation. The areas that worked well for the various disci-

plines included: increase in collaboration around planning the care of patients; timely and appropriate referrals facilitated; family issues addressed earlier; discharge plan addressed on admission; and all disciplines focused on patient outcomes. The areas that were identified for improvement included: consistent documentation; all disciplines available at same time of day; and using the time together most efficiently.

Although the quality, satisfaction, and length of stay data are impressive in terms of outcomes for the patient and the hospital, there were several other overall by-products of this process.

The registered nurses were able to articulate that their role is care coordination and not task-based care delivery. This care coordination model was used to predict staffing ratios and plans for skill

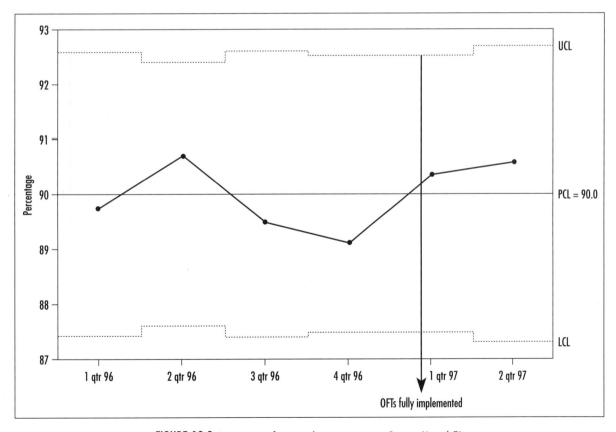

FIGURE 18-3 Inpatient satisfaction with nurse sensitivity: Percent 6's and 7's.

mix changes and hours of patient care. Role clarification assisted staff leaders to understand what tasks could be delegated to unlicensed personnel, so that the R.N.s would be available to do increased levels of care coordination. Although this allocation of time and resources is still not built into the system of charging for nursing care, the time allocated to do this service was incorporated into the staff matrixes on each unit.

In addition, the CNS and manager unit-based structure was recognized as adding value to the entire patient experience. In fact, the CNS-manager dyad model has been recognized by senior management as successful. This model will be used in four acute care hospitals that are reorganized into the metro-regional structure.

Conclusion

Porter-O'Grady (1992) contends that in these times of concentrated change, a new type of leadership must emerge. The future transformational leader needs to be committed to change, foster partnering relationships, and design systems to support the new structures. These are the very foundations for the Outcome Facilitation process.

The success of the OFT framework has been influenced by a variety of forces. The chief nurse executive challenged the leadership to recognize the changing environment and be creative in developing a model that would complement St. Luke's Medical Center's environment. Key elements that supported implementation included the high level of autonomy of the professional nursing staff, the dyad structure of the CNS and manager, and the service line leadership. The project coordinator facilitated the process by using continuous quality improvement tools to expedite the process for group decision making.

The basic framework to develop this plan includes various theories as the infrastructure. Theory gives the foundation to the nature, purpose, structure, and laws of operation, but theory does not cover the rules or procedures for applying this

knowledge to concrete, specific cases (Hanlon, 1968). Theory gives a person the cognitive tool to apply to daily practice. No theory can be considered totally valid and reliable forever because knowledge of structure and function, as well of essence and purpose, is constantly changing (Hanlon, 1968).

Which way to go? This will be our constant question in these times of rapid change.

References

American Nurses' Association: *Nursing case management,* Kansas City, Mo, 1988, American Nurses' Association.

Arnold E, Boggs K: *Interpersonal relationships: professional communication skills for nurses,* Philadelphia, 1989, Saunders.

Benner P: From novice to expert: excellence and power in clinical nursing practice, Menlo Park, Ca, 1984, Addison-Wesley. Merrill J: Defining case management, *Business and Health,* 2:5-9, 1985.

Davis K, Newstrom J: *Human behavior at work: organizational behavior,* ed 8, New York, 1989, McGraw-Hill.

Gardner BB, Demello S: Systems thinking in action, *Healthcare Forum.* Journal. July/August 1993.

Hanlon JM: *Hanlon: administration and education,* Belmont, Ca, 1968, Wadsworth.

Kast FE, Rosenzweig JE: General systems theory: applications for organizations and management. In Matteson MT, Ivancevich JM, eds: *Management and organization behavior classics,* (pp. 72-90). Burr Ridge, Ill, 1972, Irwin.

Meleis AL: *Theoretical nursing: development and progress,* Philadelphia, 1991, Lippincott.

Miller, Winstead-Fry: *Application to the work system,* 1982.

Porter-O'Grady T: Quantum mechanics and the future of health care leadership, *JONA* 27:1, 1997.

Porter-O'Grady T: Transformational leadership in an age of chaos, *Nursing Administration Quarterly* 17(1):17-24, 1992.

Scholtes PR: *The team handbook,* Madison, Wis, 1990, Joiner.

Senge PM: *The fifth discipline: the art and practice of the learning organization,* New York, 1990, Doubleday.

Wheeler C, Chinn P: *Peace and power,* ed 3, New York, 1991, National League for Nursing.

CHAPTER 19

Future Collaborative Partners in Health Care Delivery

PHYLLIS E. ETHRIDGE, RN, MSN, CNAA, FAAN

OVERVIEW

The collaboration with other health care professionals and the sharing of outcome data within the community are imperative for coming together and success as we care for individuals in the next century.

A collaborative health care model in the community is proposed for the changing managed care environment. Advanced practice nurses are in a strategic position to assist in the development and maintenance of such a model. An integrated approach to caring that encompasses a team effort to enhance quality services and reduce cost is the future expectation of consumers and payers. ▲

In today's turbulent era of economic emergence, the health care system has and continues to deny services to those in need. Nursing has recognized this deficit within our current system and has responded to many communities. This recognition of caring has placed nursing as key and pivotal to a health care system, which, according to a majority of patients and participants who have used our current health care system system, leaves much to be desired. The movement of advanced practice nurses, who are master's prepared, into clients' homes and other community entities, to manage the chronically ill as well as educate and counsel individuals after a risk assessment, has increased the consumers' trust in our profession. Advocacy for individuals in need of community health care resources and the identification of client choices have enhanced master's-prepared advanced practice nurses to lead our health care system into the future.

Nursing's progress has been monumental; however, our future impact depends upon the ability to help our health care colleagues to think prevention and wellness as opposed to acute episodic illness. The collaboration with other health care professionals and the sharing of outcome data within the community are imperative for the coming together and success as we care for individuals in the next century. The quality, cost-effective information currently available within select publications in nursing journals needs to be available to consumers and other health care professionals.

Managed care or health maintenance organizations (HMOs) have been partially successful and yet challenging in our present health care delivery system. The data from the Carondelet Nursing HMO indicated that the majority of members (80 to 85%) within a managed care program do not use an acute care facility (Carondelet Health Care Corporation, 1990 to 1992). Participants within a managed care environment have either exercised their opportunity for annual physicals, used an urgent care center, had prescriptions filled, or had no participation at all. Only 2 to 20% of young adults and/or seniors use an acute care facility. Information from managed care data indicated that the users of the system are the most vocal when it comes to quality service, especially if their needs include rehabilitation or long-term care (Carondelet Health Care Corporation, 1989 to 1995).

Managed Care Concerns

Several examples of patients' and families' concerns within a managed care environment have come to my attention and are described below. The first example involves a 5-year-old child who fractured his right ulna and radius. The fractured lower arm was obviously displaced, and according to those of us oriented to the old health care system, the child needed immediate attention. However, his father took him to an emergency room that accepted a capitated payment from the health plan. After three hours of waiting for communication with the HMO, he was directed to its urgent care facility. A resident from the local medical college had the child's arm x-rayed and diagnosed a comminuted fracture. The resident contacted the orthopedic surgeon on call and was instructed to have the parents place ice packs on the wrist, have the child take Tylenol, and place a sling on the right arm. The orthropedic surgeon stated that he would see the child in the morning. An appointment was made for the child, and the next day the parent had to take his son to the surgeon's office. The orthopedic surgeon reviewed the x-rays and determined that the child's fractured arm needed to be manipulated under anesthesia. A closed reduction of the child's arm was scheduled for the following day. Apparently, this was the time the surgeon allocated to hospital surgery. To the parent, this was another day of unpaid time off. The following day the child's fracture was manipulated under anesthesia, and his arm was placed in a cast. The parent was then instructed to take the child to the surgeon's office on the next day, no doubt to check the circulation and/or assess for other possible complications.

The procedure was accomplished at the convenience of the surgeon and the HMO plan. The parent had to take three days off from work because the HMO did not consider this to be an emergency and the loss of work time was not important to the HMO. However, the parent was irate because what he thought was an emergency situation turned out to be three days of lost work for the convenience of the health care plan without regard for his son's pain or welfare or the parent's need to support a family of seven.

The second example concerns an elderly gentleman, 85 years old, enrolled in an HMO, who had a grand-mal seizure at a local swap meet. He fell backward and ended up in the emergency room of a local hospital approved by his plan. He was transferred to a local HMO clinic, examined, and discharged to his home. The pain in the patient's back became excruciating, and he sought the services of a chiropractor. After manipulation his back pain became worse, and he returned for another treatment. His pain continued after two treatments with no relief, and he ended up in the emergency room of a hospital approved by his plan. He was admitted, and x-rays revealed a thoracic fracture of the spine. After several months, his back was no longer the problem; however, he had nerve damage to his anterior thigh. One wonders if a simple back x-ray at the time of the injury might have prevented this permanent injury to his upper thigh, which now requires narcotics for pain control and a walker to maintain his mobility.

The third example is that of a 50-year-old state employee with a malignant brain tumor. His wife worked in order for the household to survive. The patient was quickly discharged from the hospital and instructed to have radiation and chemotherapy. He drove himself to the outpatient facility on the days he was scheduled for treatment. The patient had no idea how he arrived for his treatments or how he drove home. How he spaced out with each treatment and then drove home without an accident is a miracle.

During his dying days, the HMO sent out an attendant two times a week to care for his needs. The registered nurse for the HMO appeared to collect necessary information and left with the patient's original living will, which had been recorded by a social worker within a local hospice. After the death of the patient and much communication between the HMO and a nurse case manager, the living will was returned to the family after his burial. Needless to say, the wife of the deceased was irate and registered a grievance with the HMO. Hospice services had been suggested to the patient's wife by the nurse case manager in collaboration with his primary physician. However, the HMO home care division made the decision that its services were adequate for the patient. After much discussion with the medical director of the HMO, the nurse case manager was able to get 70% of the hospice bill, which was $485.00 for the last 10 days of the patient's life, paid. Clergy and bereavement counseling for the family were not recognized as necessary services. Yet, the family members providing 24-hour love and sitter service for their dying father and husband, who benefitted from these needed hospice services, and prevented a hospitalization were not considered as important entities of the HMO plan.

All three of these patients and their families who enrolled in an HMO experienced common trends within our current health care system. If a person uses the services of the HMO, experiences delays in treatment, has diagnostic services omitted, and senses a lack of concern for patients and their families, satisfaction with the services represents only 15% of the total participants' opinions (Carondelet Health Care Corporation, 1991 to 1992).

These dissatisfactions of individuals within a community expecting health care services available to them prior to managed care insurances have sought services from a nursing profession that continues to care in a holistic manner. Nursing has emerged as the profession to care and advocate for children, young adults, and elders along the health care continuum. Advanced Practice Nurses will continue to be the primary caregivers for prevention, health promotion, minor illness, referral for acute illness, and care for the chronically ill and terminally ill (McBeth, Koerner, Ethridge, 1993).

It is time we share our experiences with our other health care professionals. This includes educating our colleagues, such as physicians, pharmacists, physical therapists, and dietitians, to negotiate contracts with HMOs to prevent illness, promote wellness, maintain those with chronic illnesses, and thereby contribute to a decrease in the cost of health care in the United States.

The future possibilities for our managed health care system to survive depend on nursing's ability to share and to help our health care colleagues to think prevention and maintenance of clients' health. Currently, payers such as insurance companies and state and federal entities, as well as HMOs, contract with local physicians, outpatient services, pharmacies, and hospitals. The entire system depends on capturing the most expensive entities within today's health care system. There is no originality or future plan, only the continuation of the status quo of the past.

Many HMOs and payers hold educational sessions once a month for their enrollees, and this becomes known as prevention. Only a select few attend, and the majority are healthy individuals seeking more knowledge. The sessions are usually held at a central location, often in the evening, which is convenient for the payer but may not be convenient for elders who may have difficulty driving after sunset. The sessions are seldom presented in local areas where there may be individuals at high risk who could benefit from the topic being offered. Presentations during weekends at churches are not an option. Health risk assessments of new enrollees to determine immediate needs are nonexistent.

The Community Nursing Organizations (CNOs), currently funded by the Health Care Financing Administration in Washington, D.C., who enroll Medicare patients are agencies that care about a person's present health status. Others seek multimembership and quantity which outweighs any indication of quality of service. To determine each new participant's risk is a must in order to allocate community services prior to an expensive hospitalization or nursing home placement, which might be avoided with home health services.

According to an article published in a recent issue of *Seniority Magazine* (1997), 12.8 million Americans need ongoing care for activities of daily living. Approximately 19%, or 2.4 million, are cared for in long-term-care institutions at an annual average cost of $46,000. An estimated 7 million are being cared for by families or friends. The remainder have no support system or identified caregiver. Unfortunately, the number of individuals who have benefitted from nurses' interventions is not available. However, these patients are definitely labeled by payers as high-risk enrollees who will potentially overutilize services within an acute care facility, especially if a crisis occurs or caregivers need respite (Ethridge, 1991). According to the current Medicare health care finance statistics, the majority of spending on seniors for health care continues to occur in the last year of life (Group Health Care Statistics, 1991 to 1994). Advanced Practice Nurses can have an impact upon this dilemma as well as support these individuals and caregivers so that death is an outcome of a process that includes love, respect, and dignity.

The future of health care within a national managed care environment depends upon Advanced Practice Nurses' willingness to evaluate their services from both a quality and a cost effective methodology. These outcomes can be shared with other health care professionals, consumers, and payers to promote the need for a reverse approach to caring. Instead of placing dollars toward illness and crisis, upfront monies for health promotion, illness prevention, and maintenance of patients with chronic illness would not only benefit these participants but also possibly increase the managed care entities' profits. The satisfaction of their enrollees is bound to increase as health care professionals are assigned to educate clients and families, assist in caring, and present options available in order that knowledgeable client and family choices with support are evident.

Health Care Models

Imagine multiple independent, futuristic community professional health care models of collaborative practice in which health care professionals are accountable for illness prevention, health promotion, treatment of minor illness, maintenance of the chronically ill, and securing a primary physician for diagnostic and acute illness. The model initially cares for a 5000-participant negotiated contract at 10% of the gross payers income per participant (Figure 19-1). Incentives or a percentage of the increased profits after an evaluation of patient satisfaction and cost outcomes for the managed care payer would be shared by all professional health care providers within each successful model. Monies would be allocated by the independent health care professional contracted entity for home care and respite support for caregivers. The number of health care professionals in each model would depend upon whether the managed care enrollees are seniors or considered participants under the age of 65 years. The 5000 enrollees should be located within a geographic location that would be accessible for health care professionals in each entity to render services in a cost-effective manner (see Figure 19-1).

The town, city, or county could be divided according to the number of enrollees within the plans. This would allow each model to expand according to the needs and the number of participants being cared for. The problem with expansion to other payers for contracted services becomes a conflict with the original managed care entity that competes with others. Collaborative health care organi-

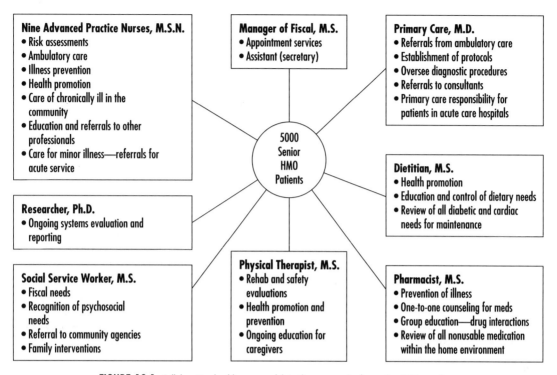

Nine Advanced Practice Nurses, M.S.N.
- Risk assessments
- Ambulatory care
- Illness prevention
- Health promotion
- Care of chronically ill in the community
- Education and referrals to other professionals
- Care for minor illness—referrals for acute service

Researcher, Ph.D.
- Ongoing systems evaluation and reporting

Social Service Worker, M.S.
- Fiscal needs
- Recognition of psychosocial needs
- Referral to community agencies
- Family interventions

Manager of Fiscal, M.S.
- Appointment services
- Assistant (secretary)

Physical Therapist, M.S.
- Rehab and safety evaluations
- Health promotion and prevention
- Ongoing education for caregivers

5000 Senior HMO Patients

Primary Care, M.D.
- Referrals from ambulatory care
- Establishment of protocols
- Oversee diagnostic procedures
- Referrals to consultants
- Primary care responsibility for patients in acute care hospitals

Dietitian, M.S.
- Health promotion
- Education and control of dietary needs
- Review of all diabetic and cardiac needs for maintenance

Pharmacist, M.S.
- Prevention of illness
- One-to-one counseling for meds
- Group education—drug interactions
- Review of all nonusable medication within the home environment

FIGURE 19-1 Collaborative health care model in the community for senior HMO enrollees.

zations that contract to care for patients in the community must be aware that inclusive contracts for services could inhibit their future growth. Therefore, initial negotiations should be left open in order that successful outcomes can be shared by other consumers and payers.

As 10% of the Senior HMO's income, approximately $40 a month would be allocated to this model or $200,000 per month. Each of the collaborative professionals would be paid a base salary of $7000 a month including benefits. The secretary or assistant to the fiscal manager would be paid $2000. Additional income depends upon the team's ability to reduce the payers' expenses and enhance the enrollees' satisfaction with all services. After rent, electricity, equipment, and so on, approximately $50,000 remains for home care respite services and other professional entities that may be necessary to provide care to the participants on a monthly basis. Ongoing support monitoring and education become crucial to primary caregivers' ability to continually review contracted services and their ability

to function within set parameters. Ongoing evaluation for effectiveness by means of chart outcomes is essential for success of the model.

Conclusion

The ability of advanced practice nurses to document and share future opportunities to care for the majority of enrollees within a managed care environment is imperative for collaborative health care independent practice models to be established. The sharing of knowledge and patients' community needs allows other health care professionals to recognize their importance within a team entity. Managing of care can be delegated to those health care professionals who have the necessary expertise to educate and assist the client and family in their immediate needs. Physical therapists, dietitians, pharmacists, and social service workers can be used to manage the care of individuals who will benefit from their services. The outcomes of all health care services should be the main focus of evaluation,

from both quality and cost-effectiveness perspectives. This collaborative effort will determine
failure or success for the future models and/or independent practice within a managed care environment. An integrated approach to caring that encompasses a team effort to enhance quality services and
reduce costs is the future expectation of consumers
and payers.

References

Carondelet Nursing HMO, Carondelet Health Care Corporation: Unpublished data, 1990 to 1992.
Carondelet Nursing HMO, Carondelet Health Care Corporation: Unpublished data, 1989 to 1995.
Carondelet Nursing HMO, Carondelet Health Care Corporation: Unpublished data, 1991 to 1992.
Ethridge P: A nursing HMO: Carondelet St. Mary's experience, *Nursing Management* 22:22-27, 1991.
Group Health Care Statistics, Washington, DC, 1991 to
1994.
Home health services: key to long term care dilemma, *Seniority Magazine* 9:14, 1997.
McBeth A, Koerner J, Ethridge P: Advanced licensure/
mandatory credentialing: a nurse executive point of
view, *Nursing Management* 24:45-47, 1993.

CHAPTER 20

Leading Change One Step at a Time

PAM L. BROMLEY, RN, MSM, **and KAY W. GARCIA**, RMT, MBA

OVERVIEW

A learning organization grows from feedback concerning both mistakes and accomplishments.

To successfully implement change, leaders must take an active role in identifying a methodology that will work within health care institutions. Within the health care industry change is taking place at an ever-increasing pace. Theories are important and provide us with a foundation to develop our own methods of accomplishing work. In order for leadership to accomplish change, it is necessary to take the theoretical concepts and mold them into a system that will be successful in a given environment. This chapter will assist the reader in understanding the basic change theories, adapt them to a change model, and apply the model to two change projects ▲

What Is Change?

Much has been written about change management and the leadership characteristics necessary to implement change. Theories are presented as neat packages. In reality, change is usually difficult and messy. We invent it as we go along. Although theories are important in guiding us, it is our ability to combine them with creativity, sensitivity to others, and openness to new ways of thinking that determines our success.

We know that one of life's constants is that things do not stay the same. John Lennon said life is what happens when you have other plans. Change management consultant Darryl Conner (1993) says change is what happens when you have disrupted expectations.

The impact of this disruption, this change, depends upon our perception of its magnitude. Our ability to cope with it depends upon our flexibility. As leaders we not only respond to change, but we also plan and orchestrate it, meaning we plan disruption for ourselves and others. To do this successfully, we must help others cope and help them become flexible. This demands creativity, sensitivity, and openness to new ways of thinking (to "coloring outside the lines").

Change Methodologies

The range of available methodologies for managing change and its consequences is large. Most provide us with some sort of model and suggest skill sets for us to develop. Many of these can be found in the major works of people like Deming (1994), Juran (1993), and Senge (1990) and also others such as Champy and Hammer (1993), Buchholzl and Woodward (1987), Conner (1993), and Collett and Melum (1995). Not all these methodologies are identified as change methodologies per se; however, application of them helps us manage change.

At times, criticism has been leveled at various methodologies for failing to deliver. In reality, the failure problem is usually *deployment* of the methodology and not the methodology itself.

We have found common threads and similar tools in most of these methodologies, and that has led us to define the basic elements for success. We suggest that leaders "cherry-pick" from methodologies the techniques that fit their organizational or project needs, while adhering to some basic tenets.

BASIC CHANGE MANAGEMENT TENETS

- Leadership manages and is responsible for successful change. Pivotal to ensuring the success of implementing a change is that it must be managed by the appropriately defined leaders.
- *Significant* change must be driven by and supported by top leadership. This must emanate from the *top* of the organizational authority lines touched by the change. Within a department, it is the department manager or director. Across departments, it is a senior director or vice president. Across VP lines, it is the CEO. The top person does not necessarily implement the change, but must sanction and *actively* support the change by giving and communicating the necessary power and resources to accomplish it.
- The person(s) implementing the change must possess the power and resources to make it happen and to manage the consequences. This comes from clear top-level support. Many failed projects owe their demise to what Conner (1993) would call unclear sponsorship. For example, the person wanting the change did not really have the clout necessary to make it happen and/or did not build the appropriate connection to that power.
- The message about what is changing must be simply and actively communicated to those affected by it throughout the duration of the change effort. The consequences of making the change and of not making the change must be certain.
- Leadership must be clear about what is different (gap analysis) between where they are today (current state) and where they want to be (future or desired state). In addition, they must understand and accept the cost of the change, both in traditional financial terms and in human cost. Although clarity develops as change evolves, success can be seriously jeopardized if leadership does not take the time to do this early work well.
- Task goals must be balanced with human goals. Task goals require planning, analysis, teamwork, and setting measurable outcome targets. Human goals require analysis, understanding, and two-way communication concerning the impact on the people involved. Too much emphasis on one to the detriment of the other can torpedo a project. We recommend using a *sys-*

temic implementation methodology, statistical tools for data display and analysis, and group decision-making tools for team management. It is nearly impossible to communicate too much.

- Leadership must *walk the talk*. There must be solidarity at the top. If middle management is expected to model teamwork and think systemically, it needs to see these things demonstrated by upper management. Frequently this requires senior leadership to reevaluate its behaviors and communication patterns and to change them.
- Resources must be provided for managers to learn new skills. This is often new learning. A critical mass of managers with the *skills* and *mental models* for implementing and managing change is necessary.

CHANGE BASICS

A *basic model for change* has these minimal elements, each of which utilizes various processes, models, and tools:

- *Understand the current state*—clarify and analyze.
- *Clarify the desired state (future state)*—determine assumptions, develop vision, etc.
- *Do gap analysis*—identify the gaps (to move from *current state* to *future state*):
  - Identify the major events (goals to be achieved) that must occur to close those gaps; set broad priorities.
  - Identify the stakeholders and analyze the impact on them (determine the extent of the impact, decide how to involve them, develop Communication Plan, and determine how the impact on them will be managed).
  - Align leadership and secure authority for change.
  - Develop ongoing reporting or feedback loops.
  - Develop Implementation Plan—determine how each major plank of the gap analysis will be achieved (means, methods, targets, measurable indicators, timelines, resources, and responsibilities). A Gantt chart is useful for this purpose. Balance these task goals with human impact goals.

Case 1: Implementing Change—Case Management System

At the beginning of the 1997 calendar year, an organizational restructuring offered the medical center an opportunity to redesign its existing case management system. The *current state* configuration for case management used Continuing Care Planners (Discharge Planners) to discharge complex patients and perform utilization review, and it used Episodic Case Managers for planning and coordinating care of the acute/complex patients. A Community Case Manager worked with congestive heart failure patients. During a recent reorganization, Continuing Care Planners moved into the Division of Patient Care Services, where Episodic Case Managers resided. The *desired state* was to eliminate redundancy, maximize the best features of each group, improve patient satisfaction, and meet the needs of an emerging integrated delivery system. The gap analysis indicated that merging the functions of Continuing Care Planners and Episodic Case Managers would be the first phase of a work redesign evolving into a case management system designed to meet the needs of an integrated delivery system.

To achieve the desired-state outcomes, an oversight or steering committee was configured to create the vision, validate goals, and ensure support for the project. The membership of the oversight committee included the vice presidents for Patient Care Services and Finance, the director of Patient Care Services, and the director of the Continuing Care Planners. The vice presidents were identified as the ones with the power and resources to sanction the change, so they were secured as sponsors. The two directors were assigned to lead the project. An ongoing reporting link to the vice presidents was planned to ensure their continued support. Those affected by the potential change were included at the very beginning.

The steering committee determined that a benchmarked foundation for the project was needed. This was developed through a literature search, phone interviews, and on-site visits to places identified as having model case management systems. After completion of the research analysis, a Task Force was formed for the purpose of actualizing the first phase of the project: to create and implement a new case management role merging the functions of utilization management, discharge planning, and episodic case management. The new role would support the service lines' goals of improvement in clinical outcomes, enhancement of patient satisfaction, and achievement of a cost reduction target of $200,000.

Task Force membership included key stakeholders: Episodic Case Manager, Continuing Care Planner, service line director, unit director, and social worker. The team size was kept small, with each member responsible for representing and communicating with his or her constituency.

The gap analysis evolved into the Implementation Plan. Attention was given throughout the process to developing means and methods for both task goals and human impact goals. A Communication Plan to broader constituencies was established as part of the Implementation Plan. A modified Gantt chart was used to organize, visualize, and continue to facilitate the work of the Task Force. It helped to document and focus the implementation process. Its major elements were designed to understand/clarify the utilization review function

and evaluate current related job descriptions and to redesign and develop new role and job descriptions. An outline of key elements of the Gantt chart follows:

I. Define and agree on organizational structure for case management
   A. Agree on reporting relationship/structure to support the new position
   B. Define stakeholders
   C. Verify top-level sponsorship
   D. Identify changes that need to occur with new role
II. Define and agree on job description/scope of role
   A. Agree to merge cost, quality, and patient satisfaction responsibilities
   B. Define and determine case load: scheduling and coverage
      1. Define patient population
      2. Develop work complexity tool
      3. Define case management and the care delivery model for this role
      4. Determine outcome measurements

BOX 20-1
Case Management Task Force Summary

Mission statement	Best possible quality of care in most cost-effective manner
Purpose statement	Create and implement a new role, which merges the functions of utilization management (UM), discharge planning (DP), case management (CM) to support service line goals of cost containment, improvement of clinical outcomes, and patient satisfaction
Boundaries	Create a new role for clinical care coordination, including educational plan, transitional plan, hiring and interviewing new staff
Task Force membership	Leaders: Directors of Patient Care Services and Utilization Review Members: Key Service Line Directors, Quality Improvement Director, Key Utilization Review Staff, Case Managers
Major outcomes and key quality characteristics	When these happen, we know we are successful: 1. Define and implement the new role 2. Hire staff into the new role 3. Train and debrief staff
Roles	Sponsors: VP for Patient Care Services; VP for Finance Agents: Steering Committee and Task Force Targets: List includes all those affected by the change, those who will have to make changes because of this new role
External targets	Insurance companies; community vendors
Cost analysis	$200,000 savings in labor

III. Market to key stakeholders to gain input and support (Communication Plan)
   A. Physician support
   B. Management support
   C. Staff support across the organization
   D. External constituencies
IV. Implement
   A. Address stakeholder and target issues
   B. Plan to transition to desired state
   C. Education and training program
V. Information resource needs
   A. Hardware/software
   B. Training
VI. Conflict management plan for case manager role

To develop the Implementation Plan, each of these areas was worked in detail on a modified Gantt chart. Multiple levels of Gantt chart were used, each becoming more detailed. The process of creating the Gantt charts further clarified and reaffirmed the desired state, as illustrated in Box 20-1. Table 20-1 is an example of the format and detail used for the Gantt charts, reflecting the first level of detail and planning. Figure 20-1 depicts the medical center's process for utilization management.

Input was elicited from in-house experts, and a series of interviews of key stakeholders gathered information about the current roles. A separate set of questions was prepared for each type of interview conducted; the results of the interviews were compiled and evaluated by the Task Force. They became the basis for the new role.

The work of the Task Force continues to be productive. It has met timeline goals and is on track in meeting identified outcomes for task and human impact goals. The new combined job description has eliminated duplication. The proposed staffing pattern indicates a $200,000 savings in salaries.

Case 2: Implementing Change—Scheduling System

In late 1993, a Scheduling Task Force was created to identify an automated scheduling system for the medical center. The goals of that Task Force were to complete a needs analysis; select an automated system that would parallel the future strategic vision and direction of the hospital; and determine the costs of purchasing and implementing such a system. The Task Force consisted of mid-level managers from admitting, operating room, information resources, and preadmitting. The immediate tasks were to complete a needs analysis and to determine whether other departments with scheduling requirements should be involved in the project. It was not clear where the authority or resources were to accomplish this. It was also not clear who was the actual leader of the effort.

The initial Task Force lost momentum and failed to meet established goals. Although there had been six months of inactivity, capital had been allocated for an automated system, so the Chief Information Officer renewed efforts, and in the spring of 1994 the previous Task Force was expanded, incorporating previously established goals. This time the Task Force planned to identify a vice president as process owner. In addition, a third immediate task was added to the previous two: to view scheduling as a process that will ensure that the patient arrives where he or she needs to be. Weekly meetings were scheduled to facilitate prompt completion of the tasks and goals. Even though the Task Force identified the need for a process owner, a vice president did not step forward.

The Task Force met weekly for approximately two months. It completed a work process flow analysis of the scheduling system, and identified and analyzed customer needs. In May it was discontinued by a directive from the CEO stating that any project without a vice president process owner would be put on hold, emphasizing the importance of securing senior leadership support.

In January of 1996 the group reconvened with goals similar to those in the past. This time the tasks included a request for a proposal to implement an automated system, development of a business case plan for the system, and completion of the capital requisition process to finance it. The renewed Task Force identified the Manager of Registration as the team leader and the Vice President for Finance and acting CEO as the process owner. Two facilitators were assigned. The membership for the Task Force remained the same as in the 1994 group. A completion target of three months was established, and weekly meetings ensued. Work was completed for the Request for Proposal (RFP). The membership expanded to include the scheduler from the operating room, who was the communication link to the

TABLE 20-1

Gantt Chart Format and Example of Level One

ITEMS (OBJECTIVES)	TIMELINE	RESPONSIBLE PERSON(S)	COMMUNICATION (STAKEHOLDERS)	TASK FORCE INTERACTION	TOOLS FOR FACILITATION	MEANS AND METHODS
I. Define and agree on organizational structure	Sept 15	Task Force	Service Line Directors, continuing care planners (CCP), case managers (CM)	Meet with each group; Director for Patient Care Services to serve as coach	Organizational Development Resources (ODR) assessment tool; negotiations model: *Beyond Re-engineering* Hammer (1996); criteria matrix; consensus tools	
A. Agree on reporting relationship						Identify criteria; develop relationship structure
B. Identify stakeholders						Task Force to identify; develop CM service agreement
C. Verify sponsor						Secure continued sponsor support through meetings and feedback
D. Identify necessary changes for new role						Identify differences and needed changes; develop role through consensus

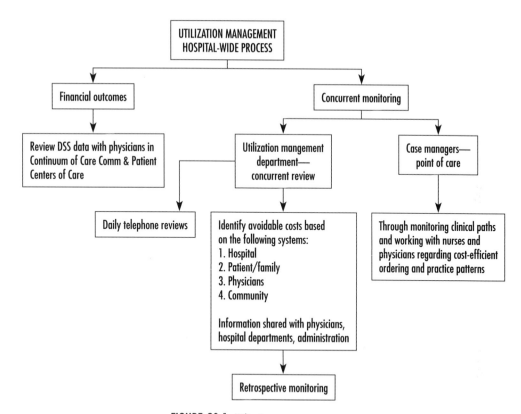

FIGURE 20-1 Utilization management process.

whole OR. Then the OR director left his position. The scheduler did not communicate with the new director. As the Task Force continued to meet, the new OR director was not included.

After completion of the RFP, the Task Force began an Implementation Plan. The still outstanding issue of centralized versus decentralized scheduling had not been resolved, proving to be a fatal flaw.

At this same time, the medical center initiated several work redesign initiatives, led by the Vice President for Human Resources. The Scheduling Task Force met once with the Vice President for Human Resources to ensure alignment with the redesign effort and to ensure that the scheduling implementation would not have to be reworked at a later date.

The Vice President for Human Resources told the Task Force that it was empowered to make the decision, stating that centralization, decentraliza-tion, or a combination of both would be in alignment with the work redesign efforts. On the basis of this input, the group determined that it was empowered to make a decision on the centralization question, and decided to implement centralized scheduling house-wide. Minimal communication and input to and from stakeholders and the rest of senior leadership were received or sought by Task Force members.

In August of 1996 the identified process owner, the Vice President for Finance and acting CEO, approved a new position for a Scheduling System Administrator. The underlying premise of the Task Force was that in a centralized system, each department would have control over its own area and would also be able to view the whole organizational schedule from its department. A vendor contract was signed and an implementation team designated, with a September kickoff target.

In January of 1997 a permanent CEO was hired. The implementation team decided to use the vendor's quick-start implementation method. February of 1997 was the designated "go live" date. As that time approached, many problems and issues surfaced. The list included: lack of buy-in for centralization; inadequate preparation of personnel; depth and complexity of the system not realized; and hardware and software issues. After several meetings with key stakeholders, the decision was made to implement the system as decentralized and then reclarify the decision and deal with the problems during the implementation.

There have been several delays; the system is functioning in radiology and laboratory for outpatient scheduling. The success in those two areas can be attributed to scheduling noncomplex cases that do not require extensive coordination of additional services. Work time and energy continue to be spent discussing a continuing list of problems, including the centralization/decentralization issue. Because this project affects the entire organization, the whole senior management team needs to become involved, determine whether it wants an automated scheduling system, determine whether the system should be centralized or decentralized, communicate and support the decisions throughout the organization, identify the person charged with implementing the project, and insist that necessary planning and problem solving occur before further "go live" situations in departments.

Conclusion

The defining differences between the processes used by the teams in the two cases involve:

1. Clarity and understanding of the desired state
2. Detailed understanding of the gap analysis
3. Ongoing top-level support and authorization for the team goals
4. Identification of, involvement of, and communication with key stakeholders to address impact issues at the beginning of the process

TABLE 20-2
Change Implementation Comparison

ELEMENTS	CASE MANAGEMENT	SCHEDULING SYSTEM
Understand/know current state	Understood and analyzed	Understood and analyzed
Clarify the desired state	Well defined	Poorly defined
Do gap analysis	Well defined	Poorly defined
Identify stakeholders; analyze impact	Identified; brought into process early; included in problem solving	Poorly identified; late into process; not included in problem solving
Align leadership	Aligned and support secured	Not aligned or secured; not clearly authorized or supported to make implementation decisions
Develop Implementation Plan (ask how each plank of gap analysis will be achieved)	Work in progress; so far this has been thorough	Not thorough enough to anticipate and mitigate problems
Develop Communications Plan	Work in progress; so far, well planned	Not planned or implemented
Determine how transition from current state to desired state will be managed (balance task goals with human goals)	Work in progress	Was not done

Other issues that arose in Case 2 could have more easily been mitigated, had these elements been addressed.

A learning organization grows from feedback concerning both mistakes and accomplishments. Some mistakes are expected as we evolve. Our major learning comes through comparing the key characteristics of both our successes and our failures. In the future we will see that the application of a consistent methodology will assist us in navigating the waters of change, while at the same time we remember to think systematically enough to make use of creativity, openness, and sensitivity to broader organizational and human issues that affect change.

References

Buchholzl S, Woodward H: *After-shock.* New York, 1987, John Wiley & Sons.

Champy J, Hammer M: *Reengineering the corporation,* New York, 1993, Harper Collins.

Collett C, Melum MM: *Breakthrough leadership,* 1995, American Hospital Publishing, Inc.

Conner D: *Managing at the speed of change,* New York, 1993, Villard Books.

Deming WE: *The best of Deming,* 1994, SPC Press.

Hammer M: *Beyond reengineering,* New York, 1996, Harper Collins.

Juran JM: *Quality planning and analysis,* New York, 1993, McGraw-Hill.

Senge P: *The fifth discipline,* New York, 1990, Doubleday.

CHAPTER 21

Practice Innovations in Academic Nursing

Targeting Outcomes

MADELINE WAKE, RN, PhD, FAAN, **MARY ANN LOUGH,** RN, PhD, and **CHRISTINE R. SHAW,** RN, PhD, CS, FNP

OVERVIEW

The education-service dichotomy is as out of place in today's world as mind-body dualism.

For the twenty-first century, outcomes of academic nursing have dual dimensions. One dimension is student outcomes, a traditional aim of educational programs. Another dimension is client outcomes, the positive changes in the health of individuals, groups, and communities. Integration of teaching and practice and the creation, by students and faculty, of new ways of delivering care target both outcome dimensions. This chapter provides examples of such efforts in practice innovation. ▲

Practice is an essential dimension of academic nursing. In the past, those in education and service were two distinct subgroups in nursing. The education-service dichotomy is as out of place in today's world as mind-body dualism. The physical dimensions of health and illness are no longer treated in isolation. Realization of holism has permeated our health consciousness. Likewise, the notion of integration of education and service has grown over the past decades. Evidence of this change rests in the increases in numbers of academic nursing centers (Barger, Bridges, 1990) and faculty practice models (Potash, Taylor, 1993; AACN, 1996). In the past, nurse educators have created the future through the nurses they prepared. Today, nurse educators also shape the future through practice innovation. A similar logic applies to the nurse scholar's mandate to expand the body of nursing knowledge. Knowledge generation in nursing includes practice development as well as traditional scholarship. Ideally, faculty share with students both when conducting research and when creating practice innovations.

With the acceleration in the rate of change in health care, the practice world will change in the years it takes to complete baccalaureate nursing education. Therefore, it is essential to prepare new nurses for roles as system builders and change agents, as well as providers of care. Preparation for these roles has implications for curriculum and for the design of learning experiences.

Marquette University College of Nursing

Marquette University College of Nursing enrolls nearly 400 undergraduate students as well as 200 graduate students as MSN and post-master's students in six program options. Over its long history, the College has stressed clinical excellence. The essential integration of teaching and practice is firmly rooted in the institutional memory of Marquette University College of Nursing (Machan, 1980). Given that history, it is not surprising to see a faculty collective committed to nursing as a practice and an academic discipline.

STRATEGIC PLAN

The Marquette nursing faculty have developed a strategic plan designed to realize a vision of creating healthy, caring communities through excellence in nursing education, practice, and research. Several components of the plan address practice innovation, including curricula, clinical settings, and nursing center. One of the six goals of the plan is: "To provide leadership which impacts on the health of the community as well as the shaping of health care, nursing care delivery systems, and the nursing profession."

CURRICULUM CHANGE

Recent curriculum revisions for the undergraduate and graduate programs have shifted emphasis to community settings and addressed new roles. The number of hours spent in community clinical learning increased from 120 hours to a range of 280 to 400 hours. In addition to increased community-based experiences, the BSN program includes a course in primary health care that stresses the comprehensive, multisectorial perspective essential for healthy communities. An introduction to nursing case management and increased content on population assessment and interventions were added. All seniors conduct a needs assessment on a population in the community. Graduate curriculum also includes content geared to different student outcomes. The master's program requires content in creating nursing care systems, program development, and case management for all students in advanced practice options (nurse-midwife, nurse practitioner, clinical nurse specialist) as well as the nursing administration option. Advanced practice nurses graduate with competencies in system management as well as in direct primary care. Box 21-1 lists desired student outcomes.

FACULTY

The faculty of the College of Nursing share a common investment in student and client outcomes. Faculty commitment is integral to the success of the practice innovations that lead to targeted outcomes. Design and implementation of innovations require creative vision and courage. Practice sites may be created through grant proposals, negotiations with

---

BOX 21-1
Selected Student Outcomes of Practice Innovations

- Ability to design client-centered care
- Knowledge of organizational factors of care delivery
- Competence in health screening
- Growth in negotiation skills

BOX 21-2
Selected Client Outcomes of Practice Innovations

Satisfaction with health care and trust in providers
Ability to access health care
Increased knowledge of health promotion
Decreased use of emergency services
Earlier identification of acute problems

---

community partners, and collaboration with other faculty. The practice innovations require faculty-student practice. College administrators give the additional support needed for faculty to practice what they teach.

CLINICAL SITE SELECTION

In selecting clinical learning sites, Marquette faculty place priority on sites where we can deliver care to culturally diverse, underserved people while teaching and learning. The goal is to effect client outcomes through our innovative practice models. To us, our city is not an urban laboratory in which we study life in a detached manner. Rather, we are committed to collaboration with the community in our urban environment. Because our College of Nursing exists, Milwaukee should be a healthier community. The desired client outcomes are listed in Box 21-2.

It is essential to measure outcomes to evaluate program effectiveness. Tracking outcomes in culturally diverse, underserved populations is challenging. Individuals may move frequently and may not have telephones. They may seek treatment only when acute health problems have escalated. They may not return to the same health care provider for subsequent care. Evidence of growing trust and return for follow-up care may be early outcomes. Faculty care providers address barriers such as financial constraints, transportation issues, and lack of culturally competent care. By celebrating small successes and minimizing the barriers to care, faculty and student providers work toward the ultimate goal of improved health outcomes.

For example, a community health faculty member and a group of RN to BSN completion students worked with community leaders to develop health and social support systems for a newly established safe house for abused children. Another example is a community health group of undergraduate seniors who completed a community assessment of an underserved segment of a hospital's service area. The study provided the hospital with valuable data regarding the population, their health needs and concerns, their environment, and community agencies used by the clients. The data were used for a grant proposal to provide additional perinatal services to the population. In addition to partnerships with 80 existing health care agencies, we have College-initiated and operated practice sites.

Practice Innovations

The Marquette Nursing Center was established in 1982 to provide students with community-based learning and area residents with direct access to nursing care. Whereas health insurance leaders talk of point-of-service plans, we have coined the term "point-of-living" care delivery for our nursing center outreach activities. We have initiated service at community settings as opposed to dedicated health care institutions. In the midst of this, we have formed logical and unlikely partnerships. In 1991, the College established a nurse-managed clinic in partnership with a distressed community. Faculty developed primary care services in which community health students participated in care delivery. Faculty worked to develop a community board and turned the clinic operations over to the board as planned in 1995.

Marquette has a Parish Nursing Institute, which has prepared over 600 parish nurses from 40 states and three countries. A faculty member who is the director of the institute has partnered with an urban medical center to support parish nurses in inner city churches. One intended outcome is reduction of inappropriate use of emergency services by inner city residents. One parish nurse has a dual position of 50% parish nurse and 50% emergency department nurse. He models care across settings to undergraduate students.

Two years ago, the school board of a nearby county requested consultation from Marquette on school health care. This eventually resulted in a faculty practice contract for a clinical faculty member as supervisor of health services for the district of 22,000 students at 38 schools. Undergraduate and graduate nursing students have had clinical placements in the system. They have worked with the nursing staff to improve the health knowledge of teachers and the health status of the children.

Three projects in practice innovation warrant extended description. The first project converted a medical residency training site into a site for interdisciplinary training. The others established health services in a homeless shelter and in a school-parish community.

COMMUNITY EDUCATION CENTER

Background. Interdisciplinary training is exemplified by the Community Education Center (CEC) model, in which health professions students from various disciplines—for example, medicine, nursing, and social work—learn by caring for underserved clients affiliated with a Family Practice Center (FPC). The clinical learning and care are designed for maximum relevance to the target population, with an emphasis on access and cultural competence. Continuity and consistency are provided by key faculty of represented disciplines. These faculty case manage clients while role modeling interdisciplinary collaboration.

The purposes of the transformation of the medical residency program to the CEC site were to identify more effective health care programs for high-risk populations and to set collaborative practice patterns early in health professional development (Lough et al, 1996). The FPC client population pro-

file, coupled with student program objectives, led faculty to select two target client groups for the CEC: young, pregnant women and chronically ill elders.

Description. Maternity clients who receive care at the FPC were selected for student home visit follow-up. The purposes of the home visits were to assess antepartal risk factors, provide anticipatory guidance, complete a social risk factor assessment, and discuss any health issues of import to the clients. All of the maternity clients resided in the central city and were diverse with regard to race, ethnicity, education, and family composition. Prior to client contacts, students discussed with faculty what assessments were required and then were encouraged to think about what interventions might be offered, knowing that the treatment plan could be changed as a result of new client input or unforeseen changes. Upon completion of the visits, students gave an oral report and prepared an interdisciplinary note. Students completed follow-up activities when possible and referred to FPC staff if necessary. During the interdisciplinary case conferences, students discussed their assessments, plans of care, and how the patients and families were involved. Complex health problems discussed included use of drugs during pregnancy, poor weight gain, a failure-to-thrive baby, and sickle cell disease. In the conferences, faculty emphasized the importance of client/family/community strengths, health promotion, advocacy, and continuity of care between the patient and the FPC staff.

Chronically ill elders, the second population, were referred to the CEC program either by referral from the FPC residents or by the hospital discharge planners. Home visits were scheduled to reevaluate the treatment plan and to assess for additional needs that may have surfaced since contact with the primary physician. The majority of these elders had multiple medical diagnoses, polypharmacy issues, limited resources, poor nutrition, and declining social supports. Prior to home visiting, students had conferences on topics such as aging, depression, and delirium and dementia, and on conducting assessments regarding cognitive functioning, nutrition, activities of daily living, medication knowledge and compliance, and caregiver issues. In addition to learning about management of chronic illnesses in the elderly, students also learned about the impact of other issues on these problems. Examples included caregiver stress, fears associated with neighborhood change and crime, abuse, living arrangement conflicts, exploitation by relatives, and nursing home placement issues. Interdisciplinary student teams planned their visit activities, determining who would assume which responsibilities. Faculty were available throughout this process to clarify the client situation and/or answer questions, as well as validate that students were well prepared for the client contacts. During the interdisciplinary conferences, students participated in case analysis by developing a problem list, refining the treatment plan, and arranging for follow-up contacts.

Case Example. A case example demonstrates the relationship developed with the CEC care providers. A student team went to visit an elderly client, Rose, who had been kept in the community through the CEC efforts for three years. Rose was 68 years old and had several medical diagnoses, including chronic renal failure, congestive heart failure, and tertiary syphilis. She lived alone in the central city in subsidized housing. Her closest relative, a daughter, lived 90 miles away. Rose was currently being followed closely for home safety issues, nutrition deficits, cognitive impairments, and limited social support in the immediate geographical area. Upon arrival at Rose's apartment, students observed police and rescue squad members outside the apartment preparing to transport Rose to the county mental health complex for confusion and disruptive behavior. The emergency team reported that she had been throwing objects out the window, locking herself in her apartment, and refusing help. The student team, an FPC resident, a nurse, and a social worker, discussed the situation with the rescue team, and requested that Rose be transferred to the hospital that was her usual source of medical care. However, because of ambulance protocol, Rose was transported for evaluation to the hospital adjacent to the county mental health facilities. As the CEC team began the case conference immediately following this incident, the students expressed discomfort with her hospital placement, since the client was well known at the FPC-affiliated hospital. The physician telephoned the receiving emergency department, described the cli-

ent's clinical situation in detail, and accepted responsibility for her transfer to her usual hospital. Contact was made with the client's daughter, who lived 90 miles away, and with whom the team had regular contact.

Within a short time, the client was transferred to her usual hospital and cared for by her regular FPC physician. Once she became medically stable, there were discussions with her daughter regarding the necessity of making a change in living arrangements. Clearly, the client's health condition had changed, and she could no longer live alone. Determination of Medicare coverage and of eligibility for placement in a nearby long-term-care facility was made. The daughter expressed relief that the CEC team had responded to her mother's crisis situation and was ready to assist with nursing home placement for her mother. This case demonstrates how the core values of this clinical program were taught to students. They learned about case management, interdisciplinary collaboration, teamwork, family involvement, and the importance of effective communication skills.

Students have gained tangible and intangible benefits from participating in a CEC program. They gained a clear appreciation for the role, values, expertise, and importance of other disciplines. Using an interdisciplinary, community-based approach in their clinical courses has helped them to see firsthand the interplay of the multiple variables influencing a client's health. The aforementioned client contacts provided students with the opportunity to design health care plans with client input. They considered socioeconomic issues in designing care and were given many opportunities to engage in cultural skill development. Caring for selected populations, such as chronically ill elders and/or young, high-risk pregnant women offered students the challenge of determining what needs exist and what needs have been met, a chance to identify gaps, and an opportunity to intervene in a timely manner. They observed their respective faculty members modeling a collaborative, interdisciplinary approach to education and practice.

The clients have benefited from this program in several ways. For example, they received additional attention at home and had more time to speak with a health care provider, in a family environment. Student visitors made pertinent observations and assisted with the identification of health-related and social or environmental factors affecting the client's health. Clients further benefitted from measurement of health status over time, which can facilitate early intervention. They learned to recognize symptoms that need to be reported to care providers. They demonstrated changes in eating habits based on nutritional counseling. Finally, clients have been assisted with timely access to the health care system. Information and findings from home visits are reported to the primary provider in writing or, if necessary, immediately by phone. Use of a multidisciplinary approach has resulted in development of comprehensive treatment plans specific to individual needs and appreciation of contributions from various disciplines. The clients cared for by the students benefited from home visits and community-based services not available to other FPC clients. Overall, the clients have responded positively to the student providers, as evidenced by the many positive anecdotal comments given to faculty and staff members, and the clients' willingness to interact with the students, even on a repeated basis.

HOMELESS SHELTER CLINIC

Background. For years, college faculty have provided episodic services to homeless individuals through Nursing Center programs. In May 1995, the Nursing Center director met with the executive director of a homeless shelter near the Marquette campus to discuss health needs of the residents and potential collaboration. In academic year 1995-1996, two undergraduate clinical groups offered health promotion programs at the shelter and a graduate student conducted a comprehensive health needs assessment. Changes in local public health funding as well as in state legislation on welfare resulted in an increase in unmet needs for women and children. The shelter director identified clinic services for women and children as the top priority and requested assistance. Her goal was congruent with our need for clinic sites for our growing advanced practice programs. Funding for the clinic was sought from a local foundation and received.

Description. The Clinic for Women and Children operates as a half-day per week primary care clinic throughout the year. The clinic also offers on- and off-site health promotion programs on a regular basis.

The staff for the clinic include a faculty project director, who established the infrastructure and links to other agencies; two nurse practitioners, one of whom was a faculty member; a nurse case manager for follow-up; and a shelter staff person as coordinator. Undergraduate and graduate students have clinical placements in the clinic, and the clinic is linked to groups of students who do health education for women in the shelter.

The uninsured patients who receive care at the clinic and participate in the health promotion programs are primarily African American women and their children. Some are homeless and have no incomes, while others are working poor with no access to affordable health care.

Complete physical examinations for well women who are seeking employment or entrance into substance abuse programs constitute approximately half of the weekly case load. The other 50% of the women present with acute health problems, most commonly vaginitis and sexually transmitted diseases or uncontrolled hypertension. The care provided these women is holistic, going beyond a cursory history and physical to include assessment of coping, nutrition, sleep, exercise, and substance use as well as safety issues. Children are seen for annual physical examinations and for acute illnesses. Growth and development and parenting skills are addressed with all parents.

An emphasis is placed upon enhancing the dignity of the clients. Adequate time with a nurse is given high priority. Relationships are developed with patients through an assessment interview with either a student or a registered nurse. This nurse remains with the patient throughout the history and examination by the nurse practitioner. The undergraduate student often participates in the physical evaluation of the patient in conjunction with the nurse practitioner and is an integral part of the interventions instituted to treat the client. This duo of student nurse and nurse practitioner provides ongoing case management for the client.

Students, with guidance from faculty, also assess aggregate needs and plan health promotion programs to meet them. The students conduct the programs and evaluate their effectiveness. Examples of programs include hypertension screening, breast cancer awareness, foot assessments, and sexually transmitted disease prevention and recognition sessions. Breakfast is served, and program incentives appropriate to the topics are provided.

All clients are asked to complete level-of-satisfaction and intent-to-change-behavior evaluation instruments. The collection and analysis of this data contribute to the evaluation of patient outcomes.

Case Example. Samantha is a 25-year-old woman who came to the homeless shelter clinic for a severe headache of four days' duration. She was assessed by a student nurse and a faculty nurse practitioner. Although the description of the headache was classic for an acute sinus infection, Samantha was not satisfied with this diagnosis and was very concerned that she had a brain tumor. There was a clear discrepancy between the young woman's physical appearance of mild distress and her very anxious voice and behaviors.

Samantha's history offered some explanation for the discrepancy. She had a history of severe unexpected illnesses and minimal social support. Essentially, Samantha had been living on her own since age 12 because of her mother's history of multiple personality and her father's chronic hypochondriasis. Her father had died recently after a rapid decline due to pancreatic cancer. Samantha felt a considerable amount of guilt and fear in regard to her father's death.

She had her first child at age 17 and, after being abandoned by the baby's father, was homeless for the first year of her son's life. Subsequently, she had several emergency hospitalizations for severe infections. These infections had started as simple problems that, because of lack of access to care, exploded into serious ones.

Samantha also had a two-year history of green drainage from the nipple of her right breast. She had sought a diagnosis at the onset of the problem but had an unpleasant interaction with a health care provider that caused her not to return for diagnostic studies. Clinical depression with previous hospitalizations was also in her history. She had not been able to afford her antidepressants and had not taken them in the previous three months. To further complicate matters, Samantha was now 2000 miles from home, having arrived in Milwaukee two weeks ago with her children, ages 3 and 8, to live with the father of

her second child, a man she had seen twice in the past year.

Samantha was very anxious about her own health, partly because of her history of minor illnesses escalating into near catastrophes. Her lack of a dense network of support in this new city and the lack of consistency and longevity in her current support system also contributed to this anxiety. On the basis of the assessment of the student nurse and the NP, it was hypothesized that Samantha, though intelligent and resilient, became easily frustrated if health care providers did not understand her needs and would respond with anger and withdrawal from the system. It was essential that Samantha be provided with the supports she needed in order for her to return to the clinic for follow-up care.

To treat her sinus infection, Samantha was provided with an antibiotic and analgesics as well as nonpharmacologic approaches to pain reduction. More important, she was given the pager number of the nurse practitioner and the assurance that she would be assisted in accessing care for her multiple concerns. Samantha paged the nurse practitioner six times in the four days following her initial visit to the clinic. Though this number of contacts would be seen as excessive in a traditional health care setting, it was recognized that Samantha was testing the trustworthiness of the clinic nurses. If they passed the test that previous health care providers had failed, she might continue her care. In these calls, she sought reassurance regarding her headache and depression as well as her breast drainage, and she received positive reinforcement from the nurse practitioner. This fostered the nurse-patient relationship and encouraged Samantha to return for her follow-up appointment.

Samantha did continue to return for care over the next several months. The interventions instituted by the nurse practitioner and the student nurse over the course of Samantha's health problems included helping her to analyze her coping strategies and her strengths, teaching her relaxation exercising, and enhancing her social support through conference calls between Samantha, her mother in California, and the nurse practitioner. Resources external to the clinic were also arranged to provide services outside the scope of the clinic. Through these interventions, Samantha's acute problems resolved and her long-term ones are being managed.

URBAN PARTNERS FOR HEALTH

Background. In 1992, the Urban Partners for Healthy Children Program was created as a partnership between the College of Nursing and the Central City Catholic School System. Public Health Nursing services were being reduced in all schools, which concerned the school administrators, who subsequently requested that the College become involved with the schools. Faculty and their students provided limited nursing services in all three schools. The faculty of one K-8 grade school was especially committed to collaboration. Funds were sought to enhance nursing in the school and expand health services through the sponsoring parish.

In the proposal to a religiously sponsored foundation, the Catholic grade school and parish were conceptualized as hubs of health care in a low-income, multicultural neighborhood. The family focus in the school promoted parents' investment in the health program. Nursing services were provided by a school nurse, a parish nurse, an advanced practice nurse, and nursing students.

Description. The advanced practice nurse, the school nurse, and nursing students provided nursing services at the school two days a week. The nursing activities were related to health promotion, health screening, and illness management for the children, teachers, and staff. Undergraduate students planned and participated in classroom health education programs and health and fitness days, and conducted development, vision, hearing, and communicable disease screening. Graduate students provided sports physicals to student athletes and follow-up otoscopic examinations of children who failed the hearing screening.

Population Served. Demographically, the school is diverse. The majority of the children (60%) are African American, with the numbers of Asian and Hispanic children being equally divided at 15% each. Less than 5% of the children reported being Caucasian. More than half of the children live in families whose annual income is below the poverty level. Although tuition is modest, approximately 95% of the children receive some form of tuition assistance through private grants and the archdiocese.

Outcomes. The school principal credits Marquette with delivering health services to children who do not have primary providers. As part of health services, all immunization records were reviewed for immunization compliance, meaning that students have the necessary immunizations and have the record on file at school, or that the parents have signed a health waiver, which is also kept in the school file. Early in the school year, the compliance rate for the school was 85%. At the beginning of the second semester, the rate was 96%. The response rate increased as a result of multiple efforts initiated by the school nurse, such as repeated follow-up notes and numerous phone calls to parents. Because this project is an academic/community venture, there is more time, with the use of student resources, to do in-depth follow-up with families. Thus, several families who might otherwise have been referred to the district attorney's office for noncompliance were spared this experience because of the service/learning model employed in this project.

Case Example. One family with three children was referred to the nurse and the social worker on a regular basis for absenteeism and a possible infectious skin condition. The nurse and the graduate nurse practitioner student attended a school/family meeting arranged by the social worker, and followed up with three home visits to the family to provide education about medication administration, management of asthma, and utilization of the emergency room for a primary care provider. In addition, the family was uninsured, temporarily not receiving Medicaid, and in need of expensive asthma and infectious disease medications. We purchased these medications through the grant. Targeted outcomes for this situation included assisting the mother and the child with early recognition of symptoms associated with asthma so that medication therapy could be instituted and possibly result in reduced school absenteeism.

Conclusion

Practice is an essential dimension of academic nursing. Practice innovations within academic nursing support both faculty and student development and contribute to the advancement of nursing knowledge. Through implementation of innovative prac-

BOX 21-3
Case Study   A New Graduate Prepares for Case Management*

Although most newly graduated nurses take traditional positions as hospital staff nurses, I am preparing myself for a year of volunteer service as a Nurse Case Manager at the Rose Brooks Center for Battered Women and Their Children in Kansas City, Missouri. Rose Brooks presently provides sanctuary and intensive therapeutic services to more than 500 battered women and their children each year. As a Nurse Case Manager for women living in the shelter, my position will entail answering the crisis hotline; completing medical intakes and providing crisis intervention services to women upon their entrance to the shelter; developing and teaching a weekly women's health group; providing nutrition and HIV/AIDS seminars; conducting health, immunization, and infectious disease screenings; providing prenatal, STD, and psychological counseling; registering clients for health care; transporting clients to health care appointments; providing clients with basic health education and generalized nursing care; and acting as a health care advocate for all clients and their children.

My training as a registered nurse with a Bachelor's of Science in Nursing degree has prepared me well for a position as a Nurse Case Manager. Aside from learning the clinical skills of physical assessment and medication administration that are essential to case management, my BSN education taught me that we must treat each of our clients as a whole person, not merely as a person subdivided into little parts. In order to be effective case managers, we need to address not only our clients' physical needs, but their emotional and spiritual needs as well. Nursing school also taught me the importance of teamwork and utilizing resources within the community in order to aid our clients in obtaining an optimal level of wellness. It is this ability to "branch out" and draw from the knowledge of others that makes case management so effective.

Through my BSN education, I learned how to properly use the nursing process of assessment, diagnosis, planning, implementation, and evaluation in order to address the needs that are a priority for the client. I was also able to develop critical thinking skills in order to increase my level of functioning as a registered nurse and Case Manager. Even though I have not had years of experience in nursing or case management, I have been given the necessary tools to analyze critical situations and determine the priority diagnoses and outcomes for each client. Finally, while I was in nursing school, I was able to observe and participate in nursing case management firsthand, thus increasing my awareness and understanding of what it takes to be a successful case manager. Case management is not an easy task, especially in nursing, but if approached with the proper knowledge and openness to teamwork, it can be highly effective.

*Written by Sheri Michele Carson, BSN, RN, and 1997 graduate of Marquette University.

tice models, such as those previously described, faculty can teach state-of-the-art nursing while delivering needed care to underserved populations. These models provide students with the opportunity to understand the changing health care system, which is rapidly becoming a community-based model, and to witness the effects of these changes on clients, families, and communities. Students are able to become familiar with and utilize technological innovations, noting the many questions related to financing, ethics, risk-benefit decisions, and quality-of-life issues. Students are afforded the opportunity to learn the importance of practicing as a member of an interdisciplinary team, which includes both professional and community participants. To assist students with learning these important skills, faculty need to consider macro and micro level issues. At the micro level, we have emphasized "point-of-living" care in homes, schools, and shelters, focusing on critical thinking skills and the use of effective communication techniques to assess, diagnose, and intervene. We have incorporated health promotion and disease prevention, analyzing important factors that influence health outcomes, such as social, economic, cultural, psychological, environmental, and physical variables.

Educators have the responsibility to prepare their graduates for practice in the changing health care environment (Box 21-3). Ways to accomplish this are selected in light of individual philosophy and mission statements of nursing programs. Our practice innovations are contributing to preparation of providers for the year 2000 and beyond.

References

American Association of Colleges of Nursing (AACN): *The power of faculty practice,* Washington, DC, 1996, The Association.

Barger SE, Bridges WC: An assessment of academic nursing centers, *Nurse Educator* 15(2):31-36, 1990.

Lough M, Schmidt K, Swan G, Naughton T, LeShan L, Blackburn J, Mancuso P: An interdisciplinary model for health professions students in a family practice center, *Nurse Educator* 21(1):27-31, 1996.

Machan L, ed: *The practitioner-teacher role: practice what you teach,* Wakefield, Mass, 1980, Nursing Resources.

Potash M, Taylor D: *Nursing faculty practice: models and methods,* Washington, DC, 1993, National Organization of Nurse Practitioner Faculties.

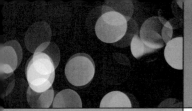

PART THREE

New Rules
Parameters of the Playing Field

Partnerships will maximize efforts, share accountabilities and ownership for processes that impact the health of the entire community by involving all constituencies in improvement activities.

TONI C. SMITH and ANN MARIE T. BROOKS

AS THE NEW HEALTH CARE INDUSTRY EMERGES from chaos and begins to take form, we can expect to experience new controls by regulatory agencies, industry, payers, and the practitioners themselves, the latter in the form of clinical guidelines. What part will the consumer, government, and the practitioners play in these developments? This section discusses some of the regulatory, legal, and consumer issues as rules, laws, and standards emerge. Some authors argue for more consumer involvement in this process, while others describe the impact of new rules on providers, or the expectation that laws will continue to follow practice. ▲

CHAPTER 22

Redefining Quality

Designing New Partnerships for Consumers and Providers

TONI C. SMITH, RN, EdD, **and ANN MARIE T. BROOKS,** RN, DNSc, MBA, FAAN, FACHE

OVERVIEW

The creation and nurturing of a strong consumer-provider relationship will be the major driver to define quality and service options based on consumer needs in the future.

Changes in the makeup of society in America necessitate changes in how health care organizations and systems decide what is service, price, and quality health care. It is time to stop using "palliative" approaches to involve consumers in determining what services are needed to meet their health care needs. This chapter discusses a needed renewed focus on the customers to redefine quality health care services on the basis of their diverse health care needs. ▲

Customer choice and informed decisions made by health care consumers will be based on indicators not considered today as elements important to quality health care services. Although there will always be a need to examine and monitor patient outcomes, service delivery methods, and access issues, consumers will play a major role in determining what information they need from providers as partners in care. Consumers will no longer be passive recipients of services and will be able to change providers that do not help them meet their health care needs and expectations. Americans are as diverse in their health care needs as the country is diverse in its ethnic composition. Predictions regarding the growth of various ethnic subgroups by 2020 indicate some major shifts of minorities, with Hispanics showing the most substantial growth. Just as education is considering how to address this shift from a language, socialization, and community perspective, health care providers must address this projection as well if they are to remain committed to the mission of improving health care services provided to customers. Although health care services have traditionally focused on acute care and specialization, the need to focus on prevention and keeping people healthy to maximize their functioning in light of irreversible conditions or chronic illness will be the key to success in providing quality care at the lowest possible cost (Sofaer, 1997).

To stay abreast of the changing marketplace, health care organizations have adopted many management tools from business, used by management engineers, to eliminate waste and redundancies and to reduce variation and errors and unnecessary complexity within their systems. As providers of health care services merge, expand, and form new alliances or systems, these new organizations will increasingly focus on market share, profit margins, building networks, and strengthening organizational performance. This growth in the number of health care provider systems has given rise to agencies and services trying to provide quality information to consumers. This new industry has caught the attention of payers and providers because of their desire for standards and recognition of differences among providers.

Management of health care quality is currently controlled by regulatory agency mandates and expectations of quality by professionals. The basis of

health care system reviews is prescribed by standards set forth by these agencies, which are based on industry- and discipline-specific standards and recognized practices. These regulatory agencies, both private and governmental, monitor health care and other services delivered by health care organizations and systems. The criteria used are based on a variety of sources and have changed markedly over the past decade. Now providers of care are setting objectives and goals for the populations they serve and developing models of care they deem to be appropriate and necessary, based on many factors and data. Old measures and standards must be revised. In the past, input from consumers was frequently sought; however, past efforts to get customer feedback fall short in providing data to ensure understanding of, and the ability to meet, the diverse needs of customers who will be enrolled in managed care systems of the future.

Health Care's Quality Reporting Dilemma

Public reporting by accrediting agencies of their findings has generated report cards, survey results of provider systems, and score cards that are packed with information deemed valuable to the public. However, these score cards, report cards, regulatory surveys, and so on, focus on current systems and processes and do not provide the context for understanding the results by consumers and how the information affects care delivery. Most consumers who hear about or read the information remain puzzled and do not usually seek further information or clarification. Managed care organizations use these reported performance measures to publish statistics on their performance and to demonstrate quality within their organizations, and they use the information as leverage to negotiate rates with providers. The preparation for these rating activities by external agencies usually diverts considerable time, energy, and resources from the organization and detracts from true customer-focused redesign improvement efforts.

Currently, there is pressure for health care organizations and systems (managed care plans, medical groups, hospitals) to disclose measurement data on utilization patterns and organizational performance in delivering health care services. These data are based on preset patient outcomes, and results of patient satisfaction surveys and services received. This type of public disclosure reporting is based on the notion that the public is interested and will use this information to make choices about which health care plans or services to select. Solberg, Mosser, and McDonald (1997) discuss two types of measurement: measurement for accountability and measurement for improvement. As linkages are formed between managed care organizations, medical groups, hospitals, and others, clarity is needed about the purposes, means, and uses of measurement data. Historically, organizations have used unified data collection methods to collect information for internal process improvement activities and for external reporting purposes (Solberg et al, 1997). Providers of clinical care remain concerned that data collected for process improvement activities could be misused to judge the quality of their services if reported by the government or purchasing groups to the public. There is also concern by providers that information will be used to reach conclusions that exceed limitations of the methods used to collect it.

However, as consumers drive demand for new and different types of services, less data collection and measurement activity will take place without being based on the values and voices of the consumer. In the past, consumers have been peripheral or superficial to health care planning. As consumers assume more financial responsibility for health care services that they use, their decisions are now being made on the basis of out-of-pocket costs and coverage options. Their interest in knowing how their monies are being spent is increasing. The onus is on care providers and systems to provide information to consumers in methods understandable to them and relevant to informed decision making to meet their own health care needs. The creation and nurturing of a strong consumer-provider relationship will be the major driver to define quality and service options based on consumer needs in the future. By fostering this relationship and accountability to develop and improve care delivery systems, providers can meet their responsibilities to the public for implementing improvement activities to provide quality health services at affordable costs in an efficient and satisfying manner to all.

The New World Order

Health care providers need to create strategies to examine and address differences in the world views of consumers and provider systems. These views are based on belief systems, and are exhibited by overt and covert behaviors, verbal and nonverbal communication signals, and intentions and actions of both parties. There needs to be a bridging of any differences through effective communication and positive interactions blending the cultures and belief systems of providers and consumers. Administrators and providers of health care plans should acknowledge that defining high-quality performance is a value-driven activity. The critical question that remains is: whose values will prevail in determining quality, value, cost, price, and access to services that are provided or that need to be provided?

There can no longer be separate and noninteractive activities to plan and deliver health care services by providers. Partnering with consumers to link long-term strategies to short-term actions to improve consumer satisfaction is imperative, according to Kaplan and Norton (1996). When providers create partnerships with consumers by using the strategies delineated in Box 22-1 to provide continuity of care throughout a community, isolated competitive models of care delivery will be eliminated. Thus, duplication and redundancies in services can be avoided. Partnerships will maximize efforts and share accountabilities and ownership for processes that affect the health of the entire community by involving all constituencies in improvement activities. These new partnerships will reform the health care industry's efforts of trying to mass produce "individualized care." Providers and consumers need to allow adequate time to plan, deliver, and receive appropriate services that are patient population specific to meet the needs of each consumer. It is through collective planning that a framework to stimulate growth through creation of new products and services will be achieved. Gaps in services for consumers can be eliminated through cooperative efforts to identify needed services and setting priorities that can be translated into new initiatives to meet consumers' needs along the health care continuum (illness to wellness programs). Adoption of customer-focused, service-oriented behaviors (see Box 22-1) by care providers is directly linked to consumer sat-

BOX 22-1
Strategies for Health Care Professionals to Create Provider-Consumer Partnerships

- Create processes to ask:
  "What do you need or how can I help you?"
  and
  "How did I do (to meet that need)?"
- Provide answers to consumers' questions and concerns with responses tailored to meet their needs and levels of understanding.
- Utilize interactive opportunities with support and self-help groups, thus creating the ability for consumers to network with others who share common problems, issues, and concerns.
- Foster the right-to-know concept (consumers have a right to information even if the information is technically difficult to understand).
- Commit to implementing ways to increase your awareness, sensitivity, knowledge, and skills related to management of diverse populations.
- Enhance your listening skills to show respect and to establish the basis for a partnership characterized by open, honest, and direct communication channels.
- Provide consistent service; recognize your professional strengths and weaknesses.
- Encourage involvement and participation of family members in care planning and treatments.

BOX 22-2
Sources of Information for Consumer Health Care Choices

Family and friends
Employer
Physicians and other health care providers
Health care rating organizations
Health care delivery systems
Government: local, state, federal agencies

isfaction, as evidenced by consumers' subsequent personal choices regarding health services used, compliance with prescribed therapies, participation in care, return visits, and the divulging of pertinent information that could affect health care needs.

A major issue that needs to be addressed by provider organizations is the assumption that consumers will make choices to improve or maintain their well-being, if they are given what providers in the health care industry and their independent raters deem as appropriate and adequate information to make sound health care choices and decisions. However, health care consumers generally make their decisions independent of this information and/or rely on the expertise, choices, or recommendations of others independent of information provided by health care providers and regulatory agencies. As shown in Box 22-2, health care providers are no longer the sole source for health care–related information. Also, the traditional reliance on the physician as the most reliable and informed source for health care information has changed. Care providers and systems are seen to possess power and thus the ability to determine which issues move from private to public domains for action. Thus, this can be seen as advancing their own issues or determining what (if anything) can be done to meet the health care needs consumers present, and therefore the views of the care provider may seem to be in conflict with those of the user (Lang, Shannon, 1997). However, there is an information explosion, due to advances in communication technology, which gives people greater access to traditional and alternative forms of health care information. Physicians and other health care providers are under the gun to respond in a timely, caring (Box 22-3), non-self-serving manner (e.g., statistics about the efficacy of health care interventions, health promotion programs, new treatment modalities). In addition, it becomes imperative that health care providers have access to and utilize the new sources of information in their practices and systems that can be shared community-wide. Health care systems will need to identify and understand what patients and families do not want, as well as identify what is needed by them to be safe,

BOX 22-3
Consumer Interactions

Dehumanizing Actions	Positive Encounter
Avoidance	Respectful engagement during interactions
Negation of worth	Caring body language, posture
Rejection	Mutual communication
Minimizing needs of others	Maintaining or restoring integrity

BOX 22-4
Pitfalls

- Not analyzing patterns of health plan services used in order to determine customers' preferences on the basis of variations in services accessed or missed appointments.
- Failure to recognize the importance of, and build on, consumer-provider relationships. . . . "build ties that bind, creating loyalty."
- Not creating an infrastructure focused and centered on the consumer to produce and provide customized care and decrease plan switching.
- Not educating consumers on how to use and access aspects of the plan or system.
- Not creating methods to evaluate consumer preferences, usage patterns, and needs.
- Failure to honor commitments or tell the truth.

secure, and comfortable. Health care systems must find open, efficient communication channels to share information at a community-wide level.

Customer-Focused, Quality Decision Making

American health care consumers will face having a wealth of data that they are supposed to use to stay abreast of changes and make decisions regarding health care services. As we are well aware, the amount of reading that Americans do is limited, and the interest of people in having or needing information varies greatly. In addition, access to computers or interest in using technology to obtain information varies across age, socioeconomic, and cultural groups. The majority of individuals 50 years of age and older are not computer literate and do not require technology for decision making. As our children get older, the requirements for communication will shift dramatically because their standard method of learning is based on technology and other innovations. A recent survey shows that most consumers agree that there is some degree of quality variation among hospitals, health care plans, and medical care providers (Robeusch, Brodo, 1997). However, many consumers may not have many health plan choices to make at this time and lack familiarity with how to interpret comparative health care quality data or feel intimidated by the system.

Choices, decisions, and behaviors reflect learned beliefs and values (Kavanagh, Kennedy,

1992). Engagement between providers and consumers to define quality health care services must be based on direct intervention, mutual open communication, and respectful engagement. In addition, opportunity must exist for reassessment of any situation and its accompanying decision(s). Providers must be prepared to be sensitive to consumers' needs before they ask intrinsic questions or assume they know what is best. Common pitfalls, as shown in Box 22-4, must be avoided if a true, durable, and collaborative relationship is to develop. There cannot be denial or negation of issues, avoidance, or the creation of a perception of invisibility by the providers. Finally, another aspect to be recognized and avoided is any perception of coercion of the consumer by the provider as a result of the inequity of power within the relationship. Coercive tactics limit options of the consumer within the relationship and erode the strength of the partnership.

There continues to be debate about what are ideal quality measures of health care by providers and regulators. In the past, measures of health care quality have included client-focused indicators that spanned the care delivery continuum. These measures also addressed organizational performance, issues of patient access to services, and costs of providing care as the drivers for organizational decisions. However, consumers need to better understand the meaning and relevance of any health care plan, based on their own health care needs and on choices and services provided. The new context and content of health care quality information will be determined by the user, and the decisions may be made by the patient, family member, or caretaker, all of whom could have different expectations for information or services required (Lang, Shannon, 1997). The existence of these different needs implies that different decision support structures or intermediaries will be needed to help the consumer to make health care decisions (Jennings, Miller, Mateena, 1997). Health care consumers have not only different needs, but different decision styles, based on their attitudes, geographic locations, and social/psychological dimensions. Also, consumers will take note of their families, friends, and their own personal experiences within a health care system, and services accessed or denied to them will influence their health-seeking behaviors and subsequent health care plan choices.

Methods to determine, and then prioritize, customer expectations based on the values and needs of the customer rather than those of the care provider are now required. Consumers' ideas about health and illness come from experiences, and social and cultural contexts. Traditionally, providers have not offered enough, if any, opportunities for clients to discuss their beliefs about illness and wellness or their perceptions of quality health care services. Culturally competent care, which is the goal of the future, involves decisions and actions that are acceptable and reasonable to the consumer, thus preserving the consumer's original perspective (Kavanagh, Kennedy, 1992). Providers must ask the customer "How can we assist you?" and then go beyond that question to assist in achieving the expectation. Care providers must move beyond the symbolic gestures of providing consumers with information determined by the providers and managers of health care systems. Information must be provided at the level of understanding of the consumer, based on his or her needs, knowledge base, and past experiences, so that or future actions and decisions will be based on a level of understanding and buy-in. Administrators and regulators of health systems and plans, and governmental agencies, will need to acknowledge the fact that increased investment in provider-identified measures of performance for the purpose of informing consumers may mean little to consumers (Jennings et al, 1997). Health care delivery systems have wasted a lot of energy on looking better to the public rather than becoming better health care providers, which should be inherent in all the time spent on most data collection activities today by providers. Health care providers must become promoters of timely and relevant information, creators and sharers of knowledge, always mindful that the final judges of performance are the person and family helped in the process.

Structure, Process, and Outcome Targets to Improve Customer Relations

The following areas are opportunities for organizations and providers to make corrections and change directions, using a structure, process, outcome framework to identify activities to break through the boundaries of entrenched attitudes and practices, avoiding obsolescence. Providers must address the following areas:
- Structure
- Process
- Outcome(s)

STRUCTURE

- Promote and use the Internet; the Internet as a source of health care information will continue to grow. "Chat" self-help groups for information abound and will continue to grow. In addition, there are Internet sites of health care information established by nonprofit consumer groups, state and federal governments, and national regulatory agencies.
- Plan (and implement) systems that provide structures for widespread customization of health services to get closer to the needs of patients and their families.
- Eliminate and minimize cultural, environmental, or attitudinal barriers in the provider system.
- Decrease the number of dimensions or elements of a provider system that a consumer has to evaluate.

PROCESS

- Promote or implement quality data collection efforts built around continual dialogues with consumers, and not a review of system "ratings," as the best way to share information geared to meet or exceed customer expectations, not just needs and expectations of providers.
- Formulate ways to partner with consumers to decrease waste and identify areas for improvement and innovation in plans and systems.
- Create a loyal customer base by going beyond what the customer expects. If a customer has experienced some delay, disappointment, or poor-quality service, ensure that he or she experiences prompt, swift, and thorough repair. Kavanagh and Kennedy (1992) describe the "replace plus one" concept used by high-class organizations, under which the customer receives more than he or she lost as a form of apology and to acknowledge the loss and show respect for the proper use of the customer's time.
- Empower employees closest to the customer to do whatever it takes to restore faith and loyalty. (If these instances are tracked and monitored, they may become areas for investigation to implement long-term improvements and/or create new products or services.)
- Eliminate pain and fear in consumers served; pain and fear produce anxiety for the helper and the helpee, so stay focused on the needs and goals of the consumer (helpee).

OUTCOME(S)

- Create methods to measure effects of information given to consumers, based on the consumer's actions, attitudes, and health status.
- Implement a set of holistic interventions to meet widely diverse and changing requirements of consumers.
- Establish partnerships with consumers that are based on reducing demand for services as a result of improved consumer knowledge and personal health care skills, and not on restricting or limiting access to reduce costs and increase profits.

• • •

Providers must put the consumer at the center of efforts to improve health care. They need to create systems that support and enhance consumer participation in health care delivery and maintenance systems. Health care professionals need to expand their knowledge and skill base for continued professional growth and to learn how to involve consumers in the care delivery process as partners.

The Future of Health Care Quality Determinations

Provider systems will continue to create and use statistical methods and performance measurement systems to define quality services within available costs. Members of managed care systems continually move around; quality data reported for selected periods can only reflect interventions for persons within the plan at that time. Parker and Wenneker (1997) discuss the fact that screening rates for new members are not informative about the effect of interventions on all members, since some members were not involved at the interventions' inception. The discussion by Parker and Wenneker points out serious limitations in current quality data submitted using existing performance measures, because of the inability to compare and identify changes in performance over time as a result of consumers leaving or joining plans. This serious limitation substantiates the fact that new measures are needed that reflect consumer satisfaction, values, and concerns about services received. There will be new alliances between public and private sector organizations to work collaboratively on defining health care services and practices for the community. As these partnership activities move forward, creating ways to involve consumers in these planning partnerships to improve services in health care delivery is essential.

Care providers, managed care systems, and community-based employees need to identify and address barriers to involving consumers in defining services and quality in meaningful ways. It is obvious that the members of the partnership will have different interests driving their participation and valuing of the process. However, consumer needs and access issues identified by the consumer will have significant impact on planning and evaluation of the quality of health services in the future. To develop and strengthen partnerships with consumers, providers of managed care systems and their employees must:

- Address territorial issues of power, control, and management based on service delivery models in which providers and administrators were decision makers.
- Challenge all old boundaries, values, and world views.
- Teach consumers how to participate and plan as true partners and provide them with the tools to be active participants.
- Examine and change how resources of the provider system are allocated (based on the physical needs of patients) and reallocate resources to address the subjective, interpersonal, or caring needs of patients (Milne, McWilliams, 1996).
- Recognize that this type of change will take time and that they must become facilitators and leaders in planning and implementing and focus on consistency in establishing and maintaining partnerships.
- Design mechanisms to acknowledge that the capability of the consumer to participate in the partnership will benefit them and their families.

Conclusion

A service delivery model that focuses on the consumer will evolve in stages, moving from one-way encounters, focusing on service needs of people, problems, and process improvement initiatives, to complete involvement of patient, family, and community to identify their needs, preferences, and desired organizational outcomes. Box 22-5 lists behaviors of providers that are critical to creating an "inclusive" atmosphere to integrate consumers from diverse backgrounds and with varying needs, skills, and education.

A recent survey by Robeusch and Brodo (1997) shows that family and friends are ranked as the highest sources for information on health care quality by those making health care decisions. This study reflects the fact that although American consumers may value information about quality, currently they do not use it as the sole factor in making health care choices. This finding supports the notion that quality measures that address consumers' experiences (often overlooked by organizations)

BOX 22-5

Creating an "Inclusive" Customer Atmosphere

- Consumers feel welcome and accepted regardless of lifestyle, race, or cultural differences.
- All segments of consumer populations served are represented in the provider system as providers/employees.
- At the time of patient/consumer meetings the session is not dominated by either party.
- Variety in dress and grooming are acceptable and the norm of the employees within the system.
- Sensitivity to and awareness of different customs and religious or ethnic holidays are demonstrated by providers.
- Provider flexibility exists to accommodate reasonable personal preferences and behaviors.

---

will continue to be important to Americans when they need to make choices. Consumers' preferences and concerns will bring about new notions of quality. Consumers will no longer be passive recipients of professional care, and many may resist top-down information. Professionals will shift into a coach/facilitator role rather than act as know-it-all authority figures. New measures of quality will define future provider-consumer relationships. Competence and skill by the provider are important; however, buy-in and participation of the consumer to identify his or her needs and subsequent quality measures across the continuum are needed. Jeddeloh (1997) states that the provider-consumer relationships of the future will reflect pooled or jointly secured resources. It is incumbent on provider systems to create ongoing measurement methods that identify and address patient expectations. Providers must be the drivers in identifying and responding to customer requirements, even in the absence of a true participatory relationship, which will take time to cultivate. Brown et al (1993) postulate that a personal relationship linking providers and consumers will become the heart of quality care.

Cyberspace will link consumers worldwide. These linkages will change forever the amount, type, and availability of information used by consumers to determine what constitutes quality health care practices used to make health care decisions. It is a responsibility of health care providers to involve consumers in efforts to redesign quality improvement methods and measures in order to elevate the consumer to the role of partner.

References

Brown S, Nelson AM, Brankesh S, Wood S: *Patient satisfaction pays: quality service for practice success*, Gaithersburg, Md, 1993, Aspen Publishers, Inc.

Jeddeloh R: Establishing the parameters for patient participation in care, design, delivery and evaluation. In American Organization of Nurse Executives: *Patient as a partner: the cornerstone of community health improvement*, Chicago, 1997, American Hospital Publishing, pp 1-12.

Jennings K, Miller K, Materna S: *Changing health care: creating tomorrow's winning health enterprise today*, Santa Monica, Calif, 1997, Anderson Consulting Knowledge Exchange.

Kaplan R, Norton D: Using the balanced score card as a strategic management system, *Harvard Business Review* January-February 1996, pp 75-85.

Kavanagh K, Kennedy P: *Promoting cultural diversity: strategies for health care professionals*, Newbury Park, London 1992, Sage Publications.

Lang LA, Shannon TE: Patient's perspective conference overview, *Journal of Quality Improvement* 23(5):231-238, 1997.

Milne H, McWilliams C: Considering nursing resources as 'caring time,' *Journal of Advanced Nursing* 23:810-819, 1996.

Parker R, Wenneker M: The quality improvement ratio: a method to identify changes in screening rates, *The Joint Commission Journal on Quality Improvement* 23(6):299-311, 1997.

Robeusch S, Brodo M: Understanding the quality challenge for health consumers: the Kaiser/AHCPR survey, *Journal of Quality Improvement* 23(5):239-244, 1997.

Sofafer S: How will we know if we got it right? Aims, benefits and risks of consumer information initiatives, *The Joint Commission Journal on Quality Improvement* 23(5):258-264, 1997.

Solberg L, Mosser G, McDonald S: The three faces of performance measurement: improvement, accountability and research, *The Joint Commission Journal on Quality Improvement* 23(2):135-147, 1997.

CHAPTER 23

Interdisciplinary, Collaborative Team Practice in Managed Care

The Provider Perspective

VIVIEN DE BACK, RN, PhD, FAAN

OVERVIEW

Without an educated consumer and an involved provider, the system of managed care cannot be successful. By its very nature, effective managed care requires the cooperation and true partnering of those delivering the service and those receiving it.

Insights were obtained on provider perceptions of the effect of change on their practice and client outcomes, through an interview process with six teams of health care providers who practice in managed care arrangements. In the midst of dramatic and rapid changes in health care, providers describe the most critical issues to be addressed in the near future. They include effective communication throughout the system; education of consumers, providers, and managers; and integrated information systems that support clinical practice. ▲

The words *managed care* conjure up strong emotions in many who are involved in health care, including managers and providers of care, businesses that buy health care packages for their employees, and clients who receive care. Depending upon your vantage point, the emotions range from total rejection to complete acceptance and everything in between. New systems of managed care are continuing to emerge as redesign and reengineering take place all across the American health care scene. The changes that have been made to create today's managed care environment have been substantial and far reaching as organizations and providers work to develop a comprehensive range of health services for their clients. The influence of the business model and the capitalistic spirit on the health care system has changed how providers practice, which includes changes in skill mix to bring more efficiency and effectiveness into the system.

Managed care allows health insurance companies and providers to manage or have greater control over how health care is dispensed to their enrollees, which helps to control costs. Managed care organizations control costs by creating networks of providers, which contract to provide services for a negotiated fee or which provide a comprehensive range of services to an enrolled population for a fixed sum of money paid in advance. Three common characteristics used to describe contemporary managed health care systems are: quality, coordinated, and cost effective. In the 1980s the buzzword was cost containment as employers who purchase health care packages negotiated for inexpensive insurance plans. In the mid-1990s the driving force in health insurance selection is quality. As this shift from a focus on cost to a focus on quality in health care takes place, questions are being raised about how to determine "quality."

The growth of managed care has been phenomenal. At the end of 1995, nearly 60 million Americans belonged to health maintenance organizations (HMOs), an increase over 1994 of nearly 15% according to the American Association of Health Plans, in Washington, D.C. (Rubin, 1996). Predictions for the future suggest that HMO enrollment will more than double in just six years. At present, more than two thirds of HMO members have the opportunity to choose from at least two plans. These figures do not include other managed care arrangements, such as preferred provider organizations (PPOs) and physician hospital organizations (PHOs). Another area of growth in managed care has been in the Medicaid population. The Health Care Financing Administration (HCFA) reported in 1995 that between June of 1994 and June of 1995 Medicaid Managed Care (MMC) enrollment increased from 7.8 million to 11.6 million (Guyer, 1996). Throughout this growth process, managed care organizations or agencies, hospitals, and other provider groups have focused heavily on structure (reorganizing the systems) and process (redesigning the methods of providing care). Strategies used have included increasing rates, reducing hospital stays, discontinuing coverage for selected groups, and increasing enrollment. Areas of the country (Midwest and West) that pioneered managed care arrangements soon found the ability to increase enrollment diminishing as managed care agencies saturated the market.

J.C. Goldsmith predicts that "as markets mature, managed care plans will be forced increasingly to actually manage care as a vehicle for generating earnings growth" (Goldsmith, 1996). In his description of the evolution of managed care, Goldsmith describes three stages in the process: Stage I, event-driven cost avoidance; Stage II, value improvement; and Stage III, health improvement. Event-driven cost avoidance is a historic strategy for generating earnings in managed care by avoiding hospitalization of subscribers after they have become sick (Goldsmith, 1996). Value improvement is the stage in managed care when organizations are forced to take a much more detailed and aggressive look at how to maximize the value of their product (Goldsmith, 1996). The health improvement stage is described by Goldsmith as cultural change that "enables managed care plans and systems to actually improve the health of their subscribers" (Goldsmith, 1996). He further identifies specific organizational behaviors that reflect each stage of evolution (Table 23-1). It was expected that through an exploration of these potential "outcomes" of the reengineering process through the eyes of the health care providers who were interviewed for this chapter, an understanding of the implications of change would emerge.

Goldsmith's stages of evolution were used as an initial framework to design questions for interviews with providers in managed care arrangements. A second organizing framework for the in-

TABLE 23-1
Managed Care: Stages of Evolution

	STAGE I	STAGE II	STAGE III
	EVENT-DRIVEN COST AVOIDANCE	VALUE IMPROVEMENT	HEALTH IMPROVEMENT
Objective function	Price	Value/customer satisfaction	Health status improvement
Cost targets	Inpatient days	Resource intensity	Health risks
Locus of control	External	Peer driven	"Contract" with family
Focal point	Inpatient hospital	Physician network	Home/neighborhood

Modified from Goldsmith JC: Managed care comes of age. In Bezold C, Mayer E, eds: *Future care: responding to the demand for change*, New York, 1996, Faulkner & Grey, p. 144. Reprinted with permission of Faulkner & Grey.

terviews was aimed at the effectiveness or usefulness of the *team* as provider. The purpose of the interviews was to determine primary care providers' perspectives on the managed health care systems in which they deliver care day after day. A second purpose was to ascertain providers' perceptions of the effect of multiple system changes on client outcomes.

The evolutionary process that the nation has been going through for several years has been most often examined by "bottom line" analysis. At this point in the reengineering process a number of different questions are being raised, such as: What effects are downsizing, restructuring, team development, and case management having on the recipients of care and the providers of that care? How well is the system working for providers and clients? What outcomes of care are being evaluated? Physicians, nurses, physician assistants, psychologists, and others have strong opinions on the environments in which they work and the impact of the changes in those environments on client care.

Six different teams of providers from the Midwest and Western regions were interviewed over a three-month period, January through March, 1997. All groups worked in managed care settings or were contracted with managed care agencies to deliver care. The total number of providers interviewed was 15. Questions were submitted prior to the interviews (Box 23-1), as well as background on the purpose of the interviews. Two persons were interviewed individually. All others were in group

BOX 23-1
Questions Submitted to Interviewees

1. What effect has the integrated team concept had on your delivery of care?
2. What specifically makes the integration of care an efficient system for you to practice in?
3. What is the effectiveness, in your opinion, of multiple providers in a single setting?
4. How is the quality of life of clients improved because of interdisciplinary teaming?
5. What actually happens as a result of partnering?
6. The literature describes integration of care as the "right provider for the right client at the right time." Is this really how it works?
7. What are the challenges and future changes needed to make the system more effective?
8. Are there other issues related to "team" or "managed" care that would help us understand the state of the art today?

interviews. The average interview time was 90 minutes. Interviewees were candid in their responses and throughout the interview process. To protect the confidentiality of individuals and organizations, no identification of participants or agencies is made.

Team Concept

For those practitioners who work in teams, the arrangement appears to be both satisfactory and efficient, as described by providers interviewed. They describe *"respect"* for one another and helpfulness to each other as key ingredients of a well-functioning team. Opportunities to consult with other professionals were considered an important benefit of working with multiple providers under one roof. Although few individuals described drawbacks in working in *their* teams, most providers related problems in the evolution of the team concept in their organizations. Chief among these was *"lack of definition of roles"* for providers in the group. This issue was most frequently referred to by nurse practitioners (NPs) and physician assistants (PAs). They believe that clearer definitions of roles and responsibilities would improve utilization of all health care providers. There was also concern that PAs and NPs were perceived by patients to be *"second-choice"* providers, to be consulted because the doctor was not available. Some providers discussed their positions in the teams as single providers working in parallel with other providers. They believe that the more efficient configuration would be to focus on the *"team as provider,"* although to move in this direction would require additional support such as access to all client information on-line. Furthermore, consumer education on acceptance of the team rather than *only* an individual as the provider of health care would be needed. A considerable emphasis on consumer education would suggest that an organization has evolved to Stage II of Goldsmith's managed care configuration.

Other issues related to health provider team success were ability to select team members, peer review, and common philosophies of delivery of health care. For example, a nurse practitioner described her heavy focus on family health education in her practice. She is teamed with a primary care physician who is medical model oriented (diagnose, treat, cure). The time she spends in health education is not valued by her team member, which results in some tension between them. *"He's a wonderful doctor and is good at what he does for sick patients. But I should not be teamed with him, since I believe in health promotion, health maintenance, and disease prevention as the most important aspects of my practice."*

Primary care providers who work in a team believe that they are providing a *"fail-safe"* mechanism for clients and families. *"There is always some-*

one there to take care of an emergency, and you know it's one of your team whom you respect and trust."* This reality provides an increase in the quality of care available to every family and individual who is served by the interdisciplinary team. The perception that clients are served well by teams is supported by satisfaction surveys that providers indicated were given to clients regularly and reviewed by them.

In some clinics, providers work side by side but not necessarily as team members. One provider described the relationship among the members of the team as *"parallel providers who share an office."* He believes this is an efficient method, since each of them has different approaches and philosophies to providing care. *"We still have the advantage of talking and consulting with each other, which we do daily."* The integrated, interdisciplinary team, functioning as a single well-developed group of health care providers, is still evolving in the teams interviewed.

What Works Well and What Does Not

Over and over again, providers describe the importance of coordinated, comprehensive care. They believe that the managed care system is an improvement over the fragmented system of the past, even though it has problems yet to be addressed. *"In most cases, I can identify a problem, refer my patient, and know within a reasonable time that the patient is seen by a specialist. From a quality-of-care point of view, this is what is working. However, getting feedback to me about this patient is not as smooth, because the return loop is not as well established"* (Primary Care Provider, 1997).

Nurses who work as case managers to effect a system of coordinated care see the problems of implementation differently. They describe provider *"lack of knowledge"* about managed care as the single most important issue in their daily work. *"Primary care providers do not understand the extent to which we can help them and their clients in creating the seamless system of care. Once they have experienced the case management system with a client, they become advocates and we hear from them often"* (Nurse Case Manager, 1997). To ensure proper use of a managed care system, physicians, physician assistants, nurse practitioners, and others need to be educated to community resources that are available. More important, nurse case managers believe, managed care will become most effective when everyone takes responsibility as a member of the team within a well-understood system of care. This would result in a shift in the locus of control, which Goldsmith describes as Stage II in managed care evolution.

Some providers believe that the reason the system is not as well developed as it could be is that they, as providers, are not consulted about changes or future plans. *"Often we hear of changes in referral providers or methods of practice or even hours of service* after *the contracts have been signed or change process is in effect. We are informed rather than consulted. Yet we have a pretty good idea of what is going to work and what isn't"* (Nurse Practitioner, 1997). Still, there are other providers who do not want to be involved in the multiple changes in the system: *"Just let me see my patients and keep me out of it* (changes in the system). Directors of managed care argue that without provider understanding and support of the system, efficiency and effectiveness cannot be achieved. Whether they are desirous of involvement in system design or not, it is clear that two key players in the managed care operation are providers and clients, both of whom are seriously underrepresented in the decision making and day-to-day management of the organization.

Throughout the interviews, two words kept appearing in the discussion of the managed care system with providers. They were *"hopeful"* and *"harried."* Most were hopeful that the system would continue to evolve toward a better, more efficient entity. *"Managed care has enormous potential for developing into the caring and efficient system we all believe in"* (Nurse Case Manager, 1997). Most providers are willing to *"hang in there"* and wait out the redesign process because they believe a health care system with a major focus on *health* will emerge (Psychologist, 1997). When asked why they believe this, they cite the strides in health care over the past five years, from a heavily fee-for-service system to managed care. Providers who are working in managed care are believers in the system or at least believe that the direction of the evolution is the more acceptable one. One provider summed up her perception of health system change: *"Early on, the concern was managing cost and as providers we were less involved. The accountants made decisions without us. Now the focus has shifted to managing the care, or the patient, or the disease, or the family. This I can get involved in. For me it means the right care at the right time"* (Primary care physician, 1997). At the same time that physicians and nurses describe hopefulness, they talk about their harried existence: *"I just wish I had more time." "I want to review the chart more carefully before seeing my patient." "I go home every night and fall asleep on the couch."*

All of the teams and individuals interviewed described their harried existence in delivering health care in today's environment, although they had various expectations about work load (expectations ranged from an average of 16 clients per day to 26 per day). There were also significant variations in the severity of client conditions and the types of patients seen, such as Medicare patients, children with chronic disease, and patients with mental illnesses. Whatever the work load, every provider felt *"pressed"* for time. *"The system is not helpful to us. Technology helps the organization in tracking client appointments and gathering satisfaction data and crunching the financial numbers. But little technology has been applied to the day-to-day care of clients. We are literally buried in paper. We have charts three inches thick. Where is the technology to help us?"* (Physician Assistant, 1997)

Communication

By far, the most discussed topic by providers was communication: how much they know about the systems within which they work, when they get to know about changes, how the new information is communicated, and what effect changes will have on their practice and their patients. Providers are not well versed in the organizational structures in which they work. They are not knowledgeable about the processes their patients go through once a referral has been made. Providers described this lack of knowledge, but few suggested ways to improve their situations or to obtain information. Clearly, errors can be made and frustration increased when people do not understand the system they are working in. On the other side of the coin, case managers are frustrated with primary care providers who are unwilling to become familiar with the system. *"Managed care is complicated. It needs to be studied to be understood. It is changing to accommodate the needs of providers and patients, so everyone, providers of care and clients, needs to learn about the system. We learned it"* (Nurse Case Manager, 1997). One physician who is trying to keep up with changes in the system spoke about his involvement: *"I read everything I can get my hands on. Yet health care contracts are so out of control that every day brings new developments, new pressures. Only an individual devoted full time to the subject could keep up."* Several providers discussed the overwhelming amount of information that comes across their desks and their inability to sort out or identify the critical information. Most believe that technology will help them solve this problem, although they could not describe how that might be done.

"We need to improve our communication with patients and families, but this takes a lot of time. Who is going to pay for that?" (Primary care physician, 1997). There was considerable frustration by physicians about communication issues with clients and families. *"How can we be true partners in care with patients if they are not knowledgeable?"* One provider says, *"Consumers have a responsibility to seek and use information regarding health care. The responsibility is not all ours."*

Communication is key to effective dialog, exchange of information, and knowledge transfer. Yet the providers of health care who were interviewed expressed a lack of effective communication in their systems and a lack of time and ability to address the subject. In this critical area of human discourse, providers described innumerable barriers to improving communication in their settings.

What to Eliminate, Keep, and Add

At the conclusion of each interview, providers of care were asked three questions. The purpose of the questions was to elicit specific actions that could be taken by organizations or individuals to improve the systems in which they work. The questions asked were:

1. If you could *eliminate* three things in the health care system today, what would they be?

TABLE 23-2
Interviewee Responses to Questions of What to Eliminate, Keep, or Add to the Health Care System

ELIMINATE	KEEP	ADD
Focus on cost	Accessibility to the system	Education of clients and providers
Employers as sole decision makers	High value on health promotion	Providers who know and value the system; involve consumers in decision making
Disrupting a team that has created a strong working relationship	Comprehensiveness: easy access to multiple providers	Focus on "team as provider" rather than an individual
Dropping a member in midtreatment (employer decision to change)	Seamless system for providing health care	Provider satisfaction as a measurement of the system
Role confusion of various health care providers (for consumers and providers)	Teams of providers	Clinical information systems, on-line, for all providers of care
Ill-defined areas of responsibility	Focus on appropriate utilization of resources	Improved data collection to support clinical practice
	Peer review	Client outcomes as system measurement
	Respect for varied health care providers	Clear definitions of various providers
		Strong team between management and providers, with provider input into system's change

2. If you could *keep* three things in the health care system today, what would they be?
3. If you could *add* three things to the health care system today, what would they be?

Not surprisingly, it was easier to add or to keep than to eliminate. Commonalities in responses emerged from the participants and were placed under common headings. The responses are found in Table 23-2.

Lessons Learned

Interviews with providers in several settings offer insights into how far managed care has evolved over the past ten years. The most lasting impression received after all interviews was the acceptance of managed care as the best (or only?) method for delivering health care in this country. Every person interviewed supported the managed care concept and the need for further development of the system. Of course, all of them are *"inside"* the system we are asking them to critique. Still, none of them would accept returning to earlier models of care, which they saw as *"wasteful"* and *"professional rather than patient focused."*

Several themes emerged during the interviews: an educated partnership, communication, and information systems to support clinical practice.

EDUCATED PARTNERSHIP

Without an educated consumer and an involved provider, the system of managed care cannot be successful. By its very nature, effective managed care requires the cooperation and true partnering of those delivering the service and those receiving it. Such partnerships do not appear to be mainstream practice, which again suggests that managed care systems have not totally evolved to Stage II of Goldsmith's evolutionary description. The education needed for primary care providers and their patients to understand the managed care system is clearly lacking. The concept of partnership with the organization is underdeveloped. *"There is little knowledge or loyalty to the organization"* (Case Manager, 1997). Only through education (seminars, inservice and conferences) will primary care providers in managed care organizations become integral partners in the system. When asked why education is so obviously lacking at a time of such great need, one nurse stated: *"At a time of intense financial pres-*

sure in the system, the first area to be eliminated is education. It doesn't make any sense, but it is a universal phenomenon."

IMPROVED COMMUNICATION

Managed care will be improved when each provider is informed about the way the system works and when and why changes in the system are made. The agencies that deliver care will benefit from improved communication with providers as they seek various perspectives on services offered. Unfortunately, most communication in the system is described by practitioners as one way, from manager to staff. Communication as *"dialogue"* has yet to be fully developed in many health care arenas.

TECHNOLOGY DIRECTED TOWARD IMPROVED PATIENT CARE

An investment in an institution's infrastructure can bring about streamlined computerization of its clinical data and affiliations with other facilities and providers. Such an investment is expected to improve the use of resources, which in turn ensures the delivery of appropriate services to a patient and improved and more efficient use of providers. Yet all interviewees indicated a lack of MIS support for clinical practice. More disturbing is the belief by most providers that clinical support systems are *"a long way off."*

Conclusion

The purpose of interviews with health care providers in managed care was to obtain a verbal snapshot of the effect of changes in the system on the individuals themselves and their perception of the effect of these changes on their clients. The results of this convenience sample of interviewees suggest that the continual changes within the system take their toll on primary care providers. All describe busy, hectic days of providing care, returning phone calls, and keeping up with *"hoards of mail"* and the literature. Becoming aware of new changes in the system is not a high priority. Few if any rewards are given to those who do keep abreast of new policies and procedures. *"I'll hear about it if it's important,"* one provider said.

Change continues. Some providers believe that they have had little input into how the system is being designed. Yet they are confident that they have much to offer in future changes. No one spoke about how he or she would implement a plan to effect change or have his or her ideas included in the process. It appears from these samples of providers that in the Midwest and West, managed care is slowly entering Stage II of Goldsmith's stages of evolution of managed care. The shift from "event-driven cost avoidance" to "value improvement" is most clearly seen in the categories of organizational objectives and cost targets. The major strategy here is to avoid or reduce hospitalization of subscribers. There is little resistance by providers to accomplishing this through substituting ambulatory care for inpatient services or practicing under a utilization review system. Resource utilization awareness and cost avoidance are known entities of primary care providers in managed care. Recently, another phenomenon has occurred. Providers, encouraged by their agencies, have been forced to take a more detailed look at how to increase the *value* of their products or practices to the consumer. This shifts the objective of managed care from a focus on price to a focus on increased customer satisfaction. Primary care providers express an interest in this change and a desire to be involved in its development. Concomitantly, providers describe an increased pressure to collaborate on a multidisciplinary team level. Decisions such as these are seen as *"top down"* directives and result in the perception that the locus of control continues to be external rather than peer driven. Clinical practitioners are eager "to engage in active, data-based dialog about the best and most cost-effective clinical practices" (Goldsmith, 1996). When and how managed care plans make use of the investigative skills of practitioners will determine the plans' ability to move fully into the value-improvement stage of managed care evolution. The primary care physicians, physician assistants, nurse practitioners, psychologists, and case managers who were interviewed expressed an interest in becoming part of the change process. The deterrents to entering into this process include their perceptions of control, time (real and perceived), and clinical leadership.

Perhaps the next step is intense recruitment and education of primary care providers who are interested in leadership positions in the organization. This is not an easy task. In an *Issue Brief* of March 1997, the following observation was made: "There is an inadequate supply of qualified people who have the breadth and depth of skills needed for a changing health system that demands not only the ability to manage costs, but to manage care as well . . . The limited supply of provider executives, plus organizations that do not know how to use them effectively, does not bode well for organizations that want to develop more cutting-edge aspects of care management, such as programs and services that can change practice patterns and be linked to outcomes of care for enrolled populations" (Center for Studying Health System Change, 1997). There appear to be clear steps to take in the continuing change process, some of which, as described by health care providers, are listed in Table 23-2. In addition, and based on this series of interviews, a final recommendation is offered. *Continued evolution of the managed care system requires a massive, coordinated educational effort that results in:*

- *Provider and customer input into change*
- *Teams that function well together*
- *Effective clinical leadership*

Acknowledgments

We have a great deal to learn from health care providers who are both caring for patients and designing the new systems of managed care. To all of the individuals interviewed for this chapter, I would like to express my thanks for their time and their willingness to share their wisdom. Because managed care in all its forms is growing and influencing every aspect of the health system, the perspective of providers of care must be sought after, considered, and incorporated into future changes.

References

Center for Studying Health System Change: *Issue Brief,* no 7, March 7, 1997, pp 1-2.

Goldsmith JC: Managed care comes of age. In Bezold C, Mayer E, eds: *Future care: responding to the demand for change,* New York, 1996, Faulkner & Gray, Inc, pp. 139-154.

Guyer J: Trends in Medicaid managed care enrollment and plan arrangements, Center for Health Care Strategies, MMCP, World Wide Web Home Page, pp. 1-2, June 30, 1996.

Rubin R: Rating the HMO's, *U.S. News and World Report,* September 2, 1996, p. 52.

CHAPTER 24

Promoting Self-Management of Chronic Illness

Possibilities for Outcome Evaluation of Case Management

MARILYN J. RANTZ, RN, PhD, FAAN, NHA, **and JILL SCOTT,** RN, PhD(C)

OVERVIEW

Through long-term, helping relationships, health care professionals help people become expert in the management of their illnesses.

This chapter will focus on the new paradigm of self-management of chronic illnesses, how case management is inherently designed and ideally positioned to promote self-management of chronic illnesses, outcome measures for effective management of chronic illnesses, the use of standardized assessment information to measure outcomes and quality, and the need to develop a case management delivery system for long-term-care services that promotes the new paradigm. Self-management skills are critical to successful care outcomes for persons with chronic illnesses. ▲

Chronic illness and its management consume major amounts of time as well as financial, emotional, and professional resources. Not only is chronic illness management of major concern to persons with chronic illnesses, but it is also of major concern to their families, close friends, and employers. Finding new and more effective ways of managing chronic disease can result in reducing pain and suffering, maximizing independence, maintaining employment (if possible), improving perceptions of health, and reducing the use of costly health care resources. Case management is ideally positioned to facilitate these important outcomes.

Chronic Illness

Steadily, factors such as an aging population, advances in medical technology, and diseases such as AIDS have increased public awareness and the prevalence of long-term, medically complex health problems (Beaulieu, Hickman, 1994). Chronic illnesses are one of the most salient issues facing society in general, and health care professionals specifically, as the twenty-first century approaches (Lancaster, 1988).

Acute illnesses have traditionally consumed the bulk of resources and attention within the health care system (Thorne, Robinson, 1989). Acute illnesses are typically sudden and dynamic in onset, with signs and symptoms related to the process itself. Usually, episodes end shortly with either recovery and resumption of previous lifestyle or death (Lubkin, 1986). Conversely, chronic illnesses are slow and insidious in onset. Months or years may be required for signs and symptoms to alter lifestyles. Chronic illnesses are irreversible, progressive, and characterized by periods of exacerbation and remission (Hwu, 1995). The effects of chronic illnesses influence all of human existence (Lancaster, 1988). Chronic illnesses are defined as an impairment or deviation from the norm having duration of more than three months and characterized by irreversible pathological change (Hwu, 1995).

Chronic Illness and Self-Management

Currently, knowledge of chronic disease is becoming more pluralistic, representing different combinations of ontology (view of persons) and episte-mology (nature and aims of the science). This pluralistic approach to the study of chronic illnesses is revealing substantive areas of consistent concern related to day-to-day living, self-management, fatigue, uncertainty, hope, control, managing regimens, access to information, social support, and family adjustment (Conrad, 1990; Dluhy, 1995; Mischel, 1988). Unlike acute illnesses, which require predominantly physical types of care, chronic illnesses' management must deal with the mind and body interacting and being interdependent with the environment (Suppe, Jacox, 1985).

According to Corbin and Strauss (1988), chronic illnesses may be thought of as traveling courses or trajectories. Chronic illnesses may be considered as probable paths, yet the actual paths of chronically ill persons may bear little resemblance to those first conceived. Just as it appears that the course of a chronic illness is under control, contingencies related to the illness and the chronically ill person's life alter that course. Often these alterations are the result of changes directly influencing the chronically ill person's abilities to self-manage. Trajectory refers not only to physiological unfolding of chronic illnesses, but to the total organization of work, or self-management, to be done and the impact on those involved in self-management work, its organization, and its consequences (Glaser, Strauss, 1968; Strauss, 1975; Strauss et al, 1984).

Consideration of trajectories of chronic illnesses provides focus to the active role chronically ill persons must have in shaping courses of chronic illnesses. Courses are shaped not only by chronic illnesses but by chronically ill persons' unique responses and their abilities to continue the work of self-management (Corbin, Strauss, 1988). Conceptualizing chronic illnesses as trajectories captures not only self-management skills, but the temporal orientation of chronic illnesses, the interplay between health care providers and chronically ill persons over time, nonmedical features of self-management, and relevant medical features of the progression (Corbin, Strauss, 1988). Finally, consideration of chronic illnesses as trajectories acknowledges the challenges of managing chronic illnesses multidimensionally, and creates legitimate implications for consideration of chronic illnesses in terms of self-management and nursing support. Supporting and improving self-management skills are keys to successful care of chronically ill persons (Scott, Rantz, 1997).

Self-Management Paradigm Shift

Sparked by growing interest in finding new and more effective ways of managing chronic diseases, cost containment efforts driven by capitation and managed care, societal belief that health care consumers have a right to know about their care, and societal commitment to ensuring that persons with disabilities are involved in society to the fullest extent possible, a paradigm shift is underway. The old paradigm that persons with chronic illnesses assume passive, dependent roles and accept being cared for and treated by health care professionals who "manage their chronic illnesses" is being replaced by a new paradigm. Now, persons with chronic illnesses are encouraged and expected to take active roles and assume responsibility for management of their illnesses by their own actions or by directing others who agree to assist them in the management of their illnesses. It is not at all unusual for persons with major chronic illnesses to become expert in the management of their conditions and to continue (or begin) productive and rewarding careers or make major societal contributions with service or volunteer work.

Case management as a care delivery system is inherently well positioned for the paradigm shift. Assisting persons with chronic illnesses to develop self-management skills is a key component in case management. Through long-term helping relationships, health care professionals help persons become expert in the management of their illnesses. Best possible outcomes are achieved for persons and families as well as for the health care system and team.

tation of care, and decreasing consumption of health care dollars. Scott and Rantz (1997) propose a model of nurse case management that emphasizes self-management skills.

A macro-perspective of the health care system, found in Figure 24-1, suggests that primary health care providers and health care organizations have influence over self-management capabilities, ultimately determining how much consumption of individual health care resources occurs. The addition of the nurse case manager to the current set of relationships influences not only self-management capabilities but also the interaction of the primary provider and the health care organization with the chronically ill person. The resulting alteration in relationships leads to changes in the amount and type of health care resources consumed. The ongoing continuum-based relationship between the chronically ill person and the nurse case manager is critical to altering the trajectories of chronic illnesses and, hence, health care consumption.

Consideration of primary diagnosis, severity of illness, and number of secondary diagnoses is antecedent to creating a continuum-based relationship (Figure 24-2). The relationship significantly influences self-management capabilities and the ability of family support to influence how effectively chronically ill persons can and do self-manage. The relationship between severity of illness and self-management skills is a critical junction at which the nurse case manager (NCM), working with a patient over time, can make a significant impact.

Nurse Case Management and Evolving Self-Management Skills

Case management remains critical for the growing population of chronically ill persons. Case management is evolving in complexity and effectiveness. In many parts of the country, contemporary health care systems continue to struggle as they deal with chronic illnesses as a series of events rather than a trajectory of illness requiring systematic support of self-management skills and care coordination across the continuum. Nurse case management as a strategy supports the ability of chronically ill persons to maintain self-management skills while increasing coordination of care, decreasing fragmen-

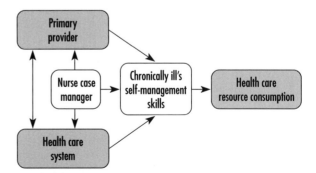

FIGURE 24-1 The role of nurse case manager within the context of the larger health care system. Nurse case managers work to enhance the self-management skills of the chronically ill.

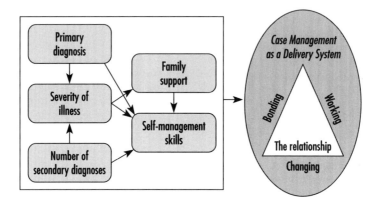

FIGURE 24-2 Antecedents of a continuum-based relationship to support the chronically ill.

Supportive, Longitudinal Relationships Lead to Self-Management

Lamb and Stempel (1994) investigated the relationship between NCM and patient, identifying and describing growing together as insider-experts. The process develops through affective, cognitive, and behavioral changes. The following three interpersonal phases emerged: bonding, working, and changing (Lamb, Stempel, 1994). Figure 24-3 illustrates the multidimensional nature of the continuum-based relationship between nurses and chronically ill persons, the primary focus of which is developing self-management skills as described by Scott and Rantz (1997).

BONDING

Initially, chronically ill persons see the NCM in the role of expert, monitoring their physical status and teaching them how to care for themselves. Over time, bonding occurs between NCM and the chronically ill persons, allowing them to feel known and cared about as individuals (see Figure 24-3, *A*). Bonding allows a person to think differently about his or her situation and gain confidence. Increasing confidence allows greater acceptance of responsibility for performing the insider-expert role.

Bonding is reported by chronically ill persons as moving from "the NCM knowing her stuff to the NCM knowing me." The roles of insider and expert are distinct (Lamb, Stempel, 1994). Often, early in

the bonding phase the chronically ill person continues to be physiologically unstable and focused on physical status. This physiological instability is seen as wide swings in the person's physical and mental condition within the trajectory of the chronic illness. As physiological stability occurs, the relationship focus shifts to emotional and spiritual concerns; sharing and bonding result. Bonding facilitates trust. Trust allows for acceptance of NCM strategies as meaningful; thus, the insider role develops.

WORKING

During the working phase of the insider-expert relationship, the NCM provides a sense of consistency and dependability in the face of chronic illness unpredictability (Lamb, Stempel, 1994). Chronically ill persons begin to identify attitudes, reactions, and behaviors exacerbating their illnesses and barriers preventing effective and efficient health care system use. Key to the working phase is demonstrated concern by the NCM.

CHANGING

In contrast to bonding and working, which emphasize affective and cognitive changes, changing refers to actual behavioral changes, also noted in Figure 24-3, *A*. Two major categories of change reported by Lamb and Stempel (1994) are doing more things for oneself and accepting help when needed. The role of NCM becomes one of supporter and encourager of new efforts. As chronically ill persons

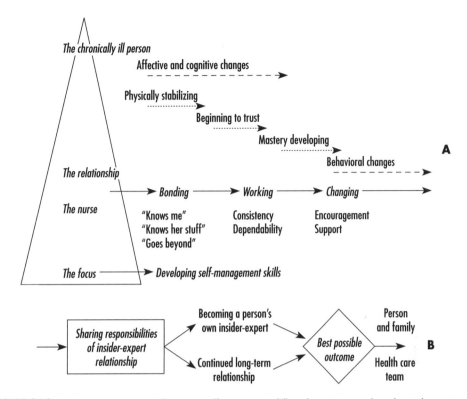

FIGURE 24-3 Nursing case management focuses on self-management skills and promotes growth as the insider-expert. **A,** The multidimensional nature of the continuum-based relationship. **B,** The continuum-based relationship evolving into the best possible outcomes through the development of self-management skills.

and NCMs continue to work together, relationships vary in the extent to which chronically ill persons can refine their self-management skills. Refinement of self-management skills creates opportunity for chronically ill persons to become their own insider-experts (Figure 24-3, *B*).

Paramount to improvement in self-management skills is development of a therapeutic relationship based upon trust and mutual respect (Papenhausen, 1996). NCMs uniquely provide for development of self-management skills as NCMs and chronically ill persons together develop insider-expert relationships. Supporting development of self-management skills is an aspect of continuum-based care that nursing truly provides most effectively. The essence of what nurses provide for chronically ill persons is embedded within the content of the relationship as supporting self-management skills development.

Outcome Measurements for Case Management and Chronically Ill People

Outcomes related to management of chronically ill persons are multidimensional. Quality, cost, and access are often cited as the standards for health care outcome measurement. Nurse case management demonstrates maximal quality, management of costs, and enhancement of appropriate accessibility (Bower, Falk, 1996). Case management is a means to quality, cost, and access measurements, not the goal.

Outcomes are anticipated, desired conditions of the patient at specific points along the continuum. Outcome measurements suggested by the model found in Figure 24-4 are within two categories: chronically ill persons-families and the health care team. While the outcome measures are oriented to

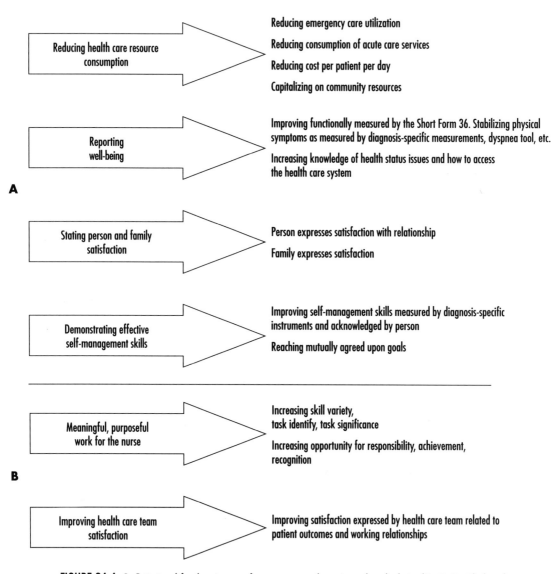

FIGURE 24-4 A, Patient and family outcomes of a nurse-managed, continuum-based relationship. **B,** Provider-based outcomes for health care teams.

continuous monitoring over time, strategically determined periodic measurements make these valuable outcome measures. Outcome measurements for chronically ill persons and their families include a cross-sectional examination of resources consumed, typically expressed as emergency and acute-care service consumption, cost per patient per day, and use of community services; reported well-being is typically measured in terms of functionality, stabilization of physical symptoms, extent of self-management abilities, knowledge of the illness and the health care system, and satisfaction.

Although the outcomes suggested by the Scott and Rantz (1997) model are appropriate initial outcomes to measure the effectiveness of the NCM and chronic illness management, the evolving health care system will require more sophisticated monitoring and evaluation of outcomes. Alternative data sources need to be explored. Large data sets of assessment information hold much potential to provide for analysis of the effectiveness of relationships between NCMs and chronically ill persons and the resulting self-management skills.

LARGE DATA SETS AS SOURCES FOR OUTCOME MEASURES

Determining outcome measures for effectively managing chronic illness is a challenging line of inquiry for clinicians and researchers. Since they are plagued with incomplete descriptions of the trajectories of chronic illnesses, determining at the individual level when appropriate outcomes are reached can be more than a small problem. However, when large amounts of data about persons with chronic illnesses can be aggregated, interpretations about outcomes are possible. Using large data sets with standardized assessment information at the level of individual persons with chronic illnesses holds much promise for outcome evaluation. If these assessment data can be combined with satisfaction data collected from the same persons, there will be extraordinary possibilities for outcome evaluation.

One health care setting serving more than 5 million persons with chronic illnesses that has implemented standardized routine assessment is our nation's nursing homes. What has been learned from the efforts to develop key indicators of outcomes of care in nursing homes can be applied to other settings. An example using the nursing home setting follows. Suggestions will be advanced for using a similar approach to care across the continuum.

DEVELOPING INDICATORS OF QUALITY OF CARE AND OUTCOME MEASURES FOR NURSING HOMES

There has been a major national effort in nursing homes to develop key indicators that could be used to assess quality of care delivered to residents and outcomes of care. These have centered on the concept of sentinel health events, such as accidents, transfers to hospitals, medication usage, infections, decubitus ulcers, catheters, contractures, tube feedings, restraint usage, or lack of participation in ac-

tivity programs (Phillips, 1991; Zinn, Aaronson, Rosko, 1993). The Health Care Financing Administration (HCFA) has a basic strategy to develop a system of quality indicators across the full range of services paid for by the Medicare and Medicaid programs (Gagel, 1995; Jencks, 1995). To develop these indicators, resident-level assessment data will be used, as well as admission, discharge, and transfer data.

USING STANDARDIZED ASSESSMENT DATA TO DEVELOP OUTCOME MEASURES

Most of the current effort for quality indicator development for nursing home care is focused on determining indicators of quality (QIs) from resident-level assessment data routinely collected in nursing homes. Much of the work toward this goal is being accomplished through a major multi-state, multi-year study sponsored by HCFA: the Multistate Nursing Home Case-Mix and Quality Demonstration Project (NHCMQ). The QIs were developed through a systematic process involving extensive interdisciplinary clinical input, empirical testing, and field testing (Ryther, Zimmerman, Kelly-Powell, 1994; Zimmerman et al, 1995). The most current version includes 30 QIs, measuring areas such as fracture, falls, incontinence, physical function, skin care, cognitive function, behavior, medication use, activity involvement, weight loss, infections, dehydration, and decline in range of motion. (Details of the QIs are available from the authors.)

The QIs are derived from assessment data from the standardized Minimum Data Set and Care Screening (MDS) instrument. To determine quality and outcome measures using MDS data is of interest, since these data are routinely obtained for all nursing home residents upon admission, at times of significant change in condition, and annually as mandated by OBRA 87 for facilities participating in Medicaid and Medicare. Selected MDS items are collected and reported quarterly. Analyses from the NHCMQ indicate that it is possible to make judgments about quality on the basis of MDS information for a specific resident, a specific nursing home, and nursing homes in aggregate (Gagel, 1995; Ryther, Zimmerman, Kelly-Powell, 1994; Zimmerman et al, 1995). The MDS data provide a mechanism that can be used to generate many pertinent resident outcomes (Kane, 1995; Karon, Zimmerman, 1996). This will be especially relevant as data become available nationwide in the near future. Many states have been collecting these data and compiling them into large data sets. All states will be required to transmit their MDS data into a centralized national data system in 1998. Although the QIs are limited to measuring care quality and resident outcomes on the basis of the assessment items of the standardized MDS instrument used across the nation, the potential for developing methods that can be readily transferred nationwide to measure and improve care far outweighs the limitations (Glass, 1992; Kane, 1995).

Determining Resident Outcomes: Missouri Nursing Homes

The multidimensional resident-specific aspects encompassed by MDS data items have much potential for directly measuring quality of care and resident outcomes, rather than depending upon measuring outcomes indirectly via other, proxy measures. Evaluating outcomes by using standardized MDS assessment data of residents with multiple chronic illnesses has been the focus of ongoing research by our research team at the University of Missouri—Columbia (Rantz et al, 1996; 1997a; 1997b; 1998). The methods developed in the NHCMQ for determining QIs from MDS items have been applied and further developed in studies using Missouri MDS data. Our research team is a multidisciplinary group committed to conducting research that will help nursing homes deliver high-quality services. The team has been testing those QIs that represent serious quality problems that can affect resident well-being, are related to well-documented common quality problems in long-term care, represent diverse aspects of quality care, and are amenable to clinical practice intervention. Several have been identified as potentially useful for measuring care quality and subsequent resident outcomes. (Again, details and algorithms are available from the authors upon request.)

Key to the efforts of measuring outcomes of residents in nursing homes is having resident-level assessment data from a standardized assessment instrument. If each nursing home, or each state, were using different instruments with different items

that could *not* be cross-walked to each other, meaningful comparisons could *not* be made. With standardized resident-level assessment data, meaningful outcome (quality indicator) interpretations of chronic illness management are possible. For example, if nurse case management were implemented in a sample of nursing homes, outcome evaluations of the residents receiving and not receiving NCM could readily be done to determine the effect of NCM on resident outcomes.

Standardized Assessment Instruments

Much of what has been learned in nursing home evaluation of outcomes can be applied to home and community settings as standardized instruments are developed and implemented for those settings. There are standardized instruments under development for home care, home- and community based services, and acute care. Recently, HCFA published a proposed rule to require the use of a standardized assessment data set, the "Outcomes and Assessment Information Set" (OASIS), for evaluating adult, nonmaternity patients for home care services (*Federal Register,* 1997). When this proposal is implemented, data will be collected that will enable outcome evaluation of patients with chronic illnesses who are using home care services, just as with the nursing home MDS data. Key to the evaluation process is that data are routinely collected for each patient so that individual outcomes can be analyzed over time. Aggregate outcomes can be analyzed to characterize the effectiveness of the services provided by individual agencies or groups of agencies. Again, the impact of case management implemented in a sample of these agencies could readily be determined by evaluating patient outcomes (or quality indicators) from the assessment data.

Another standardized home care instrument that is being developed and tested is the MDS for Home Care (MDS-HC). The MDS-HC was designed by interRAI, an international group of academics and clinicians committed to standardized assessment to improve care of elders. The MDS-HC was designed as a parallel instrument to the MDS for nursing homes (interRAI, 1996). The instrument is to be used for initial and ongoing assessment and care planning for persons needing home care services. As with the MDS for nursing home residents, patient outcomes and effectiveness of services can be evaluated over time by using patient-level assessment data.

Several states have recently developed (e.g., Virginia, Ohio) or are in the process of developing (e.g., Michigan, Idaho) uniform assessment instruments to assess functional and cognitive disabilities of Medicaid clients accessing the long-term-care systems in their respective states. The states are replacing (or planning to replace) the many existing evaluation instruments for their various long-term-care services. The intent is to better evaluate services, client outcomes, and treatment and rehabilitation plans, and in some cases determine the amount of money authorized for services. Through the use of a uniform assessment instrument, each state will be able to evaluate client outcomes and service effectiveness. A serious disadvantage is that states are developing unique instruments so that state-to-state comparisons will be difficult.

However, having assessment data for all persons within a state needing long-term-care services will greatly enhance understanding of the trajectories of chronic illnesses and the range of outcomes experienced by these persons. Persons needing long-term-care services will most likely have multiple chronic illnesses. Through initial and periodic assessment of functional and cognitive abilities, it will be possible to evaluate individual outcomes and outcomes of groups of clients receiving different service packages.

Extraordinary outcome evaluations would be possible if these assessment data could be linked to satisfaction data from the same persons. Again, standardization of the satisfaction instrument is critical. One possible option is a version of the Health Plan Employer Data and Information Set (HEDIS) that includes a satisfaction survey that participating health plans must administer annually to their adult commercial members (Grimaldi, 1997). HEDIS instructions indicate that a health plan may not alter any of the questions, or rearrange their order or response categories. Questions include information about health plan membership, satisfaction with the plan and services, health status and activities, and sociodemographic characteristics. Although the current system does *not* link

HEDIS survey participants to their individual outcome information that may be contained in other data sets, using a standardized satisfaction instrument such as HEDIS would provide the potential for possible linkages.

Case Management Delivery System for Long-Term-Care Services

A strong case has been made to use standardized assessment and satisfaction instruments to evaluate the outcomes of persons with chronic illness, the effectiveness of services they receive, and their satisfaction with the services. Of equal importance is our proposal that case management be incorporated into all long-term-care services. Although some states and counties do have case management systems, they are primarily focused on managing health care resources. The case management delivery system that we envision emphasizes the new paradigm of helping persons with chronic illnesses to become expert in the management of their illnesses. If best possible outcomes are to be achieved, the shift from passive, dependent roles for persons with chronic illnesses to active self-management roles must occur.

In the proposed case management system for long-term care, all persons with chronic illnesses would have access to a nurse case manager for ongoing evaluation and support. The case manager would be permanently assigned to a group of persons and would function as an advocate for each person as he or she uses services in a variety of health care settings across the continuum. The case manager would help each person become the expert in managing his or her individual care, and enhance each person's self-management skills. Periodic and ongoing assessment using standardized instruments to measure functional abilities, health status, service needs, and satisfaction with services would be implemented. Analysis of outcomes and services provided, based on the assessments, would be required to measure effectiveness. Because enhancing self-management skills is integral to the design of the proposed long-term-care case management system, it is likely that the outcomes of care and satisfaction with services would be improved.

The Future

We propose embracing the paradigm shift to self-management of chronic illness through the NCM delivery system. We hope the model that we have delineated will help clarify how the NCM helps the chronically ill person develop expert self-management skills as well as suggest outcome measures to determine the effectiveness of NCM. We strongly suggest that case management be incorporated into all long-term-care services. We propose that standardized assessment of persons with chronic illnesses be routinely completed and used to evaluate patient outcomes, the effectiveness of services, and the effectiveness of providers.

References

Beaulieu JE, Hickman M: Rural case management: a pilot study, *Home Health Care Services Quarterly* 14(4):69-85, 1994.

Bower KA, Falk CC: Case management as a response to quality, cost, and access imperatives. In Cohen E, ed: *Nurse case management in the 21st century,* St Louis, 1996, Mosby.

Conrad P: Qualitative research on chronic illness: a commentary on method and conceptual development, *Social Science Medicine* 30(11):1257-1263, 1990.

Corbin JM, Strauss A: *Unending work and care,* San Francisco 1998, Jossey-Bass Publishers.

Dluhy NM: Mapping knowledge in chronic illness, *Journal of Advanced Nursing* 21(6):1051-1058, 1995.

Federal Register: Medicare and Medicaid programs: use of the OASIS as part of the conditions of participation for home health agencies, *42CFR Part 484, 62(46):11035-11064,* March 10, 1997.

Gagel BJ: Health care quality improvement program: a new approach, *Health Care Financing Review* 16(4):15-23, 1995.

Glaser BG, Strauss AL: *Time for dying,* Chicago, 1968, Aldine.

Glass AP: Resident assessments: a new tool for measuring and improving nursing home quality, *JHQ* 14(3):24-30, 1992.

Grimaldi PL: Are managed care members satisfied? *Nurse Management* 28(6):12-15, 1997.

Hwu YJ: The impact of chronic illness on patients, *Rehabilitation Nursing* 20(4):221-225, 1995.

interRAI: *MDS Assessment Batteries,* University of Michigan, Health Services Administration, September 20, 1996.

Jencks SF: Measuring quality of care under Medicare and Medicaid, *Health Care Financing Review* 16(4):39-54, 1995.

Kane RL: Improving the quality of long-term care, *Journal of the American Medical Association* 273(17):1376-1380, 1995.

Karon SL, Zimmerman DR: Using quality indicators to structure quality improvement initiatives in long-term care, *Quality Management in Health Care* 4(3):54-66, 1996.

Lamb GS, Stempel JE: Nurse case management from the client's view: growing as insider-expert, *Nursing Outlook* 42(1):7-13, 1994.

Lancaster LE: Impact of chronic illness over the life span, *American Nephrology Nurses Association* 15(3):164-168, 1988.

Lubkin IM: *Chronic illness: input and intervention,* Boston, 1986, Jones & Bartlett.

Mischel MH: Uncertainty in illness, *Image: Journal of Nursing Scholarship* 20(4):225-232, 1988.

Papenhausen JL: Discovering and achieving client outcomes. In Cohen E, ed: *Nurse case management in the 21st century,* St Louis, 1996, Mosby.

Phillips CJ: Developing a method of assessing quality of care in nursing homes, using key indicators and population norms, *Journal of Aging and Health* 3(3):407-422, 1991.

Rantz MJ, Mehr DR, Conn V, Hicks LL, Porter R, Madsen RW, Petroski GF, Maas M: Assessing quality of nursing home care: the foundation for improving resident outcomes, *Journal of Nursing Care Quality* 10(4):1-9, 1996.

Rantz MJ, Mehr DR, Popejoy L, Zwygart-Stauffacher M, Hicks L, Grando V, Conn V, Porter R, Scott J, Maas M: Nursing home care quality: a multidimensional theoretical model, *Journal of Nursing Care Quality* 12(3):30-46, 1998.

Rantz MJ, Petroski GF, Madsen R, Scott J, Mehr DR, Popejoy L, Conn V, Hicks L, Porter R, Zwygart-Stauffacher M, Maas M: Setting thresholds for MDS quality indicators for nursing home quality improvement reports, *Journal of Quality Improvement* 23(11):602-611, 1997a.

Rantz MJ, Popejoy L, Mehr DR, Zwygart-Stauffacher M, Hicks L, Grando V, Conn V, Porter R, Scott J, Maas M: Verifying nursing home care quality using minimum data set quality indicators and other quality measures, *Journal of Nursing Care Quality* 12(2):54-62, 1997b.

Ryther BJ, Zimmerman D, Kelly-Powell M: Using resident assessment data in quality monitoring. In Miller TV, Rantz MJ: *Quality assurance in long-term care,* Gaithersburg, Md, 1994, Aspen, pp I26-I28.

Scott J, Rantz MJ: Managing chronically ill older people in the midst of the health care revolution, *Nursing Administration Quarterly* 21(2):55-64, 1997.

Strauss A: *Chronic illness and the quality of life,* St Louis, 1975, Mosby.

Strauss A, Corbin J, Fagerhaugh S, Glaser BG, Maines D, Suczek B, Wiener CL: *Chronic illness and the quality of life,* ed 2, St Louis, 1984, Mosby.

Suppe F, Jacox AK: Philosophy of science development of nursing theory. In Werley HH, Fitzpatrick JJ, eds: *Annual review of nursing research,* vol 3, New York, 1985, Springer Publishing.

Thorne SE, Robinson CA: Guarded alliance: health care relationships in chronic illness, *Image: Journal of Nursing Scholarship* 21(3):153-157, 1989.

Zimmerman DR, Karon SL, Arling G, Clark BR, Collins T, Ross R, Sainfort F: Development and testing of nursing home quality indicators, *Health Care Financing Review* 16(4):107-127, 1995.

Zinn JS, Aaronson WE, Rosko MD: The use of standardized indicators as quality improvement tools: an application in Pennsylvania nursing homes, *American Journal of Medical Quality* 8(2):72-78, 1993.

CHAPTER 25

Automated Outcomes Management

Criteria for Selection of Information Systems

ROY L. SIMPSON, RN, FNAP, FAAN

OVERVIEW

The challenge surrounding information management is not a lack of data collection within the health enterprise; rather, the problem is the inability to present relevant clinical information collected across the enterprise to the caregiver at the appropriate time.

This chapter presents a basic model for selecting a clinical information system for outcomes management. Specifically, both the chapter and the model address five key system evaluation criteria:

1. Vendor stability and leadership
2. Functional depth and breadth of the application
3. Integration with other systems across the enterprise
4. Performance of the technology platform
5. Vendor installation, education, and support services. ▲

Managed care continues to impose major structural change upon health care. The most compelling change—a demand for fiscal accountability—makes the need for outcomes management data more critical than ever.

Managing outcomes means managing length of stay, tracking clinical and financial outcomes, improving quality of care and controlling costs. The organization that manages outcomes effectively will gain a significant competitive advantage in this new marketplace. But managing outcomes also means managing information.

The challenge is not too little data. Rather, it is the inability of many systems to collect data across the enterprise and then present it to the caregiver at the appropriate time.

In today's typical hospital, caregivers cannot review patient encounter information outside the acute care setting. Physicians and nurses cannot review current inpatient clinical data from private-practice offices or clinics. Home care providers cannot look at a recent acute care visit or an ongoing treatment directed by a primary care physician or specialist. The result? Duplication of effort, delayed diagnoses, and increased treatment costs.

Then there's the problem caused by the move to patient-centered care delivery models. When a patient care *team*—as opposed to a single provider—is handling multiple patients, there is an even greater need to communicate and coordinate clinical information.

To remain competitive, the health enterprise must become more efficient and deploy tools that satisfy the information demands of both managed care organizations and nurses, physicians and other caregiver groups. Just as Medicare and DRGs called for patient accounting, billing, decision support, and case mix systems, today's managed care model demands a new breed of clinical information system.

This new type of system must not only address new types of information—like outcomes management data—it must also do so in different ways for different constituencies. Nurses, physicians, therapists, dietitians, and other caregivers need advanced systems that support quality care delivery and allow more time with patients. They need tools that integrate clinical guidelines, point-of-care documentation, exception-based charting, order communications, and variance reporting. Adminis-

trators and managers need systems that empower their organizations to define standards of care, measure outcomes, examine variances, and make logical changes to the care process to improve outcomes and lower costs—systems to guide the decisions that drive the organization's strategic business plan.

Effectively deployed, such solutions make improved communication and information exchange a by-product of care delivery. In addition, the right solution should provide these tangible benefits:

- Improved quality of care through process improvement
- Improved guidelines management
- Reduced risk of adverse health events
- Increased caregiver time with patients
- Reduced charting time

Clinical tools also improve the ability to comply with Joint Commission on Accreditation of Healthcare (JCAHO) requirements and lay the foundation for a computerized patient record.

The required solution is an advanced clinical system that optimizes information management and improves the efficiency of the caregiver team. The challenge is to select the right system and the right vendor partner. The system must meet the functional requirements of the health care organization, and the vendor must be strong enough to lead this changing marketplace.

The model shown in Figure 25-1 was designed to simplify the selection process. It thoroughly examines automated clinical information systems in terms of five key factors:

1. Vendor stability and leadership
2. The functional depth and breadth of the application
3. Integration with other systems across the enterprise
4. Performance of the technology platform

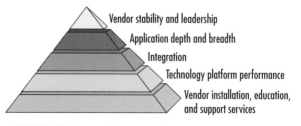

FIGURE 25-1 A model for evaluating a clinical information system.

5. Vendor installation, education, and support services

This model examines clinical solutions in terms of technology, integration capabilities, and functional benefits. Furthermore, it examines potential vendors on the basis of their staying power and service organizations. More specifically, these criteria include:

- *Vendor stability and leadership:* The vendor should be committed to the clinical information systems market and to the overall health information management industry. To keep pace with the changing regulatory environment and industry consolidation, a vendor must have both financial stability and a strong balance sheet to fund new research and development.
- *Application depth and breadth:* Today's caregivers and health care administrators need multidisciplinary tools that span both the acute care and extended acute care settings. These tools must integrate clinical guidelines, point-of-care documentation, charting, and order communications; provide powerful exception-based charting and variance reporting; and allow an organization to define its own standards of care, measure outcomes, examine variances, and make logical changes to the care process to improve outcomes and lower costs.
- *Integration:* The clinical information system must eliminate redundant data entry across care settings, streamline processes, and simplify access. It must also integrate clinical and administrative data across multiple disciplines and into other enterprise settings.
- *Technology platform performance:* The clinical information system should be built on an open-systems architecture that incorporates industry standards and allows for robust data management, exceptional hardware versatility, and economies of scale. The architecture must support substantial numbers of users, both nurse-station-based and point-of-care.
- *Vendor installation, education, and support services:* The vendor's service and support offering should incorporate both experience and flexibility to successfully meet the unique needs and strategies of each health care organization. The breadth and depth of its support

organization and experience with clinical information systems are important considerations.

Vendor Stability and Leadership

Health care has changed significantly over the past several years thanks to a number of factors, from a broad-based shift of risk to the health care organization, to a major change from fee-for-service reimbursement to capitation and managed care. And these changes have had a profound impact on the way health care consumers interact with the health care delivery system.

At the same time, these changes place tremendous pressure on the software vendors that serve the health care industry. Just as health care organizations have undergone buyouts, consolidations, mergers, alliances, and affiliations of every kind, so, too, have software vendors. As a result, many vendors are now out of business, leaving their customers with outdated software they can neither support nor enhance. Other software vendors hang by a thread, reporting dismal earnings and poor performance.

The continued success of a health care organization depends on the continued success of its software vendor, so it is imperative to choose a vendor with a bright future. The vendor must deliver superior products and services and have industrywide acceptance, as well as the infrastructure and financial strength to integrate, enhance, and support its products for years to come. Consider the following minimum requirements for choosing a vendor as your information systems partner:

Solid Financial Strength. The vendor should have a strong balance sheet. A thorough review of the vendor's annual revenues, operating income, and long-term debt can help reduce your organization's risk, while meeting its future needs.

Commitment to Research and Development. The investment your organization makes in software must be protected by the vendor's ability to enhance that software. Research and development funding is a strong indication of a software vendor's ability to meet the future needs of customers. To remain competitive and ensure future needs are met, ask for the number of dollars allocated annually to R & D.

Comprehensive Product Offering. In today's integrated delivery environment, it is not enough to offer products for just a few niche areas of the enterprise. Successful software vendors offer products for the full dimension of the enterprise, from core systems to clinical information systems, financial systems, and systems for risk management, schedule management, medical records management, enterprise management, home care and other areas of the extended enterprise.

Growth. The company should not only be financially stable and strong today but also have a favorable outlook for the future. Look at the company's past growth—revenue growth greater than 20% per year for the past five years is desirable.

People Assets. The vendor is only as good as the quality and quantity of its human resources. To successfully develop and support software to benefit an organization, the vendor must be able to attract the most talented and motivated individuals in the industry and maintain "critical mass" resources.

Clinical Competency. To meet the needs of patients and clinical users, the vendor should employ clinicians from multiple disciplines who can rely on firsthand experience to design applications and drive product requirements. In addition, the vendor should demonstrate experience and success with point-of-care computing.

Leadership in Technology. The vendor should demonstrate experience with open systems, client/server applications, wireless technology, and Windows-based solutions.

Extensive Experience. The vendor should have more than 10 years' experience in clinical information systems and employ staff with experience in all facets of clinical information systems.

Market Acceptance. The vendor's products must have widespread acceptance in the United States and international markets in a broad spectrum of settings, ensuring continual product shaping by users. The vendor's clinical information systems should be installed and demonstrable in enterprise sites.

Regulatory Compliance. The vendor should have a department dedicated to monitoring and acting upon regulatory issues and changes.

Proven Enterprise Capabilities. The vendor should demonstrate success with information sharing and communications, among other applications and care settings, as well as an ability to work with foreign systems.

Application Depth and Breadth

Today's caregivers and administrators need a multidisciplinary tool for acute-care and extended acute care settings. This tool must integrate clinical guidelines, point-of-care documentation, charting and order communications, while providing powerful exception-based charting and variance reporting. It should empower an organization to define standards of care, measure outcomes, examine variances, and make logical changes to the care process to improve outcomes and lower costs.

The multidisciplinary care team needs electronic flowsheet charting, comprehensive critical pathways support, and a number of specialized clinical applications that make communication and information exchange a by-product of care delivery. The following are minimum requirements for an application:

Guidelines. The system should integrate clinical guidelines, order communications, order management, order charging, results reporting, clinical documentation, and automated variance tracking and reporting. It should also provide a user-friendly query tool that allows an organization to create a continuous quality improvement (CQI) loop for each episode of care.

- An organization should be able to define its own standards of care, objectively measure outcomes, automatically analyze variances against those standards, and make logical changes to the care process to improve outcomes and reduce costs.
- The system should support hospital-designed clinical guidelines, as well as those developed by third-party organizations.
- Guidelines must be divided into user-defined phases of care, not just days of care, each of which has its own outcomes and interven-

tions. Users should have the option to carry elements of one phase over to the next phase.

- The system should automatically capture and report interventions not performed, documented, or included in the clinical guideline.
- The system should allow entering of nursing and interdisciplinary documentation against each element of the guideline, standard of care, and/or teaching plan.
- Guidelines should automatically generate and execute clinical interventions subject to caregiver confirmation.
- The system must allow the caregiver to customize a guideline for a particular patient.
- The system should support multiple guidelines for a single patient and report conflicts and duplications between interventions.
- The system must support multidisciplinary clinical guidelines and nursing care plans simultaneously or independently.
- The system must provide preformatted variance reports and also a user-friendly, SQL-compliant ad hoc reporting tool.
- The system should allow use of all guidelines, orders, documentation, and variance analysis capabilities at the point of care on a real-time basis.
- The system should support clinical guidelines that span care settings and individual departments.

Order Entry and Management. The system must provide a clinically oriented multidisciplinary order entry tool that streamlines the order entry process and increases the efficiency and effectiveness of physicians and other clinicians.

- The system must provide a user-friendly, Microsoft Windows–compatible graphical user interface and be accessible on-line at the point of care.
- The system must provide a physician order entry capability with a familiar, intuitive graphical interface. Physician order capabilities must also include enhanced order selection, order review, medication order entry, order sheets, real-time order alerts, and electronic signatures.
- At the point of order, the system must provide caregivers with immediate access to lab results, medication administration records, vital signs, intake and output data, order re-

view, progress notes, and cost/charge information.

- The system must provide a single screen where users can view orders and activity schedules and view results and document against the order.
- The system must allow users to automatically convert clinical guidelines to an appropriate series of discrete clinical orders for executing and documenting progress against the guideline.
- The system must offer preferred and departmental service lists and combine orders for multiple services on a single screen.
- The system must have user-defined order sets and order panels and must support easy addition to and deletion from these sets and panels.
- The system must support data elements showing start time, stop time, frequency, and duration of orders. It should also develop patient schedules and department work lists from orders

Clinical Documentation. The system should include a comprehensive clinical documentation component that links appropriate documentation back to the order and the guideline. Documentation should be functionally rich and cover the broadest possible range of patient care settings. The system should offer an intuitive, clinician-friendly user interface that provides easy access to information at the nursing station, an ancillary department, or the point of care.

Charting by Exception and Knowledge Bases. The system must support exception charting, whereby an abnormal value drives the user to chart more detailed and specific information through the use of a knowledge-based engine.

Flexible Charting Protocols. The system must allow an organization to configure assessment information to support each unit's charting protocols and provide tools that enable users to make any necessary changes.

Medication IV Charting. The system must provide an on-line MAR and use advanced bar-coding technology to integrate with the main pharmacy system and ensure that, at the time of administration, the correct patient receives the right medication in the correct dose, by the ordered route, and at the right date and time.

- The system must produce an on-line MAR accessible for data entry and review on both point-of-care and nurse-station-based workstation devices. It should also include the ability to review medications given at the patient's bedside.
- The system should display medication orders at the point of service and provide for administration of IV medication drips. Charting IVs should automatically update the I/O calculation.
- The system should provide a drug dosage calculator integrated with the drip medications to provide an electronic titration chart. When the dose is changed, a new rate is automatically calculated and indicated in relationship to the unit's configured minimum, maximum, and average doses.

Intake and Output Calculations. The system should automatically calculate all intake and output totals and produce on-line graphical shift summaries, daily summaries, and overall fluid balances.

Assessments. The system must allow assessment data to flow from one discipline assessment to the other, eliminating the need to ask repetitive questions of the patient.

Automate the Workflow Process by Making Information Available at the Point of Care. All disciplines should have a view of the patient path or plan and the ability to measure progress toward outcomes at the point of care.

- The system should support all data needs and reports without redundant data entry. Information entered at the point of care must be routed appropriately and automatically.
- The system must allow a nurse to validate and automatically record vital signs and other patient data from site-specific monitoring equipment.

CLINICAL DOCUMENTATION: RANGE OF PATIENT CARE SETTINGS

Medical/Surgical Care. The system should allow the multidisciplinary care team to chart in real time at the point of care while automatically posting to the

multidisciplinary record of care. Information must be instantly shared with other care team members, enabling them to plan, implement, document, evaluate, and coordinate patient progress on their individual guidelines and/or plans of care.

- The system should automatically transfer the guidelines, orders, care plans, and all relevant clinical information when the patient transfers from one area of the hospital to another.
- The system should provide instant access to accurate, updated information from all departments (such as laboratory, radiology, pharmacy), clinics, nurse stations, the bedside, or other sources throughout the health care enterprise.
- The system should allow the care team to do assessments, vital signs, intake and output documentation and calculations, flowsheet charting and reporting, and physician review screens.

Critical Care. The system must allow a critical care specialist to view a flowsheet with information specific to his or her specialty, including integrated laboratory, medication, IV, and patient assessment information.

- The system must automatically interface with and collect information from patient monitors and ventilators through a comprehensive and reliable data acquisition system. The data must be stored as discrete clinical information for analysis, graphing, and other purposes.
- The system must provide a graphical electronic flowsheet that is flexible and allows the organization to define hospital- and unit-specific normal values for vital signs and other parameters.
- The system must be able to collect data from disparate systems, collate and relate the data, and comparatively graph and trend the data (e.g., vital signs, lab results, medications, and other parameters).

Emergency Care. The system must provide a quick-admit triage capability that creates a skeletal patient record to capture all clinical information even before a clerk performs a full admission.

- The system must immediately start tracking length of stay, assigned treatment room, chief complaint, triage category, acuity, and other vital information and display this information on the electronic tracking board for viewing by all staff members.

- The system must support clinical guidelines, orders, results, and documentation that can be associated with the patient on an ongoing basis as the patient moves through the hospital.

Obstetrical Care. The system must capture and retain prenatal information (such as adverse reactions to medications) from other care settings across the enterprise to give the caregiver all the relevant information from the beginning of the care episode.

- The system must automatically maintain a mother-baby link and allow a clinician to easily chart on both.
- The system must allow real-time fetal monitoring and simultaneous charting and fetal strip archiving on the same integrated workstation.

Pediatric Care. The system must support the collection of pediatric-scaled information, such as weight and intake and output, in fractions of kilograms or millimeters. The system must support the capture of results specific to pediatrics, such as fontanel and cry assessments.

Respiratory Care. The system must allow respiratory therapists to efficiently organize care delivery and document procedures, treatments, and patient responses through a single flowsheet shared with other disciplines.

- The system must permit the respiratory therapist to generate respiratory charges as a by-product of documentation and eliminate the need for a separate charge sheet.
- The system must support ventilator interfaces to speed workflow and provide joint data reviews and reports across disciplines to help meet JCAHO requirements.

CLINICAL DOCUMENTATION: OTHER FUNCTIONS

Clinical Profile. Organizations today require in-depth, foundation clinical information, not tied to a specific episode or time period, concerning high-risk populations within their covered lives. The system must collect and display discrete coded "encounter-independent" information, including medical problems, adverse reactions, and medications taken.

- The system must collect other patient health history information across visits and allow the caregiver to confirm or modify the information without redundant data collection.

Multiple Encounters. The system must provide long-term storage of detailed clinical information from multiple encounters or provide data collection for a clinical data repository.

Clinical Query. The system must provide an ad hoc data retrieval and reporting tool that reports clinical information, uses an intuitive graphical interface with flexible output criteria, and exports information to other applications.

Audit Trail. The system must create an audit trail of all transactions—including corrections—and be able to create a report or audit trail of exceptional events by nursing unit and individual patient for daily use by physicians, case managers, nurse managers, charge nurses, and CQI teams.

Point-of-Care Capabilities. The system must provide real-time, on-line access to the complete electronic patient chart (including results) and be able to display this information graphically at bedside and nursing station on PC workstations or portable wireless devices.

Clinical Rules and Alerts. The vendor must have a strategy to support clinical rules and alerts across the continuum. Key elements of the strategy should be:

- Rules and alerts applied to a longitudinal repository using ASTM and industry-standard Arden Syntax, which allows an organization to develop its own rules or take advantage of rules developed at leading institutions throughout the world.
- The ability to use duplicate and conflict checking during the ordering process, including orders generated at the point of care.
- The ability to integrate external rules databases (such as Micromedex) into the ordering process.
- Rules and alerts must operate independently of ancillary systems.

Integration

A fully integrated solution set is essential to providing the best possible care across the entire continuum of the patient's experience. An organization must be able to access, control, analyze, integrate, and share financial and clinical information throughout the enterprise wherever and whenever it is needed. This requires the following:

INTEGRATION REQUIREMENTS

- Clinical information systems and automated patient monitoring devices like hemodynamic monitors, fetal monitors, ventilators, and IV pumps must be tightly integrated.
- Individual modules of the clinical information system must be integrated so that guidelines drive clinical interventions, interventions are updated by results and clinical documentation, variance tracking is automatic, and all data are accessible by a sophisticated reporting capability.
- The clinical information system must be integrated with other systems, such as ADT, billing, medical records, and ancillary systems such as laboratory and radiology.
- Information from inpatient settings must be integrated with information from other care settings, such as physician offices, home care agencies, and long-term-care facilities.

INDUSTRY STANDARDS FOR INTEGRATION

HL7 Compatibility. Compliance with HL7 level 2.2 or higher standards ensures integration with other HL7-compliant systems throughout the enterprise.

SQL Compatibility. Databases and query tools that are SQL-compliant allow users to access and analyze information with industry-standard tools. Data may be exported to PC data management applications such as word processors, spreadsheets, and database management programs like Microsoft Word, Excel, and Access.

Linking the Health Enterprise. The system should be designed to share information and processes with other applications and settings of care, allowing the organization to manage patients across the continuum.

Desktop Integration. End users may access information from multiple applications. The clinical information system integration must support published APIs that permit end users to log on once, select a patient and navigate seamlessly between applications as required to meet their information needs.

Technology Platform Performance

Evaluating technology advances and system architecture is a critical part of selecting a clinical information system. Organizations need a versatile, expandable information infrastructure. Client/server technology and relational databases provide a computing framework that mission-critical clinical information systems can depend on for high system throughput, dependable database management, exceptional hardware versatility, and economies of scale. The minimal criteria for evaluation:

Open-Systems Architecture Philosophy. The vendor should protect your organization's investment in existing systems and information technology by allowing information exchange and integration with legacy solutions from other vendors.

- The system should utilize an industry-standard, nonproprietary operating environment such as UNIX or Microsoft NT.
- The system should support a variety of industry-standard communications environments, such as Ethernet, Token Ring, TCP/IP, and Novell NetWare.
- The system should have a proven history of interfacing with other solutions and integrating information into common records, reports, and flowsheets. At the least, it should interface with ADT, laboratory, radiology, and pharmacy systems, as well as all major patient monitors and ventilators.

Hardware Platform Independence. The system should have a successful track record of installation on a variety of hardware platforms from industry-leading hardware vendors. The platforms should be highly scalable and include high-end servers such as the Hewlett Packard K, T, and V series; Data General 4800 and 5800 series; and IBM R50 and R60 series systems.

Database Management System. The system should be built around an industry-leading ODBC and SQL-compliant RDBMS architecture such as Oracle or Sybase. Ultimately, systems should be RDBMS-transparent.

Graphical User Interface. The system must take advantage of advanced graphical user interface (GUI) technology, allowing the user to simultaneously open multiple pathways to the product, easily invoke and switch between them, and provide field-level assistance. This makes the system easier to learn and use.

Client/Server Architecture. Unlike host/dumb terminal environments, distributed processing technology should be scalable and portable from one platform to another.

Point-of-Care Support. The vendor should have extensive industry experience with wireless technology, delivering interference-free, on-line, real-time access through portable devices.

- A track record with portable wireless devices.
- The system should offer device options including hand-held, cart-based, and fixed devices.
- The system should employ nonproprietary RF technology to protect the customer's investment.
- The system should offer automatic battery chargers integrated into wall mounts and automatic locking devices to secure the equipment.
- Radios and antennas should be integrated into the portable units to eliminate broken external wires and connectors.

Vendor Installation, Education, and Support Services

Your relationship with a vendor does not end when the contract is signed. The vendor you select should develop a long-term business partnership with your organization, based on the following:

Implementation Services. The vendor must have the depth and breadth of experience gained through years of effectively managing the transition from paper-based to automated processes.

Education and Training. Your organization must have access to ongoing training classes that will prepare users to effectively and independently use the system.

Productive Use and Transition to Support. A structured methodology must be in place to bring the system to productive use and transition your organization to ongoing support.

Telephone Support. Your organization must have access to a 24-hour response center. The vendor should be able to provide specific information about response time issues, the classification system, and support processes.

Online Issues Reporting. Communicating application issues should be quick and easy. The vendor should provide information on reporting software defects and whether users can enter and track issue status on-line.

Account Executive Program. The vendor should provide a representative who regularly visits your organization, understands its strategic plans, advises and assists with any issues, keeps an up-to-date written account plan, and acts as its advocate.

User Groups. User group meetings provide a friendly atmosphere for learning and exchanging information and ideas, obtaining assistance, voicing opinions, and finding new ways to take full advantage of the clinical information system.

Conclusion

These requirement lists are neither exhaustive nor exclusive. Reviewing your organizational requirements on the basis of this model, however, should give you great direction and insight into choosing a system and a vendor partner to help manage information and outcome data across the continuum.

CHAPTER 26

An Integrated Electronic Assessment Process

From Concept to Application

KAREN A. PRUSSING, RN, MS, CS(ANP), CNN

OVERVIEW

Uniting the professional talents of multiple health care professionals with goals of maximizing patient care outcomes and minimizing use of limited health care resources across the continuum of care requires that pertinent information be available to all members of the health care team.

With the movement toward managed care, the ability to communicate among members of a multidisciplinary health care team is becoming increasingly important as health care delivery systems refocus from the provider-centered fragmentation of health care seen in the past to a more coordinated patient-centered perspective, which requires multiple services operating within distinct organizations, each with its own set of patient databases and site-specific patient follow-up. Efforts need to focus on integrating inpatient and outpatient delivery systems into one comprehensive continuum of health care services with easy access to all providers, shared information, and providers collaborating in the management of an individual's entire condition (Krause et al, 1996).

This chapter will discuss the rationale for providing integrated care management through an electronic patient record system, and present one health care system's concept of a "virtual community" brought about by utilizing a shared computerized patient assessment database among providers in a physician-hospital organization (PHO). ▲

The movement toward integrated delivery is being fueled in part by the growth in managed care. Although capitated financing provides the incentives for clinicians to better manage care across a client's conditions, it does not automatically lead to mechanisms that will integrate care.

Hospitals and physicians are also moving toward further collaboration, including the development of outcome studies and the sharing of technology (Anderson, 1992). Uniting the professional talents of multiple health care professionals with goals of maximizing patient care outcomes and minimizing use of limited health care resources across the continuum of care requires that pertinent information be available to all members of the health care team.

Furthermore, patients with chronic conditions are now receiving care from multiple providers and from multiple sites and/or services. Unfortunately, the planning and management of a patient's care tend to be limited within that discipline or site. A patient-centered focus, rather than an episode or discipline focus, allows patient data to be used across time (to support a longitudinal patient record) and across settings (to support continuity of patient care throughout all delivery settings) (Patterson et al, 1995). As defined by Evashwick (1987), "A continuum of care is an integrated, client orientated system of care composed of both services and integrating mechanisms that guide and track clients over time through a comprehensive array of health, mental health, and social services spanning all levels of intensity of care." It is this need that has prompted many health care entities such as ours not only to incorporate computerized data systems into the areas of direct patient care but also to merge the large amount of information from separate data systems into an integrated system of patient care.

Reasons for an Integrated Information System

The need for computer-technology support in the management of data is becoming increasingly obvious. In our physician-hospital organization (PHO), as in many other health care organizations, a complete array of services expected in a continuum is available. Often these services are not integrated in a system of care (Evashwick, 1987). Patients should

not have to repeatedly give the same information each time they access the health care delivery system because health providers in different sites duplicate their efforts by not sharing patient information beyond their sites or services.

There has also been a striking shift of responsibility for care from the solo practitioner to organized forms of group practice (Barnett, 1984). An accompanying greater need has been access to and documentation of the services used in our medical center and PHO, both of which provide inpatient and outpatient services. It became apparent to various categories of providers that the demographic and assessment parts of the medical record are some of the principal instruments used to ensure quality care across the continuum. Furthermore, this information must be accessible to all providers to ensure efficient and integrated patient care.

Providers should have to collect information only once for many uses. This requires a "platform" on which data are captured as a by-product of the care through electronic records of every encounter in a health care system, whether inpatient or outpatient. Technological changes can make such a public-private partnership work if there is agreement on core data elements and standardization of how they are held and transmitted (Donaldson, 1994).

St. Alexius Medical Center

Rather than being concise and easy to follow, our patient records at St. Alexius Medical Center in Bismarck, ND, had become a collection of the documents of multiple disciplines. Patients were initially interviewed and assessed by multiple disciplines on admission. Many of these disciplines use their own assessment forms and care plans, some of which were not kept in the patient chart.

A Process Improvement Team was formed to evaluate, revise, reorganize, and better coordinate the initial assessment process and assessment information into a clinical database that could be shared by all disciplines within the medical center and eventually all care providers throughout our PHO, with an option for referral to areas needing further assessment during a hospital stay. In addition, the challenge to provide integrated, efficient, and cost-effective care encouraged us to search for an alternative to separate assessments by each discipline.

Recognizing that any change would affect all departments and services, all disciplines were involved. Team members included representation from physicians, dietetics, nursing, occupational therapy, physical therapy, social services, postanesthesia, emergency, home care, operating room, pharmacy, quality review, lab, and radiology. At different phases of the project, representatives from administration, information systems, patient software and hardware vendor representatives, and the PHO were involved.

To address these problems, the committee agreed that the system would:

- Provide easily accessible patient data to all care providers, and be cost and time efficient
- Retrieve and report data in a flexible manner
- Limit the number of disciplines directly assessing patients on admission
- Integrate all care plans by different disciplines into one individualized plan of care
- Facilitate patient-focused care across the continuum
- Ensure patient confidentiality of electronic records
- Allow for flexibility depending on the assessment requirements of patient encounters throughout the Medical Center and the PHO

Finally, to make the project more manageable, it was divided into seven phases:

Phase I	Evaluate current assessment process and assessment forms
Phase II	Develop assessment "tool" and propose an assessment process
Phase III	Test assessment "tool"
Phase IV	Technology configuration
Phase V	Pilot implementation of the "tool"
Phase VI	Evaluation
Phase VII	Continue implementation of "tool" and electronic interface in medical center and PHO

The Assessment "Tool"

In order to understand our assessment process, all assessment forms utilized by different disciplines were collected. The patient admission through initial assessment was then flow charted (Figure 26-1), and staff and patient interviews regarding the assessment process were conducted. Finally, a record

review for documentation of compliance with Joint Commission on Accreditation of Healthcare Organizations (JCAHO) assessment standards was conducted, as well as a mock survey. Several problems were immediately apparent.

A review of over 30 assessment forms used by different disciplines throughout the medical center revealed that many questions were asked repeatedly. Aside from duplication and inefficiency, patients were noted to express dissatisfaction by the third or fourth time they had been asked the same or a similar question.

Second, our patients were interviewed and assessed by many people on admission, which proved to be time consuming and inefficient. Furthermore, each discipline utilized its own assessment form and filed it in a different section of the patient's chart, where it might or might not be looked at by other care providers.

Last, it was noted that assessments did not carry over to subsequent encounters. In one instance a patient had three emergency trauma visits in 24 hours, and the Demographic and History sections of the initial assessment process were completed on each visit. This was not only time consuming for the providers but also extremely frustrating for the patient.

A final part of the evaluation included a mock survey using JCAHO standards. The findings indicated "a lack of evidence of collaborative and integrated assessment of needs and prioritization of needs, based on the assessment, that should occur on the interdisciplinary plan of care." This was confirmed by chart review as well.

The "Assessment of Patients" standards introduced in the 1995 Accreditation Manual for Hospitals (AMH) provided a guideline to reorganize and better coordinate initial assessment information into a clinical database shared by all disciplines, with an option for referral to areas needing further assessment. In addition, the process of forming a PHO consisting of several structurally separate major clinics, and our medical center, provided us with further incentive to access and update the same assessment information, whether inpatient or outpatient.

The team concluded that one, interdisciplinary, initial assessment form would improve our process and eliminate repeated requests for the same information from the patient. After a literature search, it

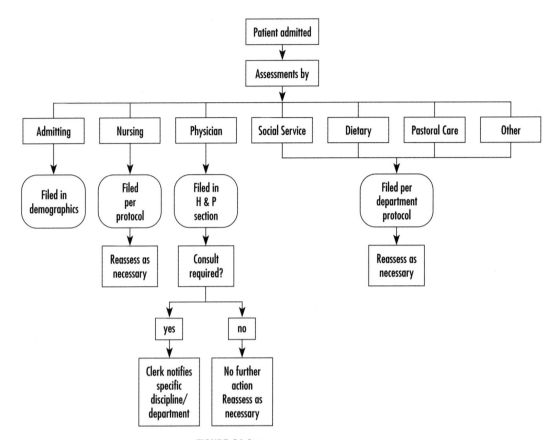

FIGURE 26-1 Current assessment process.

was concluded that excellent tools had been tested and used primarily in outpatient settings, but that they would not comprehensively meet inpatient assessment needs. One interdisciplinary, hospital-based, manual initial assessment tool was documented in the literature by Zappia and Watrous (1995), which used "trigger" questions to prompt further assessment.

Because our system required that the assessment database would eventually be computerized and integrated throughout a large PHO, it was decided to design a computerized multidisciplinary assessment database that could be updated at each encounter. The database would include three major headings: Demographics, Assessment, and Education (Box 26-1).

To ensure confidentiality and usage, each user in the PHO system is provided with a personal iden-tification security code number and a barcode number, which are entered along with his or her name, the date, and the time. This permits only authorized users access to patient records and to only those portions of the records that are relevant to their particular functions. Confidentiality statements are signed by users to acknowledge their knowledge of the legal and institutional requirements. Termination of access numbers occurs upon employment termination.

The 1995 AMH standards still require physician and nurse assessment for every patient. The nursing assessment still contains the review of systems, but because any previous encounter comes up on the computer screen, the questions need only to be verified and updated. Having the most recent past data on screen provided the nurses an opportunity to note any significant changes since the last inpa-

---

BOX 26-1
Features of the Integrated Electronic Medical Record

Demographics

Personal information	Medical history
Immunization/aller- gies	Medications
Advanced directives	

Assessment

Nursing history	Health habits
Systems review	Spiritual
Abuse/neglect screening	Psychosocial
Activity/exercise	

Education

Learning assessment	Nursing diagnosis by priority
Education needs by priority	Discharge plan initi- ated

---

tient or outpatient visit. The idea of "trigger" questions was converted to a computerized format, with key questions submitted by each discipline to electronically prompt further assessments by that discipline.

It was proposed that the initial assessment template would be electronically entered by the admitting staff. The same template would then come up on the screen to be completed by nurses as the primary patient care coordinators with 24-hour accountability, responsibility, and authority. The "nursing" plan of care would become a truly integrated, "multidisciplinary" plan of care based on the assessments completed by nursing and various disciplines as ordered or "triggered" from the initial assessment. Care needs would be documented on the patient's plan of care by all nonphysician disciplines.

The Demographics section included some questions that were already asked or updated by admitting and billing personnel. Medical center admitting and billing personnel would continue to verify information upon admission. Nurses would then electronically complete the rest of the Demographic

section, as well as the Assessment and Education sections, via PCs in the patient's room.

As the initial assessment process itself was fragmented and duplicative, an alternative assessment process geared for the use of the new assessment tool was proposed by the team (Figure 26-2). Finally, discharge planning was integrated into the assessment process, with prompts for initiation or deferment.

The "tool" was manually tested and approved for content in both inpatient and outpatient settings. A nursing staff survey regarding the concept and layout of the tool was also encouraging.

Technology Configuration

To manage care across sites and services efficiently in an integrated continuum, our information system required the capacity to input and access clinical information across multiple sites. St. Alexius Medical Center's integrated information system is composed of separate systems that are accessed through an Ethernet fiberoptic "backbone," as illustrated in Figure 26-3. The fiberoptic "cable" is the conduit for rapid data transfer between systems. It is also the most reliable means of communication utilized throughout the industry today. A flat network such as ours allows all systems to have access to each other on the Ethernet fiberoptic "backbone" (see Figure 26-3).

With the development of a newly formed PHO, a clinical respository that contains data from a single site is no longer sufficient. Individual patient data are now spread across multiple sites in spite of a centralized management—that is, a PHO. Users require an integrated view of clinical data across multiple sites (Marrs, Kahn, 1997). Moving from a repository that contains data for a single facility to one that contains data from multiple facilities is not always straightforward. Many syntactic and semantic issues were addressed in regard to mapping to the repository schema. Data are retrieved daily from the medical center's information systems, mapped to a global schema, and merged with existing data in the repository (Marrs et al, 1994).

We chose to implement a physical, instead of a logical, repository for several reasons: technical and administrative access issues; predictability of performance; availability of the data; and ability to provide data abstractions. The assessment "tool" is

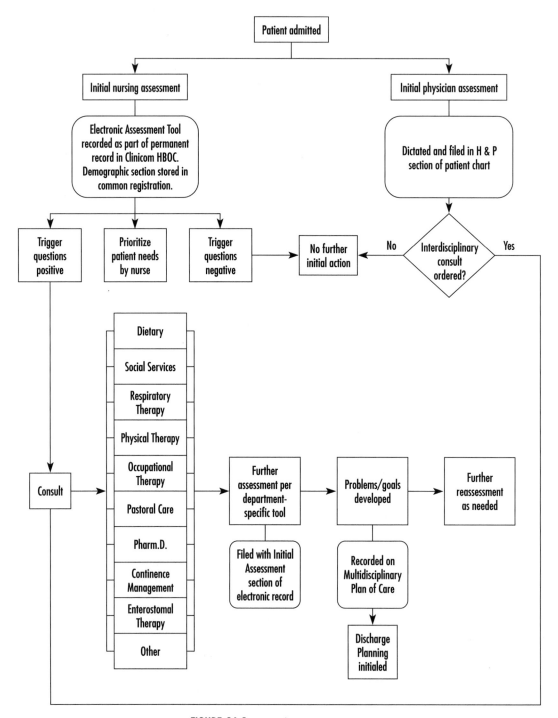

FIGURE 26-2 Proposed assessment process.

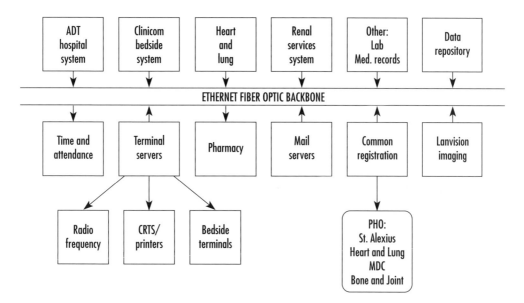

FIGURE 26-3 St. Alexius Medical Center PHO network configuration of information systems.

part of the common registration process. It ensures that accurate demographic information is available throughout the PHO. It also creates a unique identifier for each patient's chronological data.

With a physical repository, data abstractions can be integrated directly with the base data, providing the users with unique views of the data (Kahn, Marrs, 1995). A physical repository also provides us with predictable performance, since all operations are local and need not be transformed to operations on possibly multiple underlying systems. Finally, the availability of the data is dependent only on the availability of the repository, not on the availability of any underlying system.

The physical repository architecture has drawbacks as well. Unless expensive database replication tools are used, the repository can be a bottleneck and presents a single point of failure (Deutsch et al, 1994). Our repository is sufficient for most decision-support applications. To accommodate data from additional sites, each entity in the global schema of the repository was extended with an additional property identifying the facility from which the data came. All data is in one repository, allowing queries over multiple sites. Each entry by a health care provider is tagged with time, date, and provider code to allow for a continuous, chronological history of the patient's care, and to ensure confidentiality of access to the patient record.

Other than the fiberoptic cables, the entire system is exceptionally cost effective and cost efficient. No additional hardware, other than fiberoptic cables in remodeled space, or software is required, as we are utilizing terminals or PC's and therefore have access points throughout our entire campus wherever fiberoptic cables are in place.

Evaluation

Subsequent evaluation of the tool and process revealed that the time required for updating the process was decreased from 60 to 90 minutes to 20 to 30 minutes, depending on what system reviews were performed for the admitting diagnosis. For example, a patient came into Emergency Trauma Department with a broken leg, he had demographic data completed, as well as components of the system review such as cardiac, musculoskeletal, and respiratory. The general surgical nursing staff then completed the rest of the assessment. This entire process triggered further evaluation by other disciplines if appropriate.

The information was felt to have the potential for higher accuracy when we are dealing with elderly or confused patients who have established databases, or who are unable to offer any significant amount of information. Patients were pleased at not being asked questions repeatedly. Patients and families also commented that they felt as if they were known customers, because rather than being asked redundant questions, much of the information was simply verified or updated at various encounters throughout the medical center.

Prioritization of patient needs was found to be easier when completed by nursing, or other "triggered" disciplines, and immediately transferred to the patient plan of care after analysis of the assessment. This resulted in an individualized plan of care. All disciplines utilized the admission assessment and found that it was an integral part of planning care.

Another valuable feature we have found is the computer system's ability to respond to direct, on-demand inquiry, made at a computer terminal, into any part of the patient's record. This inquiry capability is especially important in caring for the "walk-in" patient or in responding efficiently to a patient's telephone call (Meyer, 1992).

Last, as an additional benefit to the patient, the patient may be given, upon request, a personal updated paper copy of a current database at any point of encounter in the PHO. By providing the patient with his or her health information, the patient is encouraged to be an informed participant in his or her health care.

Pending a positive evaluation and staff, physician, information systems, and PHO endorsement, this new system will be implemented throughout the medical center and the PHO. The effectiveness of the assessment process and its use throughout the PHO will be continually evaluated to maintain improvements in patient care.

Conclusion

There has been a striking shift from a system composed of independent solo practitioners to organized forms of group practice offering a complete array of services expected in a continuum. Along with this shift, there has been progressive inclusion of electronic record systems into daily practice;

however, they do not necessarily integrate the evaluations and interventions of multiple services to meet patient needs without duplication and fragmentation (Holle et al, 1995).

This chapter has described one health care system's approach to the integration of an initial assessment process into a "virtual community" as a computerized database management system. The initial evaluation of this work in progress has confirmed the initial goals and outcomes of the project: decreased duplication and greater efficiency in the use of human resources; improved patient and staff satisfaction; increased accessibility to on-line "key" information to all providers in a PHO; and improved continuity of care by continuous, longitudinal updating of on-line information by each provider. All of these benefits contribute to the ultimate goal of improving patient care.

Many challenges to the complete integration of patient records into one common medical record remain. Success will require cooperation and coordination, along with some sacrifice and compromise, but we are convinced that the outcomes will be worth the effort. These challenges to the development of a "virtual medical community" will occupy many of us for much of the foreseeable future.

References

Anderson HJ: Hospitals seek new ways to integrate healthcare, *Hospital* 66(7):26-36, 1992.

Barnett OG: The application of computer-based medical record systems in ambulatory practice, *New England Journal of Medicine* 310(25):1643-1650, June 1984.

Deutsch L, Fisk M, Olson D, Bronzino J: Building a children's health network: city-wide computer linkages among heterogeneous sites for pediatric primary care, *JAMIA Symposium Supplement,* pp. 536-540, 1994.

Donaldson MS: Gearing up for health data in the Information Age, *Joint Commission Journal on Quality Improvement* 20(4):202-207, April 1994.

Duplantis JW, Kobs A, Carlin J: Assessment of patients and care of patients: key issues and topics, *Joint Commission on Accreditation of Healthcare Organizations Video Conference Series,* Oakbrook Terrace, Ill, June 11, 1996.

Evashwick J: Definition of the continuum of care. In Evashwick J, Weiss L, eds: *Managing the continuum of care,* Rockville, Md, 1987, Aspen Publications, pp 23-26.

Holle ML, Rick C, Sliefert MK, Stephens K: Integrating patient care delivery, *Journal of Nursing Administration* 25(7/8):32-37, July-August 1995.

Kahn MG, Marrs KA: (1995). Creating temporal abstractions in three clinical information systems. Submitted to *Symposium on Computer Applications in Medical Care,* New York, 1995 McGraw-Hill, pp. 644-648.

Krause CR, Westdorp JM, Coonen DA, Jenks DL: Forming an integrated documentation system, *Nursing Management* 27(8):25-26, August 1996.

Marrs KA, Kahn MG: Extending a clinical repository to include multiple sites. In *Section of medical informatics,* Washington University, St Louis, 1997, pp 1-16.

Marrs KA, Steib SA, Abrams CA, Kahn MG: (1994). Unifying heterogeneous distributed clinical data in a relational data base. In Clayton C, ed: *Proceedings of the Symposium on Computer Applications in Medical Care,* New York, 1994, McGraw-Hill, pp 644-648.

Meyer C: Bedside computer charting: inching toward tomorrow, *American Journal of Nursing,* pp 34-45, April 1992.

Patterson PK, Blehm R, Foster J, Fuglee K, Moore J: Nurse information needs for efficient care continuity across patient units, *Journal of Nursing Administration* 25(10):28-36, October 1995.

Zappia P, Watrous J: Designing an integrated, initial patient assessment, *Joint Commission Perspectives,* pp 13-16, January-February, 1995.

CHAPTER 27

Computers Across the Continuum

ALICE P. WEYDT, RN, BSN, **LINDA HERTZ**, RN, BSN, **LAURIE FRAHM**, RN, BSN, and **JULIE FREDERICK**, RN, BSN, MBA

OVERVIEW

Computer technology supported the client–health care team partnership. There was better utilization of health services, resulting in enhanced adherence to the medical regimen and improved client-provider satisfaction.

Health care providers in south central Minnesota are using computer technology to develop an integrated regional health care system that includes primary, secondary, and tertiary care. The goals are to improve health status and decrease costs. Organizations are partnering within regional areas to enhance clinical outcomes and maximize utilization of resources. The guiding principle for health delivery systems must be one that values and improves the quality of life for the people served.

Clinical nurse case managers are following clients across time and settings as clients access care throughout the region. They coordinate care and ensure that relevant client information is communicated to all members of the health care team. Regionalization, nurse case management, and computer technology promote analysis and facilitate communication of clinical information to measure and improve outcomes at Immanuel St. Joseph's–Mayo Health System. ▲

Integrated Electronic Medical Records

The established electronic documentation system at Immanuel St. Joseph's–Mayo Health System in Mankato, Minn., provides open and timely communication between the nurse case manager, the physician, and other members of the health care team. The electronic medical record accompanies clients across time and health care settings, linking client health information to providers in various regions, counties, communities, providers, and client homes. Computer technology promotes communication, resulting in coordination of other needed treatment plan changes as well as more timely medication adjustments, which may prevent an extra office visit or a costly hospital admission. In all cases, improved communication and nurse case management interventions have significantly decreased the frequency of phone calls by the client to the physician's office.

Goals of Computer-Based Electronic Medical Records

It is necessary to set clear expectations about what a computer system is to achieve before selecting and designing a computer process.

There are three goals of a computer-based clinical data management system. The goals are to enhance communication, to support clinical decision making, and to provide clinical and financial data.

The first goal of an electronic computer system is to enhance communication of clinical information. In an increasingly complex and fragmented health care environment, computerized processes facilitate communication by providing access to clinical information. Every member of the client's health care team has the same information. The client is spared the stress of relying on memory and repetitious inquiries.

The second goal is to support clinical decision making. An information processing system must selectively retrieve all information and summarize it in a timely, legible, and organized fashion in order for the health care team to analyze the impact of their interventions on desired outcomes. Critical thinking is enhanced when all the relevant information is known by appropriate care providers. Today, there is increased demand for continuous

quality evaluators (Nordstrom, Gardulf, 1996). Knowing what makes a difference in clinical care and the ability to measure the difference result in enhanced outcomes.

The third goal of the electronic system is to generate individual and aggregate data. These data then facilitate clinical review that optimizes resource allocation and reimbursement. Correlating clinical and financial outcomes is vital to accountability in health care for providers as well as clients and families. Careful consideration is needed in determining data elements to meet goals that maximize the care process. This is the basis for developing a computer-based clinical data system that links clinical and financial outcomes. For computer technology to enhance client care, the health care team must be clear about its expectations and goals.

In order to achieve these three goals, collaborative planning is required by the providers using the system. Merely computerizing a process does not guarantee that these goals will be met.

Enhancement of Nurse Case Management by Electronic Medical Records

At Immanuel St. Joseph's–Mayo Health System clinical nurse case managers establish the client case management record, which is integrated into the client's established medical record. Through this system, nurse case managers are automatically notified when the client utilizes any health care service that is electronically linked to the hospital-based system.

Initially, each nurse case manager worked with information systems to build client-specific contact screens. After numerous modifications, the contact screen was standardized for all clients. The contact screen developed consists of the following: type of contact, time, mileage, interventions, outcomes, and utilization of health care services. The items on the screen can be sorted by client name or date. Planning and evaluating the effects of new forms or screens increase efficiency and save time (Congdon, Magilvy, 1996).

Each nurse case manager designed diagnosis-specific computer flow sheets. These flow sheets can be faxed directly to another member of the team or accessed if they are "on-line." A narrative note can be written if necessary.

When a client is hospitalized, hospital staff has access to the nurse case manager notes. The nurse case manager also has free access to the inpatient notes. All disciplines chart in the same "progress note" section.

Not all physicians desire or have the capability to utilize computers at this time. It is strongly believed by the nurse case managers that those physicians who are willing to establish this communication system with the nurse case managers have clients who are better served and more satisfied.

Future studies will be conducted to determine any correlation between client satisfaction and providers' use of computer technology in the client's care. Differences in outcomes will also be explored.

Clinical Nurse Case Manager Outcomes

Outcome measurements of nurse case management are possible because computer technology gathers and organizes data for analysis and comparisons. Outcomes measured include clients' perceptions of their functional status, financial activities, and client and provider satisfaction.

Site-specific client data are easily retrievable through the computer system. However, outcome measurement proves challenging when computer systems do not interface. Aggregate data are difficult to obtain. As systems span the care continuum and become integrated, aggregate data will better reflect trends and patterns.

To measure health status of clients, nurse case managers at Immanuel St. Joseph's–Mayo Health System utilize the Health Status Questionnaire 12

(HSQ-12) (Radosevich, Pruitt, 1995). The HSQ-12 is a self-administered health status measurement instrument. Twelve questions related to physical function, role limitations attributed to physical and mental health, bodily pain, health perception, energy/fatigue, social functioning, and mental health are asked. The HSQ-12 provides a breadth of measures needed for quality assessment.

Nine nurse-case-managed clients were administered the HSQ-12 upon admission to nurse case management and again seven months later. Statistical testing showed that there were no significant changes in any of the areas. It is interesting to note that seven of the nine clients experienced further health deterioration because of their chronic diseases and/or major life changes during the study. However, the clients' perceptions of their health status did not change. It is concluded that the nurse case manager's involvement was the common variable that influenced the health status results. The nurse case manager's caring behaviors helped buffer the impact of the deterioration and major life changes. The relationships that the nurse case managers have with their clients provides constancy in uncontrollable situations. It is also believed that the nurse case managers facilitate clients and their families, managing and adapting to the stressors in their lives.

Other outcomes of nurse case management facilitated by data collection via the computer reflect changes in resource utilization. Hospital admissions continue to occur; however, there are fewer admissions and there is a longer time span between the admissions. Average lengths of stay decrease when nurse-case-managed clients are hospitalized.

Table 27-1 reflects the financial activity for 126

TABLE 27-1
Financial Activity

	SIX MONTHS BEFORE	SIX MONTHS LATER	LAST SIX MONTHS (12-10-96 TO 6-10-97)
Inpatient hospital admissions	134	58	41
Total inpatient charges	$1,076,331.00	$348,514.00	$318,910.00
Total outpatient charges	$ 138,802.00	$151,151.00	$183,400.00
Total ER charges	$ 27,941.00	$ 20,030.00	$ 24,738.00
TOTAL CHARGES	$1,243,074.00	$519,695.00	$527,048.00

nurse-case-managed clients for an 18-month period. The "six months before" column represents charges and hospital admissions for the six-month period prior to these clients being nurse case managed. The "six months later" column indicates financial activity and hospitalizations for the same 126 clients in the first six months following their being nurse case managed. The "last six months" column reflects the charges and hospitalizations for these same clients for a recent six-month period.

The 126 clients include a broad range of ages and diagnoses. There are 17 chemical dependency clients, 41 medical-surgical clients, 40 behavioral health clients, and 28 obstetrical and pediatric clients represented.

Total inpatient charges decreased; however, outpatient charges increased, suggesting that utilization of this type of service was more appropriate after nurse case managers were involved. Total charges had a significant decrease in the first two time frames but had an increase in the last six months because of several clients who had high outpatient activity related to exacerbation of symptoms.

Careful interpretation of financial reports is necessary. For instance, a nurse case manager intervened early when a behavioral health client was suicidal. Through timely computer communication between the nurse case manager and the psychiatrist, the client received a series of outpatient electroconvulsive therapies, thereby averting an acute care admission.

Computer-generated reports reveal that this behavioral health client incurred $35,000 in outpatient charges from December through June. These services were vital to the client having a positive outcome. To measure success on the basis of finances only is a disservice to the clients served as well as to members of the health care team. There are times when resource utilization increases. Exacerbation of symptoms is part of the chronic disease process. Appropriate resource utilization ultimately provides long-term clinical and financial benefit. The clinical benchmarks are an important measure for success. Financial analysis must be done in combination with the clinical review.

Individual and aggregate client data are sorted by the computer for detailed analysis by the health care team. Resource utilization correlates with the electronic medical record, which details clinical outcomes (Box 27-1).

A patient classification system is being explored for nurse case managers to prioritize their client contacts and to quantify changes in client health status. "The patient classification system is a method of sorting patient populations into homogenous groups based on pre-established criteria along a continuum" (Van Slyck, 1996). This system has been utilized in the inpatient setting. Acuity is a measurement of the risk and severity of illness. It can offer an additional view of clients as they receive care across the continuum. After hospital discharge, patient classification provides the mechanism to sort patients by degree of acuity, identify resources needed, and calculate the costs associated with the required resources for each client per acuity level on an ongoing basis. This can be done in a variety of settings, including a clinic or the client's home. Because acuity correlates with the amount of nursing resources required to meet client needs, costs can be better understood and controlled. This information will be important when negotiating reimbursement contracts.

The electronic medical record will eventually have acuity tied to nursing interventions. When nurses document their interventions, acuity information will automatically be generated.

Satisfaction surveys of 76 nurse case managed clients are overwhelmingly positive. The clients indicate that they no longer "feel so alone with their illness," and that they have an advocate who helps them navigate a complex health care system. Provider satisfaction is also very positive. Physicians as well as other members of the health care team comment on the quality of the nursing care that the nurse case managers provide. The trusting relationship between the nurse case manager and the health care team has resulted in a collaborative approach to achieve desired outcomes.

The Electronic Medical Record and Regionalization

Regionalization occurs as health care systems evolve. Integration drives relationships rather than organizations developing systems in isolation. Figures 27-1 and 27-2 represent a regional health care

BOX 27-1
Case Study   Medical-Surgical Case Management Scenario

Chester is an 88-year-old man with a diagnosis of spastic bladder, hypertension, and congestive heart failure. Chester's name appeared on a computer report that lists clients' readmission to the hospital in the last 30 days. In addition to being a frequent visitor to the emergency room, he also made multiple phone calls and visits to his primary physician and the physician's colleagues. The nurse case manager coincidentally received a referral from the emergency room physicians and the primary physician on the same day that Chester's name appeared on the computer report.

Chester met criteria for nurse case management because of his chronic illness, frequent hospitalizations, greater than six prescriptions or medications, and minimal support system. The nurse case manager reviewed a computer screen of his hospital history, which gave a report of all the hospital services Chester had accessed over the years. The report indicated that Chester was frequently admitted to the critical care step-down unit. His admissions were for acute hypertension, hyponatremia, and exacerbation of congestive heart failure symptoms. His recent emergency room visits were related to his difficulty with self-catheterization and hypertensive episodes.

Copies of the inpatient admission sheet and the discharge teaching form from his last hospitalization were accessed through the computer. The nurse case manager utilized the information as a baseline for comparisons, assessments, and teaching opportunities.

Information at the nurse case manager's fingertips facilitated the process of data collection, resulting in a response within a 24-hour period. The nurse case manager planned to call Chester the fol-

lowing day; however, Chester presented to the emergency room with difficulty in performing self-catheterization. The nurse case manager introduced herself in the emergency room and explained her role as a nurse who could partner with him. Chester agreed to nurse case management. For the next two and a half years the nurse case manager was known as "Chester's Nurse."

Through the course of the relationship the nurse case manager utilized the computer for all documentation. When Chester was admitted to the hospital, the nurse case manager was immediately aware of his utilization of hospital services. On admission, Chester frequently forgot his medications or was incoherent and unable to communicate the medications he was taking. This vital information was always instantly available to the health care team via the electronic medical record.

Chester continued to require occasional hospitalizations. During these episodes, the nurse case manager utilized the computer to send and receive referrals from home care services. Upon discharge from home care, the nurse case manager received and viewed the discharge summary via the computer.

Computer technology supported the client–health care team partnership. There was better utilization of health services, resulting in enhanced adherence to the medical regimen and improved client-provider satisfaction. Chester, his primary MD, and the nurse case manager developed a plan with realistic parameters. The outcome was a 90% decrease in emergency room visits, and client calls to the physician's office decreased by 75% (McBeth, Schweer, 1998).

model being created in south central Minnesota that includes primary, secondary, and tertiary care. Integrated computer systems will link the levels of care by transferring clinical and financial data between settings. The computer system will also provide the mechanism for a client's medical record to be accessed by care providers at any site within the regional network.

The electronic medical record will span the care continuum with the Enterprise Master Patient Index (EMPI), which is represented in Figure 27-1. The EMPI includes the medical record numbers identifying individual clients. Source modules store client information by medical record number. When the electronic medical record is accessed, all the data sources are tapped to retrieve desired in-

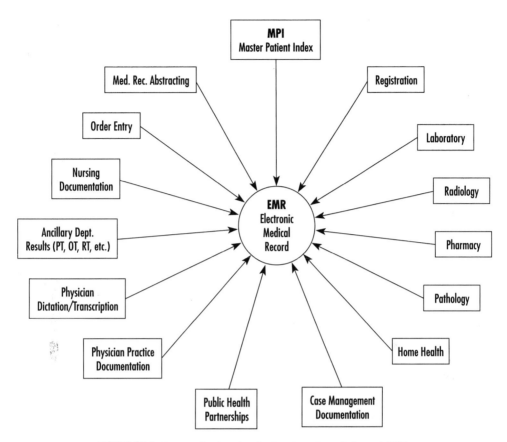

FIGURE 27-1 Sources of patient data for the electronic medical record (EMR).

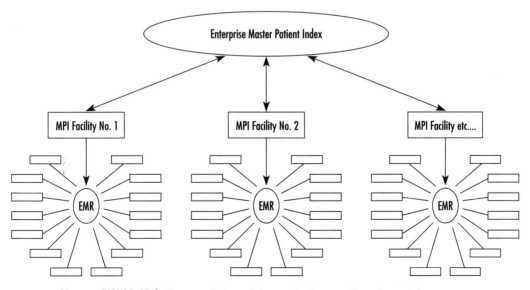

FIGURE 27-2 Sharing medical record data via the Enterprise Master Patient Index.

formation. The information retrieved is therefore the most current.

All data are tied to the EMPI, which cross references client medical record numbers from different sources, including facilities, organizations, and/or health care networks. Cross referencing facilitates the core referencing system of the electronic medical record to retrieve client information automatically, creating a seamless transfer. This can occur as long as security is maintained and confidentiality is protected, and client permission is obtained.

There is a host of complex and operational issues as early adopters try to manage computer-based client records (Kincaide, 1997). Issues of confidentiality, system interdependence, and information ownership must be addressed; however, "efforts need to focus on finding ways to protect/maintain privacy rather than opposing the use of technology in health care" (Leary, 1997).

"What we are trying to do is look at each type of case or disease so we can manage it from start to finish," (Appleby, 1997). Episodic, fragmented approaches to care management are costly and increase provider and consumer dissatisfaction. Care no longer starts and stops at the hospital door.

It is imperative that the electronic medical record exist beyond acute care as care extends across the continuum. Initially, the electronic medical record may be part of a single delivery system but will ultimately have to span multiple delivery systems and organizations. Interfaces will thread systems together. The systems will include primary care, home health, long-term care, rehabilitation services, retail pharmacies, dentists, governmental agencies, schools, alternative health practitioners, and nurse case managers. The goal is to deliver appropriate information based on client needs. Information required to measure outcomes is decided in advance, with consideration given to the users of the information. "Clinical integration requires a knowledge of existing needs. Decisions must be made about where the technology will be housed, which systems will be integrated, and who will provide the necessary resources" (Weydt, 1997).

Delivery systems will be under one umbrella as organizations and information are integrated. All the health care components will be tied together, with the "crossover focus" on clinical aspects rather than administrative ones. "An enterprise limited to its own organization does not cross over, and isola-

tion from the systems will serve no one in the future. The pay back is long term and limited short term. However, the expense can be reduced by investing in technology that meets the needs of many" (Weydt, 1997). The technology that is a key factor to providing an integrated delivery system is the central data repository. The repository facilitates the transfer, analysis, and storage of information that is necessary to support the continuum of care in addition to supporting outcomes measurements and practice analysis.

An evolution is occurring in physician practice that parallels what hospitals have experienced. Traditional physician practices have been internally automated to support the scheduling and billing aspects, but automation has been clinically limited. Integrated delivery networks require a shift in physician practice to electronically communicate clinical information. Relevant clinical information at any intervention site is readily available in the computer system, reducing the necessity to duplicate tests and the risk of missing pertinent clinical data. This results in enhanced diagnosis and treatment. Opportunities to enhance quality with lower utilization of services are also created as technology is used to complement and extend health care resources.

Conclusion

As healthcare moves beyond the walls of the institution, national information networks will link nursing information systems to clients in their own homes (Simpson, 1993). New approaches, supported by computer technology, are being used to strengthen partnerships between care providers, clients, and families. Outcome measurement is facilitated when an integrated electronic medical record is readily accessible to the health team, regardless of time or setting.

Computer technology can never replace critical thinking or caring behaviors. As computer technology revolutionizes health care, nursing's challenge is to stay focused on the caring behaviors that bond clients, families, and nurses. Caring is a concept that is based in relationships and is facilitated through communication. Computerization is not synonymous with communication. "It is only in watching nurses weave the tapestry of care that we grasp its integrity and its meaning for a society that

too easily forgets the value of things that are beyond price" (Gordon, 1997). Computer technology
can enhance care but cannot replicate or replace human interactions that are the foundation of nursing
practice.

References

Appleby C: Cyberspaces, *Hospital and Health Networks*
71(5):30-32, March 5, 1997.

Congdon JG, Magilvy JK: The changing spirit of rural
community nursing: documentation burden, *Public
Health Nursing* 12(1):18-24, 1996.

Gordon S: What nurses stand for, *Atlantic Monthly*
279(2):81-88, 1997.

Kincaide K: Web-based records spin closer to reality, *Telemedicine and Telehealth Networks* 3(1):26-33, 1997.

Leary W: Panel cites lack of security on medical records,
New York Times 146, p A1 (L), col 1, March 6, 1997.

McBeth A, Schweer K: *Building Healthy Communities—the
challenge of healthcare in the 21st century*, Manuscript accepted for publication in 1999, Allyn & Bacon.

New York Times: Electronic threats to medical privacy, p
A22 (L), col 1, March 11, 1997.

Nordstrom G, Gardulf A: Nursing documentation in client records, *Scandinavian Journal of Caring Science*
10(1):27-33, 1996.

Radosevich D, Pruitt M: Twelve-item health status questionnaire (HSQ-12) cooperative validation project: comparability study (Abstract), AHSR & FHSR Annual
Meeting Abstract Book 13:59, 1995.

Simpson RL: Case-managed care in tomorrow's information network, *Nursing Management* 24(7):14-16, 1993.

Van Slyck A: *A system strategy for success in managed care*,
Phoenix, Ariz, 1996, Van Slyck and Associates, Inc.

Weydt EA: Personal communication, August 11, 1997.

CHAPTER 28

Cost and Quality

Joint Imperatives for Case-Managed Care

ANN VAN SLYCK, RN, MS, CNAA, FAAN, **and DEBORAH CRIST-GRUNDMAN**, RN, BSN

OVERVIEW

True economies occur when patient care requirements are met through appropriate utilization of resources.

There is no escaping the reality that health care is big business. Some estimate that health care represents in excess of 18% of the gross national product. Principal health care drivers are quality care and service, satisfaction, and cost; in which all stakeholders, clinicians, patients, and payers have an investment.

Case management is one vehicle health care institutions are using to improve coordination of care in such a way as to ensure that desired clinical outcomes can be achieved, in a cost-effective manner. Whether clinicians are working with an individual patient or populations of patients, information, available at the point of care, is key to ensuring that interventions provided by clinicians make a difference. This chapter illustrates that cost and quality are clearly joint imperatives. Case studies from several health care settings demonstrate how case-managed care on a practical level is successfully working to achieve the mission of quality, affordable health care. ▲

Health Care's Fiscal Imperatives

Whether health care providers are involved in the concurrent care management of an individual patient's acute episode of care or in case managing aggregate patient populations, there are three fiscal imperatives:

- Know your costs.
- Evaluate your costs.
- Manage your costs.

The reality is that managed care is not going to happen "some day" . . . it has already happened.

Prospective and prescriptive reimbursement schemes obligate hospitals to identify their true costs of care. Successful identification of "true" costs fundamentally begins by objectively measuring clinical services provided. There is not a health care environment, regardless of the actual managed care penetration, that is not influenced by the need to effectively manage its cost of care. Essentially, knowing costs is contingent upon knowing the clinical picture. Evaluating costs requires assessing the effectiveness of clinical interventions; and ultimately, only by managing the clinical course can costs realistically be managed (Crist-Grundman, 1997). Today, consumers of health care expect that providers will be stewards of their health care dollars. Case management is proving to be an effective vehicle for achieving quality care outcomes while satisfying cost imperatives. Multidisciplinary case management processes achieve a purposeful and controlled connection between the quality and the cost of care (Freeman, 1997). They improve care by decreasing fragmentation and containing costs (Simpson, 1993). Certainly in health care today, more than ever, it is critical that a cooperative alliance exist between clinicians and their finance colleagues.

A pivotal issue for most health care institutions is linking patient-specific information with financial data. Successful case management is contingent on developing a database of patient information capturing both intervention and outcome measurements. Aligning appropriate resources and interventions to achieve optimal outcomes is a principal purpose of case management. Whether institutions embrace complex case management models or integrate core principles into every aspect of care decision making, quality moves forward and costs decline.

Cost Implications of Case-Managed Care: In Practice

How are hospitals ensuring that information necessary to daily, minute-by-minute clinical decision making is available to providers on a "real-time" basis? A number of hospitals are using nursing-generated patient information, in the form of patient acuity, as a valid measure of services consumed by the patient and his or her significant other(s). Through the process of legally charting nursing services provided, the patient population can be sorted into homogeneous groups (acuity levels), based on pre-established criteria, along the bedded continuum of care utilizing the proprietary Van Slyck & Associates Patient Classification System (Van Slyck, 1982). Patient acuity thus allows an institution to objectively sort its patient volume (i.e., patient days, number of deliveries) by severity. In the hospital-based case studies presented in this chapter, all use a systems approach for determining patient acuity. The patient classification (acuity) system they utilize sorts patients into seven acuity levels. The criteria used to sort the patients reflects a multidimensional weighting of services, based on:

- *Risk* to the patient
- *Complexity* of the service
- *Skill level* required (licensed vs nonlicensed, novice to expert)
- *Frequency* and *time*

This is a critical distinction and differentiates these hospitals' professional practice methodology from industrially engineered systems that use a unidimensional weighting based solely on time (Van Slyck, 1991). By the integration of patient data into care management processes, clear information needed to achieve case management objectives is available.

The experience of the Community Nursing Organization (CNO) of Carondelet Health Care Corporation in Tucson, Arizona, demonstrates that timely intervention by nurse case managers has resulted in chronically ill patients entering the hospital at less acute levels, lowering length of stay and bypassing critical care units (Ethridge, 1997). Ethridge indicates that ultimately this type of data was utilized for managed care contracting. Case management cost benefits occur not only as a result of decreased length of stay or level of care. True economies occur when patient care requirements are met through appropriate utilization of resources.

At Eliza Coffee Memorial Hospital in Florence, Alabama, new clinical pathways were developed to facilitate the provision of care to open heart patients. For nursing's part, common services consumed by 80% of this patient population were identified down to individual care categories, as reflected on the patient care records. The care categories identify services rendered in the areas of nutrition, hygiene, mobility, medications, behavior, state, and treatments/procedures. "Using this information, services were outlined and used as a starting point to measure variance" (Brackeen, 1997). In addition, acuity information is being used to determine resource deployment for the newly created coronary step-down unit. The goal was to determine if some of the patient care requirements could appropriately be met at a lower level of care. Eliza Coffee has achieved a 50% reduction in postoperative length of stay for its open heart patients, while sustaining favorable patient clinical outcomes and satisfaction (Brackeen, 1997).

Kay Buitenveld, Director of Oncology Patient Care Services at Harrison Memorial Hospital in Bremerton, Washington, indicates that patient acuity documentation is consistently used as a tool during multidisciplinary team care conferences. All patients are evaluated in terms of their progression (improvement) to the next lower acuity level. In this way, acuity is used as an indicator in discussions on readiness for discharge and as one of the criteria for patient placement decisions (Buitenveld, 1997). Appropriate progression of a patient along the care continuum from admission to discharge and patient placement (critical care versus general acute care) can significantly impact the cost of care.

For Augusta Medical Center in Fisherville, Virginia, nursing case management and nursing-generated patient information in the form of acuity are evolving along parallel tracks. Their focus is on case managing the chronic, complex patient populations, prone to readmission or other ongoing use of health care resources. In some instances, there may be an acute care episode (e.g., stroke) wherein it is determined that intervention by a case manager could positively affect the path and outcomes of the patient. Nurse case managers are assigned to patients hospital-wide to coordinate all aspects of care. Augusta is now looking at the evolution of pa-

tient acuity in the home health arena. Case managers hope to show, as they track patients across the continuum, whether interventions provided at home are working—in other words, improving the health status of the patient. By having available both baseline and longitudinal patient acuity data, the facility can ultimately determine cost-of-care implications, which are of particular value as managed care penetration increases within Augusta's market. While a key segment of population is case managed, Augusta embraces the value of concurrent care management for individual patients experiencing acute episodes of care. For these patients, an attending nurse is identified to oversee the care management of the patient while on the unit. This registered nurse coordinates and facilitates resources in conjunction with the health care team. Patient acuity information is used to deploy resources, with the goal of aligning the appropriate care provider(s) with the right patient, at the right time. Key decisions surrounding how the nursing care team will be composed for a specific set of patients affect the cost of care being rendered. At a broader level, acuity information about patient populations served by specific units is used as an indicator for driving budget—specifically, allocations for the number and type of FTEs (Lucente, 1997).

Memorial Medical Center in Gulfport, Mississippi is in the beginning stages of formal case management. They have designed a "point-of-service" model, with demonstration targeted for the Oncology Division. This model focuses on accountability for improved decision making, thereby improving the quality of patient outcomes. Multidisciplinary Division Councils will be accountable for patient management, clinical coordination, development of pathways, and outcomes. They embrace the view, as literature suggests, that not all patients need a pathway, but all do need clinical coordination. The RN responsible for clinical coordination is using acuity information to identify patients consuming high-level, professional nursing services. Given this information, RN assignments are made to align the novice to expert skills among the various RNs staffing the unit. Concurrent care management occurs at a broader assignment level as well. Using acuity data, nursing leadership looks at both the number and the type of resources needed to be allocated on a daily basis to best meet the needs of patient populations being served. In Memorial's current environment, managed care penetration is about 12%. The executive leadership believe it is critical that the facility get a clear picture of what it truly costs today to deliver care, in preparation for evolving managed care contracting. Critical to this initiative is the generation and use of patient information in the form of acuity. Memorial embraces incorporating into pathways and clinical coordination, patient acuity information, as a cue for intensity of services needed and consumed by specific patient populations.

In addition, Memorial is trending patient acuity levels along the hospitalization course from admission through discharge. If a patient's acuity level is high on entry to the hospital, the question case managers ask is what could have been done on the front end to intervene either to avoid admission or to bring the patient into the hospital at a lower acuity level (Bishop, 1997).

Marketplace Realities

It is imperative to recognize that reduced unit payment from all health care purchasers (private and governmental), for all services rendered, is creating a need for greater efficiency and cost effectiveness among all providers (Callaway, 1997). There simply are not "more" resources available. To ensure that affordable health care remains available, clinicians must guarantee that appropriate allocations of health care resources are made to meet today's demands, so there will be adequate resources available to meet tomorrow's needs. Quality care outcomes and affordability are complementary, not competing, variables. All organizations are having to look closely at the economic implications of existing practices and policies. "Case mix information allows health care executives to answer 'what if' questions to determine how changes in patient volumes will affect service costs, quality, and profits. Financial managers can use case mix data to assist in negotiations, revenue analysis, case-based budgeting, and physician analysis. Quality Assurance professionals can use it to analyze the misuse and overutilization of resources, and nursing managers can use case mix information to predict staffing utilization and recruitment and training needs" (Simpson, 1991). David Lawrence, MD, Chief Executive Officer of Kaiser Permanente, is quoted as saying, "The way

you drive costs down is by improving quality and service; that's been shown in every industry. And in health care, it's true in ways that are even more staggering" (Lawrence, 1997). It is therefore not unreasonable to ask clinical experts the question, is what you are doing making a difference? If variance exists, why, and what does it contribute of value to desired outcome(s)? This does not suggest that there is a single course that every patient must follow. Case management correctly embraces the notion of benchmarking better practices that achieve optimal clinical outcomes. In this way, quality care is ensured while cost is reduced. It is true then that nurses and others on the health care team make a difference by managing one life at a time.

References

Bishop S: Interview with Sandra Bishop, RN, MSN, DNSc, Division Manager, Oncology Services, Memorial Medical Center, Gulfport, Miss, August 1997.

Brackeen S: Interview with Steve Brackeen, RN, BSN, Director of Nursing, Eliza Coffee Memorial Hospital, Florence, Ala, June 1997.

Buitenveld K: Interview with Kay Buitenveld, RN, MBA, ONC, Director, Oncology Patient Care Services, Harrison Memorial Hospital, Bremerton, Wash, July 1997.

Callaway M: Integration in the real world, practical aspects of integration in three diverse markets, *Healthcare Forum Journal*, vol 22, March-April 1997.

Crist-Grundman D: Patient acuity: a viable methodology for linking patient and financial data, *Aspen's Advisor for Nurse Executives*, vol 12, August 1997, pp 4-6.

Ethridge P: The Carondelet experience: historical perspective, *Nursing Management* 28(4):26, 1997.

Freeman S, Chambers K: Home health care: clinical pathways and quality integration, *Nursing Management*, vol 28, June 1997, p 45.

Lawrence D: Taking the heat, *California Medicine*, vol 22, July 1997.

Lucente B: Interview with Betty Lucente, MSN, RN, Vice President, Patient Care Services, Augusta Medical Center, Fisherville, Va, August 1997.

Simpson R: Case managed care in tommorrow's information network, *Nursing Management*, vol 24, July 1993, p 14.

Simpson R, Clayton K: (1991). Automation: The key to successful product-line management, *Nursing Administration Quarterly*, Winter 1991, p 37.

Van Slyck A: A systems approach to the management of nursing services—part II: patient classification system, *Nursing Management*, vol 22, April 1991, pp 23-25.

Van Slyck & Associates, Inc. Phoenix, AZ, January, 1982.

CHAPTER 29

Managed Care

Legal and Policy Issues

ELLEN K. MURPHY, MS, JD, FAAN

OVERVIEW

The challenge for consumers and providers who are currently uncomfortable with managed care organizations' practices is not to look to the law for answers but to help the managed care organizations recognize that what is good for customers is good for business.

Managed care has fundamentally altered health care delivery. Without a regulatory or statutory framework tailored to guide the changes in health care, the legal system is in a reactionary mode. Some people and groups are looking to the legal system for redress of perceived wrongs under managed care and as a source of authority to structure a system of "patient rights." Others argue that governmental interference with market forces will prevent managed care from most effectively achieving its goals of quality and efficiency.

Without a national consensus, the law is ill equipped to accomplish the expectations some hold for it. Laws of negligence, contract, and employee benefits, established long before containment mechanisms were even conceived, will continue to be applied to current situations with sometimes unanticipated results. Market forces can be expected to continue driving health care reform because comprehensive legislation is politically unlikely. ▲

An adage frequently heard in law schools is "sometimes the law leads; sometimes it follows." The Clinton administration attempted to pass a comprehensive Health Security Act, in essence an attempt to use the law to lead health care reform. That effort collapsed for a variety of political, economic, and social reasons (Broder, Johnson, 1996). Meanwhile, market-driven changes and reforms have accelerated without the benefit—or, as some would argue, without the burden—of a systemic legal or regulatory framework. As often has been the case in a rapidly evolving field such as health care, the legal and regulatory systems follow rather than lead practice and delivery changes.

Legal principles involving negligence, antitrust, employee benefits, fraud, contract, and so on were established long before managed care or case management was even remotely contemplated. These same legal principles are now being applied to the previously unanticipated health care delivery mechanisms with sometimes unanticipated results (see *Effects of ERISA* discussion on p. 259). The law is being looked to as a mechanism to curb the more egregiously perceived excesses of managed care, such as legislation mandating 48-hour stays for normal deliveries or requiring inpatient care for extensive mastectomies. These single-issue proposals, sometimes derided as "legislation by body part," are usually introduced and passed as a reaction to media coverage that brings the public attention to specifically identified practices that the public is unwilling to accept despite its demand for cost containment. Legislation by body part or other single-issue proposals, such as the anti-gag rule or prohibition against denials of emergency care treatment, have compelling appeal with consumers (read "voters"), but single-issue proposals are not practical. They require too much legislative time, require constant returns to legislatures for remedies, and do not often work.

Other, more systematic changes in statutes, administrative regulations, and case law can be anticipated as society gains more experience with the evolving reforms. Thus, in managed care and case management, a situation exists where the law is following and, in some cases, playing a bewildering game of catch-up.

Like the traditional health care system, the legal system is circumscribed and episodic. This is especially true of the court system, which is designed to examine one fact situation at a time and adjudicate a time-limited resolution. But even legislatures rarely take a broad, comprehensive, integrated view of a societal issue. Indeed, when they do, they are rarely successful because too many interests are threatened and thus too many incentives to opposition arise. Even when a common goal can be identified (e.g., confidentiality, safe patient care), the devil resides in the details of how to reach it.

Nurse authors are careful to distinguish case management from managed care. Clearly, nursing case management can and does occur outside a managed care system; however, nursing case management is increasingly a component of a managed care system, and managed care is altering the legal context of nursing case management.

This chapter includes discussion of how principles of negligence and contract law have been applied to claims against managed care organizations (MCOs) brought by patients who experienced negative outcomes. It also includes a discussion of the unanticipated consequences of the Employee Retirement Insurance Security Act (ERISA), issues of confidentiality of health care records within managed care and case management systems, and likely recommendations from the Federal Advisory Commission on Consumer Protection and Quality in the Health Care Industry.

Negligence and Malpractice

Negligence and malpractice causes of action provide an avenue of redress for persons injured because of the unreasonable or imprudent actions of others. As a policy matter, negligence and malpractice law acts as one type of quality control mechanism. Specifically, negligence and malpractice law provides a financial incentive for health care professionals to provide care in a manner consistent with professional standards so as not to cause injury to others. Some would argue that such incentives are properly placed by the respective professions rather than by an outside force such as the legal system and that, additionally, legal and financial incentives are not needed to motivate health care professionals. Negligence and malpractice laws have endured substantial criticism as promoting defensive medicine and overtreatment rather than promoting quality.

Malpractice liability exposure is one of the few current financial incentives for some MCOs to invest in the staff, expertise, equipment, and programming to avoid negative outcomes. Lawsuits provide a more immediately visible effect on public relations than do the patient satisfaction surveys and outcome publications that for some managed care organizations are not yet available. Whether these theoretical policy incentives play out in reality has not yet been demonstrated. As Hall et al (1996) concluded, very few disputes arising in managed care settings have made their way to the courts—perhaps because patients are not aware of coverage decisions being implicitly enforced or because patients find it too expensive or too difficult to pursue a claim through the judicial process.

Negligence and malpractice law only provides remedies (i.e., compensation) for measurable injury. Although patients have occasionally successfully sued for emotional distress, almost always a successful suit will require physical injury. Thus, the law provides remedy for injury but provides no redress for failure to achieve many of the desired outcomes of nursing case management (e.g., improved functional status or effective parenting). Evidence of positive or negative outcomes, such as parenting or functional status, might be manifested elsewhere in the legal system (e.g., workers' compensation or disability claims, domestic neglect and/or abuse, or juvenile delinquencies), but studies to establish even a correlation between nursing case management and frequency of compensation claims or corrections cases have not been done.

Medical malpractice case law in the United States has evolved within a context of strong societal values based in individual autonomy of patients and their right to choose freely their physician providers. Physicians rightfully weighed individual patient interests most heavily in recommending courses of treatment. Any concomitant duty to conserve society's resources was certainly secondary. Individual patients (or estates) could sue a provider for unreasonable care that results in individual injury; there is no recognized cause of action for "society" to sue a provider for imprudent use of resources.

Under most managed care plans, the emphasis on the individual continues—framed by the contract for benefits with the plan. However, unlike fee-for-service plans, managed care has other incentives to conserve resources (i.e., reduce costs) as well. Treatment decisions are still made within the individual patient-provider relationship, but that relationship exists in a far different context from that provided by fee for service and free choice of physicians. Theoretically, treatment decisions and plan incentives to reduce costs are separate transactions, since plan coverage is not intended to drive treatment decisions, and denial of plan coverage does not preclude patients from obtaining a desired treatment, as they are free to buy the treatment elsewhere. However, as Hirschfield and Thomason (1996) point out, considering coverage and treatments as separate transactions ignores reality and fails to place restraints on overzealous denials of coverage, which may lead to a lower quality of care than our society may find comfortable. They argue that the law must recognize the role coverage plays in treatment decisions and develop new mechanisms to balance society's interest in constraining health care expenditures with individual patients' interests in receiving quality health care.

The court system, where negligence and malpractice law are seated, by design deals with individual circumstances and events. It is not suited as a quality mechanism or as an avenue of redress for population or aggregate outcomes, properly the focus of nursing case management.

Managed care organizations can be held directly liable for their own negligence as a business entity and/or vicariously liable for the negligence of others under their control (e.g., employees). Negligence cases that have been brought against managed care organizations have tended to group under the following theories: (1) direct liability for negligent performance of utilization review (denial of payment, no treatment authorization); (2) direct liability for selection and supervision of staff; (3) vicarious liability for the negligence of employees; and (4) vicarious liability for the negligence of non-employee physicians under apparent or ostensible agency doctrines. The latter three theories have been applied to hospitals in traditional systems as well (e.g., *Johnson v. Misericordia*, 1981; *Darling v. Charleston*, 1965; *Schlotfeldt v. Charter Hospital*, 1996).

NEGLIGENT PERFORMANCE OF UTILIZATION REVIEW

The lead case recognizing potential liability for negligent utilization review is *Wickline v. State* (1986).

Third party payers of health care services can be held legally accountable when medically inappropriate decisions result from defects in the design or implementation of cost containment mechanisms as, for example, when appeals made on a patient's behalf for medical or hospital care are arbitrarily ignored or unreasonably disregarded or overridden.

The patient in *Wickline* had had aortic surgery. Medi-Cal had authorized an initial ten-day hospitalization but granted only four days of a requested eight-day extension. Within days after returning home, she developed a blood clot in her leg, which ultimately necessitated amputation. Medi-Cal was not held liable because, among other reasons, the patient was stable at discharge and the physician had failed to further object to the four-day extension. The case is most famous for its dictum about physician responsibility:

However, the physician who complies without protest with the limitations imposed by a third party payer, when his medical judgement dictates otherwise, cannot avoid his ultimate responsibility for his patient's care. He cannot point to the health care payer as the liability scapegoat . . .

Other widely referenced denial of treatment/payment cases include *Wilson v. Blue Cross* (1990), which found that a plan could be sued for an anorexic patient's discharge after 10 authorized days despite her physician's recommended four weeks and in which the early discharge could be seen as substantially contributing to the patient's suicide. In *Muse v. Charter Hospital* (1995) the hospital was liable for an ex-patient's suicide after discharging him when his insurance benefits expired. Neither *Wilson* nor *Muse* involved managed care organizations but illustrate that liability can be imposed on organizations or agencies for denial of treatment. The managed care industry was stunned in 1993 after the widely publicized *Fox v. Healthnet* $89 million verdict for refusal to pay for a $100,000 bone marrow transplant (Reuben, 1996). Reuben reported that managed care insurers have begun stocking their reserves in anticipation of a wave of denial of treatment-related claims.

EFFECTS OF ERISA

The liability for selection and supervision of staff and the vicarious liability for negligence of employees and some nonemployee physicians are not unlike the liability exposure held by traditional hospitals. What is different for managed care organizations is the availability of a defense usually not available to hospitals. As a totally unanticipated consequence of a federal law intended to protect employee pension plans, some managed care organizations have been shielded from liability exposure to injured patients.

The Employee Retirement Insurance Security Act was enacted in 1974 as a response to Congress' concerns about private employee benefit plans. ERISA's purpose was to protect employees by ensuring that promised retirement, medical, or other benefits would actually be available when needed. Congress wanted ERISA uniformly applied and enforced in all the states. To ensure this would happen, Congress included a sentence in the statute that reads: "[ERISA] shall supersede . . . all state laws . . . as they . . . relate to any employee benefit plan." This is called a preemption clause, because state law no longer applies to lawsuits brought against benefit plans; only ERISA applies. This means that ERISA makes it impossible to sue MCOs that are part of a qualified benefit plan under state law or in state courts. Health care negligence and malpractice are matters of state law. The ironic result is that MCOs cannot be sued by injured patients for health care negligence or malpractice, and any incentive to deliver safe care that is usually provided by liability exposure is negated.

As the judge in *Kearney v. Healthcare* summarized:

Claims against an ERISA plan party premised on a failure to provide promised benefits or a misrepresentation of what benefits would be provided are preempted. A claim that participating primary care physicians were restricted or discouraged for economic reasons from referring beneficiaries to specialists or hospitals or from using the most state of the art diagnostic tests merely ascribes to a defendant a motive for failing to provide certain benefits and is preempted. A claim that an operator or administrator of a plan failed to use due care in selecting those with whom it contracted to perform services relates to the manner in which benefits are administered or provided and is preempted. (p. 187)

Thus, MCOs that are part of a benefit plan covered by ERISA cannot be sued by patients for injuries resulting from denial of treatment, lack of access to specialists, or negligent selection of care providers.

Federal courts are not unanimous in finding

ERISA preemption in cases against managed care organizations, however. The trend is toward holdings that ERISA does not preempt vicarious liability for managed care organizations' physicians' negligence. However, direct liability for withheld benefits (e.g., denial of treatment authorization) remains subject to ERISA preemption.

Some courts and legal analysts are suggesting that language in a 1995 U.S. Supreme Court case, *New York Blue Cross v. Travelers' Insurance*, indicates that the preemption clause will be further limited (Wethley, 1996). In *Pappas v. U.S. Healthcare* (1996), a Pennsylvania appellate court stated: "We, too, do not believe that Congress can have intended, prior even to invention of the cost containment system which inheres in [defendant managed care organizations'] review process, to foreclose recovery to plan beneficiaries injured by negligent medical decisions." Nevertheless, as Rothschild et al (1997) have concluded, "ERISA laws will have to be changed so that managed care organizations are held proportionately responsible for the administrative delay or denial of necessary medical services."

It should be noted that ERISA shields apply only to the managed care plan. Patients can proceed against personal assets and insurance coverage of the individual professional providers.

POSSIBLE FUTURE CLAIMS

As previously discussed, most of the negligence cases that have been brought against managed care organizations arose from fact situations similar to those resulting in suit against traditional hospitals (with the notable exception of denial of treatment determinations). More unique types of negligence cases can be foreseen because of managed care's restriction of physician choice and because of the large databases and outcome data being amassed by managed care organizations that were not available to providers under fee for services.

One possibility is a next generation of cases brought under an informed consent theory. Informed consent theory allows a patient to successfully sue providers for negligence if the patient can prove (1) that the provider failed to reasonably disclose the risks, benefits, and alternatives of a recommended treatment; (2) that the patient would not have consented to the treatment had the patient known the risks, benefits, and alternatives; and

(3) that the patient was injured by the treatment. Several permutations due to managed care arrangements suggest themselves.

One, and perhaps the most obvious, is the gag clause that some managed care organizations have placed in their contracts with physicians that prohibit full disclosure of treatment options. Like denial of treatment decisions, gag rules place physicians in the middle of a tension between their professional duty to individual patients and their personal source of livelihood. Arguably, nursing case managers employed by managed care organizations can be similarly placed as they guide clients to the right treatment in the right place.

Many states and the federal government (in the FY 98 budget bill relating to Medicare and choice) have enacted anti-gag laws. However, managed care organizations can circumvent these laws by removing the clauses from the contract, as required, but enacting a system of one-year contracts. Thus, rather than explicitly terminating a relationship with a physician for disclosing too many options in violation of the contract, the managed care organization can choose not to renew the contracts of physicians who do not follow implicit expectations.

Another possibility is suggested by a 1967 informed consent case, *Fiorentino v. Wenger* (1967). In *Fiorentino*, the court held that a hospital had no legal obligation to make certain the patient had given informed consent to an unusual spinal operation that the surgeon had performed only a few times, with mixed success, and that was being performed by no other surgeon. The court premised part of its rationale on the fact that the patient had chosen the surgeon, and to impose any duty upon the hospital to become involved in the informed consent interaction would meddle with the physician-patient relationship. Subsequent cases have repeated that eliciting a patient's informed consent to surgery is the legal responsibility of the patient-chosen surgeon not the hospital; however, now that patients are dependent on managed care organizations' selected physician panels from which to choose, that may change.

In other cases, hospitals have been found directly liable to patients injured by surgeons if the patient could prove the hospital failed to use reasonable care in its credentialling process when extending privileges to the surgeon (e.g., *Johnson v. Misericordia*, 1981). The patient's restricted choice of surgeon and the extension of *Misericordia* responsibilities to managed care organizations could be combined to place an informed consent obligation on managed care organizations that has never been recognized in hospital fee-for-service plans.

Given managed care organizations' capacity to collect data on individual physicians' practices and outcomes, the managed care organization may have some exposure to liability if it retains physicians with poor outcomes within its network. (Retaining physicians on the basis of their effect on the managed care organization's finances, sometimes called economic credentialling, is another issue.) The question of whether the managed care organization has a duty to inform patients of the physician's track record is also raised.

In *Johnson v. Kokemoor* (1996), a state supreme court concluded that information regarding the physician's experience in performing a particular procedure (cerebral aneurysm clipping), the physician's risk statistics compared with other physicians who performed the procedure, and the availability of other centers and physicians better able to perform that procedure would have facilitated the plaintiff's awareness of the alternatives available to her and aided her exercise of informed consent. (The court cautioned that the decision will not always require physicians to give patients comparative risk evidence, but in this fact-specific case, the physician had chosen to explain the risks in statistical terms and did so erroneously.) The *Kokemoor* court's conclusion suggests future possible causes of action on an informed consent theory of negligence against managed care organizations with large amounts of physician performance data and restrictive referral clauses.

STANDARDS OF CARE AND PRACTICE GUIDELINES

Another policy argument that has surfaced, at least in the legal literature, is whether managed care will or should equal a lower legally recognized standard of care (Malone, Thaler, 1996). Traditionally, the malpractice law has recognized that the requisite standard of care is that which reasonable and prudent professionals employ. Malone and Thaler note that "as managed care establishes practice guidelines, we may be faced with the creation of new standards driven by actuaries and cost containment rather than physician-based reasonable

care standards." Malone and Thaler conclude that, for those who can afford it, "a higher standard of medical care will be available for purchase, but for those limited to lower cost plans, a lesser standard of care will be all that is available." Meanwhile, Kinney (1996) advocates more inclusion of physicians in development of coverage policy for a plan as a strategy for avoiding patients' grievances.

It is curious that under current laws, individual patients cannot waive their right to sue for negligence, in essence cannot agree to accept a lower standard of care. (Courts have found hospital forms requiring patients to waive the right to sue as a condition of admission invalid or against public policy.) But it may be that employers are able to do so on patients' behalf by contract with managed care organizations. Malone and Thaler (1996) buttress their conclusion that a lesser standard will be available with language from the *Dukes v. US Healthcare* (1995) court, which speculated: "It may well be that an employer and an HMO could agree that a quality health care standard articulated in their contract could replace standards that would otherwise be supplied by the applicable state law of tort."

The conclusion that a lower standard of care will be legally required or expected from managed care organizations is of course premised on the assumption that plan coverage drives treatment decisions. Arguments that a lower standard of care will result are also premised on assumptions that managed care organization–generated practice guidelines, from whatever source, will constitute a lower standard than physician- or profession-generated standards. This assumption may be logical for cost-driven managed care organizations but is empirically unsubstantiated. Furthermore, current practice guidelines are used as but one source of evidence as to what a reasonable and prudent provider should have done. Other evidence, such as expert witness testimony, administrative rules and regulations, professional standards, and the literature, can also be considered.

OUTCOMES

Case law does serve as one, however crude, source of data regarding reported negative managed care outcomes. Reported case law cannot be regarded as comprehensive, since most negative health care outcomes do not result in suit. The Harvard Medi-

BOX 29-1
Selected Managed Care Cases

Haas v. Group Health Plan
875 F. Supp. 544 (S. D. Il. 1994)

Plaintiff suffered a punctured eardrum and resulting permanent disability after HMO employee technician irrigated ears pursuant to nurse practitioner's conclusion that the "closed feeling" in her ears was due to wax buildup and recommended irrigation. This case was allowed to proceed against the MCO for the alleged negligence of its employees.

Ricci v. Gooberman
840 F. Supp. 316 (D. NJ 1993)

Radiologist checked incorrect box on mammogram test result so as to indicate normal results. Mammogram had in fact shown a small mass. Reviewing radiologist failed to detect incorrectly completed report. One year later, plaintiff was diagnosed with breast cancer and had a mastectomy. The Federal District Court held that ERISA applied; the patient could not sue the managed care plan for the alleged negligence of the radiologists.

Pomeroy v. Johns Hopkins Medical Services
868 F. Supp. 110 (D. Md. 1994)

HMO denied payment for diplopia surgery and treatment for chronic back pain, facial tic, and severe depression. Patient maintains that as a result, he became addicted to Percodan and HMO denied payment for drug dependency treatment. Patient was not allowed to proceed because of ERISA.

Visconti v. U.S. Health Care
857 F. Supp. 1097 (E. D. Pa. 1994)

Plaintiffs claim obstetrician negligently ignored typical symptoms of preeclampsia, resulting in stillbirth. Parents sued HMO for negligent selection and oversight of obstetrician. Suit against HMO was not allowed to proceed (ERISA preempted).

Dukes v. United States Health Care
57 F. 3d 350 (3rd Cir. 1995)
(Reversing *Visconti*)

Patient died after delay in performing blood tests allegedly resulted in failure to timely diagnose extremely high blood sugar level. Federal Court of Appeals allowed the suit against the HMO to proceed for the negligence of its physician.

Nealy v. United States Health Care HMO
844 F. Supp. 966 (S. D. NY 1995)

Patient had preexisting angina and was allegedly assured he could continue uninterrupted specialist care despite switching HMOs. Bureaucratic missteps delayed obtaining referral to participating cardiologist for three months. Patient died of massive myocardial infarction the day before his authorized appointment with cardiologist. Suit against HMO not allowed to proceed because ERISA applied.

---

cal Practice Study in New York estimated the incidence of adverse events during hospitalizations in New York in 1984 at 3.7%, of which 1% were due to negligence. This study also reported that eight times as many patients suffered an injury from negligence as filed a malpractice claim (Furrow et al, 1997). Of the disproportionately few claims that are filed, even fewer result in appealed cases—and

only appealed cases are systematically reported in the legal literature. While reported case law does not serve as a comprehensive source of data regarding negative outcomes, it does provide examples of such outcomes that are based on sworn evidence. A listing of selected cases brought against managed care organizations and the fact situation giving rise to each case are found in Box 29-1.

BOX 29-1
Selected Managed Care Cases—cont'd

Smith v. HMO Great Lakes 852 F. Supp. 669 (N. D. Il. 1994)	Plaintiffs allege negligence of several treating physicians and hospital for failure to properly care for and deliver infant in fetal distress, resulting in severe disabilities. Suit against HMO for negligence of physician allowed.
Elsesser v. Hospital of Philadelphia College 802 F. Supp. 1286 (E. D. Pa. 1992)	Patient was complaining of chest pain, shortness of breath, and numbness in shoulders when she consulted her primary care physician. ECG revealed abnormal waves. Physician ordered blood tests and use of a Halter [sic] monitor. Physician discontinued monitor after one day's use because U.S. Healthcare denied payment for its use. He did not read the one day's results. On August 14, the patient went to ER with chest pain radiating across her shoulders, down her arm, and up her neck. ECG showed anterior wall ischemia. Patient was given medication and directed to return if conditioned worsened. The following day patient passed out, was rushed to the ER, where prolonged resuscitation was performed. She suffered irreversible anoxic encephalopathy. Claim that U.S. Healthcare had misrepresented that primary care physician would perform all necessary treatment and claim that U.S. Healthcare breached their contract in their failure to provide a qualified primary care physician and U.S. Healthcare's refusal to pay for a Halter [sic] monitor were preempted by ERISA. (However, the claim for HMO vicarious liability for physician negligence could proceed.)

Corcoran v. United Healthcare, Inc.
   965 F.2d 1321 (5th Cir.) Cert.
   denied 113 (S. Ct. 812 1992)
	Plan denied physician's recommendation for hospitalization for a high-risk pregnancy and substituted 10 hours/day home nursing care. Fetus went into distress and died when nurse assigned was not on duty. Federal Court of Appeals held claim could not proceed because ERISA applied.

POTENTIAL EFFECT OF NURSING CASE MANAGEMENT

Managed care that includes the services of a nursing case manager and that concentrates on continuity of care, client involvement in decision making, and client satisfaction would actually reduce the managed care organization's potential for suit in at least three ways:

1. Continuity of care and involvement of a nursing case manager will reduce the potential for injuries (negative physical outcomes). A patient cannot become a plaintiff in a negligence case unless he or she suffered injury.
2. As the Harvard Project demonstrated, even when patients are injured as a result of negli-

gence, they are unlikely to sue; patient satisfaction with providers and positive rapport with treating professionals, aims of nursing case management, are recognized as reasons making patients less likely to sue.

3. Meaningful involvement by patients in decision making and participation in their health care management will increase the availability of contributory negligence as a defense should a suit be filed.

Despite these theoretical advantages of case management beyond cost-driven utilization management, managed care organizations will have fewer incentives to install comprehensive nursing case management services, since ERISA currently protects them from patient suits.

Contracts

Health care is not, and never has been, a generalized legal right. With some statutory exceptions (e.g., The Emergency Medical Treatment and Active Labor Act [EMTALA]), health care is a mutually contracted service. Either party can condition the contract on any terms it wishes (e.g., ability to pay), as long as the other party accepts the terms (and the terms do not violate other laws, e.g., racial discrimination). In managed care, the terms of the agreement (the contract) are set forth in the policy issued by the managed care organization and agreed to by the consumer, or the consumer's employer if the policy is part of a benefits package. It is perfectly legal for a managed care organization to refuse to authorize payment for a costly intervention (e.g., bone marrow transplant) if the contract excluded payment for the intervention. Less clear are exclusions for categories of treatment labeled investigational or medically unnecessary.

The same contract principles control the managed care organization–individual provider agreement. It is perfectly legal for a managed care organization to drop an individual provider from its authorized panel if the individual provider had agreed to a "termination without cause" clause in the initial agreement to provide services for the managed care organization. It is also legal for the managed care organization not to renew an individual provider upon the expiration of the contract. As Laing (1997) points out, allowing such a "deselection" of physician providers by MCOs will further threaten the integrity of the physician-patient relationship. However, one state supreme court has held that refusal to reappoint a surgeon with a ten-year history with the HMO could violate public policy and allowed his suit challenging termination, on grounds of violation of implied covenant of good faith (*Harper v. Healthsource*, 1996). If other courts follow this reasoning, it will make it more difficult for HMOs to drop providers from their panels for any reason, or for no reason.

Confidentiality

Confidentiality of patients' health care information is protected by an incomplete patchwork of state law. Comprehensive federal regulations are just now being proposed.

States have protected patient privacy though general statutes controlling confidentiality of and access to health care records or through condition-specific statutes controlling release of information related to sexually transmitted diseases, HIV-AIDS, domestic or sexual abuse, psychiatric conditions, and so on. Privacy is also protected in states' laws of evidence that create physician, nurse, psychologist, etc., privilege to refuse to disclose patients' health care information without the patients' consent. Not all states have enacted each of these types of protection, and states vary in their enforcement of the statutes they have. All of the protections that do exist are based in a public policy belief that trust between a professional provider and a patient is critical to health care treatment; that candid and complete histories are prerequisite to appropriate treatment; that fear of disclosure will preclude seeking treatment, to the detriment of the public health and safety; and that candid and complete histories and treatment-seeking behavior will be encouraged by assurances of confidentiality. Nearly all the existing state protections were enacted when health care records were hand generated and existed in only one place at any one time.

Exceptions are included in all the confidentiality statutes. Typical exceptions include access to patient records without the patient's consent for purposes of delivering care to the patient, processing or verifying billing claims, and conducting aggregate research. These exceptions reflect the impracticality of requiring signed patient releases for each person who may need access to the records for legitimate purposes. Current state law exceptions typically do not include access to health care information with employment, social standing, or insurance coverage ramifications.

Managed care has now combined with new information technologies to create yet another challenge to confidentiality and any legal protection thereof. Personal data are now collected, stored, and retrieved in multiple locations. While password entry provides some protection, the billing clerks, unbound by professional ethics, who previously had access to a particular episode of care may now have access to the entire record—including data totally unrelated to the charge under review. Moreover, managed care organizations could conceivably profit from the sale of names and addresses of beneficiaries by diagnosis to other companies interested in marketing products related to those diagnoses.

Among the provisions of the Health Insurance Portability and Accountability Act of 1996 was a directive to the Department of Health and Human Services (DHHS) to prepare proposed federal legislation to protect the privacy of health care records. In her address to the National Press Club in July, 1997, Secretary Donna Shalala deplored the fact that Americans' deepest personal health care secrets are being shared, collected, analyzed, and stored with fewer safeguards than video store or credit records.

The legislation proposed by DHHS is based on the general principle that health care information should be disclosed for health care only. Systems with access to health care records must have security safeguards against careless, unintentional, or malicious leakage. Consumers should be able to get copies of their medical records, correct inaccuracies, and find out who has been accessing them, much like what is currently the case for credit records. Persons with access, including employees of insurers and billing service companies, must be bound by the same confidentiality standards as physicians, nurses, and hospitals. Finally, the proposed federal statute would provide criminal penalties for improperly disclosing health care information or misrepresentation to gain access to information. The latter two provisions are frequently absent even in states where confidentiality statutes do exist.

Pear (1997) described the proposed legislation as charting a middle-of-the-road course, rejecting calls from some interest groups for unfettered access and from privacy advocates wanting even stricter safeguards. He described the proposal's outlook on Capitol Hill as unclear. While many lawmakers from both parties support greater privacy for health care records, few have focused on the details to accomplish that end. It is the details that will be subject to intense lobbying efforts by all segments of the health care industry.

Confidentiality of and access to health care records have constituted a difficult balance for any legislative approach, even before the advent of managed care. Clearly patient privacy must be protected, or the sensitive information needed for proper diagnosis and treatment will less likely be disclosed. That privacy interest must be weighed against the practicality of care delivery and pay-ment, since many persons must have access in order to deliver safe health care and process payment for it; against society's increasing expectation that quality improvement and evaluation studies be conducted, requiring access to data; and against society's expectation that fraud be investigated.

This balance was difficult enough to strike when the mechanics of access were far simpler than with today's information technologies; when motives for information misuse were far fewer than in today's for-profit systems, in and out of health care; and when the state of biological knowledge (e.g., genetics) uncovered far less potentially sensitive information for inclusion in the health care record. The capability of managed care organizations to amass data on literally billions of health care encounters for millions of patients within one database only exacerbates the challenge.

Without professional restraint on the sharing of these data and/or without some semblance of comprehensive federal legislation, a new variation of "legislation by body part" can be anticipated. Rather than dealing with denial of claims for specific conditions or diseases, a series of one-issue proposals that address leakages of sensitive information can be expected as emotional reactions to egregious publicized examples of confidentiality breaches.

Other Patient Protection Legislation

Many other issues that may, or may not, be amenable to legal approaches have come to light during the relatively short experience with managed care plans. Among these issues are the adequacy (in numbers and expertise) and accessibility of the provider network in any given managed care organization, availability of timely grievance and appeal procedures, whether access to an appeal system external to the MCO should be provided, presence and adequacy of MCO internal quality monitoring and improvement programs, necessity and/or desirability of requiring external quality review in addition to or in place of that provided by accreditation, regulation of provider incentives interfering with individual treatment decisions, provision of continuity of care across MCOs, and so on.

States have addressed some of these issues in their health maintenance organization statutes.

For their part, professional associations such as the American Association of Health Plans have begun to adopt position statements relating to many of these issues. Voluntary compliance among members and offering different products and services may forestall any perceived need for federal intervention.

Meanwhile, President Clinton has appointed an Advisory Commission on Consumer Protection and Quality in the Health Care Industry, co-chaired by the Secretary of Health and Human Services and the Secretary of Labor. Its 32 members are representatives of providers, consumers, purchasers, health plans and insurers, and unions. Among the consumer issues it is examining are ERISA preemption, access to specialist and emergency treatment, financial solvency, communication and disclosure between the plan and beneficiaries, due process complaint resolution, quality performance and measures. If a federal comprehensive legislative initiative can pass Congress, it is likely that the successful proposal will address similar major categories. It is also likely that some of the same forces that opposed the Health Security Act will oppose any proposed legislation as unnecessary and cost-enhancing interference in the marketplace.

Consumer protection initiatives continue to be proposed at the state level as well, either as amendments to previous legislation or as new legislation. Among these are calls for consumer report cards, direct access to specialty care, and health insurance ombudsmen. Insurance regulations are a matter of state, not federal, law. Thus, added to this already complex and intertwined health care system and regulatory attempts are the arcane complexities of federal and state jurisdiction. Even within a given state, jurisdiction disputes are predictable between and among its regulatory agencies (e.g., should patient protection regulation issue under the rule-making authority of the department of health or the insurance commissioner's office?).

Conclusion

The frenetic changes in health care delivery have thus far outpaced the legal system's capacity to respond comprehensively. Managed care has presented a variety of challenges to the application of national legal principles, both because those principles were laid down before managed care was conceived and because managed care has shifted some of the societal values upon which the legal principles were based (e.g., individual patient choice of provider; provider ethical and legal duties to individual patients to be balanced with society's interests in cost containment).

The issues raised by managed care are complex, interrelated, and constantly mutating. The legal system is ill equipped to implement policy for a society that has not reached consensus on what policy should be.

For the foreseeable future, the market will continue to drive changes in managed care. Many will argue that this is as it should be, that any quality concerns that arise will be addressed by the market without government interference in the guise of patient protection. Others will counter that government regulation is essential to balance the otherwise disproportionate market power of managed care organizations over consumers.

Legislative initiatives at the state and federal levels can be expected to be of two types: single issue and comprehensive frameworks. Single-issue legislation is easier to pass, especially if it carries broad-based emotional appeal. More comprehensive schemes that are under consideration in state and federal legislatures relating to confidentiality and other consumer rights are being developed. Even these proposed government regulations will still rely heavily on managed care organizations to design and implement mechanisms that comply with any mandated principle or category of concern. The challenge for consumers and providers currently uncomfortable with MCO practices is to help the MCOs recognize sooner rather than later that what is good for consumers is what is good for business. Until consumers, providers, and managed care organizations arrive at that consensus, the law will be only marginally effective as a tool. Managed care organizations do have a stake in encouraging that consensus as well, lest any current backlash against managed care organizations give rise to a revolt against them, which would in turn invite ever more government regulation or perhaps a revisitation of previously discarded comprehensive government-driven reform. In this country, changes in law have always followed changes in health care. They can be expected to continue to do so.

References

Broder D, Johnson H: *The system*, Boston, 1996, Little, Brown.

Darling v. Charleston Community Hospital, 33 Ill. 2d 326, 211 N.E. 2d 253 (1965).

Dukes v. United States Healthcare, Inc., 57 F. 3d 350 (3d Cir. 1995).

Emergency Medical Treatment and Active Labor Act (EMTALA). 42 U.S.C. §1395dd.

Employees Retirement Insurance Security Act (ERISA). 29 U.S.C. §1001.

Forentino v. Wenger, 227 N.E. 2d (N.Y. 1967) *or* 280 NYS 2d 373 (1967).

Fox v. Healthnet, No. 219692 (Ca. Super. Ct., Dec. 23, 1993).

Furrow BR, Greaney TL, Johnson SH, Jost TS, and Schwartz RL: *Health Law*, 1997, West Publishing: St. Paul, MN.

Hall MA, Smith TR, Naughton M, Ebbers A: Judicial protection of managed care consumers: an empirical study of insurance coverage disputes, *Seton Hall Law Review* 26:1055-1068, 1996.

Harper v. Healthsource, 674 A2d. 962 (1996).

Health Insurance Portability and Accountability Act.

Hirschfield EB, Thomason GH: Medical necessity determinations: the need for a new legal structure, *Health Matrix* 6:3-52, 1996.

Johnson v. Kokemoor, 199 Wis. 2d. 615, 545 N.W. 2d 495 (1996).

Johnson v. Misericordia, 99 Wis. 2d. 708, 301 N.W. 2d 156 (1981).

Kearney v. U.S. Healthcare, 859 F Supp. 182 (E.D.Pa. 1994).

Kinney ED: Resolving consumer grievances in a managed care environment, *Health Matrix* 6:147-165, 1996.

Laing BA: Deselection under *Harper v. Healthsource*: a blow for maintaining physician-patient relationships in the era of managed care, *Notre Dame Law Review* 72:799-861, 1997.

Malone TW, Thaler DH: Managed health care: a plaintiff's perspective, *Tort and Insurance Law Journal* 32(1):122-153, 1996.

Muse v. Charter Hospital, 452 S.E. 2d 589 (N.C. Ct. App. 1995).

Pappas v. U.S. Healthcare Systems of Pennsylvania, 450 Pa. 162, 675 A. 2d 711 (1996).

Pear R: Law targets privacy of medical records, *Wisconsin State Journal*, August 10, 1997, p 4A. (Reprinted from the *New York Times*.)

Reuben, R.C: In pursuit of health, *ABA Journal* 82(6):54-60, 1996.

Rothschild IS, Zaremski MJ, Rust ME, Levin L, Indest GF III, Schmidtke M: Recent developments in managed care, *Tort and Insurance Law Journal* 32:463-480, 1997.

Schlotfeldt v. Charter Hospital of Las Vegas, 112 Nev. 42, 910 P.2d 271 (1996).

Wethley FC: *New York Conference of Blue Cross & Blue Shield Plans v. Travelers Insurance Co.*: vicarious liability malpractice claims against managed care organizations escaping ERISA's grasp, *Boston College Law Review*, 37:813-860, 1996.

Wickline v. State, 239 Cal. Rptr. 810 (Ct. App. 1986).

Wilson v. Blue Cross, 271 Cal. Rptr. 876 (Ct. App. 1990).

CHAPTER 30

Healthy Workers–Healthy Business

Understanding and Managing the Correlation Within the Arena of Alternative Medicine

NANCY N. BOYER, RN, NP

OVERVIEW

Alternative and complementary medicine has brought to light an awareness of the ever-increasing complexity of human health and the mind/body/spirit connection.

To create, support, and manage care, providers, administrators, and employers must have access to a range of comprehensive information. Although older than the conventional approach, alternative medicine has remained powerless to become recognized as a legitimate force in maintaining overall wellness. However, in response to waves of consumer disenchantment with the conventional approach of treating the body as "parts," insurers are adding alternative and complementary medicine coverage to strategically increase market share. Providers of alternative and complementary medicine are agreeing to partner with insurers, if only to gain acceptance as legitimate service providers. It becomes imperative that oversight organizations, neutral in their composition, begin to reality test what works and what does not. The clear candidate emerges as the employer groups who have long paid for health care benefits without the necessary arsenal of information—which benefits are effective and which are ineffective in promoting healthy employees and dependents? American business certainly does not launch a new product or purchase a new service without exhaustive research and copious information. Since decisions affecting benefit administration will be made on the basis of analysis of data, it is critical that the information be clean, current, secure, and consistent between plans and states, and that analyses based upon them are credible. ▲

In this age of computer-intensive information transmission, it is almost unfathomable that no one knows for sure, on a systematic basis, what works and what does not work in effectively promoting health. Patients, providers, and payers are still in the dark about what constitutes good practice guidelines. As a consequence, the oft-quoted percentage of the Gross National Product (GNP) used for health care (15%) cannot be converted into a reality-based number. If one is employing good, solid, measurable practice protocols, should this well-known statistic be 2% or 20%? This question should be of special interest to the business community, which picks up the biggest portion of medical expenditures. Yet, surprisingly enough, American business has had minimal involvement in any decisions regarding the expenditure of these dollars. An equally astonishing fact is that feedback from the business community has rarely if ever been solicited to help ensure that dollars spent on health benefits will improve the bottom line via enhanced productivity. Measures such as Health Plan Employer Data and Information Set (HEDIS) have demonstrated process results but not linked process to health outcomes.

The expanding arena encompassing alternative and complementary medicine (ACM) cannot make the same mistake. Beneficiaries are now demanding and receiving coverage for therapies such as chiropractic services, relaxation techniques, and homeopathy. In a market estimated to be over $14 billion (Adams, Harkness, Hill, 1996, 1997), now is the time to begin focusing on methods to answer the payer question, "What have we purchased?"

Until now, a fear has dominated that research methods could not be validated or peer reviewed, since standard evaluation tools would not be useful in measuring the unconventional approach used by these practitioners to identify and cure. *Applied* research methods are necessary to capture the business/payer/patient answers. Prior to a discussion of potential methods of study, it is important to take a snapshot of the current state of affairs within the yet-to-be-defined model of ACM in contrast to conventional medicine.

Conventional Medicine's "Diary of Health Care"

In the past, conventional-medicine insurance claims forms, including the Uniform Billing 1982 and 1992 (UB 82 and 92) and the HCFA 1500 (Medicare form), were viewed merely as vehicles for approval or denial of payment by claims processors and financial wizards. It was not until the early 1990s that clinicians began to see the claim for what it really is, a "diary of health care." Despite imperfections, insurance claims do provide a means of benchmarking physicians/patient populations—total care, inpatient, office, clinic, by provider, by patient. Simply stated, it is possible to determine on a population basis, the output of care. For the employer, the output of care is the impact of a paid benefit. For example, by using the physician and/or hospital claim, it is possible to track, by provider and by treatment type, the number of diabetic patients who develop complications and the practice guidelines that were used or the correlation (if any) between the frequency of obstetrical ultrasounds and the health status of the baby at delivery. This unknown and under-appreciated offspring of the insurance industry's product, managed care, is readily available because payment for office-based services requires submittal of a claim form, complete with diagnosis and procedure code. Prior to managed care, most physicians were paid directly by the patient for care rendered in the office, and tracking output of care with ease, simplicity, and standard data fields was not possible.

Currently, providers of ACM follow the pre–managed care modus operandi—most ACM providers have never submitted a claim form. In fact, since there is no claim form, there are no nationally agreed upon data fields requiring completion prior to payment—unlike the situation with ACM's conventional medicine brethren. To complicate matters, at present, there is no consensus on what even constitutes ACM. There is not even agreement on the name, and thus the term ACM.

Boundaries, Borders, and Bias for ACM

Does ACM include everything outside the realm of Western medicine, or is it just the nouveau services such as acupuncture (needles inserted at specific points to regulate the flow of energy, or chi), applied kinesiology (muscle testing to gain information about a patient's overall state of health), ayurvedic healing (5000-year-old medicine, first practiced in India, that detects overall body imbalance), naturopathic medicine (total well-being emphasizing the body's ability to heal), or spiritual/shamanic healing (healing energy from spiritual "helpers")? For purposes of discussion, there is general agreement that ACM represents interventions not widely taught or accepted at U.S. medical schools (Eisenberg et al, 1993).

Notice that the procedures included in the ACM list date back in origin over 7000 years. In contrast, Western medicine is only 200 years old yet considered conventional. If you do not appreciate the importance of scientifically based outcome studies, consider this fact: politics and payment aside, treatments are referred to as "ACM" despite the fact that components are centuries old, because anecdotal stories about cures and other successes are not scientific enough to negate the attacks of the American Medical Association and other professional groups.

So given the lack of a suitable, inexpensive, noninvasive way to track the output of a large and ill-defined form of medical care, where does one begin? Once again, enter the insurance carrier. Insurers are recognizing that patients, in addition to wanting to become more involved with their health care, are tired of the usual and customary approach of Western medicine—namely, treat the symptoms. Eisenberg et al (1993) documented that over 425 million visits were made to providers of ACM in 1990. This translated into over $12 billion spent out of pocket for services considered to be unorthodox or ACM.

Dynamics, Demographics, and Drivers in the Market: The Baby Boomers

Historically, baby boomers have shown unprecedented interest in diet and lifestyle initiatives that promote "health." As the baby boomers age, personal care needs take on additional importance. Today, the 50-plus group comprises 35% of the population, controls 43% of the nation's disposable income, and owns 77% of the financial assets in America. Insurers eager to maintain or grow market share have identified this significant demographic target and now recognize alternative health as a potential means of addressing a boomer health care option. Providers have taken notice of this movement as well. While practitioners of alternative medicine are not clamoring to embrace the controlled, managed care model, they are eager to be a part of the "legitimized" panels because of their preferred provider status. In a study published in 1993, it was estimated that 44% of Americans had utilized an alternative health service in the prior year (Eisenberg et al, 1993). Insurers are now beginning to offer rider coverage of benefits that were once scorned by the medical establishment, because patients are demanding it. One can only wonder what the reported percentage of usage will be by the year 2000.

Directions and Decisions for ACM

Most providers agree that good, quality research in ACM must be conducted. Furthermore, if they participate, they will ultimately become consumers of the results, reaping numerous benefits. This is the critical stage that demands employer involvement. In addition, it is the clinicians who must help employers sort though the subjectivity of health care decision making in order to ascertain the correlation between productivity and benefits. In turn, the benefits offered by ACM providers will be clearly demonstrated and more easily understood.

Employers must give feedback on the format, usefulness, and depth of information analyzed and published. In the 1980s, employers were not involved in benefit decisions because of a total lack of understanding of the health care system. Hospital admissions and cost per thousand became the standard reports and, for that matter, the only reports given to employer groups. Reporting capabilities today reflect a transformation, as it is now possible to track outpatient care performed in the office, and thus track admissions *prevented* per thousand, by provider, by diagnosis. Employers today could and should have the tools to track absenteeism by diagnosis, by provider, by benefit.

So where does one begin with ACM? Given this new breed of provider and coverage, in concert with a lack of historical claims data, obtaining universally accepted data field tracking capability provides the appropriate and effective means to initiate output studies. The purpose will be to perform population-based output studies using data obtained from all payers of ACM. Presently, there are about 25 payers of ACM across the United States. Each payer is trying to get provider agreement on the type of claim form and the degree of coding that will be required prior to payment. The banking industry probably encountered similar problems when ATM machines were introduced. Can you imagine what confusion would exist if every bank had its own ATM machine for transactions? Where to go for your health information would be as confusing as where to go for your cash. The same holds true for data storage and retrieval regarding population-based studies. The larger the 'n,' the more robust the output—and the more believable the results, whatever they are. Thus the need for standardized data tracking and gathering.

Next, since ACM is patient driven, checks and balances need to be in place to prevent patients with poor treatment results from progressing to more serious and unrecognized medical problems. Credentialing the providers will give insurers and payers some degree of comfort that patients will be appropriately referred if indicated. For now, a substitute must be put into place. Numerous studies indicate that patient functionality is a good substitute for outcomes, and its evidence-based approach prevents the need for randomized controlled studies. The SF-36, developed under the leadership of Dr. John Ware, is unquestionably the most tested and reported instrument (Ware, 1994). Its validity has been demonstrated across age, disease, and treatment groups. The disadvantage is that it focuses on health concepts and does not include condition-specific assessments such as co-morbidity or acuity. The latter is important, given the frequency of multiple diagnoses within a given patient. Clinical complexity index (CCI) software systems are available and should be used to prevent cross-comparisons of patients with varying acuity levels and multiple diagnoses. The CCI uses a regression model to measure the complexity of a provider's patient population. Costs, complications, and return-to-work status are adjusted on the basis of severity and provider specialty (Boyer, 1997).

Measuring the "Intangible" With "Tangible" Tools

Many in the ACM field believe that the usual methods of study are inappropriate. Larry Dossey, MD, director of the Santa Fe–based Center for Alternative Therapies and executive editor of *Alternative Therapies*, stated "while the double-blind method of evaluation may be applicable to certain alternative therapies, it is inappropriate for perhaps the majority of them. Many alternative interventions are unlike drugs and surgical procedures. Their actions are affected by factors that cannot be specified, quantified, and controlled in double-blind designs. Everything that counts cannot be counted. To subject alternative therapies to sterile, impersonal double-blind conditions strips them of intrinsic qualities that are part of their power. New forms of evaluation will have to be developed" (Weber, 1996).

And why? Until science is able to demonstrate the power of subtle energy associated with the provider, with prayer, with thoughts that transform into matter, the impact of ACM cannot be measured in the conventional way. Physics and chemistry play too big a role and must be included in the research equation. So, here we are—about to bridge the most widespread change in Western medicine and facing the same output of care measurement dilemmas that faced the great masters of yesteryear. But if benefit coverage and medical academia acceptance require scientific proof, what is the next step in becoming a legitimate part of traditional medicine?

The Enigma: ACM Meets Science

The NIH Office of Alternative Medicine has awarded grants to 10 specialty research centers that focus on pain, stroke, cancer, general health addictions, HIV/AIDS, asthma, allergy, aging, and immunology. A recent article in the *New York Times* cited some of this research, completed by an independent panel of experts, that concluded in a consensus report that acupuncture was an "appropriate alternative or complementary treatment for some common health problems including nausea associated with pregnancy and chronic problems like low back pain and asthma, for which standard medical treatments are inadequate or costly or may entail serious side effects" (Brody, 1997). No sooner had the report been issued than the critics, including a member of the National Council Against Health Fraud, disputed the results, citing poor research design (Brody, 1997). So, if Dossey et al are correct and alternative medicine cannot be studied by using the usual and customary means of research, then what is the most suitable approach?

Deciphering Output With "Alternative" Answers

The answer lies with the employer group tracking productivity. To create, support, and manage care, providers and administrators must have access to a range of comprehensive patient-level information. Imperfect as the inputs may be, the proof lies in the outcomes—do patients receiving ACM return to work quicker and/or, by their perception, healthier? Until there is a universally agreed upon claims data set, the SF-36 and a patient satisfaction survey tool will be used. The following steps represent the avenues that are being pursued with a major payer.

PURPOSE

1. To begin documenting and measuring self-reported changes in member health status during and after alternative health services initiative
2. To begin assessing the cost and benefits of this initiative to payer and employer clients
3. To begin to collect data with a universally agreed upon format for the purpose of comparing the payer/member outcomes with the common medical database

OBJECTIVES

To compare patients receiving alternative and complementary health medicine ("ACM") and/or those receiving conventional medicine ("CM") by the following parameters:
   1. Work absenteeism
   2. Total costs
   3. Patient-reported functionality
A touch screen (similar to that of the ATM used in the banking industry) in the provider office will be used by the patient to electronically record and sub-

mit the information. Since ACM is consumer driven, it is expected that the combination of ease of use and willingness to participate in research will encourage an 85% compliance rate.

HEALTH CONDITIONS AND TREATMENT MODALITIES

The study will focus on three to five conditions for which payer members are most likely to seek ACM. The project team will examine chiropractic, acupuncture, and naturopathic services and other modalities, on the basis of available information. The payer will separate, to the extent possible, comorbid and unintended contingencies such as unplanned complications. The project team will complete the research design and data collection and analysis, and a presentation to the payer group is expected in early 2000.

Conclusion: The Awakening

It seems ironic that at the close of this century, the connection between mind, body, and health has survived in a quiet continuum to return with blatant enthusiasm. Putting aside the fact that ACM deserves recognition, the success or failure of such treatments requires a stronger understanding, given that ACM services are becoming a part of mainstream benefit coverage. ACM has brought to light an awareness of the ever-increasing complexity of human health and the mind/body/spirit connection. This interdependent-relationship mentality will revolutionize the Western approach of treating the body as "parts." Alternative therapies deemed appropriate will be legitimately incorporated into conventional medical practice. And as this movement toward patient-centered health continues to gain speed, ACM may become the discipline that helped employers determine just what it is that they have "purchased" in this product line called health care benefits.

References

Adams, Harkness, Hill, Inc: Healthy returns: how healthier lifestyles create investment opportunities, *New Hope Natural Media Research* 21:56-72, September 23, 1996.

Adams, Harkness, Hill, Inc: Supplement your portfolio: investing in the self care revolution, *New Hope Natural Media Research* 29:9-15, March 3, 1997.

Boyer N: The art of becoming an informed health care purchaser, *Managing Employee Benefits* 5:65-69, 1997.

Brody J: U.S. Panel on acupuncture calls for wider acceptance, *The New York Times*, A-4, November 6, 1997.

Eisenberg DM, Kessler RC, Foster C, Norlock FE, Calkins D, Delbanco T: Unconventional medicine in the United States. Prevalence, costs, and pattern of use, *New England Journal of Medicine* 328:246-252, 1993.

Ware JE: Data collection methods: tech notes, *Medical Outcomes Trust Bulletin* 2:3, 1994.

Weber DO: The mainstreaming of alternative medicine, *Healthcare Forum Journal* 39(6):16-27, 1996.

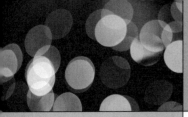

PART FOUR

New Relationships
The Power of Partnering

Primary health care concepts of access to care and programs driven from within communities with community participation are essential to any successful intervention.

KAREN A. IVANTIC-DOUCETTE AND SR. GENOVEFA MAASHAO

PARTNERSHIP HAS BEEN DESCRIBED as the key to a well-developed, coordinated system of health care, but who should the partners be? This section contains a number of viewpoints that help answer that question. One very clear expectation that is espoused is that consumers must be one of the partners in any system. Many other partnering concepts are also emerging. Individuals are partners, such as providers and consumers. Organizations are partners, such as industries and provider systems. Groups are partners, such as communities and government. Many of the authors in Part Four describe the forging of these relationships in new and different ways. The impact and global commonality of new relationships on individuals and groups, as well as the effect of subsequent outcomes, are also articulated. ▲

CHAPTER 31

Huduma Kwa Wagonjwa

An African Perspective on Case Management

KAREN A. IVANTIC-DOUCETTE, MSN, FNP, ACRN

Sr. GENOVEFA MAASHAO PHN, Nurse Midwife

OVERVIEW

Attention to relationship, spirituality, and culture is imperative to effective case management strategies and outcomes. Informal case managers arising from within communities and outside more formal structures of health ministries of a country can be utilized to provide greater access and effect.

Developing countries are seldom thought of as innovators of case management. Yet important lessons have emerged from case management models grounded in primary health care philosophy. Stories of case management outcomes in East Africa, hardest hit by the HIV pandemic, are used to capture and portray essential lessons that can further the global case management strategy and outcomes discussion. ▲

Developing countries are seldom thought of as innovators of case management, nor are they considered essential contributors to discussions of case management models and outcomes. Yet case management services are laced throughout developing countries, utilizing a variety of models and disciplines. Many of these models, grounded in the philosophy and goals of primary health care (World Health Organization [WHO], 1978), have demonstrated enhanced individual and community health outcomes contributing valuable lessons that lend to global case management discussions.

Innovative case management models have emerged in countries of East Africa that provide care to populations that have overwhelmed limited governmental health structures. East Africa is a place of immense beauty, a paradox of rich and diverse culture and extreme poverty. It provides a portrait of case management experiences of developing countries. The lessons portrayed are panoramic.

Snapshots from East Africa: An Historical Portrait

East Africa, traditionally thought of as the countries of Kenya, Tanzania, Uganda, Malawi, and Zanzibar, along the Indian Ocean, is home to generations of tribal peoples, each with unique customs and culture. Liberated from British Colonialism in the mid–twentieth century, newly created nations of East Africa, with artificial borders and blending of peoples, were left isolated to develop independent economies and implement an array of social and health programs (Basch, 1990; Falola, Ityavyar, 1992). Decades later these East African nations remain burdened with poor economies, immature governmental structures, and inadequate resource allocation to meet the increasing health burden of their many peoples.

Research indicates a direct relationship between socioeconomic and health indicators (Basch, 1990; Baum, Sanders, 1995; Graig, 1993), captured in the adage "Wealth means health and health means wealth." East African health indicators fall drastically lower than those of more developed countries, yielding a mortality rate of 16% annually compared with a rate of 1.9% in the developed world. East Africa's per capita income approximates US $170 an-

nually, with health-related expenditures averaging US $1.70 per person per year. More developed countries average US $244 annually for health-related expenditures per person (Monekosso, 1989).

At the same time that East African nations struggled toward independent national and economic development, an international paradigm shift was emerging. The international community began shifting its focus away from a world of independent economies and nations toward one of interdependent nations. All nations of the world, developed and developing, came to be viewed as partners in a new global community with the power to raise the socioeconomic and health indicators of *all* peoples.

Nations were encouraged to focus energy and resources toward the "attainment by all citizens of the world by the year 2000 of a level of health that will permit them to lead a socially and economically productive life," more formally known as Health For All by the Year 2000 (HFA 2000) (Basch, 1990). The mechanism conceptualized to achieve the goals of HFA 2000 was known as *primary health care*, consisting of essential health care delivered within communities. Primary health care encouraged culturally sensitive health care and held as a mandate the attainment of a certain level of health as a human right (WHO, 1978).

In the decade of the seventies the language of case management began to appear in social service and public health literature in the United States. Designed to provide coordination, referral, support, and direct care, these new case management programs focused on communities and addressed the needs of aggregates. Concurrently, primary health care programs, utilizing parallel structures but slightly different language, were emerging internationally (Holzemer, 1992; International Council of Nurses, 1988). Both case management and primary health care models of health care delivery promised to improve health indicators for greater numbers of people.

Looming in the shadows of global optimism and program development, destined to dramatically alter health outcomes for East Africa and the entire global community, was and remains the pandemic of HIV and AIDS. Combined with a growing disparity among richer and poorer nations, the HIV pandemic has begun to unravel the socioeconomic and health progress of nations least able to meet this new threat (International Council of Nurses, 1995; Tarantola, Mann, 1996; WHO, 1994).

A crisis of spiraling downward health indicators has forged new collaborative and comprehensive approaches to health care delivery in the developing countries of East Africa (Holzemer, 1992; Malama, 1994). Lessons are emerging from these models that may shed light on case management discussions across the globe.

Pictures and Lessons from East Africa

In Africa, it is in the telling of stories that knowledge and wisdom can be passed on. Community, relationships, and responsibilities to members of the community are valued and conveyed in the spirituality and rules of the ancestors. The community good outweighs the good of the individual. In Africa, weaving signifies a life-giving process reflecting the patterns of connectedness.

Today, 14 million African lives are becoming unwoven in the shadow of HIV and AIDS (Tarantola, Mann, 1996). Even more die of endemic illnesses. It is in the African storytelling tradition, with the weaving of patterns, that the East African case management lessons will be portrayed.

LESSONS OF RELATIONSHIP, SPIRITUALITY, CULTURE, AND INFORMAL CASE MANAGERS

In Africa, the language of case management is not easily identified. In Swahili the closest term to represent the role identity would be *huduma kwa wagonjwa*, roughly translated to mean "care of the infirmed." Case management is conceptualized as a partnership or relationship between a client or patient and a case manager (Sowell, Young, 1997), and that relationship is the vital element to effective case management services (Issel, 1997).

In Africa, relationship is the primary motivator of life and behavior. Culture identifies relationship lines and accompanying responsibilities. Maintaining honor and trust in relationships and performing one's responsibilities seriously are important to the community and show reverence to the higher power (Makinde, 1988; Khapoya, 1994). Being responsible for another is considered a great honor and should be approached with a sense of duty and

commitment. Conceptually, case management is a natural fit into African culture, more so than in cultures built upon individualism and personal responsibility. Relationship is not viewed as a job or a temporary affiliation to achieve a purpose, but holds deeper promise and effect.

In addition to the value of relationship, most Africans possess a deep core of spirituality, with a belief in a higher power and in the rules of the ancestors. Reverence for the ancestors and a higher power form a foundation of community life, spelling out guidelines for living and behavior. Symbols and rituals form an important aspect of traditional religious beliefs, while purifying medicines and sacrifices assist in removing the evilness of disease.

Huduma kwa wagonjwa is traditionally the responsibility of the family or one assigned family member, who is ready to risk life to take care of the ill person. In the wake of shattered families from HIV disease and death, responsibility lines have been shaken (Malama, 1994; Tuju, 1996). Caregivers are fewer in number, and the fear of evil spirits has prevented others from assuming their roles, setting up conflicts between traditional values and bonds of responsibility.

In the midst of the AIDS epidemic, those who provide *huduma kwa wagonjwa* are increasingly coming from untraditional places within the community. Yet, whether born of or inculturated within a given community, these new-style or informal case managers are able to bridge necessary relationship responsibilities. *Huduma kwa wagonjwa* roles are being filled by traditional healers, herbalists, witch doctors, traditional birth attendants (TBAs), religious orders, and non-blood-related friends who assume responsibility for the ill but are not assigned that responsibility by culture (Box 31-1).

Public health nurses or social welfare workers, funded by Ministries of Health, have had responsibilities for the needs of communities and have often filled the gaps in *huduma kwa wagonjwa*. But a lessening of health care allocation in most developing countries is leading to a further reduction in the availability of these health care workers.

As these informal case managers assume responsibilities once outside their domain, health indicators of mortality and morbidity, access to health in rural areas, and changes in behavior have tipped toward the positive. Although considered alternative deliverers of health care by western standards,

BOX 31-1
Case Study   The Brother's Wife
*A Picture from Tanzania**

In Africa, AIDS is believed to be a curse placed on those who have acted against or broken the ancient rules of the ancestors. It is associated with the evil spirits and not of a natural source.

A woman was married into a family where the brother of her husband came home to the village from the city with AIDS and was very sick. The whole family rejected him and wanted him to return to where he had come from, thereby taking the evil spirits with him; but he was too sick to go.

He had been working in the city when he was weakened by malaria some seven years before. The malaria left him severely anemic, and a friend donated blood to him. Several years later, the friend died of AIDS. The husband's brother tried to explain to his family that he had gotten sick through a blood transfusion, and that he had not broken the rules of the ancestors by acting unethically or immorally. Yet the family could not understand or believe him, so he stayed in a small, run-down hut somewhere nearby.

The wife of the man's brother traveled from Tanzania to Kenya to ask for my help. She was afraid, yet wanted to help this suffering man. There was no health dispensary or medicines to treat HIV or AIDS in her village, and very little information was available to her. She was advised to take care of him and instructed about HIV and AIDS. She was still afraid but she was willing.

The woman returned to her husband's village and began to support and care for the brother. She brought him food and water and cared for him when he became ill with diarrhea and when he could not reach the pit latrine. She talked to him and prayed with him. She made every effort to make him comfortable. Now the family became frightened of her as well and were afraid for her. The family did not understand her because they saw this illness as a punishment.

Toward the end of her brother-in-law's illness the woman stayed with him. He was very happy and comforted because she took care of him. He said, "At least one person can understand me! Thank you!" He died in her arms.

She prepared him for his death and burial. During the burial, she stood alone near the wood coffin. The family stayed a distance away. They did not want to attend the burial, because they were still afraid, but custom and the rule of the ancestors dictated that they must be there. After all, if they broke the rule of the ancestors, perhaps they would receive the same punishment.

After the burial, the villagers remained distant from the woman, expecting her to become ill. Even her husband was afraid and would not touch her. Yet her good health and determination remained steady. She eventually traveled to the city to have an HIV test done and was told she did not have HIV. Reassured and eager, she began to care for others in the village with HIV. Slowly the other villagers began to follow her example.

As told by Sr. Genovefa Maashao

---

informal case managers are beginning to receive international recognition and welcoming as collaborators in primary health care and case management (International Conference on AIDS and STD in Africa, 1995; Ulin, Segall, 1980).

Effectiveness in this newer role venture has been enhanced by dual considerations. First, informal case managers all arise from within a community, are part of the community, a necessary part of empowerment strategies and primary health care philosophy (Farley, 1993; International Council of Nurses, 1988). Second, they are trusted for their link to spirituality, which is vitally important to the whole person (Box 31-2).

Attention to relationship, spirituality, and culture are imperative to effective case management strategies and outcomes. Informal case managers arising from within communities and outside more formal structures of health ministries of a country can be utilized to provide greater access and effect.

BOX 31-2
Case Study   The Abandoned Woman
*A Picture from Kenya**

There was a young woman whose only shelter was on the street verandahs in Mombasa, Kenya. She had lived under these street shelters for many years, and I saw her occasionally whenever I came to the town for supplies. In Kenya there are no homes or places for people to live if they have no family. Family and community are responsible to care for the ill and abandoned.

This young woman had moved to her husband's village with his family and their three children. The husband became ill with "Slim's disease." This is how Africans refer to AIDS, because the person becomes slim like a skeleton.

When the man died, the husband's family was afraid and blamed the woman for bringing punishment upon their son. They tied her, beat her, and forced her to leave the village.

She was ashamed and ill. She could not return to her home village because it was too far away. She missed her children, who were now the property of her husband's family as tradition dictates. So she lived in the street verandahs.

One day I saw her as I was traveling with another Sister of my religious order. The woman was very ill; her whole body was full of foul-smelling wounds, and she was weak and pale. She asked us for help. We had come to town to purchase medi-

cines and equipment for our maternity ward located deeper into the bush, and we agreed to take her with us, because she would die where we found her if we left her. We took her even though we had no place for her, only beds for mothers waiting to deliver.

We made a small place for her in the corner. We cleaned and anointed her body with healing ointments. We gave her food and clean clothes. She was given love and attention, which she had not received in a very long time. Depressed and disoriented from illness, she responded by her bright smile and lively spirit, which told us she appreciated the assistance we offered.

Eventually, the woman's situation improved. She did not want to go back to the street, but she could not stay at the maternity ward. A new shelter was required. We visited the village elder, the community's chief, to inform him of this stranger's plight and ask for guidance. The woman was considered a stranger to the village, with no blood relations claiming her, so the village was not bound by customs of responsibility.

The woman stayed with us until the chief succeeded in finding her family, some 500 kilometers away. In the end, her family received her and assumed responsibility for her.

As told by Sr. Genovefa Maashao

LESSONS ON COMMUNITY AND EMPOWERMENT

"Clinical" case management is described in the literature as managing episodes of illness. Examples include primary care nursing models utilized within hospital settings, where case managers or primary care nurses are assigned to oversee the care and teaching provided to individual patients throughout the course of hospitalization. "Comprehensive" case management differs in scope, linking the social service, medical, and nursing realms together to provide ongoing care and oversight, most often in the community setting (Etheredge, 1989; Issel, 1997).

In East Africa the ratio of physicians to clients is approximately one to thirty thousand and nurses to clients, one to twenty thousand. A greater imbalance ensues as one travels rurally. Nurses and nurse midwives provide the bulk of clinically oriented case management, working in bush field stations, dispensary units, and mobile clinics. Public health nurses, grounded in primary health care practice and the wholistic practice of caring, have demonstrated that they can be gifted comprehensive case managers (Box 31-3).

HIV and AIDS have forced an increase in the need for comprehensive case management services

BOX 31-3
Case Study   The Silent Bleeder
A Picture from Kenya*

There was a woman who came to the maternity clinic in the bush. In the bush there is no communication or ability to transport to a hospital if a problem arises. This woman was in her fifth pregnancy and arrived on the day of her labor pains. She did not bring her maternity record outlining the places she had received prenatal care or how her previous births had progressed. She told us she had forgotten the record card. Her home was twenty-seven kilometers away, so we could not send her to retrieve the record card. She told us her history, which we assumed to be true, and after general examination it was certain she would have her baby within the hour.

It was a normal delivery, and the baby was in good condition. But just after the placenta was delivered, the woman started bleeding without stopping. Like a tap when opened, the blood just ran out of her body. She was given injections to stop the bleeding, but without effect. There was no sign of the contraction of the uterus. The vagina was packed to help stop the bleeding. We were able to locate a vein and gave her some intravenous glucose in water while we waited for the bleeding to stop.

I asked her if this bleeding had happened before. She said yes and that is why she did not bring her health card with her. It said she should only be delivered at a hospital. She said she was afraid to go back to the hospital, where she was sure to get AIDS from the blood transfusions. She believed she was already infected after four previous blood transfusions. She also could not afford to go to the hospital. Her family had no money, and if she bled, they would have to pay large sums of money for treatment. If she died there, her family would also have to pay money to have her body released for burial. She had no choice other than to avoid a hospital, so she came to the bush clinic and the Sisters, where she believed she would be safe.

She had bled so much that she was shivering. Her blood pressure was very low, and she was hanging between life and death. She received another injection to stop the bleeding but without success. Throughout this ordeal, she still trusted the Sisters to save her. She told the Sisters to pray for her so that the bleeding would stop. She was so weak, but there was no vehicle available to take her to the hospital some 45 kilometers away.

We gave her sips of hot tea and comforted her. We prayed with her, and told her to prepare herself for death. We tried many techniques to get the bleeding to stop, but it was a hopeless situation. I left the room to pray; I did not want to see her die. When I returned, I felt sure that she had gone, but to my surprise I found her alive. The bleeding had stopped, eight hours after it had begun.

This new mother stayed with us for one week after the birth while she recovered from her experience. I spent time with her, teaching her about HIV and how to protect herself. I encouraged her to go to the town to seek out testing and find out her HIV status, because she was still so frightened. She, like many others in the village, was afraid to know her status because of the misunderstandings about the illness and the abandonment that follows. I told her that her fear had put her at great risk of dying and had led her to make a decision to deliver her baby far from where she could get help for the bleeding.

After one year, the woman visited the maternity clinic with the baby we had helped deliver. The baby was well and growing. The mother had not gone for HIV testing and was once again pregnant. I am afraid that this time she will die.

As told by Sr. Genovefa Maashao

in developing countries, similar to the experiences in developed countries such as the United States. Descriptors of the role include intervention and evaluation, negotiation and advocacy for the development of needed services, navigation of service access, education and consultation, and psychosocial support (Wisconsin AIDS/HIV Program, 1993).

Nurse case managers arising from within communities and implementing important principles of primary health care, such as demonstrated by Grace in Akiiki's story, perform comprehensive case management services that can lead to an improved quality of death unachievable before intervention (Box 31-4). Additionally, advocating for ac-

ceptance and support for the mother and orphan by the village, through education and modeling, assisted in reshaping the community responsibilities for its members in the spirit of the ancestors (Tuju, 1996; Walker, Frank, 1995).

BOX 31-4
Case Study   Akiiki
A Story from Western Uganda

Fourteen-year-old Akiiki was quiet, her legs and abdomen swollen. She lay on a rough bamboo pad on the dung floor of her mother's mud and thatched hut and was covered by a worn, soiled sheet. Her 4-month-old baby sat quietly and attentively on the grandmother's lap, watching the goats and chickens filter in and out of the dwelling.

Yesterday, Akiiki had lain outside the hut on a bed of banana-leaf fibers waiting for death and for the evil spirits to consume her. A relative of hers had cautiously asked Brother William, a Catholic religious brother who was working on a nearby farm, to pray for this woman and remove the curse afflicting her.

Brother William had seen this plight before, during his training as a brother, when he did pastoral outreach for a mobile home care team in Kampala, the capital city of Uganda. Unfortunately he was six hours away by land rover through the bush from Kampala, too far to help this young woman. HIV disease, which was overpowering the urban areas of developing countries, was now making its way through rural areas. Although there is no testing or treatment available rurally, and it is scarce in the urban areas; Brother William recognized Slim's disease, whether it was urban or rural.

Brother William also knew of the beliefs and fears in the rural villages and of the overwhelming conflict between fear of the evil spirits and curses and the fear of displeasing the ancestors by not assuming care taking responsibilities. He traveled back to the rural town, some 20 kilometers away, and enlisted the aid of the Kabarole Home Based Care Program, a hospice program sponsored by the Ministry of Health with support of the WHO. This program was designed to deal with this type of problem.

Brother William brought to Akiiki's mother's hut a blanket, a few medicines, and Grace, a home care nurse, who would begin visiting, teaching, and helping Akiiki and the village deal with what would come next.

In the two months that followed, leading to Akiiki's death, Grace, the nurse case manager, helped the mother bring Akiiki into the hut, taught her about this illness, and attempted to assure her that the illness was not sent by the evil spirits. Grace is of the same tribe as Akiiki and her mother, although not from the same clan. In time, the mother came to believe what Grace was telling her.

Grace visited the village elder to solicit support for Akiiki, the mother, and the soon-to-be orphaned 4 month old, who were unable to support or care for themselves. Akiiki was supposed to be her mother's caregiver as her mother aged, but the role was now reversed, providing no current or future support or caregiving opportunities.

Grace's visits and her presence began to comfort and encourage trust within the village community, providing the seeds of education and understanding. Akiiki died two months later, in her mother's hut with minimal pain and with spiritual comfort. She received a proper burial, pleasing to the ancestors.

When the baby died, Grace was there again with the grandmother and the village. She ensured that the newly abandoned grandmother, who was already a widow, would be looked after by the village and the elders and would not be abandoned again from fear of association. Gradually the fear of the villagers lessened, and they began to share their meager earnings for support. The village elder took over the responsibility of oversight for the aged widow.

As experienced by Karen Ivantic-Doucette

In the developed world, patient records and control of health care information are often kept within health care systems or providers. The use of patient-controlled hand held records, such as the prenatal card referred to in Box 31-3, demonstrates a potentially effective case management tool.

This tool of empowerment, providing patient control over health information, is a strategy that warrants further discussion in developed countries as populations become more fluid in their health care. The development of hand held records for on-going treatment and education needs of persons with HIV and AIDS may provide assistance to case managers in coordinating the various team members often involved in HIV care, as well as empower the person with HIV to control his or her health care decisions.

LESSONS ON ACCESS AND PROGRAM DEVELOPMENT

Within certain geographic areas or within certain populations of people in many developed coun-

---

BOX 31-5
Case Study Pellagia
A Story from Western Uganda

Pellagia discovered she was HIV positive in her last term of nursing school when her husband died of AIDS, leaving her with four children and no means of support. Pellagia was more fortunate than many others and went on to finish nursing school in hopes of earning 30 shillings (equivalent to US $30) per month to support her children. In the end, however, no one would hire Pellagia, because they were afraid.

Sr. Ferdriana, a local Catholic Religious Sister, knew of Pellagia's plight and offered her an opportunity to work together to set up an AIDS clinic at the Catholic hospital. Sr. Ferdriana, a nurse midwife, had finished a counseling course on AIDS that was offered at the AIDS Service Organization in Kampala (similar to HIV case management education offered in the United States) and was quickly overwhelmed by the thousands of people walking from the bush and coming from the town, seeking her assistance for Slim's disease.

"Slowly by slowly," as the African saying goes, Sr. Ferdriana and Pellagia set up an AIDS program. They followed over 5000 people with HIV/AIDS in the first three years of existence of their clinic, with only donations provided by the people themselves and a bit from the European Community. The program opened a testing and counseling center, in addition to a treatment room. They also secured donated medicines and food rations. Monthly food staples of rice, oil, and beans were distributed to those unable to maintain their fields. They organized a community vegetable garden; the stronger ones helped grow food for the weaker. They organized the AIDS Fighters Association, a client support group where people could come to celebrate life while finding support. They visited the sick in the hospital and at home, wherever someone needed to be seen—especially new patients, who were often abandoned and in need of the help.

One clinic day, Ateni, a woman about 30 years old who consistently came to clinic, did not arrive. She had been staying 3 kilometers down the road in a little room that cost 1 shilling (equivalent to US $1) per month to rent. Pellagia and Sister Ferdriana, fearing that she was ill, walked to her home and found her with fever. She had no food to eat or water to drink. They bathed her, fed her, and stayed with her until she recovered.

Ateni, whose husband had died four years earlier, had a son. This son had a mental impairment and could not attend or care for her. Her own family was dead, as well; they had been lost in the war.

Over time, a community of women caring for women emerged through the efforts of Pellagia, Sister Ferdriana, and Ateni. A newly formed village community with new relationship bonds emerged. Ateni returned to take the lead in this new endeavor of the AIDS Fighters Association and reached out to others who were too frightened to be identified.

As experienced by Karen Ivantic-Doucette

tries, such as in inner cities within the United States, health access can be limited and socioeconomic and health indicators, depressed (Day, 1993; Tarantola, Mann, 1996). These areas are often referred to as "developing worlds" within the developed world, with complexities and barriers to health similar to those developing countries face.

The demographic trends of HIV and AIDS have left greater numbers of people within communities least able to afford treatment or to cope with this communicable and complex illness. Infection rates are greater in these marginalized communities, whether in developed or developing countries.

State-of-the-art HIV care and medical interventions will not work if attention has not been paid to the more basic primary health care needs of the community. Primary health care concepts of access to care and programs driven from within communities with community participation are essential to any successful intervention.

Case managers forming new programs or supporting existing community-based programs can return power to communities and facilitate access to health care (Box 31-5). Case managers attentive to primary health care directives, with an eye to social justice and equity, are necessary components to reversing the tide of HIV and AIDS and depressed health indicators, whether in developing or developed countries.

Conclusion: Summary of Lessons Learned

Case management models in developing countries, rooted in primary health care philosophy and encouraging community participation, can produce outcomes that are culturally sensitive and effective. The use of informal case managers drawn from within communities, rooted within a given community's culture, can achieve quality health outcomes at a greater rate and with longer-lasting effect. Respecting culture and cultural beliefs of a community, whether in developing countries or within one's own country, is of vital importance.

Finally, relationship is the fundamental essence of effective case management. Case managers who are able to extend relationship bonds across service provision will yield greater outcomes and satisfaction.

References

Basch PF: *Textbook of international health,* New York, 1990, Oxford University Press.

Baum F, Sanders D: Can health promotion and primary health care achieve health for all without a return to their more radical agenda? *Health Promotion International* 10(2):149-160, 1995.

Day L: *At risk in America: The health and health care needs of vulnerable populations in the United States,* San Francisco, 1993, Jossey-Bass.

Etheredge ML: *Collaborative care: nursing case management,* Chicago, 1989, American Hospital.

Falola T., Ityavyar D: *The political economy of health in Africa: monographs in international studies, Africa series, No. 60,* Athens, Ohio, 1992, Ohio University Press.

Farley S: The community as partner in primary health care, *Nursing & Health Care* 14(5):244-249, 1993.

Graig LA: *Health of nations: an international perspective on U.S. health care reform,* ed 2, Washington DC, 1993, Congressional Quarterly.

Holzemer WL: Linking primary health care and self care through case management, *International Nursing Review* 39(3):83-89, 1992.

International Conference on AIDS and STD in Africa: *Final Programme and Abstract Book: 10-14 December 1995, Kampala, Uganda,* Cleveland, 1995, Case Western Reserve University.

International Council of Nurses: *Nursing and primary health care: a unified force,* Geneva, 1988, International Council of Nurses.

International Council of Nurses: *On the continuum of HIV/AIDS care: nursing research and practice initiatives—report of the ICN conference on HIV/AIDS,* Yokohama, Japan, 6 & 7 August, 1994, Geneva, 1995, International Council of Nurses.

Issel LM: Measuring comprehensive case management interventions: development of a tool, *Nursing Case Management* 2(4):132-138, 1997.

Khapoya VB: *The African experience: an introduction,* Englewood Cliffs, NJ, 1994, Prentice Hall.

Makinde MA: *African philosophy, culture, and traditional medicine: monographs in international studies, Africa series, No. 53,* Athens, Ohio, 1988, Ohio University Center for International Studies.

Malama M: Community involvement in AIDS care and prevention in a rural hospital. In Kasonde JM, Martin JD, eds: *Experiences with primary health care in Zambia,* Geneva, 1994, World Health Organization.

Monekosso GL: The challenge: health for all Africans by the year 2000, *World Health,* Aug-Sept, pp 3-6, 1986.

Sowell and Young: Case management in the nursing curriculum, *Nursing Case Management,* 2(4):173-176, 1997.

Tarantola DJ, Mann JM: Global expansion of HIV infection and AIDS, *Hospital Practice,* October 15, 1996, pp 63-79.

Tuju R: *AIDS: understanding the challenge,* Nairobi, Kenya, 1996, English Press.

Ulin P, Segall M, eds: *Traditional health care delivery in contemporary Africa,* Syracuse, New York, 1980, Syracuse University.

Walker MB, Frank L: HIV/AIDS: an imperative for a new paradigm for caring, *Nursing & Health Care: perspectives on Community* 16(6):310-315, 1995.

Wisconsin AIDS/HIV Program: *Practice standards and administrative guidelines for HIV-related case management,* Madison, Wisc, 1993, Wisconsin Department of Health and Social Services.

World Health Organization: *Primary health care: health for all, Series No. 1,* Geneva, 1978, World Health Organization.

World Health Organization: *AIDS: images of the epidemic,* Geneva, 1994, World Health Organization.

CHAPTER 32

Community Intervention and Partnership

MARJORIE K. JAMIESON, RN, MS, FAAN

CHAPTER OVERVIEW

Increasingly, citizens are responding to their disenchantment with the inability of "big government" and other institutions to effectively address community problems by taking local action based on the principles of community association.

This case study, built upon the Living at Home/Block Nurse Program and its U.S. Health Care Financing Administration Community Nursing Organization demonstration, discusses how nurses, clients, families, and communities provide less expensive care for older neighbors that keeps them healthy, independent, and out of both the acute care and the long-term-care systems. ▲

American citizens increasingly recognize that many fundamental individual and public problems are not being effectively addressed by the programs and services provided through public and private service systems (McKnight, 1987). Going hand in hand with this public awareness, sociologists and historians have observed the re-emergence of a very important American tradition that lies at the heart of our democracy—citizens are increasingly organizing and taking action at the community level to tackle a variety of local problems through newly formed community associations (Boyte, 1989).

Widespread agreement exists across the political spectrum that the tradition of citizen action and community building has become submerged in American society. A number of key social and economic developments in the twentieth century have been cited as greatly reinforcing individualism and contributing to the overshadowing of the place of community action and participation in American life. Individuals in our society have become much more integrated into specialized spheres of social participation in a large, complex, industrial society (i.e., the workplace and the family unit) as opposed to identifying with neighborhood and community roots (Bellah et al, 1985). Individualism is greatly reinforced by the central place of competition and individual consumption in our capitalist society. Along with the emergence of the new capitalist industrial order comes an orientation away from local solutions to reliance on state and national government to solve increasingly complex economic and social problems (Boyte, 1989).

Yet the obvious failings of the service system in meeting many needs has begun to spark a revival of citizen action to restore community association. While weakened, the tradition of community action has never been completely lost. Increasingly, citizens are responding to their disenchantment with the inability of "big government" and other institutions to effectively address community problems by taking local action based on the principles of community association.

John L. McKnight, Professor of Urban Planning at Northwestern University, contrasts the effectiveness of programs that work through community association and community building with the frequent failures of the traditional service system that utilizes a production model emphasizing regulation and control. McKnight sees community building as an effort motivated by caring and carried out through the mutual consent of individuals who reflect the diversity of individuals in the community. Rather than being dominated by experts, community associations are constructed on the recognition and acceptance of fallibility, offering a place for everyone to participate. Associations center their activity on creative solutions, inclusiveness, and quick and individualized responses to needs (McKnight, 1987, 1992).

One of the most important issues facing American society is how the rapidly growing number of seniors living in our communities can best be supported to remain healthy and continue to live at home and participate in the life of the community. Family members and neighborhood residents want to enable older people to remain in the community for a number of reasons. Communities also recognize that there is significant economic benefit from enabling seniors to continue to contribute to the tax base and spend money in the community.

Older persons who live at home with chronic conditions need a variety of health and social services that can be integrated with the informal care they receive from family and friends. Tragically, the basic maintenance-custodial supports that can help seniors to meet their goal of living at home as they age are unavailable and/or unaffordable in most communities (Sharp, 1992; Harrington, 1991; Koff, 1988). Large health care institutions are generally not well equipped to work in effective partnerships with the informal resources of a senior's neighborhood.

Premature nursing home placement will become an increasingly critical issue in the coming decades. The percentage of the population that is aged 65 years and older is increasing rapidly; representing 10% of the total populace in 1990, it is projected to move toward 20% by the year 2020. In fact, people aged 85 and over are the fastest-growing segment of the population. If premature nursing home placement is to be avoided, a new strategy needs to be developed. A return to our tradition of citizen action and community building is needed.

Major Weaknesses of the Service System for Seniors

Key principles from the framework of McKnight's critique of service systems highlight the substantial problems in the system of home care services for seniors in America.

THE IMPORTANCE OF BUILDING ON CAPACITIES

McKnight indicates that health and social service systems are built on addressing a "consumer's" deficiencies and inadequacies as opposed to building on his or her capacities. In his view, the medical model carries the negative assumption ". . . that what is important about a person is their injury, their disease, their deficiency." He adds that ". . . the part of a person that is able, gifted, skilled, capable and full is not the focus of the medical model." And yet, because communities are built upon capacities, McKnight (1992) indicates that ". . . community health promotion professionals inevitably find that they must invert the medical model and focus on capacities."

In keeping with McKnight's argument, aging is viewed within the existing system as a disease process. Every intervention requires a diagnosis and a physician's order to address an identified physical acute or chronic illness. The current system of senior home care frequently misses the opportunity to support the capacity of seniors for self-care and provide early intervention in order to prevent health problems in advance of their occurrence, prevent an existing medical condition from worsening, or prevent a new medical problem from developing. The impact on the health of seniors and the economic costs to society are significant (Benson, McDevitt, 1994).

Seniors as a group are at high risk for a wide range of health problems that can be effectively addressed with health education, early identification, and health care (Rakowski, 1992; Institute of Medicine, 1990; Benson, McDevitt, 1989). Despite the importance of prevention and early intervention, the current system provides little incentive for preventive care, paying for only episodic acute medical treatment or for maintenance-custodial care under limited circumstances (Benson, McDevitt, 1994; Estes, Rundall, 1992; Gluck, Wagner, Duffy, 1989). Similarly, the existing system of services fails to recognize or support the important capacity for and

need of seniors to develop and maintain social and emotional relationships. Many seniors who come into contact with home care providers and other health care services have a range of social, emotional, and psychological needs that are frequently unaddressed within the current system (Estes, Rundall, 1992; Jamieson, 1992; Ahroni, 1989). These needs all bear directly on the course of seniors' illnesses, their ability to recover, and their ability to remain healthy. This results from the press of reimbursement incentives toward treating the presenting medical condition and away from addressing the total context of a senior's life circumstances (Benson, McDevitt, 1994).

THE IMPORTANCE OF BUILDING CONSENT AND CARING

McKnight indicates that service systems are typically modeled after corporate structures and are a tool designed to control and to produce standardized practices and outcomes. One result of this model is that the system utilizes professional experts to plan, assess needs, and provide services to be purchased by "consumers" (McKnight, 1992). In this approach, the provision of services by necessity takes precedence over the provision of caring. In addition, this orientation tends to exclude community involvement and input, which are crucial to understanding real-life needs and to accomplishing many goals. In McKnight's view, system planners view community associations and community expressions of need with suspicion at best and too often with contempt (McKnight, 1987). The expert service model of senior home care has yet to see or listen to the perspective of seniors and community members or to involve them in the planning and delivery of services.

The current system does not make available or affordable the custodial-maintenance care—support and assistance with activities of daily living and instrumental activities of daily living—that seniors need to remain in their homes. Activities of daily living (ADLs) include bathing, eating, toileting, and dressing, and Instrumental Activities of daily living (IADLs) include maintaining a checkbook, grocery shopping, and using the telephone. As many as 30% of seniors in nursing homes could live at home if these supports were available (Eustis, Greenberg, 1984).

The current home care system often lacks a mechanism to coordinate the provision of services and involvement of family and community support or to ensure that they are obtained by a senior (Benson, McDevitt, 1994). If a home care professional is concerned about social, emotional, or practical needs, there are often no local available means to identify and mobilize existing community resources (Jamieson, 1992; Kent, Hanley, 1990). Similarly, the current system does not generally provide continuous monitoring of care, so emerging needs go unobserved and are not addressed or met in a timely fashion.

The Living at Home/Block Nurse Program

LOCAL RESPONSE TO THE FAILINGS OF SERVICE SYSTEMS FOR SENIORS

In the early 1980s, community members in two separate neighborhoods in St. Paul, Minnesota, came together to develop local programs out of deep frustration with the system of services in place for seniors. There are now 15 programs, and the state provided seed money in 1997 to start up to 12 more programs.

The Living at Home and the Block Nurse Programs were organized by families, friends, neighbors, and professionals who had observed the unnecessary isolation of seniors in the community and the tragedy of seniors who experience preventable illness and nursing home placements. They observed or personally experienced the immense burden and overload placed on family members as caregivers who take on unrealistic roles in assisting their aging parents to remain in the community. They saw that the prevailing system of services is fragmented and does not provide the key supportive services that seniors need accessible or affordable. These community residents became determined to make a difference and began to undertake the efforts necessary to reshape the fundamental way that care is provided to seniors in their communities.

Community residents developed a program that would mobilize the support of the neighborhood on behalf of seniors. They developed a unique approach: the home care required by seniors to continue living at home and the support to complement the role of family caregivers would be provided by professionals and volunteers who reside in the neighborhood and be directed by a neighborhood board.

The Living at Home/Block Nurse Program (LAH/BNP), a merger of two programs, provides a strategic approach for concerned local citizens to organize a community-based network to establish a noninstitutional, long-term-care system that is unique to each community. The current model's principles and framework are based on the extensive experience of the existing LAH/BNP communities. Each neighborhood or community that initiates an LAH/BNP is charged with the responsibility of developing its own solutions. The community residents work within essential principles and framework, tailoring the approach to meet the local needs of seniors, their families, and the community.

An essential program tenet is that the LAH/BNP belongs to and is operated by the community, not a professional or government agency. The process by which an LAH/BNP is organized and governed brings diverse neighborhood residents together, operating on the principles of consent and equal participation.

The LAH/BNP is based on the principle that the capacity to care is best expressed in local communities where relationships naturally form. The principle of neighbors helping neighbors is central, where consent, caring, and mutual respect are the basis for all relationships. In order to be community based, the plans, programs, and methods are done *by* and *with* people in the community. This is in contrast to a community-oriented program, where things are done *to* and *for* the community.

The focus is on providing the coordinated care that meets the individual needs of each senior to ensure that he or she can continue to live in the community. This typically includes providing early social support, health education, and prevention-oriented nursing care, and support for daily living needs and custodial-maintenance care. Care is provided regardless of entitlements or the ability to pay. Enhancing the ability of a family to meet the needs of its own members and organizing community support when the family is not available are cornerstones of the LAH/BNP. Professor McKnight describes how the service system limits flexibility with regulations and uniformity and requires that creativity needs to go through channels. In contrast, the LAH/BNP places a premium on creative, immediate, and flexible responses. When community or neighborhood residents are seriously invited into the planning process and then challenged to carry out their plans, they become emotionally invested in the process and adopt ownership for the program. To be effective, these community-building discussions are open to consensual decision making and diversity; provide the opportunity for people to collaborate in problem solving; allow for the representation of and respect for a variety of points of view; and provide a regeneration of the community environment.

With input from the community, the organizers carefully discuss and define the following: the needs and capabilities of the community, including its values, attitudes, common bonds, and relationships; the needs and capacities of the elderly as seen by community members; the availability and use of health care and long-term care in the community; the available informal linkages and networks in the community, including senior centers, churches, volunteer groups, and others; community leaders from whom support is essential for organizing the program; communication systems, such as newspaper, radio, and television, that can be used in the community; what civic and social groups might welcome a speaker regarding the needs of seniors; and what organization in the community could be home base for the program.

Participation from local health care and human services agencies and providers is invited. These professionals often have ideas on how to work with the existing systems and adapt the professional services to a community-based framework. The group's members begin to communicate tentative plans to the community by attending community meetings and talking with friends, neighbors, and associates.

The LAH/BNP board utilizes community contacts and, if necessary, community pressure at its command to affiliate with and gain support from a local government entity such as a city district, township board, or small town. This affiliation recognizes that the program belongs to the community and yet provides the visibility, credibility, and political support that the program will need to accomplish its funding and program objectives.

AN EFFECTIVE COMMUNITY APPROACH TO CARING FOR SENIORS IN THEIR HOMES

Each LAH/BNP community's board develops the initial, informal vision into a specific neighborhood plan to provide community-based long-term care in the home for seniors. This plan always includes a unique approach that involves neighborhood volunteers working together as partners with professionals from the neighborhood to meet the long-term-care needs of any senior who needs help to remain at home (including many frail seniors). They capitalize upon the capacities of numerous neighborhood volunteers, community organizations and businesses, and family members who work side by side with professionals from the neighborhood.

The community board determines how early intervention, prevention, maintaining the health of seniors, custodial-maintenance support, and program coordination can best be accomplished. The board enters into a contract with a home health agency or a public health nursing agency and, at times, other social service agencies for the provision of care. The local board oversees the recruitment and training of volunteers and the recruitment of the nurses and home health aides/homemakers in its community, interviewing and recommending them to the agency. This gives the community a major say in decisions about the quality and delivery of care and ensures that the LAH/BNP's community-based context is firmly established.

The LAH/BNP board establishes a crucial mechanism for the coordination and monitoring of care. Communities hire an individual from the community with community-organizing skills to serve as the Community Coordinator, coordinating the extensive community volunteer involvement in the program.

The Community Coordinator and the Block Nurses (nurses who live in the community) coordinate the involvement of community volunteers and family members with the formal care. Through the local LAH/BNP, the Community Coordinator works closely with the nursing staff, family, and volunteers in a team approach to identify each member's needs. Professional staff, and frequently volunteers and family members, come together in weekly team meetings to discuss member needs and develop and revise care plans.

This close communication encourages flexibility and creativity in meeting the emerging needs of seniors. All care is provided in the context of early intervention/prevention and building strong, caring relationships and support for seniors from the community.

In one community, 85% of referrals are by word of mouth. The Community Coordinator and the Block Nurse work to involve the family and add additional community support persons. When there are no family members present, the program seeks to restore existing community ties and to build new ones for an individual. A major focus of the program is to creatively provide help and services to isolated seniors, even when they initially refuse help.

The Block Nurse typically provides each senior with regular health consultations and home-based nursing care as required. During the health consultation, a formal health assessment is carried out, personal health issues are discussed, and plans are developed for health promotion activities (e.g., diet, exercise, self-care, and basic prevention). Group classes are provided in such areas as exercise and maintaining a low blood pressure.

When providing nursing care, the Block Nurse observes and addresses each senior's complete needs. The focus is on nontraditional variables in areas that include diet (can they cook for themselves?), exercise (can they get out of bed?), daily functioning (can they wash their hair?), social relationships (are family and friends involved?), and emotional and psychological health (are they depressed?). The Block Nurse coordinates with other providers in the community, including home repair services, neighborhood pharmacies, physical therapy/rehabilitation services, and/or mental health services.

The Block Nurse monitors the client in and out of the acute care and long-term-care systems; home health aides deliver home health services, homemaking services, and chore services if doing so would be more efficient than bringing three people into the home to provide the three different services required by entitlement requirements; durable medical equipment (walkers, commodes) is collected and cleaned by volunteers and loaned to clients; travel time and mileage are minimal because staff live in the neighborhood; staff arrange for

"nonessential services" that are important to seniors, such as putting drops in a pet's eyes, telephoning the "worried well" with a call every morning, or connecting two lonely people.

The Community Coordinator is familiar with all possible sources of volunteers and supports available for seniors in the community. Groups such as scouts, service clubs, businesses, and churches are involved by the communities in volunteer support roles. A total of 2038 volunteers contributed 31,500 volunteer hours in 14 Minnesota programs in 1996.

The Community Coordinator is responsible for training and supervising volunteers and matching volunteers with seniors in a number of important support roles. All volunteers who are peer visitors and provide phone reassurance receive training in the normal aging process, listening skills, and loss and the grieving process.

Volunteers provide social and emotional support and personal encouragement through peer counseling/friendly visiting, telephone reassurance, and matching friends. This helps seniors overcome social isolation, cope with depression, and carry out health promotion and treatment plans. Community residents involve isolated persons in social and community activities and special celebrations, including involvement with former social contacts and friends—for example, church groups, dancing clubs, schoolmates, and arts and cultural events. Many isolated, reclusive seniors become reinvolved in community life. For example, one formerly reclusive senior woman is now involved in reading to children in the schools.

Each LAH/BNP designs volunteer and community services to meet specific needs: a volunteer will telephone an incontinent client who is on a bladder training program every two hours to remind her to go to the toilet; a local restaurant owner offers to deliver meals to a senior highrise on the days that Meals on Wheels are not available; a pharmacist meets with a group of seniors to discuss the drug interactions of their medications, with follow-up to physicians.

Volunteers and family members are in a key position to observe and report subtle day-to-day changes in the health and social needs of seniors, which is important to facilitating early intervention and effective care. When appropriate, family members support health care through roles that include giving shots, managing oxygen, and assisting with physical therapy. This integration of formal and informal resources within the neighborhood, and coordination with the wider community, provides an attractive and less costly alternative to institutional care.

Three separate external evaluations were done—in 1985, 1990, and 1994. The most notable evaluation, in 1985, documented that 85% of the clients would have been in nursing homes without the program, at four times the cost. The two others were similarly positive. In 1996, 14 of the Minnesota programs kept 315 people out of nursing homes for 2195 months, at an estimated savings of $3,608,928.

FINANCING THE PROGRAM

The funding of professional nursing and home health aide services is from every available source: (1) third-party payers such as Medicare, Medicaid, Veterans Affairs, insurance; (2) private payment on a sliding fee scale based on ability to pay; (3) the community.

The commitment that is generally made with the home care agency with whom the community partners is that, if the home care nursing agency will accept assignment of Medicare and other third-party payments, the community program will reimburse the agency for all costs not reimbursed through formal insurance and entitlement programs. The result is that the nursing agency recovers many of the costs that it otherwise would not have collected.

Because many of the persons served are "near poor," not eligible for Medicaid, and can pay only on a sliding fee basis, every effort is made to keep costs low. Such a financial responsibility provides the incentive for finding creative ways to provide services in the least expensive way!

Each of the 15 LAH/BNPs relies heavily on the resources of its own community to generate flexible funding from a variety of sources. Solicitations of local businesses and residents, proposals to foundations, and local fundraising events and activities at community celebrations are but a few examples. In addition, the integrated ties from the grass roots of the community generally lead to numerous examples of support and financing that are generally not available to other professional providers of care. Some examples are the use of office space in a local church at low or no rental fee, donated use of meeting rooms, and in-kind provision of printing services.

RELATIONSHIP OF THE PROGRAM TO MANAGED CARE

Although the LAH/BNPs have been able to document that people are kept out of nursing homes and to document the concomitant estimated savings because of the programs, Block Nurses have suggested that there are additional savings of thousands of dollars to Medicare and other entitlements or insurance. It is ironic that these entities receive the financial benefit of the program yet the communities have to raise money to pay for services for those who "fall through the cracks" of the system. (The average client of 81 years of age manages on $632 a month!)

In traditional home care agencies, because the agencies are paid on a fee-for-service basis, they encourage the communities to provide as many entitlement services as possible—which brings more revenue to the agencies. However, in the LAH/BNP this incentive is moderated by the need for the community board to raise money to pay for services that are normally unreimbursed, and the need to convince older citizens to pay for some services themselves. However, a more formal structure such as managed care is needed that changes the incentives.

Managed care is here to stay and has become a major approach to cost-effective health care, whether mandated by Congress or driven by the marketplace. Managed care can be defined as any mechanism that controls the provision and utilization of health services. The predominant managed care vehicle is health maintenance organizations (HMOs). Most managed care is through some form of capitation, with financial risk as in an HMO (Kerr, et al. 1997).

In regard to the differences between fee-for-service and HMO Medicare systems, the primary difference is centered in the reimbursement mechanism. It drives both the provision and the utilization of services and has tremendous impact for both providers and enrollees. Because home care and outpatient care are the predominant new service delivery modes for HMOs, the effects of capitation for home care become particularly salient.

A Community Nursing Approach to Managed Care

In 1992, LAH/BNP, Inc., a non-profit organization that advocates for and provides consultation to communities, was selected, along with sites in Arizona, Illinois, and New York, by the U.S. Health Care Financing Administration (HCFA) to be a Community Nursing Organization (CNO) demonstration site. The demonstration is in its fourth year and is expected to continue for a total of six years. The purpose of the CNO is to test whether capitated payment and nurse case management will promote timely and appropriate use of home care and ambulatory care services and reduce the use of acute care services.

The CNO provides Medicare Part A home care (usually after hospitalization) and Part B nonphysician services (outpatient PT, OT, ST, DME, and supplies), all *authorized* and *managed* by registered nurses at 95% of the "average adjusted per capita cost," or AAPCC (the usual reimbursement in fee for service based upon historical data), on a capitated, full-financial-risk basis. In other words, each CNO receives a monthly sum of money for each enrollee, based on a nursing assessment done every six months, whether enrollees need services or not, and must provide appropriate services indicated. Each CNO assumes financial risk and either enjoys the profit or suffers the loss!

In Minnesota, four new communities, two rural and two urban, were chosen; the experimental evaluation design precluded using existing sites because of the need to refuse services to the control group. The CNO has been built on the principles of LAH/BNP and provides services *not* traditionally covered by Medicare; they include:

- Services without which enrollees will use acute care (clinic visits, emergency rooms, hospitals, ambulance, etc.)
- Wellness care (health promotion, disease prevention, early intervention)
- Neighborly expressions of care and friendship (transportation, friendly visiting)
- Coordination of other programs (Meals on Wheels, Title 20 services, Foster Grandparents, RSVP, legal services, Lifeline, etc.—all based on need)

CNO nurses are gaining experience with risk-based financing of services. The Minnesota CNO is documenting "enhancements," which occur when a nurse identifies a cost saving that is achieved when care traditionally covered by Medicare is provided in a more appropriate manner or setting through effective and efficient use of resources. An average saving is estimated for each enhancement to assist in identifying the cost savings through the provision of services in the CNO compared with traditional Medicare costs. For example, in the four Minnesota communities, if an enrollee has a "medical" need, the enrollee usually calls "my nurse," who can often intervene, thus averting a visit to the clinic or emergency room. In 1996, 569 enhancements were recorded, with an estimated savings to Medicare of $129,000.

The Omaha System is used to identify members' problems, nursing interventions, and outcomes. The Problem Classification Scheme of the Omaha System provides a structure for the assessment phase. Four domains identify pertinent data, resulting in an accurate portrayal of the diverse factors that affect members' health status and service delivery. The nurse can use any of four intervention categories to develop a plan of care: Health Teaching, Guidance and Counseling, Treatment and Procedures, Case Management and Surveillance. A list of nursing interventions is used to manage the problems. A Problem Rating Scale for Outcomes measures the members' knowledge of the problem, behavior in managing the problem, and any signs or symptoms. Figure 32-1, a 1996 chart audit of the Minnesota CNO, summarizes members' improvement, maintenance, or regression, dealing with environment, psychosocial factors, physiological factors, and health-related behavior.

An evaluation is being done by Abt and Associates, Inc., an evaluation company with whom HCFA has contracted. Abt is using an experimental design in which enrollees are randomly assigned to a treatment or control group. Although Abt has not issued conclusive reports, the four national sites' preliminary data show:

- Extremely high enrollee satisfaction
- Overall lower costs than projected
- Decreased traditional Medicare home care costs
- More cost-effective mix of services
- Utilization of less expensive equipment
- Decreased use of acute care services
- Shorter duration of traditional Medicare home care

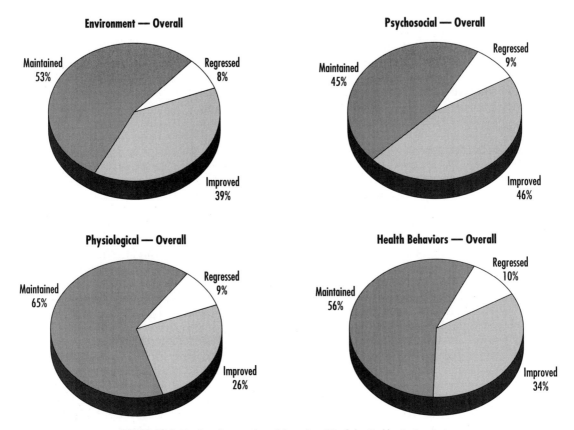

FIGURE 32-1 The four domains (i.e., Cohorts I to IV) of the Healthy Seniors Project.

Abt and Associates, Inc., has commented positively about the comprehensiveness of services provided because of the involvement of volunteers, especially when they fill service gaps not covered by Medicare.

The success of the CNO in Minnesota has been due to the cost-effective management in enrollees' homes by registered nurses, the coordination and integration of services at the enrollee/family level, and the support from the local community where the staff and volunteers live. The key is the building of close relationships and trust between the nurses and the enrollees, along with the use of volunteers and community supports. In 1996, 255 volunteers contributed 3044 hours in the form of friendly visiting, transportation, and chore services.

The major role of community nurses under capitation is to integrate the delivery and payment systems by targeting persons at risk with preventive health, education, and early intervention, which ultimately affects the bottom lines of dollars and health. Nurses promote consumer involvement in decision making and family participation in giving care, and can provide advocacy for the client. Fragmentation is reduced and appropriate services are coordinated. The issue of the lack of a single professional to coordinate services is mitigated.

The CNO has proved to be a vehicle whereby some of the excess revenue over cost that is the result of nursing case management and local community support can be made available to local communities as an incentive to enhance or rebuild a sense of community and provide volunteerism and coordination at the local level. Although the communities will still need to raise some money—and should because that makes for greater local commitment—the amount will not be as daunting as it sometimes is right now.

Interest in the CNO by HMOs in Minnesota focuses mainly on the reduction of the costs of acute care and an increased market share. Current negotiations are encouraging. Yes, managed care is here to stay. And so is the Living at Home/Block Nurse Program—because ordinary people make it work!

Conclusion

Clearly, at a time when agencies and organizations around the country are struggling to reconcile unmet needs with overdrawn budgets, the Living at Home/Block Nurse Program is a promising example of how community initiative can redesign services to make them less expensive and more effective.

References

Ahroni JH: A description of the health needs of elderly home care patients with chronic illness, *Home Health Care Services Quarterly* 10:77-91, 1989.

Bellah RN, Madsen R, Sullivan WM, Swiller A, Tiptoe SM: *Habits of the heart: individualism and commitment in American life.* New York, 1985, Harper & Row.

Benson ER, McDevitt JQ: Home care and the older adult: illness care versus wellness care, *Holistic Nursing Practice* 3:29-38, 1989.

Benson ER, McDevitt JQ: When third party payment determines service: the elderly at risk, *Holistic Nursing Practice* 8:28-35, 1994.

Boyte HC: *Commonwealth: a return to citizen politics.* New York, 1989, The Free Press.

Estes CL, Rundall TG: *Social characteristics, social structure, and health in the aging population: aging, health and behavior,* London, 1992, Sage Publications, pp 299-326.

Eustis N, Greenberg P: *Long-term care for older persons: a policy perspective.* Monterery, Calif, 1984, Brooks & Cole.

Gluck ME, Wagner JL, Duffy BM: The use of preventive services by the elderly: a staff paper in OTA's series on preventive health services under Medicare, January 1989.

Harrington C, Cassel C, Estes CL, Woolhandler S, Himmelstin DU: A national long-term care program for the United States: a caring vision—the Working Group on Long-Term Care Program Design, Physicians for a National Health Program, *Journal of the American Medical Association,* pp 3023-3029, December 1991.

Institute of Medicine, Division of Health Promotion and Disease Prevention: *The second 50 years: promoting health and preventing disability,* Washington, DC, 1990, National Academy Press.

Jamieson A: Home care in old age: a lost cause? *Journal of Health Politics, Policy and Law,* pp 879-898 Winter, 1992.

Kent V, Hanley B: Home health care, *Nursing and Health Care,* pp 234-240, May 1990.

Kerr EA, Mittman BS, Hays RD, Siu AL, Leake B, Brook RH: Managed care and capitation in California: how do physicians at financial risk control their own utilization? *Annals of Internal Medicine* 123:500-504, 1997.

Koff TH: *New approaches to health care for an aging population: developing a continuum of chronic care services,* San Francisco, 1988, Jossey-Bass Publishers.

McKnight JL: Regenerating community, *Social Policy,* pp 54-58, Winter 1987.

McKnight JL: Two tools for well-being: health systems and communities. Paper presented at a Conference on Medicine for the 21st Century, sponsored by the American Medical Association, the Annenberg Center at Eisenhower, the Annenberg Washington Program, the US Environmental Protection Agency, and the WK Kellogg Foundation, pp 1-11, February 1992.

Rakowski W. *Disease prevention and health promotion with older adults: Aging, Health, and Behavior,* London, 1992, Sage Publications, pp 239-275.

Sharp N: LTC: there's no place like home, *Nursing Management,* pp 22-25, July 1992.

CHAPTER 33

Case Management

A Strategy to Achieve Reform in Australia's Public Health Care Delivery System

MAGGIE L. BRECKON, RN, RM, B AppSc, MN,
and **BERNADETTE M. BRENNAN**, RN, Dip App Sc, FR, CNA

OVERVIEW

The case manager was considered the critical link throughout to achieve effective discharge planning, transfer to community-based care, and then transfer to mainstream community care.

The Australian health care sector is essentially funded by the Commonwealth Government. It has recently undergone a period of major change in policy, philosophy, and direction. This change encompasses major economic reforms, which have forced the reevaluation of how, where, and to whom health care services are provided. Government policy therefore is the primary driver of program development and change in service delivery models within the public sector. This chapter outlines briefly how the above has influenced the development of case management as a strategy that enables the development of new models of care delivery. It will discuss the Transition Care Packages Project and the outcomes achieved, as demonstrated through a formal evaluation process undertaken in conjunction with Lincoln Gerontology Centre, Latrobe University (1996). ▲

Background

Health care is the largest industry in Australia, with universal health care being offered to each individual. As in most other western countries, health care expenditure constitutes a significant proportion of Australia's gross domestic product (GDP) and is predicted to reach 17% of GDP by 2041 (Healthcover, 1997). Health care is currently funded by a taxation levy of 1.5% of taxable income; however, as most services are charged above the Commonwealth Government recommended fee, there is usually a gap between cost and reimbursement, which the individual pays. Less than 35% of Australians are privately insured. Those privately insured continue to pay the taxation level and are still entitled to be treated in the public system if they so elect. Despite this low level of insurance, there is a strong private sector in health care, which is driven by the private hospital groups rather than the private health insurance sector.

The previous Labour Government policies promoted privatization or corporatization of public assets to achieve efficiency savings in public health expenditure. The current Liberal Government has a commitment to public sector reform to bring health care onto a business footing. Health care is now a business! This fact has been reinforced by the formation of Hospital Networks in Victoria, which have aggregated previously independently managed hospitals into one organisation. These are managed by a board of directors whose members are appointed by the Government and drawn from the business arena. They have a corporate profile and demonstrate a corporate mentality in their operation. The effects of these policies have been significant and require a substantial paradigm shift for both consumers and providers of health care.

With advances in medical technology and care increasing the longevity of the population and the decreasing number of privately insured individuals, there is an ever-increasing burden on the health care dollar. The annual outlay on health care in Australia is $40 billion and there are sixty separate Commonwealth health programs, accounting for 43% of national spending. Each of these sixty is a separate program with its own Commonwealth-state agreement, its own eligibility rules, its own assessment process, and its own record system (Paterson, 1996).

These programs can be broadly grouped into Hospital-Related, Specialized programs such as blood transfusion cancer screening services, Medical Benefits Schedule (MBS), and Pharmaceutical Benefits Schedule (PBS). The Medical Benefits Schedule sets the recommended fees payable for all medical visits or interventions under Medicare, which covers all Australians for medical treatment, except for Health Card holders and pensioners, who do not pay. The Pharmaceutical Benefits Schedule sets the prices to be paid for subsidized prescription drugs, again with the exceptions of Health Card holders and pensioners, who pay a minimum fee.

Some programs are administered directly by the Commonwealth and others by the states; these programs are funded through program grants. For example, residential care is managed by the Commonwealth, and acute and psychiatric hospitals are managed by the state. Only two of the sixty programs, Medicare and Pharmaceutical Benefits, have no cap on expenditure and are allowed to respond to demand; the others operate within defined budget allocations (Paterson, 1996). Problems inherent in this system include its complexity, poor structural linkages across programs, poor coordination leading to duplication of service provision, and a lack of focus on those for whom the service is provided (Hindmarsh, 1997).

Because of the problems identified, there is an ability to cost shift between Commonwealth and state. For example, if a service is provided by a general practitioner (GP), the Commonwealth is responsible; if the service is provided in a hospital outpatient clinic, the Commonwealth is responsible for 50% and the state for 50%; if it is provided in a community health centre, the state is 100% responsible. This ability to cost shift has led to a climate in which the mixing of programs to provide the continuous episode of care required by the patient is discouraged. Paterson (1996) states that for those who require intensive and continuing services from multiple programs, the task of developing a package of coordinated care is extremely difficult and often not successful. The cost of this inefficiency is enormous, as this group (10% of people) consumes 50% of Australia's health care expenditure.

The Council of Australian Governments (COAG) has been formed to address these problems and is currently reviewing funding arrangements between Commonwealth and states to achieve a more efficient and responsive system. It proposes to shift from funding individual programs to funding three streams of care: general, acute (including postacute care), and coordinated care (COAG Task Force on Health and Community Services, 1995).

The above situation is further compounded by the restructuring of health care services and the introduction of compulsory competitive tendering for service provision in the community setting and has resulted in a number of operators providing a range of services. The gaps in service provision have widened as a consequence, and the need for the coordination of care (case management) across the many providers has become apparent. Programs that facilitate coordination of community-based care and appropriate, timely discharge from acute care have been developed to redress this deficiency in care provision.

Acute health care, in particular, has changed in both direction and structure since the introduction of Casemix funding based on diagnosis-related groups (DRGs) in 1993. The Victorian health care sector has experienced a period of unprecedented control of expenditure and direction in acute health care since that time. In Victoria, as in other states, the Department of Human Services (DHS) has introduced the computerized reporting systems through which all public hospitals must report patient activity on an extensive range of parameters. The information generated from this statewide database allows identification of trends, such as the state average length of stay (SALOS) for each DRG. This information is used each year to adjust, usually downward, the LOS and cost reimbursement for each DRG, which then determines the level of funding for the next financial year. The information is also used for the identification of strict performance targets and the calculation of financial penalties for nonachievement.

Analysis of the extensive Government database generated through the above mandatory reporting systems has allowed also the identification of problem areas within the system, such as extended LOS and inappropriate discharge to residential care in the aged population. This, and the economic imperative, has provided the impetus to seek alternative, more cost-efficient models of service provision. However, in the public sector, the ability to develop new programs is constrained by Govern-

ment policy and the availability of Government funding. If funding is made available for program development, it means a level of Government control over the development process, the target population, the types of services provided, and the determination of outcomes. Government-funded programs may be evaluated or monitored internally by the Government department responsible, or by independent consultants if the program is statewide or highly significant. Both business and universities have been involved in these evaluations.

Program Development

According to Hindmarsh (1997), in a paper presented at the Ninth Casemix Conference in Australia, "Packages of care attempt to articulate the total care requirements for client groups throughout an episode of care for a defined condition." An episode of care represents a combination of services and any associated elements linked to a primary diagnosis. The packages of care are designed to provide the continuum across the various environments to which the client needs access, from acute episodes of care to less acute and, finally, discharge with community-based support. Advance identification of the likely health care needs of the client means that a care plan can be developed to outline the necessary interventions and the expected outcomes throughout the complete episode of care. This concept, under a variety of titles, has been adopted by most health care sectors in Australia.

Coordinated Care Trials

This program has been initiated by COAG in an attempt to achieve greater coordination of care and funding streams. The objectives of the program are to test the hypothesis that the quality and coordination of care could be improved by pooling the different funding sources for required services to make them more efficient and user friendly. The programs have drawn case managers from a diverse range of health services, including acute care, home and community care program (HACC), Royal District Nursing Service, and GPs. The outcomes are being evaluated both locally and nationally under strict criteria, including quality, functionality, and cost, using the SF-36 tool from the New England Medical Center Hospitals, Boston,

Massachusetts. Client and carer satisfaction will be measured further by interview and questionnaire. The trials are continuing and will not be completed until June, 1999.

The Department of Veterans Affairs (DVA) is trialing a Coordinated Care Program for a target group of their clients who are the highest users of health services (Killer, 1996). It will be based on an Annual Health Care Plan, which will be coordinated by the local medical officer (GP) who is the treating doctor for each client. The DVA considered that the GP was the most appropriate case manager for this particular client groups, but accepted that different care coordinators would suit different health care requirements.

The rationale for this initiative mirrors that previously identified—that is, the provision of health care has become more complex, with multiple service providers, lack of communication, a team model, and no coordination of care or monitoring of outcomes. The objective of the trial is to reduce the cost of care by improving primary care management through care coordination; reducing the need for expensive hospitalization; preventing readmission following discharge if hospitalisation occurs; reducing unnecessary usage and wastage of pharmaceuticals and investigations; scrutinizing the use of high-cost community nursing and other services; and encouraging the client to self-help and to be involved in the care plan.

Prospective participants will be identified by the DVA high-cost database; however, participation will be voluntary. GPs will nominate clients who meet the specific care plan entry criteria and who would benefit from this initiative.

An evaluation program is being developed in conjunction with the National Centre for Epidemiology and Public Health (NCEPH). It will monitor the effectiveness of the care plan intervention on a range of indicators, including service usage, cost, and treatment outcomes, comparing homogeneous groups within the target population to a control group. In addition, it will evaluate the effectiveness of the GP as a case manager.

While packages of care will address the needs of defined case types within a specific target population, there are episodes of care which cannot be planned in their entirety—for example, emergency hospital admissions. Normal postdischarge processes and resources may prove inadequate, and a mechanism to purchase additional services from the public or private sector to meet the individual needs of the client is required. Transition Care Packages (TCP) address this need. They were developed on a national basis in 1992 with the allocation of Commonwealth funding for a four-year pilot project. The following is a summary of the outcomes achieved within the TCP project for the period September 1993 to June 1995 (approximately twenty-one months), extracted from the National Report (Charlton, 1996).

Transition Care Packages

It was identified that at some clients, primarily the aged, experiencing an acute episode of care were at risk of admission to residential care on discharge, as the existing community providers could not meet or manage the significantly higher level of services required to allow them to be discharged home. The aim of TCP was to reduce the number of inappropriate admissions to residential care, through the purchase of additional services for these clients in the short term to allow them to regain their independence after discharge. TCP aimed to bridge the gulf between the acute care episode and community care as it was recognised that there were differences in how the two service streams approached service delivery on a philosophical, practical, and professional level.

Aged Care Assessment Teams (ACAT) teams are responsible for the assessment of the need for residential or rehabilitation placement. Each team consists of a gerontologist, a nurse, a social worker, and allied health representatives. Selected ACAT in each state were identified as the fund holders for TCP and were responsible for the purchase and coordination of the required support services.

TARGET GROUPS

The initial target groups of the project were:
- Clients with a short-term need capable of resolution within a defined period, leading to a low-level need for ongoing support
- Clients likely to remain at a higher level of dependency, requiring a range of available support services in order to remain in the community
- "At-risk" older people living in the community who are in need of "crisis" support but are unable to access mainstream services.

EXPECTED OUTCOMES

The expected outcomes for clients and carers were identified as:

- Reduced inappropriate entry to residential care
- Improved quality of life for clients and carers
- Maximizing of the client's level of independence
- Ability of clients to remain in the community with normal services on exit from the program and satisfaction of client and carer with the program.

Expected organisational outcomes included that hospital discharge arrangements would improve, that linkages with other hospitals or providers would improve, and that the processes established within the model would be effective.

Guidelines were developed to define the specific criteria for client groups being targeted. These were disseminated to potential referring agencies, who then recommended clients to the program. The central process of client identification took place during the ACAT assessment. Subsequent assessments and processes often led to changes in services required, as the client's needs were reassessed and redefined. Two critical points were identified. The first was the initial visit following discharge. It was found that the assessment undertaken while the client was still in hospital often proved invalid, with some clients requiring significantly increased services and others, less service. In addition, clients often provided inaccurate information about their home environments and their ability to cope, in order to achieve discharge from hospital. This inconsistency was easily identified on the first visit and the plan of care adjusted. The second critical point was the discharge of the client from TCP to mainstream community services. This required careful monitoring to ensure that the transfer process was successful and that the client remained appropriately supported. The case manager was considered the critical link throughout in achieving effective discharge planning, transfer to community-based care, and then transfer to mainstream community care.

PROGRAM EVALUATION

The evaluation process was unusual in that it was ongoing and would be conducted over the four-year life of the project. Data were collected by the project staff members, who worked closely with the Evaluation Unit in each State. The ACAT Evaluation Units in each state were responsible for the preparation of State Reports, which were collated into a National Report (Podger, 1996).

CLIENT PROFILE

The total number of clients admitted to TCP from the six states, from September 1993 to June 1995, was 1512.

Analysis of the client population identified their main characteristics as:

- Elderly widow between the ages of 80 and 84
- Australian national
- Living on a Government pension
- Living alone in a house or flat owned by self
- Mobile
- Continent
- Mentally aware
- Recently discharged from an acute hospital following treatment for a fracture.

DIAGNOSIS

Over all projects, the most common diagnoses recorded were:

- Fracture, 21.1%
- Stroke, 12.4%
- Arthritis, 10.0%
- Heart disease, 08.5%
- Dementia, 07.5%
- Other, 24.5%.

LENGTH OF STAY

The LOS varied between states; however, these variations were accounted for with further analysis. The total number of client days across all programs was 49,995. Across all states, the mean was 39.8 days, ranging from 26.7 to 50.8 days. The median ranged from 23.5 to 57 days. The maximum LOS ranged from 74 days to 118 days (Table 33-1).

SERVICES USED

The range of services used divided the projects into two groups. One provided predominantly domestic and personal assistance to their client populations, while the other provided high levels of nursing and paramedical services. Local conditions—for ex-

TABLE 33-1
Length-of-Stay Data by State

DAYS ON PROGRAM	NEW SOUTH WALES	VICTORIA	QUEENSLAND	SOUTH AUSTRALIA	WESTERN AUSTRALIA	TASMANIA
Mean	42.3	26.7	37.9	50.8	38.4	42.9
Median	43.5	23.5	42.0	57.0	42.5	51.0
Maximum	83.0	83.0	74.0	147.00	118.0	90.0
Minimum	3.0	0.0	1.0	3.0	0.0	0.0
TOTAL CLIENT DAYS	5071	5343	5304	7316	8212	2704

TABLE 33-2
Total Cost of Program (Based on Mean LOS)

STATE	NEW SOUTH WALES	VICTORIA	QUEENSLAND	SOUTH AUSTRALIA	WESTERN AUSTRALIA	TASMANIA
Direct client costs	$1041.00	$ 679.00	$ 546.00	$ 904.00	$ 982.00	$ 795.00
Indirect costs	$ 979.00	$ 558.00	$ 678.00	$ 998.00	$ 232.00	$1564.00
TOTAL COST PER CLIENT	$2020.00	$1255.00	$1224.00	$1902.00	$1214.00	$2359.00

ample, lack of specific services, especially in rural areas, and the character of the auspicing agency—account for some variation. However, it was identified that there was variation between projects in the interpretation of the character and direction of the program. Some saw it as a rehabilitation program, and others saw it as providing initial assistance after hospitalization in areas that have proved difficult for older people in these situations. While both approaches were valid, there may have been an element of exclusion in the selection of clients if the project was skewed in one direction.

COSTS

Discrete data relating to the costs and outcomes for these clients before the introduction of this program are not available, as these data formed part of the aggregated data relating to acute, aged, and community-service programs. Data from the Pilot Projects will become the baseline to provide future comparisons between different client groups, years of operation, and other like programs.

Costs per client were calculated on the basis of direct and indirect costs. Indirect costs included other salary costs, administrative expenses, and the initial cost of capital. The capital costs were amortised over the four years of the project, and costs related to the specific evaluation period only were included. For each project, the total indirect costs and the total direct client costs were divided by the number of client days to achieve an average cost per day per client. This figure was then multiplied by the average LOS to obtain an average cost per client for the average LOS on TCP (Table 33-2).

CLINICAL OUTCOMES

The Barthel score was used to indicate the level of functionality of the individual. This score is similar to, but not as complex as, the Functional Independence Measure (FIM), which is an indicator of severity of disability. The higher the Barthel score, the greater the level of functionality. For the purpose of this evaluation, the Barthel score was collapsed into four categories:

CATEGORY	PERCENTAGE ON ENTRANCE TO TCP
Severe (0-60)	13%
Moderate (61-90)	50%
Slight (91-99)	25%
Independent (100)	12%

The average Barthel score on admission to TCP ranged from 72 to 87. On discharge from TCP the average score increased by 5 to 11 points (Table 33-3).

In some States, there appeared to be a relationship between the Barthel score as a measure of dependency and cost per episode of care. However, this trend was inconsistent across States. Costs related to age groups younger than 80 and older than 80 were also inconsistent, with some states higher and some lower.

OTHER OUTCOMES

Three different approaches were utilised to measure clients' outcomes. All states undertook a six-month follow-up of clients accepted into the program. One state conducted a randomized control study of clients recommended to TCP over the same period, and one compared client outcomes with an equivalent group of clients eligible for TCP in a different location.

When outcomes at exit and six months are compared across all States, it must be noted that data were missing for 3.1% of clients exiting from the program and 9.5% of clients were unable to be contacted at six months following exit from TCP. It can be seen from the following data that there is a decline (3.8%) in the number remaining at home at six months, an increase of 4.4% in the number in nursing homes, and a slight increase (0.9%) in the number in hostels. The number in hospital decreased by 8.8% in this period, and a further 6.9% of clients were decreased at six months after discharge. Aggregated data for all states are as follows:

DESTINATION	EXIT FROM PROGRAM	AT SIX MONTHS
Home	73.6%	69.8%
Nursing home	1.5%	5.9%
Hostel	3.1%	4.8%
Deceased	2.3%	9.2%
Hospital	9.2%	0.4%

The results of the other client evaluation methodologies were, in many instances, inconclusive, with the results being mixed across states and between control and TCP clients. However, TCP did achieve the operational goals of facilitating access to a greater number and type of community services for patients discharged from hospital to community. This was reflected in greater client satisfaction with community services (Aged Care Systems Study, 1996).

Additional data were collected by each state, using a standard questionnaire and staff interview covering a wide range of issues. They included identification of eligible clients, discharge planning, referral to services, and case management practices.

Organisation Perspective on Client Outcomes. The staffs of most programs believe that the TCP had achieved many positive outcomes for their clients, as the assessment process targeted those who were appropriate and care was based on a holistic approach to clients and their needs. The programs' flexibility, the high quality of the assessment process, and case management were considered central to their success. The ability to implement a range and level of services specific to each client was considered vital to the achievement of improved function within the eight-week period on TCP.

The most consistently identified benefit was the facilitation of a safe, timely discharge from acute care and a smooth transition to community care. It was consistently reported that TCP was successful in negating the need for admission to residential care, with more patients being discharged home. In addition, lower levels of readmission to acute care were reported.

Most considered that TCP had given the clients dignity and respect, as they were involved in the decisions regarding their care. This, in turn, increased the confidence of both client and caregivers in achieving independence and improved quality of life with appropriate support at home.

Community Service Providers' Perspective on Client Outcomes. The majority of community service providers considered the program's major achievement was reflected in the ability of clients to achieve improved outcomes. This allowed them to remain in the community on an independent basis or with mainstream service levels as their only support. There was a belief that TCP has allowed many clients to return to their original levels of functioning. In addition, the ability to convalesce at home rather than in care was considered to lead to more improved outcomes.

Community service providers also considered that there was a reduced risk of readmission to acute care and admission to residential care. They

TABLE 33-3
Preadmission and Postadmission Barthel Scores for all States

STATE	NEW SOUTH WALES		VICTORIA		QUEENSLAND		SOUTH AUSTRALIA		WESTERN AUSTRALIA		TASMANIA	
	PRE	POST	PRE	POST	PRE	POST	PRE	POST	PRE	POST	PRE	POST
Mean	83.73	89.9	77.23	86.5	86.72	—	71.82	82.7	80.85	85.5	81.59	89.9
Median	87	95	80	94	91	—	76	89	89	95	83	95
Standard Deviation	17.84	14.8	17.21	18.0	13.72	—	19.07	18.4	22.86	22.4	20.37	14.8
Minimum	19	18	7	12	26	—	15	15	0	0	5	18
Maximum	100	100	100	100	100	—	100	100	100	100	100	100
N	82	82	356	339	218	—	235	233	348	221	111	82
Proportion of total	100%	100%	93%	88.5%	100%	—	100%	99.9%	95%	60%	86.7%	64.1%

believed that the increased levels of confidence in both client and carer, regarding the ability to manage at home and achieve better quality of life, were a direct result of TCP.

Organisational Outcomes. In one state a major change in practice has been the development of "client-specific carers," who are employed on a short-term basis to provide the total home care needs of individual clients with high needs.

A home and community care provider noted that the process for clients discharged from acute hospitals to TCP was so effective that it reflected poorly on the care of non-TCP clients in relation to the continuity of care. There was a feeling that discharge planning under TCP was more flexible, better planned, and more formalized within a case management framework. Because of the one contact person who undertook the total discharge planning process, hospital staff perceived that their work load had decreased. Another advantage seen was the ability to develop a more comprehensive plan of appropriate services, which were not limited to those that were normally available.

The ability to implement the plan immediately led to the achievement of a quicker and safer discharge, with services commencing as soon as the patient was discharged, without the delays previously experienced. The continuity of care and a smooth transition from hospital to community setting boost the clients' confidence about returning to and remaining at home. Clients' functionality and other indices improve at a much faster rate, and they reach their optimal levels sooner, to achieve improved quality of life.

The process of implementing a TCP program was perceived as being central to the development of a collegiate case management model, with the ACAT assessor and the TCP coordinator working closely together. It was found that the ability to formulate care plans without the previous limitations of service availability has broadened the horizons of the case workers. There has been a definition of the role of the ACAT in discharge planning, leading to greater role clarity and a reduction in process duplication.

The case management role was considered to have achieved cost and time savings by most service providers. However, there were conflicting opinions between agencies with regard to this role and who should be driving the process. The overall view was that practice and processes had been improved by the introduction of TCP and that, with the increased case management and coordination of client requirements, there was now more communication between organizations than ever before.

Conclusion

Prior to the development of the programs facilitating the transition between acute and community care and coordinated care within the community setting, case management occurred on an ad hoc basis that was not "recognized" as case management. However, the new direction in Australian health care has led to a new classification of health care professional: the "case manager." This role is not specifically identified with nursing. Appointment is usually on the basis of primary treatment need, and a case manager may be a social worker, a physiotherapist, an occupational therapist, a doctor, or a nurse.

A selection of outcomes and the collaboration achieved by a case management model of service provision within the Transition Care Packages Project have been discussed in this chapter. The evaluation process of the Project on a broad range of indicators was undertaken as a formal and predetermined process, and the findings, in some instances, were inconclusive. However, there was some evidence, in the qualitative analysis, to indicate that improved outcomes for client, organisation, and service providers could be achieved by utilizing case management to operationalize programs such as the Transition Care Packages Project.

The future of community-based health care in Australia relies heavily on the tenets of the case management model to achieve the aims of coordinated, cost-effective care that is centered on individual clients' needs. In recognition of the expanding role of case managers in the Australian health care sector, the University of Melbourne in conjunction with the Case Management Society of Australia has introduced a Graduate Diploma in Case Management and is holding an Inaugural Conference in Melbourne in February, 1998.

References

Aged Care Systems Study: *Nineteenth progress report*, October 1996, vol 3, Latrobe University, Bundoora, Victoria, Australia, pp 79-83.

Charlton F, ed: Transition Care Packages Project: evaluation of the pilot projects, Latrobe University, Bundoora, Victoria, Australia, 1996.

COAG Task Force on Health and Community Services: Health and community services: meeting peoples's needs better, a discussion paper, 31 January 1995, Canberra, Australia.

Healthcover: "Radical measures" needed to control health expenditures, says business adviser, Healthdata Services, Sydney, 2 April-May 1997, pp 18, 19.

Hindmarsh C: Quality, continuity and cost effectiveness through packages of care, Ninth Casemix Conference in Australia, 1997.

Killer G: The ageing population: developing a co-ordinated plan of care in the veteran community, Health Summit '96: Managed Care for Australia, 18-19 March 1996, Sydney, Australia.

Paterson J: *National healthcare reform: the last picture show*, Department of Human Services, Government of Victoria, Australia, 1996.

Podger A: Best practice in the health sector, *Australian Health Review* 19(4):73-82, 1996.

CHAPTER 34

Achieving Family Health and Cost-Containment Outcomes

Innovation in the New Zealand Health Sector Reforms

MERIAN LITCHFIELD, RN, PhD, **and MAUREEN LAWS**, RN, MSc(App) (Nursing)

OVERVIEW

The major shift to the competitive, market-driven processes of the reforms underlies this fragmentation. It is antithetical to the principle of partnership that is at the core of our national identity, and it has caused confusion and public outcry.

Nurse case management is presented in this chapter as a form of health service provision that allows for the full expression of professional nursing practice. The perspective brought to the concept is inevitably shaped within the health system and the nursing development of nursing. It is embedded in the cultural, social, and political evolution of New Zealand within an international health care movement. We trace the conceptualization of nurse case management as it has evolved, in context, through a sequence of research studies, a pilot project with families, and international dialogue.

The intention of the research was to show the process of nursing practice in relation to outcome. Through the research endeavor the practice of the family nurse developed and showed how families in strife were facilitated to move toward assuming control over health circumstances, seeking and using services with discernment, and increasing connectedness as family and citizens. Considerable cost containment was identified.

An emergent nurse case management service delivery model supports this community-based practice as pivotal in an integrated package of nursing care for families as clients in the context of their everyday living. It recognizes the family nurse's knowledge, skills, and responsibilities as complementary to those of all other nurses and health and welfare professionals, wherever they provide services for family members.

The key feature of the model is the practice of a family nurse, founded in the theory of health as expanding consciousness initiated by Margaret Newman (1986, 1990b, 1994, 1996, 1997) and evolved through praxis research (Connor, 1996; Litchfield, 1993, 1997; Litchfield et al, 1994). ▲

New Zealand is a small, independent three-island Pacific nation within the British Commonwealth. In land mass it is about the size of Colorado, and it has a population of three and a half million. The Treaty of Waitangi, signed in 1840 as an agreement for colonial settlement between the British Crown and the indigenous Maori, has established a bicultural foundation for national identity and has urged a partnership approach in all social and political affairs. Immigration has increased to build a multiethnic society, and in recent years there has been a growing alignment with nations of the Pacific Rim for trade.

Hence, the principle of partnership is essential to the development of a health system that is responsive to need in the increasing diversity of New Zealand's citizens and lifestyles. It expresses cultural values underpinning our efforts to describe professional family-focused nursing practice within a nurse case management scheme, and to situate it in the reformed health service structure.

Health Sector Reform

Health sector reform in New Zealand is rooted in government policy to move the nation from the welfare state established in the 1930s, with a protected economy, to a market economy in the 1980s that is open and responsive to international forces. In 1938 New Zealand was the first country in the world to provide tax-funded universally accessible health benefits; hospital and ambulatory services were to be available free according to need (Salmond, 1997). While a small private system was maintained and a client copayment system evolved for medical consultations in the community, over 80% of total health expenditure was from the public purse until the 1990s (Laugesen, Salmond, 1994).

From the 1970s, reflecting international trend, the expanding medical diagnostic and treatment capabilities to control disease and disability increasingly focused the changes in health service delivery on its cost and the management of limited resources. Public demand together with rising expenditure eventually placed the government in an untenable position as the major health service provider within its traditional system. Reform was inevitable. Total replacement of the existing service structure was mooted by government in 1991, and

a radically new health system framework was put in place on July 1, 1993.

Health sector reform was originally envisaged by government in the same way as reform in all other sectors in a bid to control spending; consistent with trends in other countries, health was to be viewed as a commodity and its production open to market forces (Mooney, Salmond, 1994). An organizational shell for the processes of managing the public health budget was established, separating the funding from provision of services. Traditional service delivery could not continue in the same way; the provision of services was expected to develop into new configurations, with providers freed to be responsive to the diversity of need and to offer choice. The public health service would comprise contracts between purchaser and provider based on competitive tendering: the best outcomes for the least cost. Guidance in purchasing would come from the National Core Health Services Committee, charged with the definition of the basic services that all New Zealanders should expect the government to provide free of charge.

Following the reforms, the traditional institutions restructured and rationalized their services to become focused and competitive. Public hospitals began to shrink to become highly technical centers for intensive episodes of specialized care. They provide free treatment and care of life-threatening illness and injury for almost all New Zealanders (Salmond, 1997), but the condensed episodes of hospitalization mean that a considerable part of the treatment and care is expected to be in the client's home, perhaps involving highly technical and informed management. Private hospitals expanded to provide low-risk elective surgery, some of it under contract to the public purchasing bodies. General practitioners (community-based physicians) began to move into managed care arrangements in which they "take responsibility for ensuring that a given population receives a defined set of services in a coordinated fashion" (Ministry of Health, 1996); they remain the dominant providers of primary health care and gatekeepers, reimbursed for consultations from public funds and holding onto their traditional client copayment system.

In association with these changes people are delaying seeking medical attention, comply variably with prescribed treatments, and must wait for nonurgent hospital treatment. Attention is drawn to the expanding need for health care in the home and community, where people must live their lives accommodating chronic disease, disability, hospitalization, and treatment regimens. More of the responsibility for health care is being passed to the family, and for many who are already under strain this is a critical burden. In the aftermath of the health reforms, the complexity of individual health needs is beginning to be recognized by policy makers (Steering Group to Oversee Health and Disability Changes, 1997).

While new initiatives began to emerge in the new climate, the constellation of services remained fragmented and profession or institution centered, unable to address these needs. Purchasing processes perpetuated the traditional separation of primary health care from secondary and tertiary care, and accentuated divisions between medical specialties and between health and other government sectors such as social welfare, education, housing, and justice. Traditional hospital outreach community nursing has been increasingly confined by the intensifying service focus on single episodes of hospitalization and individualized protocols for treatment of medical diagnoses. Purchasing has occurred in the absence of a theory of health that would give coherence and purpose to the provision of services (Seedhouse, 1995), and further the effort to define a set of publicly funded core health services has been aborted.

The major shift to the competitive, market-driven processes of the reforms underlies this fragmentation. It is antithetical to the principle of partnership that is at the core of our national identity, and it has caused confusion and public outcry. The new coalition government at the end of 1996 agreed on a fundamental redress of the principles underlying the reforms (Steering Group to Oversee Health and Disability Changes, 1997). There is to be a change from a "competitive" to a "collaborative" approach in service development; principles of "public service" will replace "commercial profit" objectives; and the Government will resume a centralized role in decisions regarding the relationship between public and private service provision. Services will again be "funded" rather than "purchased" by one national publicly funded health authority; the focus will be on "integrated care" rather than "managed care." "Rationing" is to be

acknowledged and addressed openly in the context of accountability.

The policy makers have turned their attention to the significance of professional practice in bringing about the desired changes of effectiveness and cost containment (National Health Committee, 1996). Emphasis is on collaborative approaches for better health outcomes; national guidelines for health care are being developed, including statements of evidence-based "best practice."

Within this rather haphazard unfolding of change in health service provision, new paradigms of health and health care are called for in the reconstruction of services. Amidst the confusion, nurses are placed equally alongside their medical and other colleagues to bring their own perspectives and create the niche they require to become providers in their own right. The historical development of the professional structure, including the evolution of a theoretical foundation for practice, has positioned nurses to realize this potential to practice as fully professional clinicians with primary accountability to the client.

The Professional Structure of Nursing

A professional structure for nursing has been evolving throughout the century. Since 1973 there has been a progressive transition in the basic education of nurses leading to registration. From 1998, all nurses entering the profession with registration will have a baccalaureate degree. At the same time, post-basic education has developed as specialized clinically based courses and graduate degrees in technical institutes and universities. Holistic paradigms of health have been key in efforts to construct curricula that will provide a nursing disciplinary focus. New Zealand nursing now has the full academic structure to support the development of independent practice roles and service delivery models.

Prior to the 1993 health sector reform, nurses felt that the traditional service settings and employment conditions thwarted their efforts to operationalize the holistic frameworks for practice in which they had been prepared. In the new climate of the reforms, nurses who envisaged ways to develop their practice differently repositioned themselves to work beyond stereotyped roles. However, mostly they have done this from within and pushing at the boundaries of the traditional employment institutions already under the strain of inevitable cutbacks and restructuring. Continuation of these practice developments is tenuous. The potential of the reforms in the health sector is for innovative health care delivery models that would free nurses from the constraints of employment in services traditionally defined by medical goals.

Associated with developments in post-basic education, a clinical career structure was proposed. The first model depicted clinical practitioners, with a range of abilities and responsibilities, collectively "maximizing nursing's potential to positively influence the health of New Zealanders" (New Zealand Nurses' Association, 1976). The notion of complementarity amongst nurse roles was emerging. Then, recognizing the value of the American Nurses' Association (1983) professional social policy statement in giving direction and promoting accountability to service and practice development, the New Zealand Nurses' Association (1985) published its own statement, which further substantiated a clinical career structure. A process for certification of nurse clinicians and nurse consultants who would practice with autonomy followed (New Zealand Nurses' Association, 1988).

A national clinical nursing structure was elaborated and ratified by members of the New Zealand Nurses' Association (1991). In this, the concept of complementarity was made explicit. Each practice role was defined in terms of interdependence and considered to be of equal value, with the whole much greater than the sum of its constituent parts. The professional practitioner's knowledge, experience, and role responsibility determined the scope of practice and the extent of professional autonomy. The nature of the knowledge linked with experience related to the extent of flexibility in where, when, how, and for what purpose nursing was practiced. It was envisaged that the most highly qualified of clinical nurses, expressing a unique philosophy, could move freely throughout communities, including hospitals and medical clinics, within negotiated boundaries rather than institutionally defined boundaries. These nurses would work with clients to make sense of what was going

on for them in their lives, regardless of service setting. Consistent with the belief that one nurse cannot respond effectively to multiple specific needs, there was the expectation that consultation amongst colleagues, wherever they were employed, would continue the development and provision of client-focused practice.

In the expression of these concepts of complementarity, collegiality, and independence in the professional career structure, consistent with the principle of partnership, and supported by the education structure, nursing is well placed to contribute significantly to achieving the political goal of an integrative health care system. Nurses have the social mandate and the structures for developing the competence to respond effectively to the open invitation for different models of health care. This is the context for the development of the concept of nurse case management into an innovative service delivery model.

Emergence of Nurse Case Management

In anticipation of the new climate for innovation to be created by the 1993 reforms, a two-day national conference to explore and explicate the potential contribution of nursing in health care was organized in February 1992. The conference brought together professional nurse leaders: practitioners, executives, educators, and heads of the professional organizations. As a feature of the conference, a two-hour interactive videoconference provided for dialogue between a representative panel of nurses in New Zealand and a similar panel in the United States led by Dr. Margaret Newman at the University of Minnesota.

The focus of the videoconference was a pioneering nurse case management scheme at Sioux Valley Hospital, Sioux Falls, South Dakota. The development of this scheme involved the preparation of nurses in a service-education collaborative venture based on principles of differentiated nursing practice (Koerner, 1992). A resource for development of the scheme had been a trilevel model of nursing practice proposed by Newman (1990a) that would represent an integrative phase in the development of nursing service delivery, allowing the movement to full expression of professional nursing practice.

The wider conference discussion in New Zealand evolved around the differing cultural perspectives of practice and service development, the significance of the nursing roles in case management, the nature of the decision-making function, and the demonstrated cost effectiveness of nurse case management at Sioux Valley Hospital. Reflecting the different historical and health service contexts, the Sioux Falls concept of differentiated practice (Koerner, Karpiuk, 1994) and the New Zealand concept of complementary practice (New Zealand Nurses' Association, 1991) expressed a similar trend in each country to promote greater integration of care, making best use of the range of knowledge and skills of nurses collectively. The professional practice that involves the full flexibility in movement of the nurse according to client need could be considered in relation to access to services and their coordination.

The conference culminated in a submission to the Minister of Health of a general statement on the nature and place of professional nursing practice in health sector reform. The statement identified nursing as "concerned with people in any setting, their experience of health, illness and disability, and the ways in which they get on with life and living" (Conference Participants, 1992). Reflecting the previous conceptualization of a clinical career structure, the statement explained that when nurses in all services with their varied expertise and specialist knowledge view their practice as complementary and their roles as interdependent, nursing practice can attend to the full complexity and uniqueness of client health circumstance and family and community life. Where a range of health workers and assistants are needed, their coordination by expert nurses who have the overview of the situation would improve efficiency and client satisfaction in health care provision generally. Supporting reference was made to the success in quality and cost outcomes of nurse case management projects in the United States reported during the videoconference.

This statement heralded, in the political arena, a New Zealand vision of professional nursing as a form of nurse case management, acknowledging the significance of the practice of nurses. It would be at the core of the profession, operating beyond the traditional employment divisions of extant service institutions, and integrating the practice of nurses employed in all these settings. Within the approaching reform of the health service structure, nurse case management would provide for new scope and diversity of practice and flexibility in the ways nurses might attend to their clients. Nursing would play "a vital part in the health care within any community" (Conference Participants, 1992).

While the content of the nurses' practice for individuals and families had been identified in broad terms within this vision, the practice as the expression of a holistic nursing paradigm was still to be explicated in the context of the new health system. A pilot service was needed.

A Pilot Project to Explicate Nurse Case Management

An opportunity to realize this vision of nursing and develop the practice was provided by government funding for primary health care initiatives with potential as innovative models. The proposal for a ten-month pilot project to explore the concept of nurse case management was selected. The aim was to explicate and establish the feasibility of a nurse case management scheme that addresses the needs of families with complex health circumstances. Dr. JoEllen Koerner of Sioux Valley Hospital, South Dakota, became a consultant for the management and costing aspects. The report of this Professional Nurse Case Management pilot project (Litchfield et al, 1994) presented a descriptive framework for the nursing practice that developed through the project. It included the changes that occurred in the families, estimates of cost containment associated with the change, and a proposed niche for the nurse case management service within the new health system structure.

PARTICIPANTS

A nurse was seconded to the project to establish a new role of family nurse. She had the freedom to interact with family members anywhere and at any time in the movement of their everyday lives. The family nurse would take an overview of health experience and predicaments within the unfolding pattern of family and community life, and would work with family members as they effected change. Two researchers and a professional mentor, together with the family nurse, constituted the research group.

Families were referred by nurses from the existing Service for People with Physical Disabilities. Recruitment was according to criteria of (1) complexity in the family predicaments not being effectively addressed within current services and (2) the families' actual or potential heavy use of services. Many agencies and personnel were in contact with the families (8 to 35 per family), each making an important contribution to some aspect of their predicament, but none with an overall view of the family circumstance. At entry to the project, the families were judged to be in a predicament of strife. Families with at least one child were targeted; the custodial parent identified other persons who might be classified as "family," those concerned with the impact of the disabilities in everyday living.

Nineteen families participated, comprising 79 individuals between 3 months and 75 years old, almost half of them younger than 20 years old. There was considerable diversity in family structure, living situations, type of disability, and ethnicity, and these continued to be in flux through the 10-month duration of the project.

THEORETICAL FOUNDATION

Foundational to the project was the theoretical framework for health and the praxis research approach. The theory was of health as expanding consciousness expressed in the interrelationship of movement, space, and time, the inspiration of theorist Margaret Newman (1986, 1990). The way of living with disability is an expression of the unfolding pattern of family-environment relating. The theory evolved as a framework for the process of health patterning in nursing practice in a study with New Zealand families with complex health circumstances (Litchfield, 1993).

The framework for the praxis identified its elements in a discontinuous progression represented as interrelated themes (in bold) and subthemes (in italics):

Within a **moment of partnership** with identified *parameters of entry and closure*, where *timing* is a phase of disruption in family life, and the process of the encounter has an *informing capacity*, there is an **evolving dialogue** as a continuous *flow of unfolding and enfolding* that is *embedded in the social/political health system context*. Within the dialogue, the **recognizing of pattern** occurs as *incidental revelations* and *insight as the potential for action*, expressed in an **expanding horizon** seen in the movement from being *in the present without vision* to an understanding of *the presence of past and future*. With greater vision there was **increasing connectedness** shown as *inclusion as family members and citizens, interdependence* in the need for support, and *transformation* in the pattern of the life process.

This theoretical framework was expressed in the guiding definitions for the pilot project:

- *Health patterning* is a process by which the family and nurse in their partnership recognize pattern in the complexity of their health circumstance as the potential for action. The insight gained in the process is expressed in an expanding horizon of possibilities for future direction and increasing connectedness as family/group and citizens.
- *Health circumstance* refers to the configuration of the events, situations and relationships of significance to the family, constantly unfolding in time and place, which characterizes the particular way in which each family gets on with life and living.

METHODOLOGY

A praxis approach (Litchfield, 1993; Newman, 1990b) grounded in the unitary transformative paradigm proposed by Newman, Sime, and Corcoran-Perry (1991) directed the design of the project. With this approach, the methodology for the practice partnership of family nurse and families merged with the hermeneutic-dialectic methodology for the research partnership of family nurse in the research group. All were participant in the changes occurring in family living through the project. The family nurse became integral to the unfolding pattern of family living as together they sought to understand the family predicaments.

Through a series of weekly meetings of the research group in the latter half of the project, the family nurse shared her stories of the families and her visits to them. As we reflected together on their changing predicaments, we elaborated and worked to make sense of the picture of family living. The whole group's understanding of the family circumstance took shape in terms of how the family moved in time and place. The recognizing of pattern in the family circumstance was the potential for action in the subsequent visits with the families, and this was integral to the unfolding of meaning of the whole.

The action of the family nurse within the nurse-family partnership involved the immediate mobilization of relief services if necessary and orchestration of services as needs emerged in the partnership process of pattern recognition.

CHANGE IN FAMILY HEALTH CIRCUMSTANCE

As meaning unfolded within the dialogue, changes could be seen in retrospect in the way the family members were more open and spontaneous. They interacted in a more focused, purposeful, and cooperative way; they had not previously heard each other's experience or the meaning disability had in their individual lives. Together they worked out ways to rationalize the required tasks within the home, ways for each to extend his or her involvement beyond the home, adjusting work and home schedules and following recreational interests. Some also became involved in community action, believing that the experience and skills they had learned should be shared.

Almost all of the families showed movement in at least some of these ways. At the closure of the partnership they had developed a view to the future, a re-envisioning of the present predicament of strife as just a passing feature of the evolving pattern in family life. They could see that there were possibilities for living differently, beyond the struggle of the moment, in a more manageable and fulfilling way, accommodating disability with more freedom of movement in their respective worlds. Medical conditions and their management were just part of everyday family living.

The families' greater knowledge and awareness of their predicaments and acceptance of interdependence as family members and citizens in community life showed in their more discerning use of services and informed assertiveness in focusing the care. They were clearer in their expectations of health professionals and found their own strategies for obtaining information and being participant in clinical decision making. For a few families, ongoing involvement of a health professional was

deemed necessary, to be a consistent contact person, advocate, and coordinator. These families, with the family nurse, chose the *person* (rather than service) who would be appropriate for them.

In review of the series of weekly research group meetings, the changes in the family circumstance and the nature of the family nurse participation were described. The families had gained insight into their circumstances and moved to greater independence and control in health matters associated with the disabilities, while accepting their interdependence within family and society (including service access). This meant that they had incorporated physical disability into everyday living with more meaning in terms of a future. In retrospect, they could be seen to have become empowered. Health was expanding consciousness, integral to the activities of everyday living.

COST CONTAINMENT

Cost containment was associated with the cooperative stance and collaborative actions of the family nurse within the family and network of services. Hospitalizations were avoided because there were more integrated, timely approaches to problems as they arose and possibilities were considered before problems were manifested. The length of hospitalization was minimal when families were more informed and supported in dealing with a hospital episode as a feature of family life. The number of health professionals involved and the number of consultations became limited to what was necessary through good-natured collaborative review of how the self-identified family needs might be best attended to, in their full complexity, in the most convenient and streamlined way. While the mobilization of new services in some cases increased cost in the short term, the efficiency could be seen in all of them in the long term.

EXEMPLAR

The interrelatedness of family predicament, nursing practice, and efficiency in the use of health and welfare services can be illustrated in a case study of one participant family:

At the point of referral to the family nurse, it was two months since Bruce had been discharged from a four-month stay in hospital following serious head injury. He had recurrent nonspecific intense pain, was irascible with aggressive outbursts, was physically incapacitated in self-care, and behaved in a similar way to his nine-year-old stepson, often in competition with him. He was at home with his wife Meg and their two younger children: a toddler of 14 months and an infant born while Bruce was in hospital. Meg had decided the family needed a different house to accommodate their changed family situation, so friends had just moved the household while the family were out of town at the funeral of Bruce's father. Furniture was yet to arrive. The infants had the flu and, with Bruce, required attention at frequent intervals day and night; none could be without vigilant supervision. Meg had not managed to complete the formalities of the complex procedural requirements for urgently needed financial maintenance.

Meg described her predicament as "frozen." She was exhausted, confined to the home, had dwindling resources, and could not see how she and her family could continue. Thirteen people from a range of services were visiting the home. "I felt like it was an open house," she said, "lots of different people giving me advice but very little practical assistance."

The family nurse immediately mobilized emergency services to provide interim respite for Meg with child care. She prompted, linked, and focused the agencies concerned with the financial affairs to expedite the payment of due benefits. Then she attended to the broader pattern of family relating and living with Bruce's predicament and very young children settling into a new home. She became as if a "friend" to Meg and Bruce, taking stock of the whole family experience and circumstances. As the relationship progressed and the tension was relieved, Meg moved to bring a different perspective to her situation, to see possibilities, to choose and to direct her own affairs, including accessing services.

Together, they attended to Bruce's pain and agitation and medical prescriptions for family members within the context of home and family life, working through options and tailoring strategies to their unique situations. Bruce's agreement to participate in a Men Against Violence program was important in addressing a complexity of needs of all family members within the one action. Ways of dealing with the nighttime disturbances and unrelenting demands on Meg were trialed. In her changed life circumstance she found how to reestablish a network beyond the home for company and relaxation.

In retrospect, Meg saw the family nurse as an "interpreter" in her contacts with the array of services, "coordinator" in initially bringing together all those involved, and general "facilitator" as she and Bruce moved to recognize pattern in their reha-

bilitation, establishing new forms of relationships as family and with health and welfare personnel. Some clarity on "the direction in which we are headed" developed.

Cost containment was shown (1) in the short term as the efficiencies of the family-nurse partnership while in progress, and (2) in the longer term in relation to the anticipated public expenditure through Bruce's working life span. The short-term cost containment was shown in the comparison of the actual scenario and two hypothetical scenarios of family life through the year following the accident:

- The actual scenario concerned the use of services by the whole family associated with the changed family circumstance during the episode of Bruce's hospitalization, the episode of partnership with the family nurse, and the two months between these episodes.
- A *worst-case* scenario was derived from Meg's unsolicited comments about her predicament and what she thought, in retrospect, would have happened to the family if they had not had the family nurse but had proceeded to "inevitable breakdown."
- A *best-case* scenario concerned the earlier involvement of the family nurse with the family, starting right from the time of the accident (Figure 34-1).

From comparison of these scenarios, a short-term saving of 3% was estimated to have been achieved through the partnership with the family nurse in the actual scenario. This was the balance of savings over the additional cost of the family nurse and other services she mobilized. Cost was contained mainly through avoidance of the rehospitalization of Bruce, specialist care for Meg, and welfare care of the children.

A 13% saving might have been made over the same period in the best-case scenario if the family nurse had been involved from the initial critical time for the family at the time of the accident. Meg wrote of it: "I remember the morning of his accident as though it was yesterday. It was June 8, 1992 at 7 AM, when I received a phone call informing me of the accident. I was eight months pregnant, I had a ten-month-old daughter, a nine-year-old son, and on top of that a husband in hospital fighting for his life." The saving from early involvement was largely attributed to earlier discharge from hospital and coordination of services. Duplication and re-

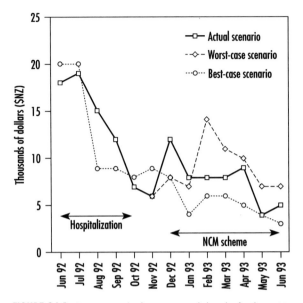

FIGURE 34-1 Cost per month of services provided to the family participant in the nurse case management (NCM) scheme comparing hypothetical best and worst case scenarios with the actual scenario.

dundant consultations with health professionals and welfare agencies were avoided while the necessary support services were focused on the challenge of accommodating the disabilities, a new infant, and altered relationships in a new form of family life.

Estimation of cost saving in the long term, within the best-case scenario of early involvement of the family nurse, was much more dramatic. Earlier consideration of the pattern in family life, and future possibilities for family living and action to shape it with the focused assistance of services, would have optimized Bruce's rehabilitation potential and chance of some form of employment. It would have facilitated the reconfiguration of relationships earlier, increased the likelihood of keeping the family together, and provided a more secure, healthy foundation for growing children as future citizens. The cost of publicly funded sickness/injury and welfare benefits to fully support the fractured, unemployed family until the usual age of retirement (for the following 20 years) might have been one and a half million dollars.

FAMILY NURSE PRACTICE

The form of partnership was the expression of a distinct nursing practice theoretically founded on a knowledge of health as expanding consciousness involving transformative change in the lives of the families, accommodating the disability and chronic illness. The family nurse accompanied the families initially as a partner, facilitating their movement to the hub of an integrated network of services to assume control of their own health matters. She attended to the whole family predicament within the partnership, explaining that she made available to the family her accumulated knowledge and expertise in the care of families living with physical disability and chronic illness. Similarly, the client's perspective of a nurse case manager's role has since been descriptively presented as insider-expert (Lamb, Stempel, 1994).

The caring relationship and a sense of fiscal responsibility were central. The theoretical perspective of health as expanding consciousness shaped, and was shaped within, the dialogue of the research group and hence was integral to the practice of the family nurse. Nurse case management involved, but was much more than, the accessing and coordination of services. Furthermore, it became clear from the stories of the families' experience that it was futile, wasteful, and thus unethical to pour money into highly technical treatments if the family and the wider context within which the disabled persons are to live out their lives are not attended to as well.

INTEGRATIVE PRACTICE

The feasibility of nurse case management with this theoretical orientation to nursing practice was further elaborated by depicting a niche for the service provision within the new health system structure created by the health sector reforms. With the focus on how the family lived with disability, and the meaning it had in their lives, their partnership with the family nurse created a new way for a range of services to become integrated. The family nurse recognized that she could not have practiced without clinical nurse specialists carrying out their specialized operations. Her involvement altered the way they practiced: they felt able to more intently focus their specialist skills and experience.

The general medical practitioners reported the

same. It could be seen how nursing practice complements the practice of other health professionals. Each provided a particular input which, in context, made sense to the client, while the family nurse had the overview and could attend to the integration of knowledge and skills in a complementary way.

We have proposed that the nurse case management scheme be situated alongside other service providers, and purchased independently within the public health system. The role of the family nurse, involving the orchestration of a package of nursing for any one family, would be to coordinate the practice of nurses employed in the range of settings of the other service providers with which the families had contact. Nursing practice, in its complementarity, would be integrated across settings with a common professional purpose and the primary accountability to the family.

Continuing Research

Elaboration of the concept of nurse case management through praxis research is continuing to develop our understanding and ability to describe the nature of the nursing practice at its core. Building on the praxis model developed through the nurse case management pilot project, Connor (1996) attended particularly to the nature of the client-nurse relationship that facilitated the process of change. She was convinced that the non-prescriptive relationship was the key feature of the nurse case management scheme and wanted to further explore how this enabled clients to "safely and honestly reveal their circumstances in a way that has meaning for them . . . [through which] the client together with the nurse can work out what is relevant to their situation" (p. 6), including the use of services. Characteristics of her partnerships with client participants were elaborated into a model of personal practice depicted by the metaphor of a web of relationship, which had four major interrelated themes: constructing context, the art of speaking to one another, building up and moving on, changing and transforming.

The foundational framework of the praxis methodology for health patterning has been reviewed and reformed into a model of the process of prac-

tice in a further study involving young families with complex health circumstances (Litchfield, 1997). The praxis experience of recognizing pattern was elaborated as a process of unfolding meaning in family health, where health is dialectic in the evolving dialogue of partnership. Concepts of health in terms of medical diagnosis, service access and use, and the implications for family living, focused the dialogue. The model expresses the reflexive nature of theory development in practice.

These studies represent the evolution of the theory of health as expanding consciousness in personal practice which underpins the distinctive conceptualization of nursing case management.

Conclusion

The pilot project was undertaken to operationalize the concept of partnership as the practice of a family nurse and to show its effectiveness and efficiency as a form of nurse case management. It provided the opportunity to demonstrate how the quality of nursing practice in addressing complex family health circumstances can be presented and the cost containment measured.

The service delivery model that was developed places emphasis on the practice of the family nurse as the integrating feature of the scheme. This nurse, free to move with family members in their everyday lives, was pivotal in the collaborative network of health care workers to link all service settings. The nature of the partnership between the nurse and families was the key to health outcomes of the case management scheme and attention to the coordination of services was just one aspect. The practice was theoretically founded in a view of health as expanding consciousness, facilitating a transformative change in family life, and a revision of how health and welfare services would be drawn upon to greatest effect. The praxis methodology for the evaluation research was also the educative process for the family nurse within the scheme. The model of nurse case management emerged through the processes of the project.

The pilot project provided a timely indication of how nurses might contribute significantly to service development in our major health sector reforms. The framework of professional education and regulation of nurses in New Zealand provided the necessary background and support for the family nurse to work as a fully independent practitioner. While particularly responsive to the New Zealand context, the project was connected within the international movement to develop nurse case managment schemes that will improve health outcomes with limited resources through the integration of health care. The next phase is a more extensive interdisciplinary pilot project through which to elaborate the model and position it within the service and funding structures.

References

American Nurses' Association: *Nursing: a social policy statement*, Kansas City, MO, 1980, American Nurses' Association.

Conference Participants: *Nursing practice in health sector reform*. Statement prepared for submission to the Minister of Health at the conference held in Wellington, New Zealand, 21-22 February, 1992.

Connor M: *The web of relationship: an exploration and description of the nature of the caring relationship in a nurse case management scheme of care*. Unpublished master's thesis, Victoria University, Wellington, New Zealand, 1995.

Koerner J: Integrating differentiated practice into shared governance. In Porter-O'Grady T, ed: *Implementing shared governance*, St. Louis, 1992, Mosby, pp 169-196.

Koerner J, Karpiuk K, eds: *Implementing differentiated nursing practice: Transformation by design*. Gaithersburg, Md, 1994, Aspen.

Lamb GS, Stempel JE: Nurse case management from the client's view: growing as insider-expert, *Nursing Outlook* 42:7-13, 1994.

Laugesen M, Salmond G: New Zealand health care: a background, *Health Policy* 29(1,2):11-23, 1994.

Litchfield MC: *The process of health patterning in families with young children repeatedly hospitalised*. Unpublished master's thesis, University of Minnesota, Minneapolis, Minnesota, 1993.

Litchfield MC: *The process of nursing partnership in family health*. Unpublished doctoral thesis, University of Minnesota, Minneapolis, Minnesota, 1997.

Litchfield M, Connor M, Eathorne T, Laws M, McCombie M-L, Smith S: Family nurse practice in a nurse case management scheme: an initiative for the New Zealand health reforms, Wellington, New Zealand 1994, Centre for Initiative in Nursing & Health Care.

Ministry of Health: *Managed Care: Options for New Zealand*. Highlights of the conference held in Wellington, New Zealand, 2-4 May, 1996.

Mooney G, Salmond G: A reflection on the New Zealand reforms, *Health Policy* 29(1,2):173-182, 1994.

National Health Committee: *Fifth annual report to the Minister of Health*, Wellington, New Zealand, 1996, National Health Committee.

New Zealand Nurses' Association: *Policy statement on nursing in New Zealand: new directions in post-basic education*, Wellington, 1976, New Zealand Nurses' Association.

New Zealand Nurses' Association: *Nursing: a social policy statement*, Wellington, 1985, New Zealand Nurses' Association.

New Zealand Nurses' Association: *A process of certification of nurse consultants and clinicians*, Wellington, 1988, New Zealand Nurses' Association.

New Zealand Nurses' Association: *A proposal for career development for nurses in clinical practice*, Wellington, 1991, New Zealand Nurses' Association.

Newman MA: *Health as expanding consciousness*, St Louis, 1986, Mosby.

Newman MA: Toward an integrative model of professional practice, *Journal of Professional Nursing* 6(3):167-173, 1990a.

Newman MA: Newman's theory of health as praxis, *Nursing Science Quarterly*, 3(1):37-41, 1990b.

Newman MA: *Health as expanding consciousness*, ed 2, New York, 1994, National League for Nursing.

Newman MA: Theory of the nurse-client partnership. In Cohen EL, ed: *Nurse case management in the 21st century*, St Louis, 1996, Mosby, pp. 119-123.

Newman MA: Evolution of the theory of health as expanding consciousness, *Nursing Science Quarterly* 10(1):22-25, 1997.

Newman MA, Sime AM, Corcoran-Perry SA: The focus of the discipline of nursing, *Advances in Nursing Science* 14(1):1-6, 1991.

Salmond G: Health sector reform in New Zealand, *British Journal of Health Care Management* 3(2):88-90, 1997.

Seedhouse D, ed: *Reforming health care: the philosophy and practice of international health reform*, Chichester, England, 1995, Wiley.

Steering Group to Oversee Health and Disability Changes: *Implementing the coalition agreement on health*, Wellington, New Zealand, 1997, New Zealand Government.

CHAPTER 35

Value-Added Outcomes

Featuring a Professional Nursing Practice Model

MARY KAY KOHLES, RN, MSW, **WILLIAM G. BAKER, Jr.,** MD, **PAM COWART,** RN, MSN, CCRN, and **JULIE WEBSTER,** RN, MN, CANP

OVERVIEW

The collection, analysis, and reporting of useful information are of major importance as responsibility and accountability for effective and efficient outcomes become the focus of all health care stakeholders, including clinicians, payers, and persons receiving services.

The Piedmont Medical Center in Atlanta, Georgia, designed and implemented Transformation in Care Delivery (TCD), a program that changed roles, work, processes, systems, routines, and services throughout the institution. This program depends on data-driven clinical management and incorporates new physician performance profiles and community clinical case management. Effective physician performance profiles are critical to improving the overall outcomes of physician services. Community clinical case management is essential to coordinating clinical care for medically complex, chronically ill, high-risk persons who utilize multiple health system resources with frequent readmissions. In this program, advanced practice nurses collaborate with key physicians to implement co-designed interventions of care for patients identified through data analysis. A new Professional Nursing Practice Model (PNPM) provides the theoretical framework and guides nursing practice. This chapter highlights the use of clinical management indicators in the TCD program, presents the components of effective physician performance reporting, and describes the PNPM. ▲

Transformation in Care Delivery

Transformation in Care Delivery (TCD) begins with individuals or groups examining current clinical and operational practices and behaviors to determine if person-centered care can achieve increased value-added outcomes. "Person-centered" is defined as the dynamic relationship between the caregiver and care receiver and the institution and all stakeholders. Person centeredness respects the concerns, priorities, wishes, needs, and expectations that the person receiving care and his or her family identify as important to their health. It also embraces respect for the diverse beliefs, values, and practices of the many persons providing care. The care providers represent many disciplines, including physicians, nurses, other health professionals, and those providing support, such as environmental, purchasing, and medical records services. Everyone at Piedmont Medical Center (PMC), clinicians and management, is responsible and accountable for the TCD program, to ensure enhanced value in an atmosphere of person centeredness.

Emphasis on Value

Health care is in a true revolution because economic and market forces are wringing decades of excess supply out of the system and the sacred and highly personal interface between the caregiver and the care receiver is being threatened. The need for proper measurement and reporting of outcomes data is becoming critically important. Although care is still given "one-on-one," the selection and contracting for that care are largely "group-with-group" in a highly impersonal business atmosphere where decisions frequently must be made on the basis of meager data. The collection, analysis, and reporting of useful information are of major importance as responsibility and accountability for effective and efficient outcomes become the focus of all health care stakeholders, including clinicians, payers, and the persons receiving services.

Contemporary health care emphasizes value. Value at PMC is defined as:

$$\text{Value} = \frac{\text{Clinical quality} \times \text{Service quality}}{\text{Cost}}$$

Payers, including managed care companies and employers who purchase health care for their em-ployees, are increasingly focusing attention on key data elements that may include:

- Outcomes, both clinical and functional
- Cost or resource consumption
- Satisfaction surveys, including appropriate access to necessary care

This new focus creates tension for clinicians who primarily seek the best clinical outcome without having to weigh cost components as a major factor in decision making. However, both payers and the clinicians increasingly are recognizing the importance of service satisfaction as perceived by the person receiving care. The clinician must be able to support and articulate clinical quality and service quality along with cost considerations, because of more prevalent use of data by purchasers of health services in choosing where they will purchase health care (Cohen, Cesta, 1997; Kirk, 1997). Data-driven clinical management is the foundation for successful reporting of value-added outcomes that achieve improved clinical and service quality at lower cost (Kohles, Baker, Donaho, 1995). *Value-added outcomes are defined as those outcomes which improve overall organizational performance and enhance quality of life for care receivers and personal and professional satisfaction for care providers.* Data enhance the ability of the clinician to explore alternatives or options of care modalities that will achieve better value for the persons receiving and providing service. These measures may include (Kaplan, Norton, 1996; Kirk, 1997):

- Current performance (outcomes)
- How the performance was achieved (process)
- How performance compares with that of peers within the institution, market area, the region, or the nation (comparative benchmarks)
- Desired performance (organizational, community targets)

The specific use of data in the TCD program at PMC has included analysis of local outcomes in comparison with national, regional, and local benchmarks provided by the Voluntary Hospital Association (VHA), MediQual, and SatisQuest. For physician performance reporting and for the selection of diagnoses (DRGs) for institutional performance-improvement efforts, a software program (Action●Point by MECON) has met the requirement for rapid access to data and conversion to useful information in a timely and attractive

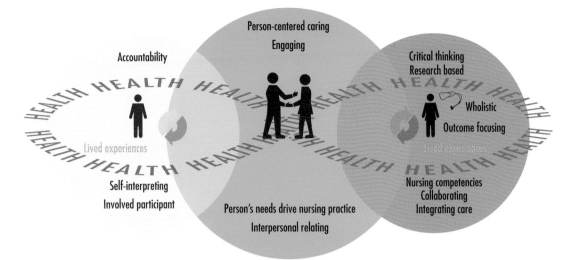

FIGURE 35-1 Conceptual model of professional nursing practice. (Redrawn from Cowart P, Webster J: Piedmont Medical Center Professional Nursing Practice Model, 1997.)

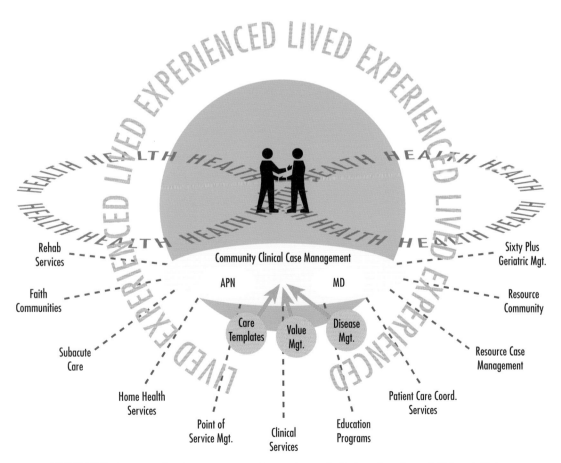

FIGURE 35-2 Community clinical case management integrated network. (Redrawn from Cowart P, Webster J: Piedmont Medical Center Professional Nursing Practice Model, 1997.)

graphical format. This program has guided physician performance reporting over the past year and is providing the focus for identification of the patients who are included in the initial phase of the community clinical case management (CCCM) program. Comparing yearly financial outcomes of the top thirty highest-volume inpatient Medicare DRGs shows that organizational income moved from a loss of $454,526 to a profit of $4,159,505 in one year of physician performance reporting. Over the same time frame, institutional income resulting from the inpatient Medicare practices of thirty-six key physician leaders moved from a loss of $831,941 to a profit of $1,245,903. These results were achieved through reducing resource consumption and decreasing practice pattern variations. A systematic process of reviewing physician performance included aggregating, analyzing, and presenting clinical and cost information based on DRG data with ongoing and regular physician reporting. Clinical pathways were selected and constructed by multidisciplinary teams for those diagnoses with wide variations in value outcomes, and community clinical case management (CCCM) patients who consumed a high number of resources were selected in DRGs with opportunities for value improvement in comparison to benchmarks.

Physicians are traditionally viewed as the ultimate locus of control within the health care system, particularly in the acute care and chronic care settings, and the responsibility and accountability for outcomes of value clearly have rested with them. However, with the emphasis on improving performance, they increasingly are delegating care to other health professionals and assuming shared responsibility and accountability with the entire caregiver team. They also recognize the importance of self-management by the person receiving care and his or her family and understand that often it is the nurse or other health professional who can best influence this outcome. CCCM nurses, in collaboration with key high-performance physicians, are defining who is responsible and accountable for which value-added outcomes. The nurse and the physician combine their knowledge bases and skills to influence a desired value-added outcome for the person receiving service. This is the basis for PMC to be able to report value-added indicators to payers who are identifying providers with the

best clinical and functional outcomes, cost performance, and satisfaction.

Principles of Effective Physician Performance Reporting

Profiles of physician performance are highly useful in improving effectiveness and efficiency of care, but only if used in the proper setting. *The most effective use of physician profile reporting occurs in an educational atmosphere of nonpunitive mutual trust and respect between the persons giving and receiving the reports.* The sending of performance profiles to practitioners without proper preparation usually has the sole effect of putting them on notice that they are being observed, and little positive behavior change results. In fact, defensive and negative reactions may ensue as a result of improper preparation. Before reports are actually sent, education regarding the health care marketplace emphasizing the increasing power of consumer choice will significantly improve physician receptivity. If physicians are convinced that patients and payers are seeking value-added outcomes and that they must learn how to demonstrate those outcomes to survive, and even thrive, they will become enthusiastic participants in the process. There are four main uses or objectives of physician performance profiles:

1. *Education:* Physicians readily accept measures that are collected, analyzed, and reported in a positive and friendly manner, with emphasis on helping the practitioner improve care. If profiles are used for economic credentialing or sanctioning, a confrontational conflict likely will ensue, with an undesirable outcome.

2. *Continuous value improvement:* Sharing information for continuous process improvement in a positive atmosphere will assist in enlisting physician involvement in initiatives underway for improving the value in health care outcomes.

3. *Financial incentives:* Many managed care organizations use outcomes data to increase physician compensation through either withholding pay to be returned or granting a bonus if predetermined performance measures are attained. In addition, more favorable capitation

> **BOX 35-1**
>
> ## Principles of Effective Physician Performance Profiles
>
> | | |
> |---|---|
> | Why? | To increase value-added outcomes |
> | What? | Clinical quality, including functional outcomes |
> | | Service satisfaction, including access |
> | | Resource consumption |
> | Data? | Correct |
> | | Current |
> | | Confidential |
> | How? | Peer-comparison data |
> | | Severity/case mix adjusted |
> | | Exclusion of outliers |
> | When? | Regularly |
> | | Ongoing |
> | Where? | Mail (general) |
> | | Personal (specific) |
> | Who? | By a respected physician |

payments usually can be negotiated by practitioners who can demonstrate effective and efficient outcomes.

4. *Marketing:* Those practitioners or provider systems who have reliable and desirable outcomes may be able to use their profiles in marketing their practices to secure more favorable contracts.

The components of effective physician performance profiles are presented in Box 35-1 and include why, what, data, how, when, and who.

WHY

The major purpose of reporting performance is to change physician behavior, resulting in improved value-added outcomes.

WHAT

To focus on value, data must include measurements on clinical quality, including functional outcomes; service satisfaction, including access (availability and timeliness); and resource utilization. These data must be presented in an attractive, preferably graphical, format with the ability to answer quickly the multitude of questions that predictably will

arise in any personal reporting session. The focus will usually revolve around financial or resource-consumption comparisons, and the ability to "drill down" to specific patient records and demonstrate how unit-level charges or costs are accrued through a personal practice pattern is the key to maintaining the physician's attention and inducing a motivation to alter long-standing inefficient habits.

DATA

Physicians quite naturally will question the validity and timeliness of the data used to construct their profiles and must be convinced that the information is correct, usually through their own efforts to confirm the statistics. Confidentiality of any practitioner-specific data is an absolute requirement, and nothing must be shared about a colleague without a specific written release by him or her to do so.

HOW

If a physician is able to see and be convinced that his or her performance in peer-comparison data is unfavorably at variance with that of his or her peers, an almost instant resolve to improve is observable. This is particularly impressive if the practitioner can identify those peers with whom he or she wishes to be compared. Another essential requirement is that the data be severity/case mix adjusted to account for the inherent selection differences in the unique population base cared for by that practitioner. In addition, as personal reports are being given, the ability to discuss patient-specific data that may indicate that the case is a true outlier or that the physician did not have complete control over the cost is vital. The discussants may agree that the individual case is a true outlier and needs to be removed from the profile results. The ability to do so and instantly recalculate the data provides an additional powerful incentive for the physician to accept and to act on the data.

WHEN

If physicians have received effective preparation and have confidence that the data are correct, current, and being presented confidentially, regular and ongoing mailed reports of general outcomes are effective, preferably quarterly. A cover letter should accompany each report, noting specific opportunities for improvement and inviting the recipient to come for a personal discussion of the outcomes, at which time more detailed patient-specific and unit-level costs can be presented.

WHO

A respected physician, preferably one who has had actual practice experience, is the most effective person to lead the performance profile initiative. Profiles for health care professionals other than physicians who are implementing case management models also are important. Computerized data elements, using software such as Action•Point by MECON, eventually will be designed to include monitoring capabilities for advanced practice nurses who are primary providers of service through the CCCM. As the development of these data elements emerges, it will be important for these nurses to identify service interventions based on nursing practice along with expected value-added indicators.

Professional Nursing Practice Model

An innovative Professional Nursing Practice Model (PNPM) was developed at PMC to provide guidance for nursing documentation of care, decision making related to clinical practice, and communication for establishing nursing practice standards. The model encompasses a unique wholistic* perspective of caring for the person, family, and important others and embraces a person-centered philosophy that respects the priorities and needs as defined by the person receiving care while valuing the priorities and needs of those giving the care. The model provides infrastructure defining the attributes that guide the practice of the professional nurse. These attributes provide the bases for the synergistic relationship between the nurse and the person receiving care as well as the relationship with other care providers, including the physician, other health professionals, and support workers.

The PNPM was developed through a compre-

hensive review of the research and writings of many different nursing theorists. The perspectives of three, whose views closely reflect the desired practice of nursing at PMC, were selected as the foundation for the PNPM. These theorists are Patricia Benner, primacy of caring (Benner, Wrabel 1989); Rosemarie Rizzo Parse, the human becoming theory (Parse, 1992); and Jean Watson, the human science of caring (Watson, 1988). Based on the perspectives of these theorists and PMC nurses about their definitions of nursing practice, the theoretical framework for the PNPM emerged. The model defines concepts of nursing, person, and health by describing the attributes of each.

NURSING

Nursing is a synergistic relationship between the nurse and the person receiving care. Persons receiving care include the family and/or important others participating in the care process. Synergy is the interaction of two persons who come together in a care process. This relationship results in a care outcome that is different from and superior to one that either the nurse or the person receiving care could accomplish alone. Nursing practice is centered around *being with* (Parse, 1992) the person in his or her lived experience of health (Benner, Wrubel, 1989; Parse, 1992). The PNPM defines the key attributes of nursing as thinking critically, practicing based on research, viewing wholistically, focusing on outcomes, nursing based on fundamental competencies, collaborating, and integrating care. These features support the nurse in providing a wholistic and systematic assessment with the person receiving care to achieve health as defined by the person receiving care (Parse, 1992).

PERSON RECEIVING CARE

Nursing approaches the person receiving care as someone who is accountable for his or her perception of health and the decisions he or she makes to alter it. A patient is a person; therefore, nurses intentionally do not use the term *patient*, which labels the person as being ill. The family and important others are also recognized as integral in caring for the person (Benner, Wrubel, 1989; Watson, 1988). Nursing practice acknowledges the person as a self-interpreting individual and an involved participant, moving synergistically with the nurse toward

---

*The spelling is symbolic of the fact the person should be seen as a whole.

maintaining or improving his or her own quality of life. Self-interpreting means that the person does not come into the world predefined, but becomes defined in the course of living his or her life (Benner, Wrubel, 1989; Heidegger, 1962).

HEALTH

Health is the lived experience perceived by the person, encompassing all of the qualities of his or her emotional, spiritual, and physical life. It is conceptualized and symbolized in the PNPM as an infinity sign because health is not a linear entity that can be qualified by terms such as more or less. A person conceptualizes his or her own meaning of health (Parse, 1992) on the basis of lived experiences, which include cultural heritage, religious or spiritual beliefs, family values, and other factors.

PERSON-NURSE RELATIONSHIP

This relationship joins the attributes of the person and the nurse in a person-centered philosophy of care. Mutual acknowledgment of each others' lived experience is desirable, but it is essential to the person-nurse relationship that the nurse acknowledge the person's lived experience. The needs and priorities of the person receiving care are recognized and honored when true synergistic person-centered caring takes place. The synergistic force of the relationship binds together the person and the nurse in an integrated, goal-oriented movement toward mutual understanding of health as defined by the person receiving care.

The PNPM provides a synergistic relationship in which both the nurse and the person have accountability for outcomes resulting from the caregiving process. The model (shown in Figure 35-1, p. 319) symbolically is represented by two smaller outer circles merging together to create a larger inner circle. The larger inner circle reflects the interaction of the nurse and the person, whose combined effect is greater than their individual effects. The model is represented by colors; the outside nurse circle is blue, and the person (involved participant) circle is yellow; these circles blend and overlap into green to symbolize the fusion of the two. Circular arrows at each interface represent the experiences that each person continuously brings and takes from the relationship.

Nursing Knowledge

Nursing care frequently is viewed as rank-ordered tasks requiring different levels of skill and having different associated costs; this view slowly is becoming a myth. Nursing practice rightly is being redefined by its own distinct body of knowledge, which provides a new basis for identifying and demonstrating the importance of the nurse-person relational process. Nurses are co-creating a new practice that increases benefits to them and the persons for whom they care. PMC nurses now confirm their unique body of knowledge by living out the person-nurse process, guided by the theoretical framework. The tasks and procedures performed by nurses are different in each care setting and constantly change as new technologies are developed and new disciplines are established. The Piedmont Medical Center PNPM emphasizes that tasks and procedures are not the core of nursing practice; the core lies in the knowledge that guides the person-nurse relationship.

Community Clinical Case Management

Community Clinical Case Management is a program that improves the management of medically complex, chronically ill, high-risk persons who utilize multiple health system resources. These persons require ongoing health assessments and psychological support. The theoretical framework for this program is grounded in the PNPM. Persons receiving care are viewed as self-interpreting individuals. Their lived experience of chronic illness is complicated by diverse elements such as health, social, emotional, economical, and spiritual issues.

CCCM recognizes and honors each individual person's lived experience, recognizing that health is the quality of life as the person defines it. The advanced practice nurse (clinical nurse specialist and/or nurse practitioner) in this role approaches care situations with a person-centered philosophy, which stimulates the creation of a healthy relationship by providing ongoing health assessment, monitoring, and education. The advanced practice nurse possesses the expert knowledge and communication skills that are essential in caring for a person across the continuum. The model of CCCM, shown in Figure 35-2, p. 319, is supported by an integrated network of PMC resources, including Dis-

BOX 35-2
Case Study

Ms. B is a 91-year-old widow who has chronic congestive heart failure (CHF), chronic obstructive pulmonary disease (COPD), Crohn's disease, diabetes mellitus, and chronic anemia. She lives alone in an independent living center for senior adults. Her only family, a son and a daughter-in-law, live over 400 miles away, limiting their involvement in her care to urgent and emergent situations. Ms. B ambulates with assistance from a walker, and, along with many oral medications, she is on almost continuous oxygen therapy. However, with the exception of bathing, she cares for herself. Commenting on feeling fatigued and short of breath following any activity, she says, "I cannot go on living like this; I want to be able to do the things I want and not be limited by my [shortness of] breath and chest pain, and be as independent as possible for as long as I can." She is very frustrated with her declining health. When asked how a CCCM nurse could be helpful, she said, "I want to be able to leave my apartment to visit my friends." Prior to CCCM visits, Ms. B was unable to leave her apartment because she could not manage both the walker and the oxygen tank. The CCCM nurse arranged with the oxygen home care vendor to provide a small transportable oxygen unit that attached to the walker, so she now can leave her apartment, meet with friends, and do other activities that are important to maintain her independence. In addition, Ms. B is on a low-salt diet. She had been relying on preprepared frozen meals because of minimal preparation requirements. The CCCM nurse dis-

cussed dietary guidelines and arranged for a telephone assessment by a cardiac dietitian. She now is selecting and preparing frozen foods that are more appropriate for her health needs, and "enjoying the food much more." She recently developed chronic myelodysplastic anemia, and the CCCM nurse arranged for monthly outpatient transfusions. Ms. B was quite reluctant to initiate phone calls or even discuss her problems in person with her primary care physician, stating: "He can't do anything more for me." The CCCM nurse encouraged calls and meets her in the physician's office to facilitate communication and strengthen the understanding by the physician of Ms. B's needs as she perceives them. Since Ms. B's family lives at such a distance, she is using home care services to transport her for transfusion and physician office visits. The CCCM nurse helped her identify these services and set up taxi transportation on an urgent basis. The CCCM nurse visits with Ms. B weekly to assess her general well-being, lung sounds, edema, and blood pressure and to titrate her diuretics as needed. Prior to the CCCM visits, Ms. B had seven inpatient admissions in seven months, with an average length of stay of 4.6 days. Weekly CCCM visits were initiated, and over the next five months, she had only one, three-day admission, to general care rather than intensive care, with four outpatient visits for transfusion, and frequent titrations of diuretics for CHF. Ms. B states, "I am more independent, and I feel like someone cares about me; I have hope now."

ease Management, Value (Resource Utilization) Management, Care Templates (Pathways), and Point-of-Service Management (acute care episode). Care is coordinated through the continuum by a collaborative approach among the advanced practice nurse, the physician, and the person receiving care.

PATIENT SELECTION

CCCM is focused on those patient populations that will benefit most from specific personal care

management as defined by prior data analysis. Initial patient groups for CCCM were identified by retrospective analysis of cost, length of stay, and multiple readmissions into the acute care setting by using the software program Action•Point by MECON. The initial two populations that showed the best opportunity for increasing value-added outcomes were persons with congestive heart failure (CHF) and persons with chronic obstructive pulmonary disease (COPD). Projections of potential cost avoidance on readmission alone in these patients were calculated by using retrospec-

BOX 35-3

Outcome Indicators After 4 Months of CCCM (N = 27 Persons Receiving Service)

Readmission—Avoidance
Medication adjustment—21 episodes
Initiated home oxygen therapy—2 episodes
End-of-life care at home—2 patients

Readmission—Decrease Acuity of Symptoms
Four readmissions to general care unit
   One COPD episode: LOS of 3 days (pre-CCCM avg. LOS 5.58 days)
   Two CHF episodes: avg. LOS of 5 days (pre-CCCM avg. LOS 5 days)
   One CHF/COPD episode: LOS 13 days (patient had a sustained admission to complete diagnostic procedures for oncology)
   One readmission to an intermediate care unit
   One CHF episode: total LOS 6 days (new diagnosis)

Point of Access—Appropriate Visit
Outpatient visits versus inpatient stays—5 visits
Physician office visit versus emergency room visits—10 visits

Community Services—Enhanced Usage
Parish nursing—1 episode
Meals on Wheels—2 episodes
Home care—2 referrals
Geriatric case management—2 referrals
Collaboration with home care and geriatric case management—22 episodes

Person Centeredness/Quality of Life—Perceived by the Person
Improve activity (ambulation, social experiences)—15 patients
Improve nutrition—19 patients
Improve medication self-administration—27 patients
Improve self-care as expressed by the person—27 patients
Improve satisfaction with living as expressed by the person—25 patients

Estimated Cost Avoidance: $75,000

tive financial data for a six-month time frame and are estimated on the combined populations to be at least $200,000 per year.

PHYSICIAN PARTNERSHIP

After target populations were selected, best practice physicians with the highest value outcomes in patients with these diagnoses were identified and enlisted as partners with advanced practice nurses in the delivery of care. The advanced practice nurses and the physicians together determined many of the CCCM interventions, such as medication adjustment, nutritional and functional assessment, oxygen therapy, health education, and use of community services. They are collaborating in the co-creation of a care management program specific to each person selected, and ongoing measures of value outcomes are being collected and trended.

CCCM OUTCOMES

The advanced practice nurse providing care through the CCCM is using data-driven clinical management reports from Action●Point to evaluate patient care outcomes. In addition to the commonly measured outcomes of cost, length of stay, and recidivism, CCCM is measuring other quantitative and qualitative outcomes, such as admission acuity, appropriateness and timeliness of health care access, matching of the person's needs with available community services, and person centeredness/quality of life, including functional and physiological outcomes and personal satisfaction. The case study in Box 35-2 exemplifies the person-nurse relationship, showing the outcomes that are valued by the person receiving service. CCCM nurses and physicians are using data-driven clinical management reports to discuss the effectiveness of interventions for the person receiving service. Although CCCM is still in an evaluation phase, the program has demonstrated a cost avoidance of at least $75,000 for PMC as shown by the outcome indicators for 17 CHF patients and 10 COPD patients over 4 months (Box 35-3). All patients express satisfaction with the services provided by the CCCM nurse, and most show an improvement in their quality of life by increased activity and socialization with others outside their living environments. As one person stated, "I feel I am not alone with my illness and somebody cares." Physicians indicate satisfaction with the collaborative efforts for many reasons, ranging from their improved performance profiles to the patient's functional status. Physician performance profiles for CCCM patients show reduced cost per admission and improved utilization of outpatient resources. Since these patients are encouraged to visit their primary care physicians on a regular basis, a physician can more appropriately manage a patient's functional and physiological status. The CCCM nurse often joins the patient during these office visits; physician, nurse, and patient together therefore are able to define the responsibility and accountability for each mutually defined value-added outcome. The advanced practice nurses also express great satisfaction with their roles, since they portray the importance of nursing knowledge as an essential component for projecting and achieving both quantitative and qualitative value-added outcomes. Interventions carried out by the CCCM nurse are guided by the collaborative nurse-physician care plan involving the person and family, thereby stressing the importance of the fact that "what care is needed" must include the patient's perspective. The advanced practice nurse plays a profoundly stronger role in this process as responsibility and accountability for outcomes are shared by the physician, the advanced practice nurse, and the patient in an environment of person centeredness.

Conclusion

Piedmont Medical Center is using data analysis and reporting to increase value-added outcomes for all stakeholders within the institution and the community it serves. Data are the basis for physician performance reporting and for Community Clinical Case Management using a new and innovative Professional Nursing Practice Model. The practical application of this model and the principles of conversion of data into information useful in achieving value-added outcomes have been discussed.

References

Benner P, Wrubel J: *The primacy of caring: stress and coping in health and illness,* Menlo Park, Calif, 1989, Addison-Wooley.

Cohen EL, Cesta TG: *Nursing case management: from concept to evaluation,* ed 2, St Louis, 1997, Mosby.

Heidegger M: *Being and time,* Macquarrie J, Robinson M, trans, New York, 1962, Harper & Brothers.

Kaplan RS, Norton DP: *The balanced scorecard,* Boston 1996, Harvard Business School Press.

Kirk R: *Managing outcomes, process, and cost in a managed care environment,* Miami, 1997, Aspen.

Kohles MK, Baker WG, Donaho B: *Transformational leadership: renewing fundamental values and achieving new relationships in health care,* Chicago, 1995, American Hospital Association.

Parse RR: *Illuminations: the human becoming theory in practice and research,* New York, 1995, National League for Nursing.

Watson J: *Nursing: human science and human care,* New York, 1988, National League for Nursing.-

CHAPTER 36

The Ethics of Case Management

Communication Challenges

ROBERT J. BARNET, MD, MA, **and Sr. CAROL TAYLOR,** RN, PhD, CSFN

OVERVIEW

Our once unquestioned commitment to patient well-being is being tested in systems that seem to value profit over care.

Trusting relationships are essential to good health care outcomes. Effective relationships are the product of good communication skills. This chapter describes the characteristics of ethical communication, contrasts models of health care decision making, explores the case manager's role in communicating to mediate ethical conflict and to secure informed consent, and concludes with a brief discussion of attitudes that impair optimal communication. Practical exercises invite reflection and the application of basic communication principles to practice situations. ▲

There is an ethical dimension to each clinical encounter. *How* a case manager chooses to communicate with a patient, patient's family member, colleague, or payer, as well as *if* a case manager chooses to communicate, can have profound ethical significance. At stake is the other party's sense of personal well-being and confidence in the health care system, valued outcomes, and our own professional integrity. Good interpersonal skills are essential for case managers. Unfortunately these skills are often simply assumed to be operative even when grossly deficient. "We are all skilled communicators, right?" "Never at a loss for words . . ." And then there is the problem of the skilled communicators caught in the demand to "work harder, smarter, and faster," who wonder if they can reconcile their desire to be successful with their commitment to good communication.

These problems are exacerbated by the conflicting roles being imposed on case managers: quality advocate and cost-cutter, gate-keeper and facilitator. Underlying the role conflicts are value conflicts. Our once unquestioned commitment to patient well-being is being tested in systems that seem to value profit over care. The communication that builds trusting relationships is often labor and time intensive. Those who value cost containment and efficiency above all else are suspicious of those committed to optimal communication. At issue is whether it is morally justified to consider optimal communication a "frill" for those who can afford to pay "a little extra" rather than a nonnegotiable of health care for all. We believe that communication is essential to good patient outcomes and central to the role of the case manager. It is unethical for case managers to be deficient in communication. Failures to use communication to adequately determine patient need, develop plans of care that are consistent with practice guidelines (individualized, prioritized, holistic, attainable, and affordable), and coordinate the multidisciplinary team's best efforts to secure necessary resources are negligent and unethical.

Optimal Communication

Communication between health care professionals and patients is important not only because patients have a "right to know" and be involved in (some

would say, "to direct") health care decision making (i.e., procedural criteria), but also because their informed participation is essential to good patient outcomes (i.e., substantive criteria). Similarly, good communication among the members of a multidisciplinary team and increasingly between the team and payers is linked to better patient outcomes. Communication in the past was generally unidirectional: health care professionals spoke and dictated a plan of action, "good" patients complied, and payers paid. Today communication is multidirectional: health care professionals offer information and may make a recommendation, payers dictate which options are reimbursable, and patients or their surrogates make choices often after elaborate consultation processes. Current factors influencing health care professional–patient communication include the public's decreased trust in medicine and the health care system, the increasing difficulty of weighing complex diagnostic and therapeutic options, and a better educated and more medically sophisticated public.

Situated as a bridge between a patient/family and a complex network of health care professionals, other resources, and payers, case managers play a vital role in promoting optimal communication on all sides. The situation described in Box 36-1 illustrates how case managers can influence outcomes by encouraging patients and family members to actively collaborate in decision making by encouraging health care professionals to truly listen to patients and their stories, as well as by inviting health care companies into the dialogue about how best to meet patient needs in constructive ways.

Ethical Communication

The characteristics of ethical communication between health care professionals and patients are described below and listed in Box 36-2. Facilitating and impeding forces are noted.

AFFIRMS DIGNITY AND PROMOTES AUTONOMY AND WELL-BEING

The nineteenth-century philosopher John Stuart Mill (1859) argued that each person is the best judge of his or her own good and ought to be free to make his or her own choice. Personal freedom is essential

BOX 36-1
Case Study Promoting Communication

Tom was a 55-year-old attorney who suffered from multiple disabilities, including life-threatening arrhythmias that were not controlled by standard medications. Unwilling to accept defeat, Tom's attending insisted that he try an experimental drug available through participation in a clinical trial being conducted at a prestigious medical center some 200 miles away. When Tom asked what would happen if he chose not to participate, his doctor refused to comment.

Tom's wife, Jill, was a skilled researcher with a doctorate in anthropology and a subscription to *The New England Journal of Medicine*. She knew the current literature better than Tom's doctor and the ever-changing medical staff.

Both Tom and Jill complained to the case manager. They rejected the idea that they should accept without question a regimen laid out without consideration for their personal values and priorities. Their case manager affirmed their desire to be active and valuable decision-making partners and invited the attending to listen to their concerns. What followed were 2 years of fruitful collaboration before Tom's death.

Tom never did try the experimental drug but enjoyed a quality of life that was acceptable to him and to Jill. Tom's attending confided to the case manager that while he was initially intimidated by Jill because she came into the office with the latest articles and a yellow notepad in hand, he learned to value their sessions and felt professionally good about the outcomes. "I've learned the importance of listening with more than a stethoscope."

Since Tom was a bit of an "outlier," his treatment never quite fit the standard plans. Ongoing communication with his managed care company was essential to securing approval for needed services.

BOX 36-2
Characteristics of Ethical Communication

Characteristics of Ethical Communication Between Health Care Professionals and Patients
- Affirms the dignity and worth of each party
- Reflects a commitment to the patient's well-being
- Promotes the patient's autonomy (right to be self-determining)
- Maintains confidentiality
- Reflects a commitment to truthfulness and trust building
- Respects diversity of values and priorities

Facilitating Forces
- Mutual trust
- Belief that good communication is essential to good patient outcomes
- Willingness to value communication process sufficiently to allocate to it scarce time resources
- Setting is conducive to the sharing of information that may at times be highly personal or private
- Staffing patterns allow sufficient time to be spent with each patient/family
- Congruence between verbal and nonverbal messages (e.g., "My body doesn't say, 'I'm busy, don't bother me' when my voice is asking, 'How may I help you?'")

Impeding Forces
- Task rather than person orientation on the part of the health care professional
- Low priority assigned to interpersonal communication
- Lack of trust
- Lack of privacy
- Staffing patterns fail to allow sufficient time to be spent with each patient/family

to being truly human. Rational beings are self-determining or self-governing. For Mill, autonomy or self-determination was essential to human development and happiness. Autonomy may be restricted only to prevent harm to others. The underlying presumption is that each individual is uniquely qualified to decide about what is in his or her best interest. This idea is rooted in the recognition of the dignity and worth of the person. To deny autonomy is to treat someone as less than a fully rational person.

RESPECTS CONFIDENTIALITY

For centuries patients expected, with good reason, that their medical histories and personal health information would remain confidential. Our obligation to respect confidential information is rooted in each patient's right to privacy. This arrangement allows patients to freely share the personal information necessary for health care planning. In recent years the maintenance of confidentiality has become increasingly difficult. As early as 1982 physician-ethicist Mark Siegler noted that as many as 72 different individuals had access to medical records in a university hospital (Siegler, 1982). Since then, there has been even greater access, with health care conglomerates depending on computerized record systems and government attempts to monitor quality and prevent fraud. Although it is increasingly difficult to maintain privacy, case managers should know the limits to privacy and ensure that patients likewise understand these limits. Without an honest sharing concerning these limits, trust is undermined. Recorded information should be accurate and relevant, and reflect concern for the privacy and dignity of the client.

IS TRUTHFUL AND BUILDS TRUST

The example found in Box 36-3 emphasizes the problems of withholding the truth, even from a child, and the importance of relationships built on truthfulness and trust. This scenario underlines the importance of finding solutions that involve open communication and trust among team members, patients, and families. It invites us to reflect on whether our usual styles of communicating invite trust and demonstrate trustworthiness.

BOX 36-3
Case Study   Truthtelling and Trust

Susi was a 10-year-old with terminal cancer. She had been on the oncology unit for 3 weeks when her physician, Dr. Moore, told her parents and the staff that he did not believe Susi had more than a month to live. He recommended that she remain in the hospital, since her palliative care regimen was complex and her parents had three younger children at home. Her parents' health plan agreed to cover this stay. After painful discussions, the parents agreed with this plan, but insisted that Susi not be told of the seriousness of her condition. Dr. Moore agreed and left explicit, written and verbal orders that Susi not be told that she was dying.

Three weeks later, Susi became very weak, had more pain, and was nauseated from her medication. She had become especially close to her case manager, Joan, who often snatched moments to visit and share a joke or simple conversation. Late one evening, Susi began to cry and told Joan, "I know I can trust you. I'm going to die, aren't I?" Immediately Joan regretted her early decision not to challenge the family and physician's decisions to withhold the truth from Susi. Joan could not lie to Susi, but this now entailed, at least implicitly, breaking the confidence Susi's parents and physician had placed in her. Joan knew that she had to confront everyone . . . and wondered what the long-term consequences would be. While Joan did not want to deceive Susi, and could not, she was also unhappy with the prospect that she might not be trusted in the future.

RESPECTS DIVERSITY

Each person is unique and makes choices in light of "goods." What constitutes an acceptable quality of life can vary dramatically from one individual to the next. Individuals differ in the need to be in control and to be comfortable, and in productivity, mobility, health, wealth, and ability to communicate. Diversity is also evident in gender, race, ethnicity, socioeconomic status, education, life experience, body size, and physical appearance. A critical characteristic of ethical communication is its respect for diversity. It is instructive to step back from clinical practice and evaluate the degree to which any kind of diversity makes a caregiver respond to a patient differently, whether positively or negatively. Are there some patients for whom caregivers are willing to go to extremes and others for whom caregivers will do nothing? If a camera captured all of your patient communication during the day, would it reveal a difference in the way you interact with different patients? Are you more or less respectful because of certain elements of diversity for which you have assigned a particular meaning?

Decision-Making Models

There are at least three distinct models to guide health care decision making. While these are described differently in the literature, we will use the designations strong paternalism, independent choice, and enhanced autonomy. Quill and Brody (1996) contrasted the independent choice and enhanced autonomy models in a recent article, and we join them in recommending the enhanced autonomy model as most suited to the objectives of case management. This model is respectful of patient freedom and obligates health care professionals to provide all the information and support necessary to ensure decision making that advances the patient's welfare. Box 36-4 compares the three models. It is useful, when you are experiencing ethical conflict about treatment goals and options, to determine whether different styles of decision making among team members and between the team and the patient/family are contributing to the conflict. A strongly paternalistic physician will inevitably spark conflict with an independent-choice-model patient. Strong communication skills are needed to mediate this type of conflict.

Physician and psychoanalyst Jay Katz (1984) explores the issues of conversation and understanding in his now classic text, *The Silent World of Doctor and Patient*. His formula for meaningful decision making includes the following four aspects:

1. The initial perspective should include not just a recognition of the patient's freedom to make his or her own decision, but also a *reflection* on those rational and irrational determinants

that are involved for both patient and physician.
2. There should be recognition that the patient is a mature adult rather than a dependent "child."
3. It is important to cultivate the *art of conversation* so as to facilitate the patient's assimilation of information. This requires an exploration of patient values and preferences.
4. There should be an acknowledgment by physicians and others in health care of the uncertainty and limitations of medicine.

Informed Consent

Informed consent began as a legal imperative that protected clinicians from charges of assault and battery. In the 1950s it received international attention because of the abuses associated with human experimentation in concentration camps during World War II. The concept of informed consent as it is understood today was strengthened by the rise in autonomy in the 1960s. It now applies not just to experimentation, but to any significant medical intervention. It is appropriate to consider formal consent when a planned procedure is intrusive, when there are significant risks, or when the purpose or expected results of the procedure or treatment are unclear or questionable.

While informed consent as a legal imperative often degenerates into a minimalist, read-this-and-sign-on-the-dotted-line requirement, informed consent as a moral imperative involves far more. The President's Commission for the Study of Ethical Problems in Medicine and Behavioral Research (1982) lists four requirements for informed consent: capacity of the patient, disclosure of information, comprehension, and freedom. Case managers have a role to play in securing each.

First, their ongoing relationships with patients enable them to participate in judgments about the patient's decision-making capacity, to ensure the documentation of these judgments, to notify the team when changes in a patient's condition impair capacity, and to secure the identity of a legally and morally valid surrogate for patients who lack decision-making capacity.

Second, case managers can ensure that patients and their surrogates receive all the information they need, in a language they understand, to make deci-

BOX 36-4
Three Decision-Making Models

Strong Paternalism Model
1. The relationship is health care professional centered and based on beneficence.
2. Health care professional knowledge and expertise dominate.
3. Health care professional control is central.
4. Health care professional experience and values, even when questioned, are rarely challenged.
5. There is no meaningful dialogue and only limited discussion.
6. The patient abdicates responsibility to health care professionals.
7. The decision is the responsibility of health care professionals.

Independent Choice Model
1. The relationship is patient or client centered and based on respect for autonomy.
2. The patient's experience and values dominate.
3. Patient independence and control are central.
4. Patient experience and values may remain unquestioned and unchallenged.
5. The health care professional is a passive informer who relates data, options, and outcomes; he or she does not seek to influence the decision.
6. The health care professional abdicates responsibility to the patient.

7. The decision is the responsibility of the patient or the patient's surrogate.

Enhanced Autonomy Model
1. The process is relationship centered, involves mutual trust, and promotes enhanced autonomy and beneficence.
2. Knowledge and expertise are shared.
3. Collaboration between the patient and the health care professional is central.
4. Patient and health care professional experience and values are brought to bear on the decision at hand; patient competence and vulnerability are acknowledged, and understanding is promoted.
5. The process involves an open dialogue with an exchange of information and values; the health care professional is an involved and active guide.
6. Responsibility is shared.
7. The decision is the responsibility of the patient or the patient's surrogate; health care professionals are responsible to provide the support and to acknowledge patients' and surrogates' need to make the decision that is right for them.

Modified from Quill TE, Brody H: Recommendations and patient autonomy: finding a balance between physician power and patient choice, *Ann Intern Med* 125(9):763-769, 1996.

sions that truly advance their interests. They should be informed of the nature of their illness, the purpose of the planned intervention, the risks and benefits of treatment options and nontreatment, and their likely prognosis with and without treatment. Most families also want to know what it will mean for them realistically to "walk down" the path of each option in light of their values and preferences. The reason the "gag rules" that characterized some managed care organizations were so morally offensive to many health care professionals was that they made it impossible to provide the information necessary for autonomous decision making. Understandably, much state and federal legislation has moved to ban gag rules that compromise adequate disclosure.

Third, case managers can ensure comprehension by inviting patients to describe in their own words what has been disclosed to them. Until they hear an accurate report, health care professionals can only hope that patients have understood what they were told. This essential step in informed consent is frequently overlooked.

Physician-ethicist Samuel Gorovitz (1982) illustrated its importance when he related the following story. A conscientious surgeon carefully explained to a mother that her child had a heart problem (septal defect) requiring surgery. He took the time to draw a schematic diagram of the heart, showing that the unnatural opening between the two heart chambers could be closed with ease. When a surgical resident visited the mother the next morning and asked her if she understood what was going to be done and why, she replied that she did. To be sure, he then asked her to explain this in her own words. Remembering the diagram, the mother replied, "The problem is that my baby has a square heart." While this mother probably understood enough to give consent, the story dramatically shows how differently a physician and a patient can interpret the same language and the same visual image.

Finally, case managers have a role to play in ensuring that decisions are truly made voluntarily. This is facilitated when one has developed the types of relationships that make it possible to detect obvious and subtle coercive forces. Coercion may result from the power wielded intentionally or unintentionally by health care professionals, family members, or other individuals known by the patient.

While informed and voluntary consent is generally considered in the context of intrusive diagnostic and therapeutic interventions and research, its underlying principles apply well to the decision making case managers facilitate when working with individuals and groups who are making choices about health plans, clinician preferences, treatment settings, and lifestyle modifications. Box 36-5 describes an informed consent situation in which a case manager might have intervened to secure better outcomes for a family.

Communication and Ethical Dilemmas

Optimal communication is also essential to the prevention and resolution of complex ethical problems. Case managers who are advocates for patients and families frequently find themselves mediating conflict between the patient and the family or among members of the health care team, the patient, and outside parties. The case manager's willingness to become involved, patience in working to uncover hidden sources of conflict, ability to tap resources, and success in getting conflicted parties to collaborate will contribute dramatically to a

> ### BOX 36-5
> ## Informed Consent
>
> The young parents of an acutely ill infant were visited by a charming and articulate surgeon, who quickly convinced them of their baby's serious condition and the need for surgery. Both parents had a tenth-grade education, and neither was working at the time. The physician was a university professor. The parents were clearly worried about their baby and acquiesced immediately to the physician's recommendation; when asked to sign a consent form, they did so without question or hesitation. The child was operated on unnecessarily and died after 14 operative procedures, many of which were painful. He spent months in the PICU. Unknown to the couple, the physician had falsified his credentials and was currently under active investigation. The legal requirements for informed consent were "somewhat" met in this situation, although there were caregivers who questioned at the outset whether surgery was indicated, and whether the parents had the support they needed to reach a truly informed and voluntary decision. Most problematic was that the hospital enforced a "conspiracy of silence" after the infant's death, and the parents' requests for information about what went wrong went unanswered.
>
> 1. If you were the case manager for this infant, how might you have intervened? How might the outcomes have been different with a successful intervention?
> 2. What specific communication skills would best ensure the success of the case manager's intervention?
> 3. Would you judge a case manager to be ethically justified in choosing not to intervene both at the outset and after the infant's death?

dilemma's resolution. Even more important, once good communication skills become the norm, a health care team is well on its way to preventing recurring ethical problems and dilemmas. It is critical to remember that good people can reason differently about what is the "right thing" to do in complex situations. Ethically relevant considerations, in mediating conflict, include the following (Fletcher, 1995):

- Balancing benefits and harms in the care of patients
- Disclosure, informed consent, and shared decision making
- The norms of family life
- The relationships between clinicians and patients
- The professional integrity of clinicians
- Cost effectiveness and allocation
- Issues of cultural and religious variation
- Considerations of power

The four scenarios found in Box 36-6 can be used to determine your skill in communicating to resolve ethical problems.

Barriers to Optimal Communication

There are numerous barriers to optimal communication. Three attitudes are discussed, because of the frequency with which they impair communication in clinical settings.

"IT'S YOUR PROBLEM."

One response, when confronted with tough clinical decision making, is to nicely throw the decision into the laps of those for whom decisions are needed. This maneuver can be done with great ethical posturing about how respectful this is of the individual's autonomy. It is also often a "cop-out" and a failure to become involved, as well as to provide the support necessary to ensure good clinical decisions. The recent mammography controversy best illustrates this.

In January 1997, the National Institutes of Health (NIH) created a controversy when it failed to recommend routine annual mammograms for women under the age of 50. There was an angry outcry from women's groups, radiologists, and the American Cancer Society when the NIH panel recommended that women in their forties review the available information and decide for themselves about the appropriateness of mammograms. There were 32 presentations given by experts. Data showed that between 0 and 10 of every 10,000

women would have their lives prolonged because of routine annual mammograms in their forties. Thirty percent (i.e., 3000) of every 10,000 women would have a mammogram reported as abnormal, with all the disruption this creates, although there would be no actual pathology. Further complicating this scenario was concern that radiologists were upset by the lack of recommendation because mammography represents a significant source of their income. Without the NIH medically justifying this procedure, it was unlikely that insurance companies would reimburse for it. Similarly, there was concern that oncologists and surgeons were dismayed by the lack of a recommendation because their emotional commitment to early diagnosis prejudices them in favor of screening for early detection, even at the cost of 3000 false positives and 3000 needlessly frightened women and their families. There are similar issues with screening for prostate cancer in men. It is unproven that early detection of prostatic cancer will prolong life. The issue is not just cost effectiveness, but, as with any disease, whether the diagnostic studies (and what follows from the initial decision) are either directly or indirectly harmful. When the incidence of a disease is low in a population, the incidence of false positives is particularly problematic.

How would you respond if you were confronted with the statement: "I'm so confused about all of this mammography information . . . what do you think I should do?" Why would you respond in this manner?

"YOU DO NOT DESERVE MY TIME AND ENERGY."

When invited to be honest and answer why they are selectively attempting to communicate with patients, one group of case managers acknowledged that they tended to give less of themselves to patients who were "not worthy" of their time and energy. Of particular interest was finding that the criteria that made certain patients "unworthy" of a case manager's time differed from one case manager to another. Popular "criteria" included age, socioeconomic status, lifestyle factors, history of self-care, personality, and level of education. Interesting criteria similarly linked to a case manager's spending less time in attempting to communicate included "small, quiet people who never asked for anything and never seemed to need anything."

BOX 36-6
Case Study   Scenarios

Elizabeth Gordon

Elizabeth Gordon is an 84-year-old woman who was placed in a nursing home 2 years ago because her daughter (an only child) felt she was no longer able to take care of Elizabeth satisfactorily at home. The daughter is a parish secretary at a local church and attends church services regularly. Elizabeth was diagnosed 3 years ago as having Alzheimer's disease. She had become increasingly dependent, very forgetful, and confused about what year it is and where she is. For the past 3 months, Elizabeth has failed to recognize her daughter. She has not been on medication. Her general physical examination has remained unchanged and unremarkable. Laboratory studies done 6 months ago were also unremarkable.

Until a month ago, Elizabeth sat up most of the day, went to the dining room for meals with assistance, and fed herself. She had lost 10 pounds in the past year. About 3 weeks ago she began to have difficulty chewing and swallowing solid food and would occasionally choke. Two weeks ago, she could not be encouraged to go to the dining room, even by wheelchair. She began to sleep 16 to 18 hours a day. When she was awake, she would periodically mumble a few words. One week ago, she began to refuse taking any food except occasional sips of juice or water. When something else was offered, she would clamp her mouth shut and lower her head. She appears comfortable and in no significant pain or discomfort. Although she is covered under Medicare, she has chosen a health maintenance organization option. Her daughter has asked the nurse about nasogastric feedings and possible medication. The question was deferred to the geriatric case manager.

As a geriatric case manager, how might you approach the daughter? What would your comments and questions be? Would you respond differently if you were employed by the managed care organization? How would you interact with the nurse re-

sponsible for Elizabeth's care? What conversation would you have with the attending physician? Should costs be a consideration? How would you deal with the managed care organization? Who should make the decision? What criteria should be used?

Anna Santo

Anna Santo is a 43-year-old, married woman who is a mother of six children (ages 8, 12, 15, 17, 20, and 25). Anna was born in Mexico, where she completed six years of school. She moved to the United States when she was 16 years old. Her primary language is Spanish. She has never been employed outside of the home.

Recently, a mammogram was conducted after Anna detected a lump. This mammogram revealed a 1.5 cm mass in her left breast. A biopsy revealed cancer. There is no evidence on physical examination of its spreading to the lymph nodes. It was anticipated that her medical care would be covered under her husband's employment-linked health insurance.

Henry Clearspeak, the surgeon to whom Anna was assigned in the clinic, explained (in English) several options to Anna and her husband. These options included chemotherapy with simple mastectomy, simple mastectomy, simple mastectomy with radiation, and total mastectomy. He acknowledged that there was no clear evidence that survival was documented as better with one approach over another. He then recommended, when asked, that the total mastectomy be done because ". . . then we will know that we probably got it all." Anna and her husband signed an informed consent form for the total mastectomy.

As a hospital-based case manager, what is your ethical responsibility in this situation? Was proper informed consent obtained? What might have been done differently?

BOX 36-6
Case Study   Scenarios—cont'd

The Egan Family

Susan, your niece, is a nurse employed by a private home health care organization. She is providing home care to 3-year-old Erin Egan, who has AIDS. The cost approaches $3000 a month. The expense, except for a deductible, is currently covered by private insurance. Erin's parents are also HIV positive. Susan has become very close to this family, especially to Erin. Erin's father is still actively employed and has a major medical policy. It is projected, however, that the costs will eventually exceed the available benefits.

A state social worker on a home visit suggested to the family that they use another health care agency, which will provide the same care at a significantly lower expense to the family. The alternative agency (Beta) is also for-profit and is "squeezing out" established firms (including the one for which Susan works). Although the total costs to the insurance company will increase by approximately $200 a month, Beta will "write off" the deductible of $100 a month that the Egans now pay. The state is concerned about rising costs and has sought to support Beta in anticipation of lower overall costs because of their "cut-rate" prices on state-funded care. The family has asked Susan for her advice. You are a case manager employed by a nonprofit community organization. Susan calls you with the following concerns:

- Susan and the family do not want to lose the relationship they have.
- Susan is concerned about her obligations to her employer, and how this might affect her position.
- She is concerned about the insurance company being exploited and her conflicting obligations. What are the ethical issues? What would you advise Susan?

Julie Henderson

You are employed as a case manager in a neighborhood health center. Last week Mrs. Henderson and her daughter, Julie, appeared in the clinic. Julie is 17-years-old and single. She is 3 months' pregnant by her 20-year-old boyfriend. Her mother is insisting that Julie have an abortion. Julie and her mother argue.

"I have a right to have my own baby," Julie says.

"You're just a child yourself. . .," her mother begins.

"I'm seventeen," Julie interrupts. "You were the same age when I was born.

"But you're not married. I was."

"Henry and I may get married before this baby is born," Julie responds to her mother's surprise. "We just haven't decided yet."

"Haven't decided yet!?! You told me that he has no intention of marrying you."

"Well . . . he could change his mind."

"And if he doesn't," her mother says, "where will you be then?"

Determined, Julie responds, "I'd quit school and get a job."

Julie's mother gives a short laugh and responds, "Doing what? Working at McDonald's? Don't forget what life has been like for me working and raising you and your brothers by myself since the divorce. Don't think I'm going to raise your child, too, because I'm not. God knows I have enough trouble keeping bread on our table as it is."

"I'm not expecting you to . . . I'll take care of this baby on my own."

The conversation continues, with Julie telling her mother she feels as if her mother is always trying to run her life. Mrs. Henderson insists that she is only worried for Julie's "own good." Finally, Mrs. Henderson turns to you and says, "You try to talk some sense into this girl, will you?"

As a case manager in this setting, how would you handle this situation?

Health care professionals then mistakenly assumed that the patient seemed to know everything necessary to know and seemed highly educated. It is helpful to try to reconstruct what it is about patients that makes us, consciously or unconsciously, more or less willing to be present to them. When injustices appear, it is important to address them.

"I WISH I COULD, BUT . . ."

A final attitudinal impediment to optimal communication is reflected in the statement: "I really wish I had the time to talk more with the Shusters, *but* staffing today just doesn't allow it." Current practice realities will almost always make it possible to find some excuse for not creating the time to communicate adequately with patients, family members, colleagues, and payers. Case managers who are committed to good communication acknowledge these problems and find ways to work around them or to change the systems creating the constraints. Even a quick review of your typical response when confronted with communication challenges should reveal whether you are content to allow external forces to absolve you of your obligation to communicate. If you characteristically accept the inability to initiate necessary communication, it may be time to reevaluate your commitment to the populations you have promised to serve.

Conclusion

Outcome-oriented case managers are quickly learning to value relational competence and communi-cation skills. The ability to successfully design a clinical pathway that responds to the needs of a complex patient aggregate, coordinate the efforts of the health care team and payers to meet the needs of individual patients, or appeal a refusal for treatment or treatment reimbursement is closely linked to the ability to communicate effectively. Working "smart" in today's health care system entails proficiency in communication. Technologically impaired (or challenged) health care professionals quickly seek resources to remedy their deficiencies or are directed to do so; likewise, relationally impaired health care professionals who are prudent and committed to patient and society well-being do the same.

References

Anonymous essay: Mill on liberty, *The National Review* 8:393-424, 1859.

Fletcher JC et al: *Introduction to clinical ethics*, Frederick, Md, 1995, University Publishing Group.

Gorovitz S: *Doctor's dilemmas: moral conflict and medical care*, New York, 1982, Macmillan.

Katz J: *The silent world of doctor and patient*, New York, 1984, Free Press.

President's Commission for the Study of Ethical Problems in Medicine and Behavioral Research: *Making health care decisions*, vols 1-3, Washington, DC, 1982, US Government Printing Office.

Quill TE, Brody H: Recommendations and patient autonomy: finding a balance between physician power and patient choice, *Ann Intern Med* 125(9):763-769, 1996.

Siegler M: Confidentiality in medicine: a decrepit concept, *N Engl J Med* 307(24):518-521, 1982.

Stand on mammograms greeted by outrage, *New York Times*, January 28, 1997.

CHAPTER 37

Sustaining Therapeutic Alliances Through the Community Nursing Organization

GRACE McCORMACK DALY, RN, EdD, FNP, CS

OVERVIEW

The Visiting Nurse Service of New York's Community Nursing Organization's community-based practice model provides the environment that fosters the development of a relationship between the client and the nurse . . . Because of the ongoing relationship, the nurse is aware of the client's coping skills, emotional and financial resources, social supports, attitudes, and receptivity to service.

The Visiting Nurse Service of New York's Community Nursing Organization has created a program that provides access to the nurse in the community and provides continuity of care through services from the same nurse over time in multiple settings. The program was designed to foster a nurse/client relationship. It creates an environment that facilitates the nurse "knowing the client" and the client "knowing the nurse." After four years of operation, our experience reveals this nurse-client relationship to be a "therapeutic alliance." ▲

The Visiting Nurse Service of New York (VNSNY) has one of the four Community Nursing Organization (CNO) sites in the country, sponsored by the Health Care Financing Administration. This capitated demonstration project came about as a result of legislation passed by Congress in 1987. Its purpose is to test the function of the nurse as case manager for Medicare Part A home care and Part B nonphysician services of enrolled clients.

Lillian Wald, who is credited as being the first public health nurse, founded VNSNY more than one hundred years ago. Today VNSNY is the largest and oldest nonprofit Medicare-certified home health agency in the United States. The public health model embodied by Lillian Wald emphasized the nurse learning about a population, a defined community, and caring for that community across the continuum of health. The CNO model was envisioned as a return to the public health model, moving away from the home health model of episodic care for acute illnesses. The VNSNY CNO practice is community based and fosters a relationship between the client and the nurse. These premises underpin our practice.

The Nurse Consultant

The community-based practice model we envisioned requires the nurse to address wellness issues with clients, promote healthy lifestyles, maintain health through assessment and monitoring, and provide the skilled nursing care required for the home health care benefits. We titled the CNO nurses "nurse consultants" to denote their availability to the client and their ability to provide information about health and wellness. We did this to reflect a broader and different role than traditionally encountered in certified home health agencies.

The nurse consultant serves as the primary care nurse for a panel of clients, which ranges between 80 and 140. Case management caseload size depends on the ratio of sites to homebound enrollees and nursing complexity. The nurse consultant functions as a case manager for his/her Medicare CNO benefits, and authorizes nonphysician services (physical therapy, social work, psychological services, durable medical equipment and supplies). In addition, the nurse consultant renders the skilled nursing care and coordinates other services when the client requires home health services.

The Practice Sites

Community sites identified in the service area serve as hubs from which the nurse extends into the community to persons who are homebound or otherwise not able to access the sites. We have twenty-five sites, located at senior centers, NORCs (naturally occurring retirement communities), community organizations, and church-based senior clubs. Each nurse consultant has scheduled hours at his or her community sites, some weekly and others bimonthly or monthly.

These site visits can be client driven, based on clients' perception of need, or nurse driven, based on nurses' perception of client needs. Whenever clients have questions, feel a need to talk things over, or want their blood pressure checked or blood glucose monitored, they can initiate contact at one of the community sites or telephone a nurse. Clients are also able to access their nurses at our storefront office, located in one of the communities we serve. The nurse consultant makes home visits, if needed.

The nurse consultants see approximately 50% of our clients at home. These clients either are homebound, do not live within accessible distances from one of our sites, or do not choose to access a site. The nurse consultants schedule routine home visits for clients "at risk," which means that they have chronic health problems that require ongoing monitoring but do not qualify for Medicare home health care. This ongoing monitoring enables us to communicate abnormal findings to physicians on a timely basis and results in early medical interventions. Many times we are able to prevent hospitalizations.

Nursing Model Assessment

The functional health patterns typology serves as the framework for our assessments. Each of the eleven patterns is an expression of the client's biopsychosocial integration. Clients' responses are influenced by cultural, developmental, and spiritual factors. Nursing diagnoses are derived from the information gathered, and care plans are formulated. The nurse consultant treats human responses to illness, not disease. Health promotion and preventive care are strong components of the program and are included in each client's plan of care. Nurse consultants monitor physiological status, medication compliance, and drug interaction responses and provide skilled nursing care. Intimate knowledge of the workings of the community and its resources enhances the nurses' ability to provide comprehensive care.

Creating the Environment That Fosters Therapeutic Relationships

The VNSNY CNO community-based practice model provides the environment that fosters the development of a relationship between the client and the nurse. The marketing for our CNO was built on accessibility to "your own nurse." Presentations to prospective enrollees emphasized that the nurse would know the enrolled client and be available for questions, problems, and referrals, as well as provide care at home, when needed. Whenever it was possible, the nurse consultant assigned to the community site was present at marketing sessions so that prospective enrollees could see and meet the nurse for that site. This approach was highly successful; 75% to 80% of eligible presentation attendees enrolled in the CNO on the spot. A large number of enrollees have joined the program via word of mouth from CNO members.

The client is assigned his or her "own nurse" upon initial enrollment. This nurse performs the initial assessment and designs a care plan based on each client's health needs. The CNO program requires clients be reassessed every six months; however, they have access to their nurses at community sites throughout the year. The nurse will contact clients who do not access sites between reassessments if their conditions or situations are of concern. Our CNO program was designed to facilitate the nurse "knowing the client" and client "knowing the nurse." Each client is treated as an individual. Because of the ongoing relationship, the nurse is aware of the client's coping skills, emotional and financial resources, social supports, attitudes, and receptivity to service. When the client's health status changes, the nurse is able to provide targeted and appropriate care because of his or her knowledge of the client, family, and community. We recently sent out surveys to our enrollees; 69% responded, and, of those, 86% felt that having their own nurses was important to them.

Clients' Stories Reveal Therapeutic Alliance

After four years of operation, our clients best express the outcome of this planned intervention of nurse accessibility and continuity of care. It is their words that reveal the profound influence of this relationship.*

"THE CARING VISITS AND THE TELEPHONE AVAILABILITY ARE PRICELESS."

One client tells of his experiences at the community site. Eighty-five years old, he had just lost his wife after 53 years of marriage when he first joined the CNO. He explains how access to the nurse has changed his health maintenance practices and how his nurse has helped him. Initially he saw his nurse weekly at the community room in his apartment complex. In addition to health guidance he also received grief counseling from his nurse consultant (master's-prepared mental health nurse).

I used to go to my doctor three to four times a year. I have cut down to three. I'd love to cut down to two now because of the work that she [nurse] does. She has been quite helpful. I have a circulation problem, and I've been treated for this for fifteen years. I take a couple of pills a day.

He went on to explain:

Doctors are not warm when you visit them; they are not warm at all. My heart specialist, I have been going to him for fifteen years; I started with him when he came out of school. He spends more time with me than any other doctor has. But he is strictly a heart specialist, and when another problem develops he wants to send me to another doctor, which he has done over the years. But my nurse's effort is greater to me than any doctor that I have ever known. I think the relaxing attitude of a visit here [community room] is much better than a visit to a doctor's office. The cost of a nursing service in comparison to the cost of a visit to a doctor is so tremendous. He does the exact same things. They [doctors] don't have the time to listen to you . . . It was she who very skillfully guided me back to normalcy. The psychiatrist recommended by my doctor would not have had the ability, interest, and patience with me . . . The caring visits and telephone availability are priceless.

---

*The following accounts are from Daly G: *A qualitative study: the client's perception of the community nursing organization,* an unpublished manuscript.

It is clear that the nurse consultant is treating his mind and body. She not only monitors his chronic health problems but also nurtures him back to "normalcy" after a life-shattering loss.

"SHE DOES EVERYTHING THE DOCTOR DOES."

This 86-year-old homebound client has a history of high blood pressure, heart failure, atrial fibrillation, osteoarthritis, spinal stenosis, and glaucoma. She describes the cost savings and stress reduction she has received from having a nurse visit her at home.

I've been relieved of a lot of stress. She has saved me about four trips to my doctor; doctor visits, you know what they cost. Well, she does what the doctor does. I have congestive heart failure; when she comes, she checks my lungs to see if there is water in my lungs. When she leaves, I feel so much better because she gives me the okay. I have very high blood pressure, and when she takes it and when she is finished I know whether I'm under control. If she finds I'm out of control, I have to go to the doctor. She does everything the doctor does for me, which I have to pay a couple hundred bucks every time I go. It is very expensive, like it costs me over a hundred dollars just for the trip [transportation.]

It has taken so much stress off me, the fact that there is someone who cares enough about my health to come and visit me from time to time to check on me.

She continued, describing other services the nurse has provided her through the program [home health aide and social worker]:

Everyone in the program is so understanding, so nice, so warm, and so friendly. It makes my day when they come.

It cheers me up because I have no family. I have no one that I can call or ask to do anything for me. I find that they do things for me that I never expected. I am overwhelmed with all the care I'm getting.

She continued:

I have a lot of stress because I never know what my pressure is, because it shoots up, it shoots down. I don't know if my lungs are filling up with water. I am never sure how I am going to be tomorrow.

She described how the nurses' monitoring has promoted her healing:

She has helped me mentally; when she comes I really feel great. And when she leaves I feel so much better, she

gives me an okay. I have very high blood pressure, and when she comes she takes it and when she is finished I know I am under control. So when she comes I feel a sense of relief. I am under a lot of stress, but when she visits me, I think all my stress goes away. I can't begin to tell you how relieved I am when I see my nurse. She is God sent, really, for me.

She explained her transformation:

I am not as nervous, as stressed out; I'm not as scared as I've always been. I was just plain scared, I was scared stiff before I met you [Community Nursing Organization of the Visiting Nurse Service of New York]. I am not scared anymore. I am not scared; all I know is you are a phone call away.

This story illustrates that access to the nurse has resulted in improved quality of life. The nurse's skilled monitoring and vigilance have provided cost savings as well as stress reduction.

"THE THING YOU CAN'T BUY IS THE NURSE."

This client sees her nurse at the site, but when she is unable to get out because of arthritis, her nurse makes home visits. She is 76 years old, and also has high blood pressure and diabetes mellitus. She relates how her nurse tries to help:

She will say, 'Can I do anything?' Sometimes she says, 'Look, try this' or 'Do that.' That is wonderful! That's something I never had because if you go into the doctor's office, he barely has time; he writes me prescriptions. He writes me a prescription for these and the refills that carry me through the year. That is the reason I go to the doctor, and even her good word, the fact that she is caring and concerned . . . that is so meaningful, to me at least.

She continues on about her nurse's attentiveness:

One Friday the phone rang; it was about five-thirty, quarter to six; it was my nurse. I figured everybody's home in their house. She said, 'I called Dr. _____.' I'm thinking, 'My God this lady don't give up.' To me this was amazing because I figured, why in heaven's name would she be so diligent?

This same client credits her nurse with encouraging her to seek out medical care:

I went to a clinic in Astoria. It was a new clinic that had opened. My nurse thought it would be a good idea if I went there and they gave me a complete checkup.

She also explained how her nurse helped her avoid a hospitalization:

When I first met my nurse, I had been having problems with my blood sugar. It just could not seem to come under control. The time I'm talking about it was 444 (mg/dl). She had me write down the food that I was eating, everything I put into my mouth, all the meals. She told me what I should be eating. I brought the blood sugar down. I would say within less than two months. I was down to 115 (mg/dl).

She explained that she was eating the wrong foods:

I was having a glorious time with candy. Chocolate was my downfall . . . I didn't have room in the refrigerator for fruits and things. I had it stuffed with Milky Ways. I would say it has been a year and a half or more that I've put a piece of chocolate in my mouth, haven't touched it!

She described her past behavior:

You know the candy aisle in the supermarket; I used to work my way in there, into the candy aisle. Oh, my eyes used to get big as marbles. I am telling you, I was like a junkie, even worse.

She attributes her behavior modification to her relationship with her nurse:

I think it started with writing down the foods, because if I ate it I would have to write it down. I told her that I would never lie. I would be cheating me, but I even considered her more; if I ate it I would have to write it, so I stopped it.

After discussing the equipment her nurse got her for an arthritic condition [cane and TENS unit], this client explained that it is the human tie and her nurse's concern that are significant:

That is important [equipment], but to me the important thing is I can go across there [community room] and say to someone, this hurts me, or this; somebody that listens and tries to help, that's very meaningful, very important.

I'm happy because an older person sometimes has illnesses that don't go away. But knowing that someone is interested, concerned, caring, whatever the word is you want to use, it is a good thing. It is a helpful thing. It is almost like taking medicine.

She summarized her experiences in the Community Nursing Organization by explaining that she could go out and buy a cane or the TENS unit:

"The thing you can't buy is the nurse."

"GO HOME! I'M ALL ALONE"

This 73-year-old client related his dilemma when the hospital discharged him with a draining wound immediately after urological surgery. He explained:

Go home! I am all alone; there is no one to bring me home. So I came home; then I called my nurse, made her aware. Religiously she was here for six weeks [wound care]. I could not have done it without her, every day for six weeks.

He went on to relate that it was his nurse who discovered his hypertension, when making daily visits to change his dressing, during his recovery from the urological surgery:

If it were not for my nurse I never would have discovered about the hypertension. She called my cardiologist, told his secretary to have him call her right back in my apartment. She was determined; she wanted me to see him.

He describes his relationship with his nurse:

"She gives me very good advice. I could talk it over with her and she would suggest what to do."

"IT WAS LIKE WINNING THE LOTTERY."

This 77-year-old client, whose regular community site was closed for the summer, was impressed when her nurse called with her summer schedule. She explained that her nurse said: "I did not see you and I was wondering about you."

She explained that the Community Nursing Organization also sent her a letter about the importance of drinking water during the hot days of summer.

Wasn't it nice that they should be so concerned, because then I drank the water. I'm not a person who drinks a lot of water. I drank it! Isn't that wonderful that they were so thoughtful?

She summarizes her experiences with the CNO:

"It was like winning the lottery."

"IF I HADN'T KNOWN MY NURSE, I DON'T KNOW WHAT I'D HAVE DONE."

This 81-year-old client explained that she had her blood pressure checked by her nurse at the local Senior Citizen Center occasionally. She told her nurse that she was having a biopsy of a breast mass. The biopsy was malignant, and she had a complete mastectomy. When she was discharged from the hospital, she was told that Medicare would not provide her any help. She remembered that her nurse had said: "Get in touch with me after you have the operation and tell me what occurs."

So I did tell her, and she said she would get me someone through her; I was able to get someone to help me (home health aide). If I hadn't known my nurse, I don't know what I'd have done. I don't know.

She explained that her nurse guided her recovery and helped her to get well:

I was told by my nurse to do breathing exercises and also squeeze the ball. I had stopped squeezing the ball because I did not think it was necessary.

She then reminisced about an earlier encounter with a visiting nurse:

When my children were born I had a visiting nurse, because I had nobody. The visiting nurse used to visit me with a little black bag, many, many years ago. That was a happy experience for me. I had nobody to help me. She was very helpful.

"IT WAS SHE WHO TOLD ME HOW TO GET BETTER."

This 87-year-old client described the weekly activity of going to the community room in her apartment complex with her friends, who are also members of the Community Nursing Organization of the Visiting Nurse Service of New York. She reported how the nurses promote wellness through their presence and teaching:

We all go down to the community room to see these nurses. They [her friends] love the attention they're getting from the nurses and the fact that they are being spoken to. They have special meetings where they talk about 'How to Take Care of Yourself,' 'How to Get Sleep,' 'How to Do Exercise.'

She explained:

The nurses always tell you if you need anything, call us immediately, we'll get back to you. We'll see if there's something we can do for you. It is like somebody who knows you and wants to help you, a friend.

She went on to say how her nurse had told her: "If you ever need any help in arranging for a hospitalization, let me know right away so I can help you with it."

When she was hospitalized for serious surgery at 86 years of age, she described how her nurse visited her at home after the surgery and guided her to recovery through her coaching and interpretation:

She came two or three times a week, and took my vital signs and talked to me. She really made feel as though I had somebody around to help me, because the doctors didn't say anything. She really helped me to adjust to this difference in my living, because I had not been really sick in a long time. I had to be independent, did everything for myself. I didn't need any help. But she helped me understand that it's more than taking care of your medical needs. You need to be told how to help yourself by getting into your own routine, by having someone help you when you need to be helped. It was she who told me how to get better, that I would get better. I kept saying, oh, I'm not getting back to where I was. She kept saying, you'll get there: it will take a little bit of time and you have to help yourself. It was through her, I feel, that I really made a recovery. Without her I would not have, I'm sure. But she kept telling me that I could do it and that I needed the help [home health aide] and I would have it as long as I needed it.

She related that during her postsurgical recovery her nurse, while monitoring her vital signs on a routine home visit, identified an abnormal heart rhythm and informed her that she had to be seen by her doctor immediately. The client was immediately admitted to the cardiac intensive care unit from the doctor's office. She remained there for thirteen days. She stated:

"If she [nurse] hadn't told me, you have to go now, I would not have gone, and Lord knows what would have happened."

Conclusion: "It Is Like Having a Friend in Court."

It is the CNO members themselves who inform us of the significance of this nursing program. These stories illuminate the variability of the role of the community nurse. They illustrate health promotion and wellness activities as well as crisis intervention during a life-threatening event. They depict access to care, connection, and continuity of care. They portray the thoughtful adaptations nurses use to meet therapeutic goals. The nurse case manager's presence, knowledge, and caring practice have improved the quality of life of these enrollees. One client put it this way: "She is more than a nurse to me; she is a friend. It is like having a friend in court." The skilled hands of the nurse reach out in nonthreatening settings and maintain contact over time. The nurses' ordinary everyday practices are transformed into extraordinary events. They touch the lives of the elderly living in the community. These stories describe the therapeutic alliance created at the CNO.

References

Daly GM, Mitchell RD: Case management in the community setting, *Nursing Clinics of North America* 31(3):527-534, 1996.

Storfjell JL, Mitchell R, Daly GM: Nurse-managed health-care: New York's Community Nursing Organization, *Journal of Nursing Administration* 27(10):21-27, 1997.

CHAPTER 38

New Partnerships in the Integrated Environment

The Brookwood Experience

JEAN NEWSOME, RN, DSN, **DEREK T. SPELLMAN**, RN, MSN, **GLENDA ETHRIDGE BROGDEN**, RN, MSN, **and BILL BRODIE**, RN, MSHA

OVERVIEW

Learning to speak a common language has long been identified as the greatest challenge between clinical and financial experts; however, understanding that all must share the common goal of balancing the quality, service, and cost equation is what now forms the bedrock for the new partnerships among components of the integrated delivery system.

As providers respond to the pressures exerted by the purchasers of health care to reduce the dollars expended for services, they are extending their reach beyond traditional boundaries and developing integrated health care delivery systems. The emerging integrated delivery systems are composed of a full gamut of services from cradle to grave. The opportunities for partnerships to emerge among players within each of the component services are often the result of process-improvement activities born from the need to enhance the transition of patients across the continuum. Because of the nature of the care delivery process, partnerships are most frequently formed between clinicians and financial experts, physicians and case managers, payer- and provider-based case managers, and hospitals and other components of the integrated delivery system. This chapter will explore new partnerships developed as staff at Tenet's Brookwood Medical Center worked toward the development of an integrated health care delivery system in Birmingham, Alabama. ▲

As providers respond to the pressures exerted by the purchasers of health care to reduce the dollars expended for services, they are extending their reach beyond traditional boundaries and developing integrated health care delivery systems. What once was considered to be a complete system for health care, such as an acute care hospital, is now simply one component of a newly defined, much larger system poised to provide services spanning the life cycle. These new, larger systems may be arranged in a variety of ways, including community health planning alliances, joint ventures, joint contracting, holding companies, merged income statements, and up to and including full asset mergers resulting in a single-owner system.

The emerging integrated health care delivery systems are composed of a full gamut of services, including primary care physician management, medical subspecialty care, diagnostic studies, outpatient surgery, home care, skilled nursing, rehabilitation, assisted living, emergent/urgent care, trauma, and hospital-based acute care. The opportunities for partnerships to emerge among players within each of the component services are often identified as the result of process-improvement activities born from the need to enhance the transition of patients across the continuum of care. As a result of the nature of the care delivery process, partnerships are most frequently formed between clinicians and financial experts, physicians and case managers, payer- and provider-based case managers, and hospitals and other components of the integrated delivery system (Barron, Westermann, 1995; Coddington, Moore, Fischer, 1994; Gilmore, Hirschhorn, O'Connor, 1994; Hudson, 1993; Pitcavage, 1994; Pointer, Alexander, Zuckerman, 1995).

A brief overview of the Brookwood inpatient model of case management is presented as a backdrop for the partnerships that developed on the path to vertical integration. Admissions Planning Nurses (APNs) are responsible and accountable for the preadmission process. Since 80% of Brookwood's admissions are scheduled admissions, the role of the APN is a critical one. Case managers are responsible and accountable for case-by-case clinical, financial, and quality outcomes for a caseload of 12 to 15 patients. Outcome managers, on the other hand, are responsible and accountable for aggregate clinical, financial, and quality outcomes for a select population of patients.

Clinical and Financial Partnerships

Learning to speak a common language has long been identified as the greatest challenge between clinical and financial experts. However, understanding that all must share the common goal of balancing the quality, service, and cost equation is what now forms the bedrock for the new partnerships among clinical and financial experts. Although this challenge may appear simplistic, much truth is contained in the perspectives gleaned from interaction with chief financial officers (CFOs) and chief nursing officers (CNOs) of the early 1980s. The primary, and sometimes exclusive, objective of the CNO was to deliver optimum care to all presenting for patient care, while the CFO had an equally narrow focus on achieving the financial objectives. Each set about to achieve his or her narrowly focused goals, with infrequent collaborative planning, resulting in de-optimization of the system. Following the introduction of the prospective payment system, fear of the unknown was rampant among clinicians and financial leaders. The shift from cost-plus to prospective payment created a situation in which the clinical and financial leaders were literally forced to communicate with one another regarding their respective domains. The need to speak a common language became apparent so that each could achieve his or her primary goals. This initial, mutually awkward, yet beneficial communication formed the basis for the clinical and financial partnerships of the integrated delivery systems of today. At Brookwood Medical Center the ability of clinical and financial leaders to speak a common language evolved to provide four major opportunities for new partnerships:

1. Prioritization of improvement efforts
2. Managed care contracting
3. Business planning and forecasting
4. Evaluation of existing and new clinical programs and services

PRIORITIZATION OF IMPROVEMENT EFFORTS

When a case management program is just beginning, or even if a well-established program exists, prioritizing improvement efforts can be a challenge. For example, in the beginning stages of implementation of the case management program at Brookwood Medical Center, clinical and financial experts collaboratively decided how existing hospital resources would be utilized to get the "biggest bang for the buck." Since the rate of future expansion of the case management program was dependent, to a large degree, on demonstrating positive financial and clinical outcomes from case management initiatives and processes, this initial collaborative decision between the CNO and the CFO was critical.

Today, nine years later, clinicians and financial experts prioritize improvement efforts on a much more sophisticated basis. In addition to identifying specific length-of-stay and variable cost-reduction initiatives within diagnostic related groups (DRGs), Outcome managers and financial staff collaborate to identify cost-reduction strategies across multiple case-types as well as initiatives aimed at clinical integration across remote sites, the development of a new program aimed at volume growth, and capital deployment that enables both growth and cost reduction.

MANAGED CARE CONTRACTING

At Brookwood, all managed care contracts are reviewed by the appropriate clinical expert(s) and utilization management specialist, in addition to financial staff. While the financial leaders are often able to identify variable cost-per-case and length-of-stay targets that will make a particular contract profitable, it is the clinicians who must identify the specific strategies for achieving those targets. Often the language of the contract with regard to preadmission certification, utilization review, and discharge planning activities has a major impact on the ability of the case managers to achieve clinical, financial, and length-of-stay targets. Questions related to contract language are important to answer prior to signing of a managed care contract, as millions of dollars may be at stake, depending on how these relationships are structured. For example, who is responsible for admission certification, concurrent utilization review, and discharge planning, and what are the identified processes for each? More importantly, the patient may get caught in the crossfire when providers and payers do not clearly delineate specific responsibilities. It has been proven beneficial to develop a case study to explore how the payer and the provider will interact and to flowchart the process after an understanding is reached.

FORECASTING FOR THE BUSINESS PLAN

Two major portions of the business plan, estimating volumes and identifying variable and fixed cost-reduction strategies, lend themselves well to clinical and financial partnerships. While the CFO may be the first to sound the alarm when changes in volume by product, case-type, or physician occur, it is the clinician who is able to explain the changes once they have occurred or forecast the changes likely to occur in the future. At Brookwood, each outcome manager prepares a list of potential practice pattern changes by payer for the CFO in preparation for completing the annual business plan. The outcome managers consider, among other things, movement from inpatient to outpatient trends, knowledge of practice pattern changes among the physicians in each subspecialty, and payer-driven utilization changes in managed care markets. Consider the following explanations provided by outcome managers at Brookwood to project or explain volume variances from the previous year's business plan:

1. HMOs requiring surgical colonization instead of hysterectomy for cancer in situ, hormonal therapy and D&C before considering hysterectomy, and Doppler venous study before precertifying varicose vein stripping.
2. Physician pattern changes such as premature labor managed at home via home infusion and postoperative thoracotomy patients placed in step-down rather than critical care units.

It is apparent that much more accurate forecasting of volume, cost, and revenue is attainable when these types of clinical and utilization data information are shared between financial and clinical staff.

The other major opportunity for collaboration between clinical and financial leaders in the development of the business plan is in the area of identifying variable cost-reduction strategies. While the CFO may be able to identify opportunities by reviewing benchmark data by case-type, it is the outcome manager who is familiar enough with the expected course of inpatient stay and the utilization patterns of admitting physicians to ensure achievement of the financial goals. In much the same way that clinical and financial staff collaborate to prioritize opportunities for improvement, they develop an annual business plan that contains case-type-specific and physician-specific variable cost-reduction strategies (Box 38-1).

While the examples provided thus far illustrate how clinical information adds to the financial information, the reverse, of course, is also true. In many instances, clinicians do not always understand the financial impact of changes in practice that they seek to implement. A good example is an outpatient congestive heart failure (CHF) clinic designed to teach chronic patients how to self-manage their disease. This type of strategy would undoubtedly reduce inpatient readmissions and emergency and physician visits, which might have a short-term negative impact on revenue. How-ever, when improved clinical and financial out-comes result, payers and patients positively influ-ence market share through channeling and referrals. While the decision to pursue an initiative or cost-reduction strategy is never based on this fact alone, the knowledge of the impact is impor-tant to any organization with quality, service, and cost targets to achieve.

EVALUATING NEW AND EXISTING PROGRAMS

Another example of clinical and financial partner-ships centers around the evaluation of new and ex-isting clinical programs. At Brookwood, the evalu-ation of programs is a joint effort of financial, administrative, and clinical staff. The following are some recent examples of this partnership at Brook-wood Medical Center.

A preliminary pro forma to evaluate the devel-opment of a long-term-care "hospital within a hos-pital" showed a net profit the first year. The CFO reviewed the pro forma and determined that the re-duction in outlier payments caused by the move-ment of patients from the acute care setting to a long-term-care setting would have a significant negative impact on inpatient revenue. The pulmo-nary medicine outcome manager reviewed the pro forma and determined that the time frame for iden-tification of potential patients (day two or three of the length of stay) was not clinically achievable. In addition, the outcome manager was able to identify significant numbers of patients who should not be considered in the pro forma volumes because of physician variance issues. When the pro forma as-sumptions were rewritten to account for these clini-cal and reimbursement issues, the bottom line was not financially feasible. A decision was made not to pursue this opportunity.

Brookwood recently evaluated the addition of a Pharmaceuticals Study Unit. After a multidisci-plinary evaluation of the proposal demonstrated strong physician interest, perceived positive ben-efits by consumers, a positive financial margin, and Institutional Review Board (IRB) endorsement, there seemed little doubt to the psychiatric outcome manager that this was a worthwhile program to pursue. Before the administrative team agreed to pursue this opportunity, however, the COO re-quested that the CFO calculate the potential nega-

---

BOX 38-1
Case Management Initiatives for the Business Plan: Pulmonary Program

The following is an example of cost-reduction incentives for the business plan developed col-laboratively by financial and clinical staff.

1. Reduce length of stay (LOS) by 2.5 days by eliminating avoidable complications in the pulmonary patient (DVT, UTI, fluid imbal-ance), as noted in the Care Management Sci-ence data.

2. Implement a medical-surgical ventilator unit on the fifth floor for "difficult-to-wean" chronic ventilator patients currently housed in Medical Intensive Care.

3. Monitor, report, and act upon turn-around times (TAT) associated with antibiotic admin-istration in the Emergency Department (ED) for all pneumonia patients.

4. Reduce asthma inpatient LOS by one (1) day and ED and acute care asthma readmission by arranging Continuing Care Clinic visits for the day of discharge and as needed be-tween acute care discharge and appointment in the primary care physician's office.

5. Reduce asthma patient TAT in the ED by training the ED nurses to assess asthma se-verity and begin bronchodilator treatments.

tive impact to Blue Cross/Blue Shield revenue. The COO reasoned that the addition of these low-cost patient days associated with drug study patients might dilute the overall cost of delivering care at Brookwood and thus lower the Blue Cross/Blue Shield per diem rate, which represents 30% of Brookwood inpatient volumes. While this was initially very confusing to the outcome manager, this information provided by financial experts was critical in determining the overall profitability of the program.

Hospitals and Physician Partnerships

The earliest partnerships created when case management began at Brookwood were those between hospital administration, case management, and physicians. Those early relationships were, at best, tentative. Whether present or not, an alignment between hospital administration and case and outcome managers against physicians can be perceived. Physicians can fear loss of control over their decision-making powers, along with a fear of negative communications about their practice patterns and outcomes.

EARLY PARTNERSHIPS

The case and outcome managers at Brookwood Medical Center were practicing clinicians prior to their recruitment into their new roles. Role confusion was therefore a threat to both the physicians and the nurses. The central focus of the case and outcome managers on enhancing clinical care coordination, along with navigating the utilization and regulatory environment on behalf of the patient, physician, and hospital, led to the realization that all would benefit from this new role. Communications about "best practice," reduction in resource utilization, and length of stay were uncomfortable for both parties. Through a process of some trial and error, shared successes, and the simple passing of time, the newness, role confusion, and threats were quietly resolved.

Positive patient, financial, and regulatory agency outcomes emerged following the initial implementation period. Physicians were made aware of overall decreases in length of stay, decreased cost per case, and enhanced revenue from a global perspective. Those conversations were introduced by referring to the case management initiatives from which those positive outcomes arose. This general approach to success laid the foundation for more individualized initiatives. As physicians learned the benefits both to the hospital and to themselves from care coordination as well as service, quality, and cost-saving initiatives, new opportunities for hospital and physician partnerships emerged. Today, hospital staff and Brookwood outcome managers partner with physicians in protocol and guideline development, interpretation and analysis of external benchmark and comparative data, managed care contract review, joint ventures, and clinic and office management.

OUTCOME DATA ANALYSIS AND DISSEMINATION

Outcome managers at Brookwood began sharing financial (charge) data with physicians in 1989. Since that time, the process has evolved to become a major strategy for managing outcomes. The typical format for outcome data includes: blinded, risk-adjusted clinical and financial data organized into a resource counsumption matrix by physician and department (Table 38-1); "best practices" by physician peer; clinical and quality outcome data; and physician-specific opportunities for improved clinical and financial outcomes.

Certain lessons had to be learned along the way to make outcome data dissemination more meaningful and valid. Some of those lessons are:

1. Involve physicians in the development of the methodology for sharing data (e.g., data systems, format).
2. Include clinical outcome data in addition to financial data.
3. Recognize and clearly communicate flaws, shortcomings, and bias in the data.
4. Benchmark both internally and externally.
5. Utilize clinicians instead of financial staff to share data.
6. Share the data in one-to-one meetings with physicians and Outcome managers.
7. Customize the reports to reflect the unique needs of each subspecialty. For example, sample size must be statistically significant, which may be difficult with internal-medicine physicians.

TABLE 38-1
Resource Consumption Matrix: Actual Variable Cost by Department; DRGs 79, 88, 89, 99; June 1996 through January 1997

	PHYSICIAN 1	PHYSICIAN 2	PHYSICIAN 3	PHYSICIAN 4
No. of cases	12	33	21	36
Average length of stay	4.67	6.76	6.19	8.67

Cost by Department (these numbers are fabricated—do not reflect actual dollars)

	PHYSICIAN 1	PHYSICIAN 2	PHYSICIAN 3	PHYSICIAN 4
Blood Services	283	0	0	354
Cancer Center	0	27	0	0
Central Stores	67	98	117	110
Diabetes Center	0	275	0	40
Diagnostic Radiology	34	36	84	67
E.R.	65	53	52	69
Eye Same Day Surgery	0	23	0	37
Lab Services	143	95	161	172
MRI	0	0	156	44
Nursing—ICU	1156	375	865	1153
Nursing—M/S	461	740	653	976
Nursing—Womens	0	0	149	214
O.R. Supplies	0	3	23	2
Other	190	256	264	419
Pharmacy	229	422	404	542
Physical Therapy	35	55	9	189
Respiratory Therapy	123	231	199	269
Same Day Surgery	0	75	0	103
Ultrasound	0	69	39	39
TOTAL	$1,326	$1,945	$2,011	$2,819

Payer- and Hospital-Based Case Management Partnerships

Health care delivery systems attempting to achieve vertical integration must ultimately achieve clinical integration. The benefits of clinical integration, both from our experience and according to the literature are: improved coordination of care and outcomes; better communication among care providers; increased patient, payer, and, provider satisfaction; and reduced cost (Conrad, Shortell, 1996; Conrad, 1993; Danzon, Boothman, Greenberg, 1995; Hunt, 1996; McQueen, Marwick, 1995; Porter et al, 1996; Stahl, 1995). Early in 1993, Brookwood Medical Center established clinical integration as a system priority. The resulting integrated health care deliv-

ery system, or Alabama Health Services, is summarized in Box 38-2.

To the hospital-based case managers, this new system priority required a change in focus from illness to health, individual patient management to population-based management, and care provided in the acute setting to care across the continuum. Clinical integration across the continuum provided many opportunities for Brookwood outcome managers to collaborate with leaders within the system's health maintenance organization (HMO). In the early stages of development, outcome managers were instrumental in the development of the vision for case management systems across the continuum. In addition to program design, the outcome managers collaborated with the payer to

BOX 38-2
Alabama Health Services

Health Care Facilities
Brookwood Medical Center
Medical Center East
Lloyd Noland
Blount Memorial (managed)
St. Clair Regional

Ambulatory Services
117 employed PCPs
  45 clinics across 9 counties
Family Practice Residency Program
3 Outpatient Surgery Centers
4 Diagnostic Centers
Home Health/DME/ Hospice
Occupational Health Programs
Health Advantage Plans (HMO)

Group Administrators, Inc. (TPA)

Specialty Clinics
Womens Medical Center
Eye Institute
Center for Mental Health
Boshell Diabetes Endocrinology
Cancer Treatment Center
Regional Cancer Institute

Long Term Care/Assisted Living
Skilled care—54 beds
Assisted living—85 beds
Independent living— 714 units
Respite care

From Alabama Health Services: a health care delivery system in Birmingham, Alabama.

design health plan benefits; develop practice guidelines across the continuum; identify health risk screening tools and processes; develop targeted screening programs by age and sex group and implement preventive care protocols; develop physician profiling and data dissemination processes; and develop processes for utilization review, discharge planning, and other components of care management (Figure 38-1).

The collaborative partnerships between the hospital-based outcome managers and the HMO staff were mutually beneficial. Brookwood outcome managers learned about new strategies, such as primary care management, epidemiologically based planning, and alternative mechanisms to reduce variation in medical care. Brookwood outcome managers, on the other hand, were able to share their extensive knowledge of individual physician practice patterns and resultant clinical, financial, and quality outcomes.

Partnerships Along the Continuum

Studying ourselves internally led to external partnerships to improve quality and service and reduce cost. Continually evaluating length of stay and other patient outcomes has led to partnerships with all components of the health care delivery system where patients are seen. Transfers to skilled nursing facilities are one of thirteen core processes continually measured, monitored, and analyzed by the Case Management Department at Brookwood Medical Center and provide an excellent example of hospital partnerships across the continuum. Outcome managers developed a statistical process control (SPC) system with more than 80 indicators to continually measure clinical, quality, and financial outcomes of the thirteen core case management processes. Case management core processes involve activities such as rehabilitation referrals, home care transfers, discharges to home, utilization review, skilled nursing facility placements, and many others. Early analysis of the SPC data revealed many opportunities for streamlining and redesigning processes that had been used for years without revision.

One of the earliest processes to be totally redesigned involved skilled nursing facility transfers. Brookwood worked collaboratively with more than 40 nursing homes across five counties to dramatically improve the skilled nursing facility placement process. Process improvement activities resulted in:

- A 30% reduction in lost days because of discharge planning problems
- An 86% reduction in unnecessary faxing of medical record information between the hospital and the skilled nursing facilities
- Reduced skilled nursing facility response time to requests for placement of patients, from 60 hours to 4 hours
- A reduction in Medicare length of stay by 1 day
- Development of a comprehensive education tool for patients and families about skilled care

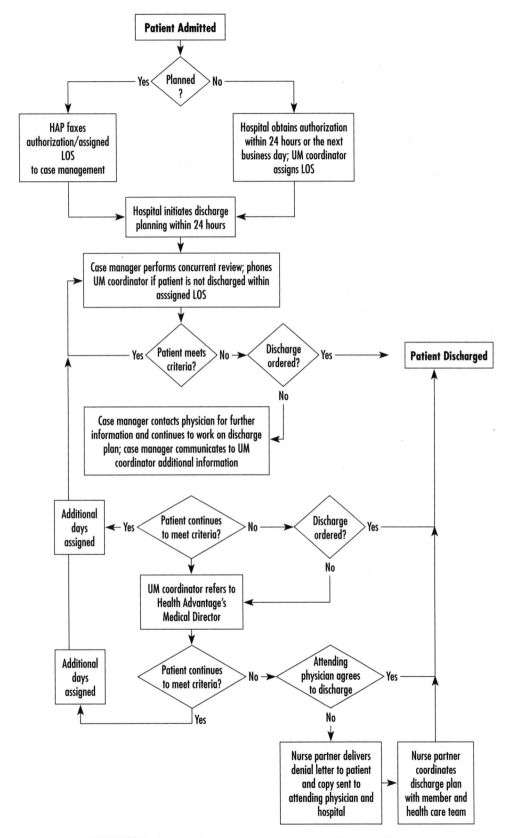

FIGURE 38-1 Flowchart of case management processes for Alabama Health Services.

- Preferred provider relationship status with select skilled nursing facilities
- Greater satisfaction with the search and transfer process among patients, their families, and the skilled nursing facilities themselves.

The Asthma Center of Excellence

The Asthma Center of Excellence (ACE) at Brookwood Medical Center provides a good example of the four types of collaboration and the new partnerships that have emerged in the integrated health care environment. Brookwood's ACE program is a comprehensive care delivery program established to address the needs of asthma patients throughout the continuum. Components of the program include all sites of care where asthma patients are likely to benefit from professional health care (Figure 38-2).

The ACE program is based on the six-part asthma management program recommended by the National Heart, Lung, and Blood Institute (National Institutes of Health, 1997). Unique features of the ACE program include:

- A dedicated full-time, master's-prepared advanced practice nurse to serve as the program coordinator

- A coordinated approach to case management that links payer- and provider-based case management processes and each component of the ACE program
- A new level of care, called the Continuing Care Clinic, specifically designed to meet the needs of patients who require intensive one-on-one training and assessment that cannot be accomplished in the physician's office or acute care setting
- A state-of-the-art outcomes management program designed to measure the individual and aggregate impact of ACE on patient outcomes
- A dedicated ACE referral and patient information line staffed 24 hours per day, seven days per week, with a "one-call" referral process and 100% callback by the ACE program coordinator

Establishment of the ACE program required collaboration and coordination among nearly all of the players in the integrated health care delivery system described in the introduction to this chapter.

Disease management programs like ACE have been shown to reduce hospital admissions, emergency visits, and physician office visits (Brown, 1997; Donahue, 1997; National Institutes of Health, 1997; Tilly et al, 1996). In an environment where

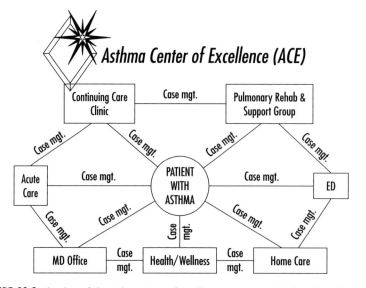

FIGURE 38-2 Flowchart of the Asthma Center of Excellence's program at Brookwood Medical Center.

payer-provider contractual relationships continue to be based on per-visit reimbursement, programs like ACE would be expected to result in reduced revenue. Balancing that reduced revenue with an overall increase in market share and quantifying the patient impact in terms of improved quality of life and service to the community became the opportunity for clinical and financial collaboration described earlier.

Opportunities for hospital and physician collaboration were readily apparent as all members of the health care team established standardized physicians' orders for the management of the asthma patient in all settings across the continuum. The establishment of the advanced practice role in the Continuing Care Clinic afforded new opportunities for physician-nurse partnerships in establishing and monitoring complex medical management plans for individual asthma patients.

Merging processes of the provider- and payer-based case managers required much dialogue between those two groups. While payer-based case managers would manage access to various components of the ACE program, hospital-based case managers negotiated to manage the acute setting as well as coordinate data collection and dissemination throughout the continuum. Partnerships based on trust and mutual respect were apparent throughout this phase of development.

The establishment of partnerships between each of the settings where care was to be delivered was a requirement of the program. One member from each component of the continuum represented each provider partner on the program steering committee. The referral process, patient education materials, and tools for patient care documentation were the results of collaboration among all members of the continuum.

Conclusion

The ACE program serves as a good example of the new and exciting opportunities for partnerships and collaboration that have arisen from the movement toward integrated health care delivery systems. Each of the component parts of the integrated system is extending beyond its tradiional boundaries to create a care delivery model that should ultimately serve to improve the health status of the community. Only time and comprehensive evaluation of the "new" system will tell if the promise of "integrated health care" will live up to its name.

References

Barron E, Westermann D: Getting it all together, *Health Progress* 76(3):38-40;48, 1995.

Brown K: Improving follow-up care for high-risk adult asthmatics, *Quality Connection* 6(1):8-9, 1997.

Coddington D, Moore K, Fischer E: In pursuit of integration, *Healthcare Forum Journal* 37(2):53-59, 1994.

Conrad D, Shortell S: Integrated health systems: promise and performance, *Frontiers of Health Services Management* 13(1):3-40, 1996.

Conrad D: Coordinating patient care services in regional health systems: the challenge of clinical integration, *Hospital and Health Services Administration* 38(4):491-508, 1993.

Danzon P, Boothman L, Greenberg P: Consolidation and restructuring: the next step in managed care, *Health Care Management: State of the Art Reviews* 2(1):221-235, 1995.

Donahue J: Inhaled steroids and the risk of hospitalization for asthma, *The Journal of the American Medical Association* 277(11):887-891, 1997.

Gilmore T, Hirschhorn L, O'Connor M: The boundaryless organization, *Healthcare Forum Journal* 37(4):68-72, 1994.

Hudson T: The rage to integrate: who will be the leaders? *Hospitals and Health Networks* 67(11):24-27, 1993.

Hunt R: Overcoming barriers to integrated health delivery, *Frontiers of Health Services Management* 13(1):50-52, 1996.

McMahon J, ed: The roles of hospitals in an evolving delivery system: living in two worlds—capitation and fee-for-service. *Report of the 1994 National Forum on Hospital and Health Affairs,* Durham, NC, 1995, Duke University, The Fuqua School of Business and The Duke Endowment, pp 64-81.

McQueen J, Marwick P: Introduction: Evolution of patient-focused care within the contextual framework of an integrated delivery system (IDS), *Journal of the Society for Health Systems* 5(1):5-9, 1995.

National Institutes of Health: *Highlights of the expert panel report II: Guidelines for the diagnosis and management of asthma* (draft for administrative purposes), Bethesda, Md, 1997, National Heart, Lung, and Blood Institute.

Pitcavage J: Integrated delivery systems: one staff's experience, *Pennsylvania Medicine* 97(4):18-19, 1994.

Pointer D, Alexander J, Zuckerman H: Loosening the Gordian knot of governance in integrated health care delivery systems, *Frontiers of Health Services Management* 11(3):3-52, 1995.

Porter A, VanCleave B, Milobowski L, Conlon P, Mambourg R: Clinical integration: an interdisciplinary approach to a system priority, *Nursing Administration Quarterly* 20(2):65-73, 1996.

Stahl D: Integrated delivery system: an opportunity or a dillema? *Nursing Management* 26(7):20-23, 1995.

Tilly K, Garvey N, Milton G, Powell E, Proudlock M: Outcomes management and asthma education in a community hospital: ongoing monitoring of health status, *Quality Management in Health Care* 4(3):67-78, 1996.

CHAPTER 39

Case Management by Design

New Roles in Acute Care

SHARON MASS, PhD, ELIZABETH JOHNSON, RN, CAROLYN E. AYDIN, PhD, and LINDA BURNES BOLTON, RN, DrPH, FAAN

OVERVIEW

The purpose of cross-preparation was to ensure a type of "one-stop-shopping" model for all of our customers.

This chapter describes the evolution of case management in one hospital from separate utilization management and medical social work departments to a single case management department in which case managers and social workers work in "dyads" and are cross-prepared to perform both functions to meet the needs of patients. The authors include their detailed curriculum plan for cross-preparation, evaluation instruments and outcomes, and describe recent experiments in rehabilitation and psychiatry units in which one individual performs the combined social work/case management role. Creative solutions for expedited discharges have also resulted in cost savings for the Medical Center. ▲

Background

The interdisciplinary case management system presented in this chapter was initiated as part of Cedars-Sinai Medical Center's 1993 to 1994 patient care redesign project to ensure the appropriate use of hospital and patient resources while assisting to achieve desired outcomes in patient care (Mass, Esquith, Johnson, 1995). Driven by the increase in managed care and the need for a more coordinated approach to the social work, discharge planning, and utilization management functions, a model of service delivery was created that would achieve a seamless level of case management. The aim of the case management system was to provide a collaborative practice model that would integrate the skills of each health care professional in the service delivery arena.

Prior to patient care redesign, the Department of Medical Social Work and the Department of Utilization Management functioned as two separate and distinct departments. The social work staff (all master's-prepared social workers) were members of a centralized department, were assigned to specific services, and had direct patient care responsibilities for psychosocial assessment, support, and intervention. They provided community resource referrals and transacted all placements of patients to alternative levels of care. Although they collaborated with patient caregivers as needed, the social worker's function was autonomous and independent of the patient care unit.

Like the social work department, the utilization management coordinators were members of a centralized department and were assigned to specific units. Their responsibilities included concurrent review of charts for appropriateness and timeliness of care, initiating discharge planning referrals to social work and home care departments, collecting data regarding quality issues and health services research, and acting as the primary contact for payer information and other related but non-direct patient care contacts. They reviewed all patients' charts, provided specific information to all payers, and communicated with physicians about specific care issues. Like social workers, utilization management coordinators functioned autonomously, although the two disciplines met daily on the patient care unit (with the unit manager and the home care coordinator, as available) to review patients' status for post-hospital needs.

In the new case management system, the utilization management coordinator's role was expanded into a case manager position. This work redesign allowed the case manager to be actively involved in developing, coordinating, and directly influencing the care process while maintaining the traditional utilization review functions. In addition, the social worker provided the discharge planning, abuse identification, and crisis intervention/psychosocial support role, supplementing the service delivery. Social workers became more integrated into the unit team, although remaining a centralized department. Social workers and case managers were partnered for a collaborative approach intended to yield a more coordinated level of post-hospital planning. This unique partnering, or "dyad," would be the basis for future service delivery enhancement.

Data Collection and Management

In addition to the social work and case management functions described above, the case management department also provides data to administrators, physicians, and unit managers that demonstrate several aspects of how different processes within the system are performing. (Figure 39-1 shows a sample report.) Currently this monthly report details the average length of stay, case mix index, top five DRGs, discharge status, number of discharge delays, reasons for delays in workup or treatment, delays in performing diagnostic or therapeutic procedures, delays in establishment of discharge plan, quality issues, location (specific service) of delay within the system, and reason for the delay. For example, the report shows whether a delay in service is attributable to physicians (i.e., no medical necessity for continued stay), scheduling gaps (i.e., scheduling issues, weekend or holiday procedures delay), delays in response to referrals, and so on. System issues are trended and shared with other areas within the hospital through various groups reviewing Medical Center performance (e.g., Utilization Review Committee, service line Performance Improvement Committees, specific departments, service line managers) for quality improvement or system enhancement.

At the monthly Utilization Management Committee meeting (a medical staff function), for example, the committee chair reviews the data col-

CASE MANAGEMENT REPORT

Unit: ALL
Month: February
Year: 1998

Vital Statistics

	Case Mgt	Pathways	U.R.
Cases	3031	132	662
%	79%	3%	17%

	This month	Last month
Discharges	2332	2539
Pt days	14606	15096
Delay days	321	190
Adj days	14285	14906
Avg los	6.2	5.9
Adj los	6.1	5.8
CMI	1.51	1.47
Avg Cost	$11,227	$9,970

Payor

Payor	Cases	%
Medicare	1041	44%
Private	99	4%
PPO	405	17%
Champus	1	
Cigna	34	1%
Free	2	
HMO Cap	131	5%
HMO non Cap	189	8%
Medical	288	12%
Misc	2	
Government	25	1%
Capitation	28	1%
Self	79	3%
Workmans	8	
Unknown	0	

Delays

	Cases
Avoided	48
Delay	147

	Case	Path	U.R.
Avoided	45	0	3
Avoided %	93%		6%
Delay	126	5	16
Delay %	85%	3%	10%

Reason Codes

THIS MONTH

#	Reason Label	Cases	Days
3	No medical necessity for continued stay	12	43
50	Proactive services involved	3	31
31	Delay in response by S.S to consult	9	30
26	Scheduling issue delay	14	25
27	Weekend or holiday proc. delay	13	23

Service Codes

THIS MONTH

#	Reason Label	Cases	Days
CDL	Cardiac diag lab/Cath/PTCA/EPS/Pacer/	7	12
CDS	Cardiac surgery all open cardiac	7	11
NEO	Neonatology	5	11
PTX	Physical medicine OT/PT	4	6
RAD	Radiology-All x-rays CT/MRI	4	6

Discharge Status

Status	Cases	%
Routine discharge	1547	66%
Short term	13	
Skilled nursing	146	6%
Other type	172	7%
Home health	254	10%
AMA	26	1%
Hospice	13	
Expired	85	3%
Unknown	76	3%

Top 5 Diagnosis Related Groups

DRG #	Drg Label	THIS MONTH Cases	LOS	Target	% Diff	LAST MONTH Cases	LOS	Target	% Diff
430	Psychoses	101	8.1	.0		103	8.3	.0	
127	Heart failure and shock	82	7.1	.0		84	6.2	.0	
112	Percutaneous cardiovasc proc.	78	3.4	.0		91	4.0	.0	
89	Simp pneum/pleur age >17 W/CC	68	6.9	.0		80	6.1	.0	
143	Chest pain	51	2.0	.0		58	1.9	.0	

FIGURE 39-1 Sample case management report.

lected by case management suggesting an observable trend (such as delays in performing diagnostic procedures on weekends or holidays). The committee members review the data and decide whether to request that the Utilization Management (UM) Chair forward this information to the department responsible for the procedure in question and request a response. Additionally, at the respective Performance Improvement Committee, the UM Chair may bring the issue to the committee's attention for further discussion/resolution. The UM Chair, as a member of the Quality Improvement Committee, will update the committee on the observable trends as reported by case management and will report on the actions taken to respond to the issues. The charts in Figure 39-2 display the Medical Affairs Department Dashboard with several of the performance indicators being tracked. The case management report also provides the information and often serves as the impetus for the various interested stakeholders to form quality action teams to work on resolving specific identified issues.

Current Issues and Education

By the end of 1996, the "dyad" (case manager, social worker) had been in place for over a year, and there appeared to be a division among many of the dyads in which individuals lacked an understanding of the dyad's function in working toward mutual organizational goals. It appeared that some case managers were still "stuck in basic chart reviews" and failed to understand the broader picture of care coordination and goals of case management. Conversely, several social workers were stubbornly entrenched against the case managers, whom they perceived as inappropriately dictating or misallocating the need for social work services to patients and families in the hospital. At the root of this identified problem was poor communication and a lack of teamwork and spirit of collaboration within the dyad.

The strategic plan for the case management model, however, was to further expand the scope of the roles between the case manager and the social worker, achieving as much integration as appropriate. This further integration meant that the traditional roles of utilization management nurses and medical social workers as discharge planners would be confronted with the even greater challenge of understanding new concepts and assuming new responsibilities. In an effort to more fully integrate the responsibilities of the case manager and the social worker to improve efficiency, reduce lengths of stay, and maximize service delivery, the department's two managers, working with an administrative intern (candidate for master's in health administration), and with input from staff, developed an education program to improve the knowledge and understanding of the respective dyad roles and provide skills enhancement education (Box 39-1).

The purpose of the cross-preparation was to ensure a type of "one-stop shopping" model for all of our customers. In this model, when a nurse or a unit manager inquired about a patient needing a service (e.g., placement, abuse identification, third-party interface), the dyad member would accept the inquiry instead of saying "Oh, that's the social worker's task" or "That's the case manager's task." The now acceptable response is "We can handle this" and the individual will then either take care of the problem or contact his or her dyad partner. Furthermore, on days when one dyad member is extremely busy the other can go ahead and make the call to the third-party payer or help place the patient or provide a more in-depth clinical assessment, which will yield enough information to assist the team. With the dyad members' new familiarity with each other's tasks, it is expected that the case management process, communication, and patient services will be more efficient and effective across the continuum of care.

Evaluating the Case Management Process

The skills enhancement educational program was presented to the combined social work/case manager staff over a ten-week period. Following the education program, 45 unit managers and faculty physicians received a questionnaire asking them to evaluate various aspects of the case management process (Figure 39-3). Thirty-eight individuals (84%) responded. The results of this survey are shown in Figure 39-4. In addition to the summarized findings, results for each service line were examined in detail. Findings were included in employees' individual performance evaluations, and managers worked with case managers and social

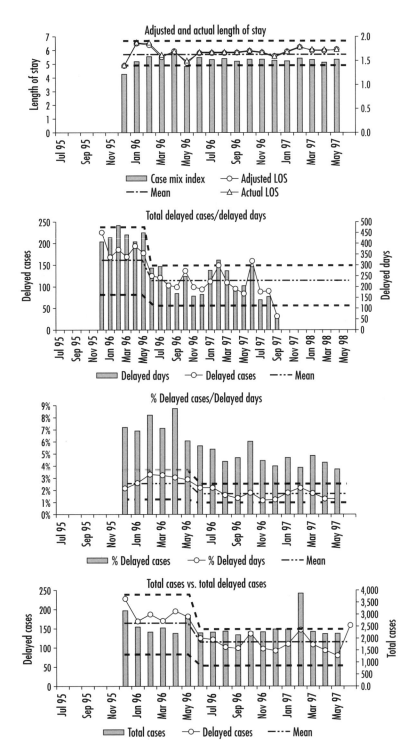

FIGURE 39-2 Medical Affairs Department Dashboard showing tracking of several performance indicators.

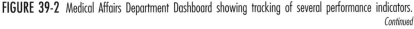

Continued

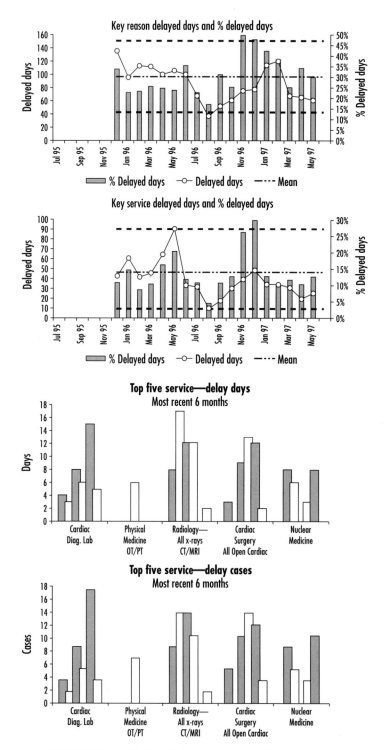

FIGURE 39-2, cont'd Medical Affairs Department Dashboard showing tracking of several performance indicators.

BOX 39-1

Curriculum Outline: Case Management Skills Enhancement Project*

I. Case Management: The Big Picture
   A. Tasks (case mgr/social worker)
      1. Assessment
      2. Planning
      3. Intervention
      4. Monitor
      5. Evaluate
   B. Integration
      1. Which discipline?
      2. Which task?
      3. Focus of dyad—separate but equal?
      4. Multiskilled
      5. Redesigned
   C. Value
      1. Improved outcomes of care
      2. Intelligent management of patients
      3. Coordination of best services available
      4. Risk management
      5. Enhanced reimbursement
      6. Safe post-hospital care planning
      7. Appropriate length of stay
      8. Replanning
II. Team Building (Outside Facilitator)
   A. Icebreakers
   B. Boundaries
   C. Fears, anxiety, anger, aggression
   D. Communication
   E. Collaboration
   F. Accountability
III. Responsibilities/Tasks/Roles
   A. Social worker
      1. Determining referral need
      2. Indicators for intervention
      3. High-risk screening criteria
      4. Clinical SW assessment
      5. Discharge planning
      6. Data collection
   B. Case manager
      1. Key aspects of CM assessment
      2. Determining level of CM involvement
      3. Care coordination
      4. Secure sponsorship (funding)
      5. Use of physician advisor
      6. Data collection
   C. Discharge coordination
      1. Levels of care across continuum
         a. Community

      b. Acute acre
      c. Acute specialty
      d. Subacute/skilled nursing
      e. Community (home health, retirement hotel, board & care, assisted living, transitional living, nursing facility, acute specialty hospital)
      2. Characteristics
      3. Funding sources
      4. Case studies
IV. Financial Aspects
   A. Definition
      1. Managed care
      2. Funding sources (indemnity, preferred provider organization, exclusive provider organization, HMO, point of service, physician practice models)
      3. Physician practice models
   B. Reimbursement models (fee for service, discount, per diem, capitation, all inclusive, risk sharing)
   C. Role plan reimbursement strategies
V. Focus of the Case Manager/Social Work Dyad
   A. Daily rounds—shared information
      1. Patient's age, name, primary diagnosis, procedures
      2. Significant medical history, premorbid living situation, level of functioning (services needed prior to hospitalization)
      3. Effects of current episode of illness on premorbid level of functioning
      4. Anticipated needs upon discharge
      5. Funding available to cover needs
      6. Existence of special programs that could assist in provision of necessary services
      7. Availability of assistance from patient's support system in providing physical care
      8. Known or anticipated transportation issues
      9. Referrals needed or already made to other hospital disciplines
   B. Identification of team member who will perform necessary action
   C. Case studies
   D. Resource directory

Dear: Re:

Our goal is to provide you with an efficient, high-quality case management process (Utilization Management, Social Work, Continuum of Care Coordination/Discharge Planning) throughout the Medical Center. Please take a few minutes to assist us in evaluating our services by completing this survey and returning it in the enclosed envelope. Your feedback is important and we appreciate your time. Thank you.

		Poor	Fair	Good	Very good	Excellent
1.	In responding to your needs, was the nurse case manager:					
	Available: How easy to reach	1	2	3	4	5
	Friendly: How cooperative	1	2	3	4	5
	Skillful: Demonstrated the knowledge and skills to meet your patients' needs	1	2	3	4	5
	Effective: Results of efforts met your patients' needs	1	2	3	4	5
2.	In responding to your needs, was the social worker:					
	Available: How easy to reach	1	2	3	4	5
	Friendly: How cooperative	1	2	3	4	5
	Skillful: Demonstrated the knowledge and skills to meet your patients' needs	1	2	3	4	5
	Effective: Results of efforts met your patients' needs	1	2	3	4	5
3.	How would you rate your overall experiences with the case manager?	1	2	3	4	5
4.	How would you rate your overall experiences with the social worker?	1	2	3	4	5
5.	How would you rate the extent to which the social worker and case manager coordinate their efforts to meet you and your patients' needs?	1	2	3	4	5
6.	How would you rate your overall experiences with case management?	1	2	3	4	5

FIGURE 39-3 Example of a questionnaire used to evaluate the case management process.

workers to improve their performance in areas that survey respondents identified as weak. The survey was then repeated in August 1997 to evaluate long-term outcomes of the enhanced integration and education program and to track improvements in the case management process. This second survey demonstrated a decrease in satisfaction within the overall case management process (explained by the need to use outside registry staff because of an unexpected and sustained high volume of patients).

Do the services provided by Medical Social Work/Utilization Management
assist you in controlling costs?   Yes____ No____

What other suggestions do you have to assist in this area?

_____

_____

_____

What do you like about the case management services? _____

_____

_____

_____

_____

What would you like to see changed/made available in case management? _____

_____

_____

_____

_____

COMMENTS: _____

_____

_____

_____

_____

Thank you for your time:

Please use the enclosed addressed envelope to return this survey to:

FIGURE 39-3, cont'd Example of a questionaire used to evaluate the case management process.

While the overall results were less satisfactory than the initial findings (Figure 39-5 vs. Figure 39-4), the information has generated discussions with unit managers on how to better serve the needs of the unit. Currently ad hoc task forces have been formed to reexamine the communication vehicles on several of the units; review the purpose of team meetings, daily rounds, and discharge planning meetings; and reach a consensus on how to better meet customer needs. The director and two managers of the department also continue to monitor and evalu-

ate progress by observing the dyads as they interact with and relate to each other and the other health care team members. Figure 39-6 shows the evaluation tool used to measure the observed levels of interaction and integration.

Measuring Outcomes

The case managers provide unit-specific information to the unit managers on a regular basis. Care coordination that is directive and timely adds value

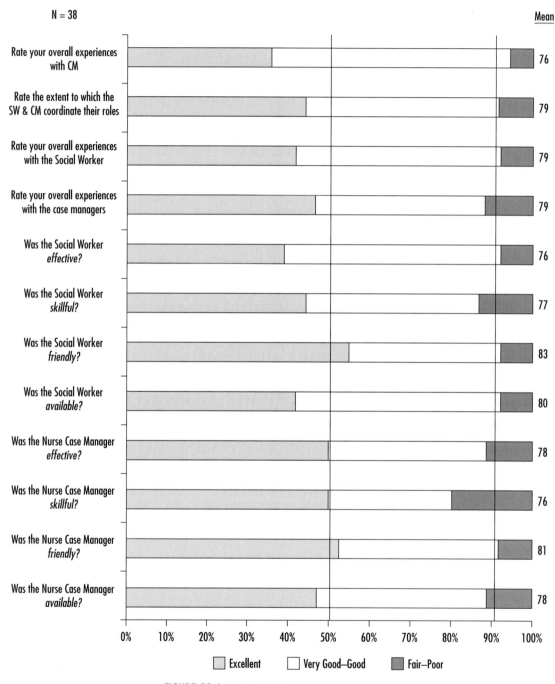

FIGURE 39-4 Results of the first survey in March 1997.

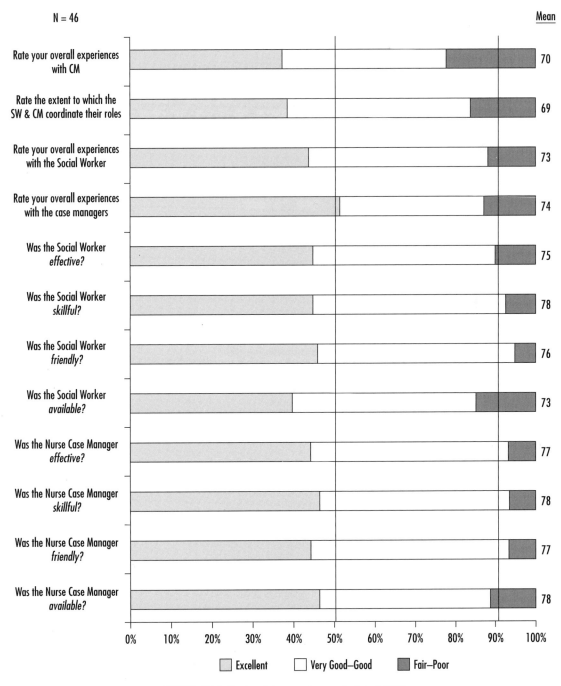

FIGURE 39-5 Results of the second survey in August 1997.

CASE MANAGER/SOCIAL WORKER
DAILY ROUNDS & COMMUNICATION EVALUATION FORM

UNIT SURVEYED:_____   DATE:_____
STAFF EVALUATED:_____
EVALUATED BY:_____

The case manager and social worker discussed the patients (including physical & emotional status,
support network, pre-morbid needs & living arrangements, high-risk factors, and projected needs)
and made appropriate recommendations and referrals. *If no, explain:*_____
_____
_____

When patients were referred for services/intervention (e.g., home care, patient accounting, social
work, etc.), there was an appropriate rationale. *If no, explain:*_____
_____
_____

The case manager had reasonable information about the patients and was able to present it in a
clear and useful manner. *If no, explain:*_____
_____
_____

The social worker asked appropriate questions about the patients to enhance the dialogue and
facilitate the referral of patients with social work needs. *If no, explain:*_____
_____
_____

When discussing patients who had been previously referred to social work (e.g., follow-up
discussion), the social worker demonstrated involvement with information that was timely and
germane. *If no, explain:*_____
_____
_____

The case manager and social worker demonstrated a willingness to work collaboratively toward
meeting patient needs. *If no, explain:*_____
_____
_____

Opportunities observed to improve the dyad._____
_____
_____

Additional comments_____
_____
_____

FIGURE 39-6 Sample evaluation tool used to measure the observed levels of interaction and integration.

to our hospital. When our system works well, we connect the correct intervention with patient and family needs and positively impact the consumer by reducing duplication and unnecessary burdens or costs. However, opportunities for improvement in service delivery still exist, and patient surveys also suggest room for improvement in efficiency and customer satisfaction.

Currently the case managers and social workers are assigned to each nursing service. Again, how well they integrate with the patient care delivery system varies by service and also with the specific interpersonal skills of the professionals and how well they are perceived as a member of the team on the unit. Outcome measures monitored by our department include length of stay, patient/customer satisfaction, and number of delay days/discharges averted because of our intervention. We also track the potential dollars saved through the adoption of creative solutions to unexpected barriers to timely discharge. Examples of some of the creative solutions being evaluated include paying for a board/care stay for a patient needing supervision while awaiting MediCal; arranging to fly a patient home to family in another state rather than have him or her stay in the hospital because of lack of funding to purchase an airline or bus ticket; transporting a patient home by taxi or ambulance, as needed, in lieu of remaining in the hospital when he or she no longer requires acute care but lacks funding for transport; purchasing needed medication or providing home visits to uninsured patients who no longer need acute care.

Case managers and social workers are aware of the department's policy of facilitating or expediting discharge of nonfunded or indigent patients, and they recognize the importance of being creative and innovative in transitioning all patients to appropriate levels of care in as timely a manner as possible. When there is an unexpected cost to the discharge, or one that either insurance or the patient cannot cover, department management will be consulted for the authorization of funding. Estimates of savings resulting from these creative solutions are shown in Table 39-1.

Using more conventional measures, data comparing 1996 with 1997 show the effects of changes in the case management system on the number of delays in patient discharge from the Medical Center (Table 39-2), as well case managers' estimates of additional delays averted by their interventions. The

TABLE 39-1
Estimated Savings from "Creative Solutions"

FUNDING FOR EXPEDITED DISCHARGES	1995	1996	1997
Number of patients served/projected days saved	15/170	22/519	12/180
Estimated dollar value (based on $300/day)	$51,000	$155,700	$54,000
Cost to CSMC (i.e., monies advanced for plane tickets, taxi fares, board/care stays, etc.)	$18,000	$ 50,900	$11,000
Cost recoverable by CSMC (deposits/ guarantees)	$12,000	$ 39,000	$ 3,000
Cost benefit to CSMC (assuming recovery of all deposits/ guarantees)	$45,000	$143,600	$46,000

decrease in total number of actual delays, as well as the increase in estimated delays averted, may be attributed to earlier establishment of discharge plans, including early contact with the patient and family by the case manager, as well as improved working relationships between case managers and social workers.

Ongoing Change

Since the cross-preparation was implemented, we have continued to move forward with further integration of the case manager and social worker roles. On our rehabilitation unit, for example, we now have a master's-prepared social worker performing the case management role. Discharge planning, treatment authorization requests, discussions with external case managers for post-hospital services, and the negotiation/broker role for special services were already within the scope of the social worker's responsibilities. We added authorization for admission and request for continued stay extensions (the utilization management piece) to enable the social

TABLE 39-2 Case Management Impacts on Discharge Delays				
	JANUARY TO JUNE 1996		JANUARY TO JUNE 1997	
ACTUAL DELAYS IN DISCHARGE	NO. OF CASES	NO. OF DAYS	NO. OF CASES	NO. OF DAYS
Delays in establishing discharge plan	389	384	211	224
Actual delays in dis- charge	338	605	223	446

	TOTAL 1995		TOTAL 1996		JANUARY-JUNE 1997	
	CASES	DAYS	CASES	DAYS	CASES	DAYS
Estimated averted delays*	551	1,333	691	1,912	840	1,890

*Based upon case manager estimates following interventions.

worker to provide full case management service on the rehabilitation unit.

In our psychiatric service line, the Director of Case Management and the Director of Mental Health also collaborated to experiment with a new model of service delivery. Instead of two separate positions (a case manager and a social worker), we have integrated each discipline's responsibilities into a new job description entitled "psychiatric case manager." When we advertised for this position, we specified the need for an M.S.W. with utilization review and case management experience. We provided training for the respective disciplines so that they could learn what was needed, and we currently have both nurses and social workers performing the psychiatric case management function on the mental health unit.

The organizational structure for case management at the Medical Center has also continued to evolve. As mentioned in the introduction, in November 1993 the Medical Social Work and Utilization Management Departments were integrated into one department under the leadership of the Director of Medical Social Work. At that time the goal was to assist both disciplines in working collaboratively in a collegial manner and to help them bridge the perceived disparity between their respective roles (e.g., UM "throws people out of the hospital, SW helps with discharge"). In February 1995, the transition to case management began with the conversion of the utilization management role to a case management role. At that time there was some integration in that both disciplines were part of one department, but it was not until June 1995, when both disciplines were housed in the same office, that the working together really began. In June 1996, a department-wide effort was undertaken to develop the curriculum for the educational program detailed in Box 39-1. This program was developed, implemented, and completed in April 1997. In August 1997, the Departments of Medical Social Work and Utilization Management were actually combined as the Department of Case Management, under the leadership of the same director. This department reports to a physician, who is the Medical Center's Vice President of Medical Affairs.

Additional Challenges

An additional challenge the department faces is the lack of education about and understanding of the case management process on the part of the physician. Physicians frequently attribute an adversarial role to any aspect of the case management process and perceive any desire to collaborate or partner as "control" or "dictating how they should practice medicine." To explore these issues, the case management department held a physician focus group facilitated by a neutral, non-department member. At this 1½-hour meeting, the consensus was that the physicians saw the department as "only interested in the financial aspects" and adversarial to their process. In an effort to address these issues, we are working with the Chief of the Medical Staff to publish articles on the case management process that illustrate the advantages of care coordination to patients and to patient care. In addition, on a one-to-one basis, each staff member is attempting to educate attending physicians to our process and the advantages to physicians of timely identification of obstacles and the use of creative solutions to smooth the discharge process.

Conclusion: Future Directions

This chapter described one hospital's experience in designing and implementing a more comprehensive delivery system for care coordination, utilization review, social work, discharge planning, and continuity of care. Our new and continuously evolving level of service provides a comprehensive approach to many of the difficult and complicated problems in our service environment and addresses the patient's need for linkage within all of the interacting levels of care.

Case management is an integral process in the overall system of care. As Cedars-Sinai expands the integrated delivery network, the role of the case manager will continue to evolve. Direct nursing care providers will assume greater responsibility for managing the processes of care to ensure achievement of the following outcomes:

- Reduced cycle time associated with the admission, transfer, and discharge processes
- Decreases in missed and delayed treatment associated with inherent system failures
- Improved multidisciplinary team coordination to facilitate patient progress and the transition to home or other sites along the continuum of care

- Care coordination processes that bridge levels of care and are managed by integrated delivery team case management experts

It is this last role, in particular, that will drive the work of today's case managers. The demand for health outcomes management across the life span will exceed our current capacity. To meet this demand, we will need case management professionals with strong clinical and acute care backgrounds and extensive experience in working with the community. Today's practice environment is preparing tertiary case managers in a market with 40% or greater managed care penetration to assume new roles as health outcomes managers. The opportunity for nurses and social service professionals to provide complementary services will continue to exist within a changing health care market.

Reference

Mass S, Esquith D, Johnson B: Patient-focused care model for social work and utilization management. In Aydin CE, Bolton L, Weingarten S, eds: *Patient-focused care in the hospital*, New York, 1995, Faulkner & Gray, pp. 133-154.

CHAPTER 40

Outcomes of Academic and Service Partnership

MARJORIE PECK, RN, PhD, **JON D. CHRISTENSEN,** RN, BSN, **and DONNA FOSBINDER,** RN, DNSc

OVERVIEW

To bring service and education into partnership requires time and support from educators, administrators, staff members, and students.

What began in 1990 as a redesign of a medical nursing unit evolved into a powerful partnership between educators, hospital-based nursing staff, and administrators. The staff of the medical unit at LDS Hospital in Salt Lake City defined a model of differentiated practice to provide optimal care for their patient population. Using the South Dakota Healing Web model as their guide, Salt Lake Community College and Brigham Young University faculties worked with LDS Hospital staff and management to bring students together from associate degree and baccalaureate degree programs to educate them for differentiated roles, mutual valuing, and collegial relationships. The outcomes were positive for patients, staff, faculty, and students. ▲

Getting Started

To describe the outcomes of this academic and service partnership, one must tell the story of the evolution of the relationship and the context in which it happened. In 1990 the 46-bed medical unit (W8) in LDS Hospital (a 520-bed tertiary hospital in Salt Lake City) was experiencing a 49% turnover of registered nurses (RNs), a 50% vacancy rate, excessive salary expenses because of the use of agency nurses, very low staff morale, and low "unit esteem" as described by the staff who worked on the unit. W8 patients were predominantly high-acuity older adults, often frail, usually with very high dependency needs. The budgeted staff mix was 90%+ R.N. with a few nursing assistants and licensed practical nurses. The department manager hired 10 to 12 newly graduated nurses twice each year, but their tenure rarely exceeded one year. A 1988 to 1989 study of patient preparation for discharge indicated that patients were not adequately prepared to manage their health care needs at home.

The nurse executive and director for medical-surgical nursing decided that the system needed a major change. The decision was made to redesign care delivery. The redesign work was accomplished by a number of teams, in two major initiatives over 7 years. The first redesign initiative had three goals:

1. A patient-centered model of care delivery. Patient centered was defined as meeting patient care needs and expectations first, and staff needs second.
2. Budgeted expenses would be at or below the 1990 expenses.
3. Staff satisfaction would increase as evidenced by reduced turnover.

The reasons for describing the first redesign initiative are, first, to introduce a collegial relationship that continues today between members of the service and academic institutions and, second, to recognize the long-term nature of the work of staff development and change implementation. The faculty-staff relationship evolved into a partnership that enriched faculty, staff, and student experiences and facilitated the development of the Utah Healing Web. In the 1990 to 1991 school year, when the redesign project began, one faculty person, the director of the graduate program in nursing administration, from Brigham Young University (BYU) offered to assist with the work of design and support for staff during design and implementation. The

faculty person and the nurse executive at LDS hospital had been colleagues in another state prior to coming to Utah. The relationship enabled continued work together to support each other, students, and staff.

Beginning the Partnership: Redesign (1990-1991)

Staff nurses, physicians, respiratory therapists, a housekeeper, a pharmacist, the nurse executive, the director for medical-surgical nursing, the director for nursing research, and a patient representative met to begin redesign of the medical unit's care delivery system. The director of nursing research interviewed patients to identify their needs and expectations. Physicians and nurses were asked to state their views about patients' greatest needs. RNs were asked to indicate what did not get done when they were busy. Time-and-motion studies demonstrated how time was spent by each discipline working on the unit. The following are highlights of the findings:

- Patients reported that they were not prepared for discharge and self/family care at home.
- Patients and nurses thought call lights were not answered quickly.
- Approximately half of the time spent with patients was spent on activities of daily living (feeding, toileting, bathing, dressing).
- Nurses reported that teaching and preparation for discharge were not done when they were busy.

CARE DELIVERY MODEL DESIGN

The redesign team developed a model that included two clinical care coordinators (episodic case manager), a bedside RN, a certified nursing assistant (CNA), unit secretary, and an environmental technician (housekeeper, greeter). They changed the staff mix to 52% RNs, 40% CNAs, and 8% unit secretaries and environmental technicians. The RNs and CNAs worked together, as a team, assigned to provide care for a group of patients during their shift.

The hospital-based nurse researcher, informal staff leaders, the BYU faculty colleague, the nurse executive, and the director for medical-surgical nursing were all actively involved in implementing the new model. The human resources (HR) department educated nursing staff about hiring practices, appropriate interview questions, and equal employment opportunity (EEO) issues. RNs worked with the department manager and HR to hire CNAs for the unit.

Orientation to the new model was provided by the manager, the director for medical-surgical nursing, the nurse executive, members of the design team, and the chief resident of the unit. All staff members from the unit were oriented in a full-day session. Staff debriefings were held every shift for two weeks. Debriefings slowed in frequency as staff expressed increased comfort with and demonstrated increasing ability to work with the new model. Debriefings were staffed by the nurse researcher, staff leaders, a faculty colleague, the nurse executive, and the director for medical-surgical nursing.

OUTCOMES OF THE FIRST REDESIGN

The following lists the outcomes of the first redesign as obtained from interviews:

- Patients expressed satisfaction with response to call lights.
- Patients knew their care providers, and they could identify who the RN and the CNA were.
- Patients' needs continued in the area of discharge preparation.
- Clinical care coordinators noted that their work load was greater than the time needed to do it.
- Salary costs per patient day, which had been over budget for months, and irregularly controlled for over two years, returned to budgeted amounts. Salary costs increased less than inflation during the next three years.

Solidifying the Partnership: Redesign (1994)

It was during the second redesign initiative that the service-education partnership blossomed. During the years between the first and second redesign initiatives, the W8 staff and manager developed unit-based shared governance. Shared governance, now the hospital's model for nursing governance, re-

quires each member of the nursing staff to accept accountability for nursing practice in his or her work area. Shared governance places decision-making authority for practice with the staff. This is significant, because it was the staff nurses who ultimately embraced differentiated practice and defined the practice needed for their population of patients. Also of significance was the continued role our university faculty colleague played as mentor for a number of staff nurses. The credibility of this faculty person with staff and administration opened doors for our partnership.

The director of the graduate program in nursing administration at BYU introduced the LDS Hospital nurse executive, the director for nursing research, and staff nurses to members of the Healing Web in Sioux Falls, South Dakota. The original Healing Web was composed of staff nurses, faculty, and administration from Sioux Valley Hospital, Augustana College, and South Dakota State University. Sandra Bunkers' description of the Healing Web follows: "This project is a model for the reconciliation and transformation of nursing. It is designed to help education and service think more clearly about the future of nursing" (Bunkers, 1992). Sioux Valley Hospital implemented differentiated practice in the late 1980s. Differentiated practice defines different and distinct roles for RNs on the basis of their education, experience, and professional goals (Koerner, Karpiuk, 1994).

One purpose of the Healing Web was to bring faculty and students in associate degree nursing (ADN) and bachelor of science in nursing (BSN) programs together to facilitate mutual valuing of roles and to heal the wounds that had developed within the discipline of nursing between educators and service, and between nurses educated in the two programs. Another purpose of the Healing Web was to support implementation of differentiated practice in nursing to provide comprehensive patient care and to recognize that more than one nursing role is required in order to provide complete patient care (Newman, 1995). Members of the Utah Healing Web worked together to implement a differentiated practice model of care delivery and to educate ADN and BSN students together as colleagues who valued the role each could play in providing patient care (Fosbinder et al, 1997).

The concept of healing the wounds of years of dissension between baccalaureate and associate degree educated staff and faculty was very appealing to the administration and faculty members involved in the Utah work. Differentiating R.N. practice, to recognize that no one person could do all that patients required, appealed to the staff of the medical unit. By 1993, the Dean and two faculty members from BYU and the nurse executive and director for nursing research from LDS Hospital met with members of the Sioux Falls Healing Web group for the purpose of developing a National Healing Web Partnership. The Utah group invited the director and a faculty member from Salt Lake Community College's associate degree program to join the initiative (Fosbinder et al, 1997). In 1994 the staff of the medical unit agreed to be the pilot unit for differentiating practice and implementing the Healing Web concepts at LDS hospital.

Teams were brought together at three levels:

1. Unit level. Members included staff nurses and the nurse manager. They defined roles and job descriptions that would meet the needs of the patient population, and developed the education program required to orient staff to the new roles.
2. Hospital level. This group included members of the unit team, administration, a system case manager, representatives from finance and home health, HR, and faculty from both the ADN and BSN programs. This group integrated the work of the unit and the colleges together and maintained a systems view of the work in order to facilitate interfaces between hospital, home health, case management, and support departments.
3. College level. Members included faculty from both Salt Lake Community College (ADN) and BYU (BSN). They were to define student outcomes and establish the curricular changes required to achieve outcomes. Faculty also coordinated student clinical experiences and postclinical conferences to facilitate integration of the two student groups.

GOALS

The goals of the Utah Web included the following:
- Define the roles needed to meet patient expectations and care needs
- Match end point student competencies with entry level competency expected for staff positions

- Mutual valuing of all roles for nurses and faculty
- Insure fiscal responsibility, defined as recognizing and adhering to approved costs within the approved budget
- Prepare staff and faculty for a new model of care delivery
- Ensure a supportive environment for students, the colleagues of the future

ROLES OF STAFF REGISTERED NURSES

The unit team defined the following three staff RN roles:

1. Care manager—nurses responsible for the patient from the time of admission to discharge. Responsibilities include care planning and coordination, facilitating interdisciplinary team conferences, and overseeing patient and family education and preparation for discharge. Integration of bedside nursing care with care planning and patient education is a hallmark of differentiated practice.
2. Clinical nurses—nurses responsible for providing care to the patient according to the plan of care on a shift-by-shift basis. Direct physical care, psychosocial care, and patient education are included in the clinical nurses' role.
3. Clinical care coordinator—a charge nurse with management responsibility for the shift. Responsibilities include making patient assignments, staffing within the context of patient needs and budget, and planning for continuous unit needs.

Other roles include CNAs and unit secretaries. Clinical nurses and CNAs continue to work in teams.

To assist RNs in deciding which role they wished to fulfill, they were asked to complete a modified version of the Role Choice Tool defined by Koerner and Karpiuk (1994). The instrument poses 36 specific statements that define the nurse's preferred method of practice. Statements focus on either shift-specific, episodic care or multidisciplinary continuum-based care. The director for nursing research and the director of the graduate program in nursing administration at BYU met with each staff person to discuss his or her interests and skills, which facilitated decision making about his or her future roles. Staff members interested in the care manager or clinical care coordinator roles applied for those positions. There initially were three care managers and fifteen clinical care coordinator positions. Staff members not applying for clinical care coordinator or care manager positions were involved in the selection process for those positions.

OTHER UNIT STAFF MEMBERS

The unit staff, through shared governance committees and the hospital team (made up of faculty, management, and staff) provided an orientation for all staff, which included:

- Information about differentiated practice and the Healing Web
- Definition of roles and role expectations
- Dialogue about mutual valuing
- Introduction of faculty
- Plans for student experience
- Fiscal expectations for the unit and the staff's role in meeting those expectations.

Faculty from the two colleges selected students for education on W8. The ADN students worked directly with clinical nurses, and the BSN students worked directly with care managers. In both cases, the goal was to introduce students to the roles for which their education best prepared them. Faculty from both programs were available to students from either program, as well as to unit staff, to answer questions about clinical care, roles, and goals of the Utah Healing Web. Similarly, staff members were available to answer students' and faculty's questions about clinical care, organizational policy, roles, and goals of the Utah Healing Web.

A major focus for the student experience was that students would be valued along with faculty, CNAs, RNs in all roles, managers, and administrators. The preparation for mutual valuing was done predominantly through discussion about the significance of each role, recollection by all involved of how they were greeted and treated as students, the deliberate description of students as colleagues of the future, and dialogue about the impossibility of any single nurse fulfilling all nursing roles. Mutual valuing of all nurses in all roles is the hallmark of the Healing Web work in Utah, South Dakota, and nationally. The ability to bring nurse educators, nurses in service settings, and students together to discuss patient needs, roles that

support patients, and how we interact with each other leads to the establishment of a powerful, positive coalition.

Outcomes

The process itself became an outcome. This group of nurses, their manager, and faculty viewed redesign as an evolutionary process that required them to continually evaluate whether they were meeting patients' needs and how they were treating and communicating with all individuals involved. Student outcomes from Healing Web sites including LDS Hospital include the following (Fosbinder et al, 1997):

- A much higher level of confidence with clinical and organizational skills
- Knowing the real value of a detailed plan of care and the effects on quality patient care
- More active participation in interdisciplinary planning
- A better understanding of the distinct roles that the associate and baccalaureate students have in care delivery
- The importance of shared learning with staff, faculty, students, other providers, and patients
- Ability to see the bigger picture, or how important integrated planning is to assist the patient with post-hospital access to care

W8 staff members understood that all students were not required to provide all care for patients, but were expected to learn specific roles in the context of differentiated practice. For example, a staff member challenged the technical ability of a B.S.N. student on the unit. Another staff member stopped the interaction, restating that this student was learning the role of the care manager, not technical skills. This on-the-spot clarification demonstrated appropriate communication, recognition of multiple roles, and valuing of different roles.

Before redesign, the W8 staff viewed themselves as having little voice in decision making about care delivery, and unable to halt the rapid turnover of staff from their unit. Now, staff members assert their control over the delivery and design of patient care on their unit. They evaluate their work on the basis of the needs of the patients and continue to identify education of students as part of their professional role.

Staff nurses planned and implemented the orientation for their peers in preparation for differentiated practice and the new student experience. In the first redesign effort, orientation planning was led by management and administration; now staff nurses see themselves as responsible for orienting current and future colleagues. In videotaped sessions in 1991 and 1995, RNs, CNAs, and nurse managers described the unit functions (LDS Hospital Media Services, 1995). In that video, staff members noted increased clarity in role expectations, the ability to get their work completed, and confidence in their ability to make decisions regarding practice on the unit.

Staff turnover dropped significantly in 1991 (26%), reaching an all-time low in 1994 (5%). In 1996, the turnover rate was 12%, still below the general hospital rate of 15%. In 1997, the department manager reported a waiting list of individuals seeking to work on W8. Reasons given for leaving the unit are no longer discontent and burnout, but other opportunities such as family and school.

Financial management became a focus for staff in cooperation with the manager. Since 1991, the salary costs per patient day increased only at the rate of inflation, with a slightly greater increase in the years 1996 to 1997, when an additional care manager (now there are four) was added. The medical unit is now consistently within budget guidelines.

System-wide measures of patient satisfaction show no significant changes in perceptions of clinical and service quality over the past four years. The system-wide evaluation tool was changed between 1990 and 1994, so comparisons of data are not meaningful. Patient and staff interviews demonstrate enthusiasm for the care provided on the unit. Physicians who normally admit patients to W8 do not want them admitted to other units; when this does occur, they request that the W8 care managers follow their patients.

Faculty and staff work as colleagues, critiquing their own work, asking how to improve it. They have continuing dialogue with each other and with students to support and improve patient care and the environment for staff, students, and faculty. At one time when the hospital group had not met for four months, a staff nurse called a meeting. The staff nurse noted the need to continue dialogue, evaluation, and celebration in order to continue accomplishing the outcomes achieved to date. The staff nurse stated that she realized she was as responsible as the nurse manager or the administrator for continuing the work of the Utah Web.

It is important to note that we are aware of many variables influencing care delivery, turnover, and education in the hospital. Differentiated practice and the Healing Web Partnership were two such variables. During the time of this project, other variables included the development and implementation of system-wide nurse shared governance, oversupply of nurses in Utah in 1994, and a corporate-wide quality improvement initiative.

The Utah Web is expanding both differentiated practice and ADN/BSN complementary education to additional settings in and out of hospitals. The sites in process at this time include the medical/step-down unit and the intensive care unit at Cottonwood Hospital and Intermountain Health Care's home health agency. Faculty from two additional schools have expressed interest in joining the Utah Healing Web. The Utah Web meets monthly to discuss the process of expansion, results of work in process, and requirements for maintenance.

Conclusion

Through an education-service partnership, staff on a medical unit were able to redesign their care delivery model and work with university and community college faculty and students in a collegial relationship. The result was an improved ability to meet patients' expectations. Given support from administration and faculty, staff nurses, those caring for patients, will actively participate in designing care and educating students. To bring service and education into partnership requires time, and support from educators, administrators, staff members, and students. There must be willingness, ability, and intent on the part of all parties to dialogue about issues of importance to the success of the initiative.

The process of redesigning care delivery led to increased staff involvement in decision making, and student nurses developing an expanded view of nursing's role and nurses' roles in care delivery. Through clarification of patient expectations and nurses' roles, faculty were able to modify teaching methods and curriculum to prepare students for the varied roles required in the service setting.

Nursing viewed from W8 is focused on patients, is supportive to patients, students, and staff, and is improving continually.

References

Bunkers SS: The Healing Web: a transformative model for nursing, *Nursing and Health Care* 13(2):68-75, 1992.

Fosbinder D, Ashton C, Koerner J: The National Healing Web Partnership: an innovative model to improve health, *Journal of Nursing Administration* 27(4):37-41, 1997.

Koerner J, Karpiuk K, eds: *Implementing differentiated nursing practice: transformation by design,* Gaithersburg, Md, 1994, Aspen Publishers Inc.

LDS Hospital Media Services: Patient care improvement: staff perspectives (video), Salt Lake City, Utah, 1995.

Newman M: Keynote address, First National Healing Web Partnership Conference, Park City, Utah, 1995.

CHAPTER 41

Haircuts and Health Promotion

A Community-Based Curriculum in a Baccalaureate Nursing Program

BERNARDINE M. LACEY, RN, EdD, FAAN, **and JEWEL MOSELEY-HOWARD,** RN, EdD

OVERVIEW

Clinical practice sites that provide opportunities for students to effectively accomplish the program objectives are interwoven with and inseparable from the broadest health issues, in which health care promotion, teaching, and related science coexist and thrive in an environment that supports the future of healthy individuals and communities.

A nursing program designed to bridge the gap between conventional medicine and less conventional health care practices is located at Western Michigan University School of Nursing. The curriculum is community based, relationship centered, and holistic in its philosophy, structures, and content. One community clinical-practice site is a beauty parlor where the focus is on involving the community in its health, rather than in its disease or illness. Selected health care services are available to clients and anyone, male or female, who drops by the beauty salon. This community nursing program has responded to the changing community distribution channels and ensures a patient base, regardless of the site or the modalities of health care delivery. Such a program has the potential for a positive impact on educational purpose, faculty balance, tenure structure, and investment priorities. ▲

The Curriculum and Community Connection

Western Michigan University's College of Health and Human Services currently has a National League for Nursing–accredited nursing program designed to bridge the gap between conventional medicine and less conventional health care practices. The program focus is relationship-centered care, coupled with the concept of mind-body-spirit health promotion. The nursing program's unique curriculum is also community based, relationship-centered, and holistic in its philosophy, design, and content. Throughout the program of studies, nursing students are required to meet program objectives as they work with individuals, families, groups, and communities. In addition to traditional biomedical skills, students are taught a variety of complementary approaches to healing, including relaxation and therapeutic touch. With the implementation of this curriculum, the nursing program has graduated practitioners of nursing who can use the appropriate instrumentation needed for a complete and integrated approach to health care delivery within any community. One pertinent issue addressed by this community nursing program is the need to respond to changing community distribution channels and ensure a patient base, regardless of the site or the modality of health care delivery.

A summary of the following eight program objectives responds to the well-understood health market and draws broadly on the institutional strengths of Western Michigan University (WMU) College of Health and Human Services. These objectives are to:

- Facilitate partnerships that improve health in families, populations, and communities while balancing cost, access, and quality in the delivery of holistic health care.
- Analyze community, group, and individual health and illness status, using system models. Plan health and illness care services to meet the needs of communities, groups, and/or individuals.
- Identify and classify the research bases that support current nursing practice.
- Support the right of individuals and groups to choose their own lifestyles and codes for living. Act as an advocate for clients in care settings where human rights are at risk.
- Demonstrate commitment to the caring principles that are integral to professional nursing.
- Analyze professional nursing's contribution to the development of health care policy at the local, state, national, and international levels.
- Integrate biological, social, and nursing science to design and deliver primary nursing services across the continuum of health care.
- Consistently use principles of therapeutic communication to establish, maintain, and end relationships while providing care to families and individuals.
- Consistently use effective group and political communication skills when working with the community and other health care professionals.
- Use information technology systems in health care.

These program objectives are neither independent from nor fully apprehensible outside the context of the School of Nursing's mission and curriculum strategy, and the culture of the community. Clinical practice sites that provide opportunities for students to effectively accomplish the program objectives, are interwoven with and inseparable from the broadest health issues, in which health care promotion, teaching, and related sciences coexist and thrive in an environment that supports the future of healthy individuals and communities.

Community as Clinical Practice Site

If nursing programs are to change community health behaviors and promote health, then the required resources must be available. In regard to the availability of such resources, there are several issues that faculty considers in selecting clinical practice sites. Examples of such issues include the following:

- Who should be in our health care coalition?
- What resources need to be in place and operational?
- How should resources be interwoven to promote collaboration?
- What is the nature of community-based health care leadership?

- How does one educate individuals for community health leadership?
- Where are the health care professionals being trained to actually make a difference in the world?

From a community perspective, these are key factors that raise additional questions. Is our starting point without existing resources, or can we build on and/or enhance what is already in the community? Where resources are present, does communication exist between and among organizations and personnel, and are they aware of each other's presence?

The concern about leadership skills of future health professionals and the context of their education are worthy of serious dialogue. Thus, we will ensure that those who promote care—for example, when trying to fulfill a public or assisted housing health initiative—do not go out into the communities uninformed, and without the appropriate technique and health science background. Feelings of pity and compassion for those who are suffering are meaningless, unless they lead to strong social action and positive change in community health behaviors.

Because of the need for changes pertinent to the implementation of the nursing program and the selection of meaningful clinical sites for practice, several faculty members addressed the issues with a creative initiative. The challenge of selecting clinical practice sites that would allow students to meet the program objectives was enhanced through the use of a community survey assessment designed to identify common health needs within the community. This community survey found that technology and clinical expertise were being rapidly disseminated from hospitals to community-based facilities. Patients were being channeled through managed care plans, with less formal hospital arrangements for illness prevention and health promotion. Information from the survey also acknowledged the facts of accelerating hospital demands manifested in continuing cost containment and constricting reimbursement. It was apparent that traditional values relevant to lengthy hospitalizations, with emphasis on the use of hospitals as clinical sites, were conflicting with economic market exigencies and the clinical role of nursing faculty.

To ensure the quality of both patient care and nursing education, as well as meet pertinent community health care needs, the faculty also recognized that despite the challenge facing the delivery of health care, they had to integrate the traditional demands of nursing education with performance standards for clinical practice. Without health insurance, individuals within the community requiring health care had limited economic resources and were unable to afford measures that support health promotion. It was clearly understood that the compelling direction and focus for health care delivery required the creation of clinical practice sites in the community.

Haircuts and Health Promotion

One example of the faculty's commitment to a community-based curriculum is found in an unusual and nontraditional clinical practice site. In early 1995, Bernardine M. Lacey, Director of the Western Michigan University School of Nursing, conceptualized the idea of health promotion activities in a beauty shop. Not only do people get a haircut and manicure, but they also receive blood-pressure screening and health care information that is specially geared to African Americans.

This program is a women's health care initiative sponsored by Western Michigan University, the Black Nurses Association, and the Mane Attraction, a beauty salon in Kalamazoo, Michigan. With the support from the salon patrons and publicity gained from an article printed in *The Western News,* a Kalamazoo newspaper, the salon initiative received a grant of $10,000 from the John E. Fetzer Institute of Kalamazoo. These funds were allocated to special workshops and development of culturally sensitive health promotion materials.

Lacey and the faculty observed that unlike conventional clinical settings, the beauty shop is a warm, friendly, nonthreatening environment. In such a setting, the women were more receptive to health care information. These women were willing to share with their beauticians some of their most private thoughts. Historically, it has been a place for women to talk about their joys and sorrows, pains and sufferings, so it appeared to be a natural place to introduce, promote, and educate individuals about health care.

The program added educational information on breast self-examination, CPR training, stress reduction, and healthy cooking and eating. Once a month, low-fat recipes featuring traditional African American fare are prepared for clients to sample.

Most of the health care services and information is provided by area nurses or WMU nursing students who are offered opportunities to establish relationships with the clients. This in turn meets program objectives of facilitating partnerships that improve health in families, populations, and communities. In reply to requests made by the women at the beauty salon, several other professional groups share their expertise and provide additional pertinent health information.

The faculty underscores the fact that this approach "is not prescriptive, but rather oriented towards health and wellness promotion . . . Clients are continually surveyed to make sure the programs offered meet their specific needs" (*The Western News*, 1997). Information is recorded and maintained on how clients view and manage their health care, allowing health providers to assist clients more effectively (*The Western News*, 1997).

The positive community impact of using the beauty salon as a clinical site has been useful as a referral base that strengthens ties to primary care physicians, local hospitals, and other available resources. Course objectives were accomplished by students as they became engaged in partnerships with a community having urgent health care needs.

POTENTIAL PROGRAM OUTCOMES

There is potential for positive impact on educational purpose, faculty balance, tenure structure, and investment priorities, which are elements inherent in this academic and clinical program.

Educational Purpose.
A community-based nursing program that is responsive to its members, coupled with an awareness of environmental change and concomitant health care opportunities, fosters cohesion among teaching and clinical practice entities and enables effective health care delivery. Structured health care workshops that include videotaped reviews and responses to simulated community and clinical situations are also useful in evaluating program objectives. They are crucial aids in making decisions to maintain or revise components of a program.

Faculty Balance and Tenure Structure.
A more flexible and balanced academic culture can be achieved when community-based nursing programs recruit faculties that are multidimensional in expertise. This approach facilitates participation by members of the faculty in all aspects of health care delivery. Recruiting expert faculty is well understood to be the foundation for program success and change. There may be a stronger need for an expanded clinical position that reflects the depth and range of the nursing program. Clinical supervisors who are prepared at the master's level are not on a tenured track; however, they are encouraged to participate with other faculty in all aspects of the program. Requisites for an expanded clinical role can be essential for the success and progress of the program as well.

Investment Priority.
Poor outcomes in health care systems are costly. In addition to the competitive advantage, nursing care that includes health promotion and illness prevention is a managerial imperative that transcends academic programming and equates to community-appropriate, cost-effective, quality health care.

Future Clinical Sites

The next community clinical practice site will be located in a large Laundromat. Women and children bring their clothing to be washed and because of convenience, carry various food items with them. Lacey observed that refrigeration of food within the Laundromat was not available. Most of the children were younger than 6 years of age and had little or no health promotion teaching. In addition, the mothers of these children did not have enough time to properly address their personal health care needs. Seldom can one find so many underserved people in one place without any planned activity. There was not even a book to read.

Lacey has begun plans for a "well-baby" clinical site that will involve participation of family members who are present with their children. Promising efforts are underway to develop a registration pool whereby families who desire health care can communicate their needs to the appropriate source.

Conclusion

The cost-benefit issues of such clinical practice sites are not as yet resolved; however, they offer families the economic means and opportunity to become supportive of health promotion without the fierce competition for more strictly limited resources. The faculty and students of this nursing program have embraced collaboration and availed themselves of one approach to maintaining a balance in health care delivery while emphasizing clinical performance and the need for a healthy community.

Reference

The Western News, Haircuts and health promotion on the agenda for initiative between WMU and local salon, vol 24, September 4, 1997, p 2.

Additional readings

Collado CB: Primary health care: a continuing challenge, *Nursing & Health Care* 13(8):1992.

Kalamazoo County Healthier Community Assessment: a report on health and human services, Kalamazoo, Mich, Public Sector Consultants, Inc, March 1995.

CHAPTER 42

Medicine, Nursing, and Public Health

Partnering to Improve the Community's Health

SHEILA A. RYAN, RN, PhD, **JANE MARIE KIRSCHLING**, RN, DNS,
RICHARD J. BOTELHO, B Med Sci, BMBS, MRCGP, **NANCY M. BENNETT**, MD, MPH,
and **MADELINE H. SCHMITT**, RN, PhD

OVERVIEW

An ideal setting for interprofessional learning is the community, where competencies can be improved for all professionals in population approaches to improving health.

This chapter describes a collaborative project that is designed to implement and evaluate community-based, behavior change programs using continuous quality improvement methods and provide community-based learning opportunities for health professions students grounded in collaborative inter-professional teamwork and continuous improvement. The project evolved from a partnership between the University of Rochester Schools of Nursing and Medicine/Dentistry (New York) and the Monroe County Health Department to improve the health of the community.

Supported in part by a Community-Based Quality Improvement Education for the Health Professions (CBQIE-HP) training grant, health professions students (including undergraduate students majoring in health and society, baccalaureate and master's degree nursing students, medical students, and master's of public health students) and family practice residents will work collaboratively in Student Improvement Teams with the support of two or three faculty members over the course of a semester. The initial four activities are responsive to the Health Department's priorities in maternal/child and adolescent health. Opportunities for interprofessional education based in the community, like the CBQIE-HP project, have the potential to improve the health of the community served. ▲

As health professionals, we must be open to interprofessional collaborative models of practice if we are to be fully responsive to the needs of our patients, communities, and society. To achieve this goal, health professions must be prepared to put aside traditional discipline-specific boundaries and engage in creative dialogue with each other. If we expect students to practice together in interprofessional teams, then it is most logical that we educate them together. During the past decade, there has been a revival of interest in the use of interprofessional teams in health care, under pressures for greater efficiency and fiscal accountability from the government and managed care organizations. Historically, one of the best institutionally based examples of a model for interprofessional learning has been the Veterans Administration interdisciplinary team training programs (Feazell, 1990). However, in recent years there has been a growing emphasis on community models, including the demonstration projects funded by the John A. Hartford Foundation, in which a variety of community-based and managed care settings are being utilized to conduct interdisciplinary student training in care of the elderly (Siegler et al, in press), and by Community-Based Quality Improvement Education for the Health Professions (CBQIE-HP) (Headrick et al, 1996).

Interprofessional education can be defined as "an educational approach in which two or more disciplines collaborate in the learning process with the goal of fostering interprofessional interactions that enhance the practice of each discipline" (Tresolini, 1994) and therefore the care to the individual, family, group, or community. Such education should be based on mutual understanding and respect for the actual and potential contributions from different disciplines, take place in both the classroom and the clinical setting, and be woven throughout many experiences. Learning together is better served by a "health" model than an illness model and is strengthened by sharing and diversity. This type of learning involves self-awareness and disclosure where individuals accept responsibility and accountability for their own actions. Most important, learning together will lead to working together. The Pew-Fetzer consensus report concludes that interprofessional learning is aided by quality improvement approaches and benchmarks to measure outcomes of learning (Walker et al,

1997). An ideal setting for interprofessional learning is the community, where competencies can be improved for all professionals in population approaches to improving health.

Background

During the 1997-1998 school year, the University of Rochester Schools of Nursing and Medicine/Dentistry (New York) established a formal partnership with the Monroe County Health Department to improve the health of the community. This collaborative effort is located in the new Center for the Study of Rochester's Health (CSRH), which is under the direction of the Deputy Director of the Monroe County Health Department, Nancy Bennett, MD, MS. The Center will foster research related to community health improvement and increase preventive and population-based approaches in health professionals' education and practice. One of the first initiatives of the director of the Center was to collaborate with School of Nursing and School of Medicine/Dentistry faculty in the second phase of demonstration projects through the Interdisciplinary Professional Education Collaborative. A training grant, CBQIE-HP, was awarded through the Department of Family Medicine from the Health Resources and Services Administration in partnership with the Institute for Healthcare Improvement.

The Interdisciplinary Professional Education Collaborative, initiated in 1994 (Bellack et al, 1997), has four educational elements: "Involvement of students and faculty from nursing, medicine, and health administration; experiential learning in actual health care settings; faculty development in continuous improvement; and interdisciplinary team-building" (p. 309). Our demonstration project represents the confluence of several initiatives in the university and the community: community health improvement, continuous quality improvement, interprofessional education, and behavioral science.

The greater Rochester community, with the leadership of the Health Department, has been engaged in a process to identify and work toward community health improvement goals. Monroe County is a large metropolitan county with a population of 716,000. While the health of the overall population is relatively good, the excellent health of the suburban population masks the generally poor health status of the 227,000 inner-city residents. The city is segregated from the surrounding suburban population and suffers from high rates of mortality from chronic diseases such as cancer and cardiovascular disease. Other classic health indicators, such as infant mortality, teenage pregnancy, and sexually transmitted disease rates, remain poor. Prevention efforts have been limited because volunteer agencies have had difficulty establishing effective urban programs.

In 1995, Andrew Doniger, MD, the Monroe County Health Director, decided to address these problems by convening a team of local stakeholders including representatives from the two major insurers, the University of Rochester Medical Center, the local health planning agency, the local consortium of hospitals, and the Health Department. This group, now formally called HealthAction: Priorities for Monroe County, quickly reached consensus on the need for a common approach to planning service delivery and improving outcomes. Five subcommittees of HealthAction (maternal/child, adolescent, adult, older adult, and environment) will use "health report cards" to assess pressing health problems in the community and will publish data every two years. HealthAction will use a community process to set and achieve specific goals and monitor progress toward some of the *Healthy People 2000* (U.S. Public Health Service, 1991) goals. This health assessment data, along with the input from the local community, will form the basis for identifying specific areas of focus for an array of community learning activities. The Center for the Study of Rochester's Health provides analytic support for moving to the next step—to implement community-based projects. The CBQIE-HP, as a subset of this work, adds another dimension to this work by fostering interprofessional learning opportunities for health professions students and providers based on continuous improvement. The CBQIE-HP project targets initiatives in areas identified as high priorities by the County Health Department.

Faculty in the School of Nursing have successfully moved half of the required clinical experiences in the baccalaureate program into the community. Developing a "learning community" has also been a central component of the curriculum revision (Ryan et al, 1997). The potential for community-based interprofessional learning experiences, which emphasize a population focus,

will broaden and strengthen our ability to foster a learning community that prepares physicians and other health care providers, as well as nurses, for the evolving health care delivery system. In addition, having students learn about and "practice" continuous improvement will better prepare them to move into practice settings where this approach has increasingly been used during the past decade. For example, the University of Rochester's Strong Memorial Hospital (SMH), which is a training site for both medicine and nursing, started to use Total Quality Management methods in 1989. SMH was one of the original participants in the National Demonstration Project on the Application of Industrial Quality Control Methods to Health Care. In 1990, SMH joined the Quality Management Network as one of over 30 organizations jointly working on total quality transformation. Leaders involved in this SMH-based initiative have been recruited as part of the local CBQIE-HP project to incorporate this learning into Rochester community sites where continuous quality improvement efforts have already been initiated as part of the HealthAction planning process.

Community-Based Quality Improvement Education for the Health Professions

The overall goals for this project are twofold: first, to implement and evaluate comprehensive, community-based, behavior change programs that use continuous quality improvement methods in work, school, and health settings (primary care, community health centers, and the public health department); second, to provide community-based learning opportunities for health professions students that are grounded in collaborative interprofessional teamwork and continuous improvement.

The Local Improvement Team (LIT), led by Richard Botelho, MD, is responsible for the overall design of the project as well as overseeing its implementation. Dr. Botelho has extensive experience in faculty development and is the Director of Fellowship Training for the Family Medicine Department. He brings behavior change expertise to the LIT. Additional LIT members include Nancy Bennett, Robert Panzer, Jane Marie Kirschling, and Madeline

Schmitt. Bennett brings expertise in public health and epidemiology, as well as experience with community intervention projects. Panzer is the Director of the Office of Clinical Practice Evaluation at Strong Memorial Hospital. In this role he is responsible for all quality-related and clinical improvement activities throughout the hospital. Kirschling oversees the academic programs in the School of Nursing. Schmitt has extensive expertise in interprofessional team education, practice, and research.

The LIT identified four activities to be initiated in January 1998. These activities focus on selected priorities (RCPs) from the first two report cards in maternal/child and adolescent. Given the complexity of the health problems selected, we expect that the activities will continue to evolve over time and that new ones will be formed. As new Student Improvement Teams are established each semester, they will build on the work of the previous teams. In addition, it is hoped that students will elect to work across semesters on a RCP activitiy and use this learning opportunity to meet additional course, clinical, or program requirements for their respective degrees.

Healthy Start: Accessing Prenatal Care in High Risk Areas involves students going into the southwest and northeast quadrants of Rochester to interview women about their pregnancy experiences. Included will be questions on where (and if) they went for care, what their experiences were like, nutrition, child care issues, and community services. The information generated through these interviews will ultimately be transformed into a quantitative interview measuring barriers to care, access to care, and satisfaction with care.

The *Adolescent Developmental Assets Activity* focuses on youth development. Developmental assets are building blocks that correlate with adolescent behavior. When an adolescent lacks these fundamental assets, he or she is more likely to engage in risk-taking behaviors (e.g., use and abuse of alcohol and drugs, violence, unsafe sexual practices). This team will review the health of adolescents in Monroe County, learn about the asset model, develop the methods to administer a survey of middle school students, and implement and evaluate the plan.

The Sticky Tar Program: To Smoke or Not to Smoke will be implemented with sixth and seventh graders. This project will use a motivational approach to enhance students' capacity to make healthy choices, in addition to addressing cigarette smoking. Team members will make presentations to students and gather feedback from students, teachers, and parents. The team will use this information to improve the materials for future presentations.

The *Childhealth Plus Program* will be the focus of the fourth Interprofessional Team. Childhealth Plus is a legislated insurance program so that all children can access health care. Faculty will work with students to evaluate the number of uninsured children in a five-county area who should be covered, as well as determine the actual number who enroll following targeted enrollment initiatives.

CARRYING OUT THESE ACTIVITIES

Two or three faculty members from across health care disciplines will guide each of these RCP activities. Residents and health professions students, including undergraduate and graduate nursing students, undergraduate students majoring in health and society, graduate students in public health, and medical students, will form interprofessional teams. The teams will work together over a period of 14 weeks, spending up to four hours a week on RCP activities. Each semester, the faculty and students involved in the designated activities will participate in a half-day training session on the core support areas for the overall CBQIE-HP project. The training session will include didactic content related to population health, quality improvement, interprofessional team development, and behavior change. In addition, members of the LIT will be available throughout for "just-in-time training," given that each activity may have unique needs related to the core areas.

Although we are early in the process, this demonstration project has the potential to help develop viable long-term training models integrated with important community health initiatives. The project also has the potential to greatly enhance the various health care professionals' educational experiences. However, we also know that the barriers that the initial demonstration have faced (Bellack et al, 1997) will require ongoing work to ensure the success of this project. Bellack and colleagues identified the barriers as:

- "general institutional inertia, resistance to change, and desire to preserve the status quo . . .
- institutional and disciplinary traditions and culture, hierarchical governance and communication structures, power imbalances, vertically organized curricula, and professional territoriality . . .
- rigid curricula . . .
- lack of understanding and/or commitment from institutional leadership . . .
- faculty lack experience with interprofessional teaching and practice . . .
- current funding structures and faulty reward systems in health profession education programs . . . undervalue the contributions that interprofessional work and team teaching make to student learning and preparation for work in the changing health care system" (p. 313).

As part of this demonstration project, we hope to alleviate several of these barriers. A systematic evaluation plan will help us improve on the outcomes as we continue to offer interprofessional learning opportunities during the coming years.

Conclusion

According to Baldwin (1996), the benefits of team and collaborative care have long been recognized in specialty teams in hospital settings and have enhanced delivery of comprehensive and continuous care to many communities, especially to underserved populations. Specific benefits have included, but are not limited to, lower mortality rates in infants and the elderly, improved patient compliance and satisfaction, increased efficiency and reduced costs, fewer broken appointments, fewer hospitalizations and emergency room visits, shorter lengths of hospital stays, and, in the elderly, fewer drug prescriptions, improved morale, and improved functional status. As we search for better answers to the continuing problems of access, quality, and cost effectiveness of care, it is clear that there needs to be more efficient and effective utilization of all kinds and many levels of health professionals through increased cooperation and collaboration. Health pro-

fessionals need to rise above the adversarial perceptions and preconditions that often separate those involved. Opportunities for interprofessional education based in the community, such as those that will be available through the CBQIE-HP training grant, have the potential to improve the health of the Rochester community.

References

Baldwin DC Jr: Some historical notes on interdisciplinary and interprofessional education and practice in health care in the USA, *Journal of Interprofessional Care* 10:173-187, 1996.

Bellack JP, Gerrity P, Moore SM, Novotny J, Quinn D, Norman L, Harper DC: Taking aim at interdisciplinary education for continuous improvement in health care, *Nursing & Health Care Perspectives* 18:308-315, 1997.

Feazell JH: Interdisciplinary team training in geriatrics program: a historical perspective on team development and implementation reflecting attitudinal change toward team training and team delivery of health care. In Snyder JR, ed: *Interdisciplinary health care teams: proceedings of the Twelfth Annual Conference* Indianapolis, 1990, Indiana University School of Medicine, pp 18-23.

Headrick LA, Knapp M, Neuhauser D, Gelmon S, Norman L, Quinn D, Kaer R: Working from upstream to improve health care: the IHI interdisciplinary professional education collaborative, *Journal of Quality Improvement* 22(3):149-164, 1996.

Ryan SA, D'Aoust RF, Groth S, McGee K, Small L: A faculty on the move into the community, *Nursing & Health Care Perspectives* 18(3):139-141, 1997.

Siegler E, Myer K, Fulmer T, Mezey M: *Geriatric interdisciplinary team training,* New York, Springer, 1998.

Tresolini CP, Pew-Fetzer Task Force: *Health Professions Education and Relationship Centered Care,* San Francisco, 1994, Pew Health Professions Commission.

US Public Health Service: *Healthy people 2000: national health promotion and disease prevention objectives,* Washington, DC, 1991, US Department of Health and Human Services, Publication PHS 91-50212.

Walker PH, Baldwin D, Fitzpatrick JJ, Ryan SA, Bulger R, DeBasio N, Hanson C, Harvan R, Johnson-Pawlson JK, Lacey B, Ladden M, McLaughlin C, Selker L, Sluter D, Vanselow N: Building community: developing skills for interprofessional health professions education and relationship-centered care. *Report of the Interdisciplinary Health Education Panel, formed by the National League for Nursing* (April, 1996), New York, 1997, National League for Nursing.

CHAPTER 43

The Best of Both Worlds

An Academic and Business Partnership in Nursing Case Management

PATRICIA CHIVERTON, RN, CS, EdD, **PATRICIA HINTON WALKER**, RN, PhD, FAAN, **PATRICIA HRYZAK LIND**, RN, MS, and **DONNA TORTORETTI**, RN, BS

OVERVIEW

A working partnership contains elements of both process and outcome in its formation. As an outcome, it reflects attainment of a mature association that is mutually satisfying and beneficial to both participants . . . Partnerships demand a circular-patterned dance of connectedness, leading each member to trust the other while exemplifying their jointly generated, shared beliefs.

As health care costs have continued to rise, one of the ways that businesses and employers have tried to control costs is through the development of partnerships. The Community Nursing Center of the University of Rochester Medical Center and Blue Cross/Blue Shield are working in partnership to provide community-based psychiatric case management services with a focus on quality and cost outcomes. This chapter describes the development of this partnership and the implementation of an outcomes-based management system. It discusses the unique positioning of academic health centers to provide leadership in the development of innovative, research-based health care delivery models. ▲

Changes in the health care delivery system resulting from health reform and market forces have placed increased emphasis on prevention, outcomes (quality and cost), population-based care, and access to care for underserved populations. New models of health care delivery designed to improve the health status of communities are receiving increased interest. One such model is a community-based case management program for a psychiatric patient population. This model is a community partnership between a payer, Blue Cross/Blue Shield, and a Community Nursing Center (CNC). This CNC is a faculty practice associated with an academic medical center. The goal of this new academic-service model is to provide outcome-based quality care through problem identification, risk reduction, and care coordination with primary care providers. This goal is consistent with the broad health goals articulated in *Healthy People 2000: National Health Promotion and Disease Prevention Objectives* (U.S. Department of Health and Human Services, 1990).

In the past decade, psychiatric hospital days have been steadily decreasing. This reduction in hospitalization has increased the need for community-based services. Studies show that intensive forms of case management, which emphasize alternatives to inpatient care, can result in fewer inpatient days, reduced costs, and improved quality of life (Semke, Hanig, 1995). Community-based case management also has the potential to promote the health of a psychiatric patient population by reducing risk, supporting patients in the community, and addressing the costly inpatient readmissions that are common in this patient population.

Several different models of case management have been described in the literature: hospital-based models; hospital to community models; and community-based models (Ethridge, Lamb, 1989; Zander, 1988; Korr, Cloniger, 1991). The partnership described in this chapter is a community-oriented case management model, managed out of an academic health center, and based on a nursing conceptual model, the Neuman Systems Model (Walker, 1996). Interventions in the Neuman Systems Model focus on three levels of prevention as intervention: primary, secondary, and tertiary prevention. The care in this case management model provides for primary prevention (counseling, sur-

veillance, and health promotion) to alter risk behaviors; secondary prevention interventions for early detection of medication noncompliance, loss or ineffective support systems, and screening for disease; and tertiary prevention interventions to promote readjustment to the community following an inpatient hospitalization.

Cost implications and benefits of new community-based programs in this changing health care environment are required if these programs are to grow and survive. Communities are developing integrated systems of care, some in partnership with payer groups, but little is known about the cost-benefit of these new models of care. While the effectiveness of these partnerships is often judged by their success in obtaining a market share of the population, this does not tell us the nature and types of services delivered, the quality of the care provided, or the actual costs of the service. There is clearly a need to demonstrate the effectiveness of new models of community-based care, such as the case management initiative, in terms of quality and cost outcomes. This chapter will explore a new academic-service partnership.

Background and Development of Partnership

As health care costs have continued to rise, one of the ways that businesses and employers have tried to control costs is through the development of partnerships. These partnerships develop for different reasons; the major reason usually is that one organization does not have the resources, skills, knowledge, and expertise to produce a particular product (Kaluzny et al, 1995). This was the basis for the development of the partnership between Blue Cross/Blue Shield and the Community Nursing Center of the University of Rochester School of Nursing.

The CNC of the University of Rochester School of Nursing was created to implement faculty practice of advanced practice nurses in community settings. Since its inception in 1991, the CNC has developed a number of partnerships and/or business coalitions for the purpose of delivering new models of community-based care. A variety of services are provided by advanced practice nurses in urban and rural settings, including in rural community hospitals, group homes for troubled teens, primary care offices, county health departments, and school-based clinics. With the reduction of inpatient hospital beds and the need to move toward community-based care, staff nurses are now included as providers of care in the community. While these bachelor's-prepared nurses are not faculty members, they contribute to the education mission of the School of Nursing by functioning as clinical preceptors in community settings.

The partnership between the CNC and Blue Cross/Blue Shield came about as a result of a pilot study that investigated the cost and quality outcomes of a program that provided transitional case management services to a psychiatric patient population. The results of this study demonstrated reduced service utilization and cost and an improvement in health status indicators (Chiverton et al, 1997). The Community Nursing Center was approached by a representative from Blue Cross/Blue Shield, and subsequent meetings with representatives from both organizations led to the development of a community-based case management program.

This program provides case management services to all psychiatric patients covered by Blue Cross/Blue Shield insurance. This has resulted in the CNC providing case management services to insured patients within the University of Rochester's integrated delivery system, and also to psychiatric patients in other area health care systems.

The benefits of this program to the consumer are related to the ability of the case managers to bridge integrated delivery systems of care. Psychiatric patients frequently obtain services from more than one system of health care. Case management programs provided within one health care delivery system are limited in their ability to move across systems. This community-based program provides case manager continuity for the patient and ensures communication among local, competing health care systems. The communication is crucial in the identification of high-risk patients who might not be identified because utilization patterns are tracked by the health care system, not the community at large.

Program Development

While the focus of most public sector case management programs has been continuity of care,

private sector case management programs strive to restrain escalating health care costs (Vallon et al, 1997). The partnership between the CNC and Blue Cross/Blue Shield focuses on both quality and cost. This program developed from Blue Cross/Blue Shield's need to coordinate services across systems of care and the ability of the CNC to demonstrate improved patient outcomes through case management. Also, leaders in the CNC were interested in demonstrating the outcomes (in cost savings) of theory-based care. In this partnership, we were particularly interested in the cost savings of primary and tertiary prevention as intervention using the Neuman Systems Model (Walker, 1996). One of the important contributions of an academic-service partnership is the opportunity to evaluate theory-based care from an academic perspective while demonstrating the value of nursing models of care in the business community.

Psychiatric illnesses, for the most part, are chronic conditions that require ongoing treatment; thus, the concept of virtual health management is supported by both the CNC and Blue Cross/Blue Shield. Virtual health management is an approach to health and outcomes maximization, cost effectiveness, and patient satisfaction initiatives that focuses on the patient's needs and concerns as defined by the patient (Meyer, 1996). Involving the patient in care decisions allows for a partnership between the patient and the case manager. In the case of a chronic psychiatric patient population, frequent communication with the patient and the development of systems to monitor and ensure compliance provide for early identification of episodes of illness and an improved quality of life. Lifetime case management includes prevention and health promotion activities and outcome-oriented programs that provide patient empowerment through education and choice in treatment options.

CONTRACT NEGOTIATIONS

Blue Cross/Blue Shield subcontracts with the CNC to provide case management services to psychiatric patients. The development of this program required contract negotiations related to enrollment, referrals, information systems including record keeping, confidentiality, quality and health status indicators, cost, and satisfaction measures. Clinical and financial representatives from the School of Nursing and Blue Cross/Blue Shield participated in the contract negotiations. The combination of clinicians and financial representatives was helpful, during negotiations, in maintaining the focus of the discussions—improved patient care. Since both parties were entering a new initiative and were committed to the success of the program, it was agreed that flexibility would be ensured and that the program would be continually revised as we gained experience in working with this patient population from a community perspective.

Enrollment. An agreement was reached that all patients receiving mental health services and insured by Blue Cross/Blue Shield would be offered case management services. Participation in the program is completely voluntary, and if patients choose not to participate they receive the original benefit package. Patients who elect not to participate continue to be tracked by the payer for service utilization patterns and health care costs. Patients who are readmitted to the hospital are again offered the services of the program. Approximately 50% of patients enroll in the program following a hospital readmission.

Referrals. At the onset of the program, patients were referred by the utilization nurse employed by the payer. All referrals were made from the hospital setting, with attention to the complexity of the patient and family needs and high-risk status of the patient. Because of their high service utilization patterns, these patients were the most difficult and costly to the system, and there was limited opportunity to demonstrate an improvement in health outcomes. Most of these patients use the hospital (secondary prevention according to Neuman) during times of stress and are intractable when it comes to developing different coping mechanisms. It was recognized that it will take time for the case managers to establish a trusting relationship with this group of patients and their primary care providers before changes in health outcomes will be noted.

The decision to enroll the "high-risk" patients also meant that the case managers would be caring for the most acutely ill patients and that the costs would not be spread across the total population. After the first two months, all patients admitted to

an inpatient service were enrolled in the program. This change reduced the high acuity of the case loads of case managers and provided an opportunity to demonstrate outcomes for an entire patient population. Future planning includes enrolling patients cared for in partial hospital and ambulatory care settings.

INFORMATION SYSTEMS

Several initiatives were required in order to develop compatible and supportive information systems. First, the development of a database was needed to track patient referral and enrollment information, patient management, service utilization, and quality and cost data. This database was developed by the School of Nursing in collaboration with Blue Cross/Blue Shield. This database provides an individual patient profile, monitors health status using the scores from the completion of standardized instruments, and collects information regarding the costs of care. Next, linkages were established between Blue Cross/Blue Shield and the CNC to provide current information regarding patients' service utilization patterns and the cost of services. This process involved several internal agency alterations, including revising the billing system to accommodate a different payment mechanism. The last initiative will be the implementation of laptop computers for the case managers who will download the information into the database.

OUTCOME INDICATORS

The quality of mental health services has traditionally been defined on the basis of setting, structure, service processes, and consumer outcome variables (Srebnick et al, 1997). While an extensive literature on outcomes assessment and measurement exists, very little practical information is available on how to implement an outcomes-based management system.

In developing the outcomes for this program, consideration was given to how the outcomes data were to be used. It was determined that the ultimate aim of the program's outcomes management system is to provide data to improve clinical performance and patient outcomes. An appropriate set of outcomes was developed on the basis of a review of the literature, discussion with consumers and expert researchers, and the experience of the program partners. The following areas are addressed: nursing care practice statistics, patient demographics, health status and quality measures, and service utilization and cost.

Nursing Care Practice Statistics. Nursing care practice statistics include not only number and type of interventions, but whether these interventions are primary, secondary, or tertiary. Nursing productivity is monitored by case load (i.e., active, tracking only) and by time spent in direct versus indirect activities. Early in the development of the program, an experienced, traditional (nonclinical) case manager was hired to assist with those activities that did not require a professional nurse. The ability of the staff to use the "right person for the right task" is one way of improving performance. The next step in the program is to determine the appropriate "nurse dose." This is an assessment of registered nurse care, factoring in the experience and educational background of this health care provider as measured by the frequency, timing, and length of program interventions (Fitzpatrick, Brooten, 1996).

Patient Demographics. Patient demographic data include age, gender, marital status, diagnosis, income level, and educational background. These data are used in the following ways: developing health prevention/promotion activities (educational classes, support groups); assisting in the management of case load assignment, especially geographic location of the patient; and projecting future enrollment.

Through the pilot study (Chiverton et al, 1997), it became evident that several associated factors required monitoring, such as home environment and safety, transportation, and access to a pharmacy or a primary care provider. These data are collected for the use of the case managers and are helpful in determining specific areas in the community that may have problems related to access to health care services.

Health Status and Quality Indicators. Adequate assessment tools have three basic characteristics: easy to use in a clinical setting; comprehensive (cover all relevant treatment and outcome domains); and have demonstrated reliability and validity (Smith et

al, 1997). Another issue to consider is generalizability, or the extent to which the information gathered can be compared with data from other settings and populations.

The health status indicators that were selected for this program were based on the need to monitor the following domains: behavior, cognition, function, mood, and severity of illness. Discussions were held with psychiatric faculty members currently involved in research to seek their recommendations regarding the appropriate selection of instruments and to attempt to coordinate the measurement tools selected so that the data collected would be useful to a variety of mental health professionals in the community. We believe it is important to have a common language and to be able to generalize results when referring to the health status of the psychiatric patient population in our own community, since this program crosses integrated delivery systems. The instruments selected are displayed in Table 43-1.

Quality indicators include patient, provider, and payer satisfaction, and demonstrated effectiveness in meeting HEDIS measures related to behavioral health.

Service Utilization Patterns and Cost. Service utilization is the quantifiable use of health care resources provided in a variety of settings, including hospitals, emergency rooms, urgent care centers, primary care offices, primary mental health settings (ambulatory, partial hospital, day treatment), or other formal sites of health care delivery. These data are obtained through administrative claims data or chart review.

For purposes of this program, service costs are defined as the quantifiable monetary prices of providing health care service, with attention to variables affecting costs such as risk sharing, capitation, copayments, and sliding-fee schedules. One of the aims of the case management program is to determine indirect and direct costs of the psychiatric case management program and to contrast these costs with service costs. In order to determine the costs of the case management program, activity-based costing was implemented. During the pilot program, we worked with a consultant (Judith Baker, C.P.A., Ph.D.) to utilize activity-based costing methodology to determine the direct and indirect costs of providing care in a hospital to commu-

TABLE 43-1

The Concepts, Instruments, Collection Method, and Time of Administration

CONCEPT	INSTRUMENT	COLLECTION METHOD	TIME
General health	SF-36 (Ware, 1992)	Self-report	Baseline—12 months
Mental health	Basis-32 (Eisen, 1986)	Self-report	Baseline—12 months
	BPRS (Overall, 1988)	Clinician scored	Baseline—4, 8, 12 months
Cognition	MMSE (Folstein, 1975)	Structured interview	Baseline—8, 12 months
Function	GAF (APA, 1994)	Clinician scored	Baseline—8, 12 months

nity case management program (Baker et al, 1997). This methodology and process of determining costs was applied to the community-based case management program. The steps of activity-based costing include:

- Estimation of resources utilized by case managers and secretary/information analyst
- Creating activity categories and activity mapping
- Designing the data collection forms and procedures
- Costing the activities
- Identification and application of activity drivers
- Considering the costs of building community partnerships in a new practice
- Calculating and reporting the results

Estimates of resources were primarily related to the mean salaries and benefits of the practitioners and support staff. The nurse case managers and the nonclinical case manager are costed out of the staffing costs separately to determine clinical versus nonclinical time. The secretary/information analyst's time is also broken out by direct patient contact and administrative time. The next step in the process is the completion of activity categories and the map of the activities of care. Activity mapping includes: duties and functions of the secretary/information analyst, such as data entry and clerical functions related to billing; activities of the practitioners related to maintaining community partnerships and marketing; and activities related to the types of services provided (telephone contacts, home visits). On the basis of our experience during the pilot project, similar data collection

forms were developed that measure direct and indirect time based on the activity. The costing of activities is completed by using the database that was developed for this program. The activity drivers are determined (full-time-equivalent employees, enrollment of patients, number of visits, etc.) and values assigned. Since this program is in the early phase, we are continuing to work with the consultant to refine our costs and project program development needs. During contract negotiations, it was decided that the first two years of the program would be cost-based and that during the third year we would move to a capitated rate based on our experience.

Typically, fee-for-service structures encourage increased utilization of services, with rapid exhaustion of annual mental health benefits. Identifying patients who use a large amount of inpatient mental health services and referring them to case management offers an opportunity to proactively intervene before patient benefits are exhausted and they are referred to public programs (Vallon et al, 1997). While this community is still in a fee-for-service structure, the move to a more tightly managed care market and a capitated environment is imminent. This program has been developed with attention to resource allocation and the determination of resource consumption.

INTERPRETING DATA

Data entry, analysis, and interpretation are vital aspects of outcomes management. Techniques such as case-mix adjustment, risk adjustment for severity of mental illness, and appropriate cost-benefit analy-

TABLE 43-2
Project Aims and Outcomes

PROJECT AIMS	OUTCOMES
Health care utilization will decrease	Reduced health care claims
	Decreased number of hospitalizations
	Decreased length of stay
	Decreased number of emergency room visits
	Decreased number of primary care visits
Appropriateness of care to risk category will increase	High-risk members will utilize more nursing interventions
Health status and functional scores will improve	Members with a higher nurse dose will have improved health status and functional scores
Appointment compliance will increase	High-risk members will have a higher compliance rate and will meet the HEDIS criteria
There will be no negative impact on provider satisfaction	Provider satisfaction surveys will improve
Member satisfaction will increase	Member satisfaction surveys will improve
Program costs will be covered by reduced health care utilization	PMPM rate will be determined

ses are necessary for meaningful data interpretation (Smith et al, 1997). The purpose and aims of the case management program are utilized to interpret the data and evaluate the effectiveness of the program (Table 43-2). The broad question to be answered is: "What is the effect of a psychiatric case management program on health care? Is it utilization, appropriateness, health and functional status, compliance, member/provider satisfaction, and/or program costs?"

Implementation

Fitzpatrick and Brooten (1996) discuss the need to shift from an event-driven to a risk-driven framework for providing and paying for health care. This case management program begins to move from an intervention following an event (hospitalization) to an intervention with those individuals meeting the criteria for "high risk."

COMMUNITY INVOLVEMENT

Since the program design involved crossing systems of care, it was important to ensure the com-

mitment of all mental health professionals in the community and ascertain that an adequate communication system was in place. The project director met with the psychiatric leadership staff in all of the integrated delivery systems to explain the purpose and design of the program and to set the stage for ongoing communication. These discussions also involved an identification of the barriers related to program implementation. For example, access to inpatient records required approval by credentialing committees. This issue was resolved through discussion and the spirit of community partnership.

STAFF SELECTION

The nurse case managers were selected through a competitive interview process. The qualities and experience that were felt to be essential were psychiatric experience in dealing with complex patient issues, commitment to the program, ability to establish relationships and to empower others, advocacy skills, translating vision of well-being into reality, and knowledge of community resources. As we continue to develop and refine the program, it is anticipated that other disciplines will be added to enrich the case management staff. All disciplines need to move across a continuum of care, and nurses need to continue to participate as members of multidisciplinary teams while demonstrating their own contributions as team members.

ROLES AND RESPONSIBILITIES OF CASE MANAGERS

The relationship between the primary mental health provider and the case manager is important, and its success depends on education, collaboration, and communication. The role of the case manager is not to provide direct treatment, but rather to provide continuity, support the treatment approach of the primary mental health provider, and coordinate services. Frequent communication during episodes of illness is essential to avoid splitting and to ensure a consistent approach to the patient. Other roles and responsibilities of the case manager include completion of a biopsychosocial assessment; evaluation of the patient's response to treatment plan/care modalities and suggesting modifications as needed; encouraging education, advocacy, and empowerment of patient and family; understanding the historical perspective of the client's covered life; and provision of health promotion and prevention activities.

The case managers are accountable professionals who follow the standards of practice for case management. Their practice is peer reviewed on at least an annual basis, and consultation is provided by a cadre of specialty-based advanced practice nurses from the University of Rochester Medical Center.

REFERRAL AND ENROLLMENT

Once a patient is referred to the program by the utilization nurse from Blue Cross/Blue Shield, the case manager contacts the facility where the patient is receiving treatment and establishes a time to meet with the identified patient. If the patient is an inpatient, this meeting takes place in the hospital prior to discharge. If the patient decides to participate, a consent is signed, and a meeting is arranged with patient, family, and primary mental health care provider. The purposes of this meeting are to establish health care goals, to define specific treatment interventions, and to discuss the role of the case manager in assisting the patient to remain in the least restrictive health care setting. A follow-up letter is sent to the primary mental health provider to review the purpose of the program and identify the case manager who will be working with his or her patient.

CLINICAL PRACTICE PROTOCOLS

All patients receive treatment based on the established protocol, as shown in Box 43-1.

A Home Safety Screening Tool is completed at the time of the first home visit. This instrument can be referred to by any person who makes a home visit and includes information related to the external living environment (parking, lighting, accessibility, animals) and the internal living environment (phone, weapons, alcohol, drugs).

A description of nursing interventions is captured in the database. The next steps in program development will be the development and evaluation of nursing interventions based on patient risk. At the start of the program, no information was available regarding the "right dose" of nursing interventions. Further research on quantifying nursing intervention is in progress.

DOCUMENTATION

At the time of enrollment, the case manager completes an admission care map. This care map includes demographic data and information related to past history, and ensures that the standardized assessment instruments are completed. The nursing process is documented on the care map. This care map is completed following each interaction with the patient. The care map incorporates the following parameters that assist with the development and implementation of on an ongoing treatment plan: biological status, individual functioning, interpersonal functioning, compliance, and health promotion activities. The interventions are coded as primary, secondary, or tertiary. The care map also tracks the time each case manager spends on any intervention.

Phone logs are maintained that indicate the purpose and length of the call, and a treatment history log is also maintained for each patient. This log is useful in capturing a patient's service utilization pattern and changes in treatment approaches.

BOX 43-1
Case Management Clinical Practice Protocol

Acute

Client identified on first day of admission by utilization log

   Case manager (on site within 24 hours of admission):

- Review record/talk with inpatient treatment team
- Open chart
- Enroll client in program

Client offered/educated regarding case management program by case manager

Client **accepts** program (if client deemed incompetent or is a minor, has legal guardian or power of attorney, primary identified person will sign consent/forms)

   Consent for Services reviewed and signed

   Client's Bill of Rights reviewed and signed

   Release of Information reviewed and signed

   Prior to discharge, baseline clinical measurements are completed and appropriate data gathered

   Follow-up home visit appointment is arranged by case manager

Client's physician(s), community case providers are notified by letter and telephone contact

If client **refuses** case management program

   Case manager will track client

   If client reappears at ED or is readmitted, program will be offered again by same case manager

Subacute/Stabilization

Case manager will be in contact with client/family at least weekly (by telephone or home visits) for eight weeks after discharge

Health Maintenance/Promotion/Prevention

A minimum of one monthly contact will occur, with comprehensive case map assessments (however, if at any time the client requires more services or home visits, the case manager will adjust interventions to those specific needs)

Four, eight, and twelve months—client will be contacted twice, with one home visit to complete onsite assessment and measurement tools

---

It was important, at the beginning of the program, that the case managers understood the difference between documentation for the outcomes program and research. When clinicians can see and use the data that the system provides about patients, they begin to value an outcomes-management system. Timeliness is also an important consideration. The turnaround time needs to be rapid if the interest of clinicians is to be maintained. The case managers also needed to understand that in order for data to be meaningful and the conclusions drawn from it valid, systematic scientific procedures need to be followed (Smith et al, 1997).

PROCESS ISSUES

Program implementation began in December 1996. In 1997, internal and external issues surfaced that needed to be addressed. Internal issues related to

the partnership between Blue Cross/Blue Shield and the Community Nursing Center involved discussions related to staffing, communication, billing, and documentation. The program was originally planned to proceed in phases, beginning with adults and expanding to include children and adolescents. Initial referrals included not only adults but also children and adolescents. The original staff hired for the program were experienced only in working with adults. In an effort to be responsive to the needs of the payer, we added a part-time nurse who was experienced in the care of children and adolescents. The case managers carry case loads of approximately 75 to 100 patients, with a combination of active and inactive (those who have refused the program and are being tracked for service utilization patterns and health care costs) patients. We have not yet determined the "right-size case load" and will be using the data we are currently collecting to assist with the continual refinement of the program. Program evaluation will be completed in January 1998.

Keys to Successful Partnerships

The success of this program has been based on three key factors: the ability to take risks, flexibility, and responsiveness. A working partnership contains elements of both process and outcome in its formation. As an outcome, it reflects attainment of a mature association that is mutually satisfying and beneficial to both participants. Because of human dynamics, true partnership continues to evolve and reconstruct for continued participant development and goal directedness. Partnership is present when the involved peers develop a trusting relationship and interconnectedness. Within a partnership, optimal relationships develop when power is shared and all members are active participants in the process. Intrinsic to relationship forming is learning about oneself and one's potential when in partnership with another whose talent, skills, and resources are beneficial to each one as well as the collective. One needs to believe that interconnectedness and involvement will be growth producing and important to goal attainment.

Partnerships demand a circular, patterned dance of connectedness, leading each member to trust the other while exemplifying their jointly generated shared beliefs. The development of a partnership firmly based in trust allows risk taking. Taking risks with attention to community needs and building relationships between many organizations have been a hallmarks of this union. Both partners developed trust so that the risk of initiating a program that would span hospital systems to better serve patients with psychiatric illness would be minimized.

Crucial to the success of this partnership is the role of the nurse as care provider, program innovator, and researcher. Health care reform literature describes the critical and crucial role of the nurse in leading change within, and external to, institutional settings. The goal of the nurse is to ensure that the composite of activities and functions results in a net advantage to the patients and facilitates enhanced or normative outcomes (Porter-O'Grady, 1994).

The partners' flexibility is the second key success factor. Each partner had individual, well-developed skill sets with needs; each shared a common vision and the determination to achieve improved patient care for this population. Underpinning a successful partnership are the investigation and development of a strategic direction and the synergy to sustain that journey. In any partnership, the ability to change course to improve the potential for a successful outcome is paramount to success.

Finally, responsiveness to the needs of the partners as well as the needs of the patients is critical. The program coordinators demonstrated their responsiveness through changes in staffing to accommodate the admission of children and adolescents into the case management program, revisions of care plans for these diverse populations, and integration of databases to meet each partners' organizational needs.

Inherent in the establishment of any partnership is the committed belief by all involved parties that this union or merger will be sustained and enhanced by the passage of time. Partnerships are not short-lived marriages of convenience, but enduring nourishing affiliations that require commitment, energy, and perseverance to maintain and develop.

Conclusion: Role of an Academic Health Center in Community Care

Academic health centers are uniquely positioned to provide leadership in the development of innovative, research-based health care delivery models. As leaders in the practice of health care, academic health centers have purchased or developed clinical practices as part of integrated delivery systems. With the development and acquisition of primary and specialty care practices, academic health centers have the ability to initiate new care models with attention to measuring outcomes and designing new practice patterns. As centers for research, academic health centers provide leadership in the development of theoretically based studies. Partnerships with other entities, such as payers, furnish new ground for clinical research ranging from the design of intervention studies to the evaluation of practice models. Finally, as providers of education, academic health centers serve as the training grounds for future clinicians. Through unique partnerships, like the one described in this chapter, opportunities exist for clinical placements of undergraduate students with preceptors providing care, for graduate students majoring in health care administration or aspiring to become psychiatric clinical specialists, and for doctoral students in the design, development, and analysis of research projects.

Through partnerships or direct participation as managed care providers, the introduction of capitation to an academic health center encourages research and practice responsibilities. Shine (1997), suggests that academic health centers have an opportunity to determine how to intervene in maintaining the health of a population and to create a laboratory and a classroom that would be useful in assessing the community. Quality, cost, and health status outcomes are integral to the success of managed care plans; education, research, and patient care are values of academic health centers. Blending these institutions and their talents through active partnerships will only serve to strengthen our health care delivery system.

References

American Psychiatric Association: *Diagnostic and statistical manual of mental disorders,* ed 4, Washington, DC, 1994, American Psychiatric Association.

Baker J, Chiverton P, Hines V: Psychiatric case management costing and capitation, *Journal of Health Care Finance,* 1997.

Chiverton P, Tortoretti D, LaForest M, Walker P: Bridging the gap between hospital and community care: cost and quality outcomes (in press).

Eisen SV, Dill DL, Grob MC: Reliability and validity of a brief psychiatric report instrument for psychiatric outcome evaluation, *Hospital & Community Psychiatry* 45:242-247, 1994.

Ethridge P, Lamb GS: Professional nursing case management improves quality, access and costs, *Nursing Management* 20:30-35, 1989.

Fitzpatrick JJ, Brooten D: Managed programs of healthcare: evaluating effectiveness, *The American Journal of Managed Care* 2(8):1133-1134, 1996.

Folstein MF, Folstein SE, McHugh PR: Mini-Mental State: a practical method for grading the cognitive state of patients for the clinician, *J Psych Res* 12:189-198, 1975.

Kaluzny AD, Zuckerman HS, Ricketts TC: Partners for the dance: forming strategic alliances in health care. In Walton GB, ed: *Strategic alliances: a world wide phenomenon comes to health care,* Ann Arbor, Mich, 1995, Health Administration Press.

Korr WS, Cloniger L: Assessing models of case management: an empirical approach, *Journal of Social Services Research* 14:129-146, 1991.

Meyer LC: It's about time: virtual health management, *TCM,* pp 53-68, 1996.

Overall JE, Gorham DR: The Brief Psychiatric Rating Scale: recent developments in ascertainment and scaling, *Psychopharmacology Bulletin* 24:97-99, 1988.

Porter-O'Grady T: The real value of partnership: preventing professional amorphism, *Journal of Nursing Administration* 24(2):11-15, 1994.

Semke J, Hanig D: A state management planning system for addressing high levels of use of inpatient psychiatric services, *Psychiatric Services* 46:238-242, 1995.

Shine K: Challenges facing academic health centers and major teaching hospitals, *JONA* 27:21-26, 1997.

Smith GR, Fischer EP, Nordquist CR, Mosley CL, Ledbetter NS: Implementing outcomes management systems in mental health settings, *Psychiatric Services* 48(3):364-368, 1997.

Srebnick D, Hendryx M, Stevenson J, Caverly S, Dyck DG, Cauce AM: Development of outcome indicators for monitoring the quality of public mental health care, *Psychiatric Services* 48(3):364-368, 1997.

US Department of Health and Human Services: *Healthy people 2000: national health promotion and disease prevention objectives,* Washington, DC, 1990, U.S. Government Printing Office.

Vallon KR, Foti MG, Langman-Dorwat N, Gatti E: Comprehensive case management in the private sector for patients with severe mental illness, *Psychiatric Services* 48(7):910-914, 1997.

Walker PH: Blueprint example: an integrated model for evaluation, research and policy analysis in the context of managed care. In Walker PH, Neuman B, eds: *Blueprint for use of nursing models: education, research, practice and administration,* New York, 1996, NLN Press.

Ware JE, Sherbourne CD: The MOS 36-item Short Form Health Status Survey (SF-36): conceptual framework and item selection, *Med Care* 30:253-265, 1992.

Zander K: Nursing case management: strategic management of cost and quality outcomes, *Journal of Nursing Administration* 18:23-30, 1988.

CHAPTER 44

Bridging the Gap

Collaborative Partnerships Between Academia and Service

JUDITH PAPENHAUSEN, RN, PhD, **CAROL BRADLEY,** RN, MSN,
ELEANOR G. FERGUSON-MARSHALLECK, RN, PhD, **LINDA BURNES BOLTON,** RN, DrPH, FAAN,
CAROLYN E. AYDIN, PhD, **and JO ANN WHITAKER,** RN, MS

OVERVIEW

Within both education and service, there is a consensus that collaboration is a highly productive and desireable behavior. . . . However, the consistent application of true collaborative behavior proves to be a challenge in the rapidly changing health care environment, in which each institution has its own traditions, politics, financial motivations, and entitlements.

This chapter describes the collaborative implementation of service-academic partnerships between California State University, Los Angeles, and two major health care providers in the Los Angeles area, Huntington Memorial Medical Center and Cedars-Sinai Medical Center. These partnerships were designed to provide baccalaureate and higher-degree education to employees of the two major medical centers through an on-site educational program specifically designed to meet the needs of the full-time employed nurse. The benefits and difficulties encountered during development, implementation, and operation of this on-site educational model are summarized, including the specific outcomes achieved, from the perspectives of both the educational and the practice settings. ▲

Marketplace Drivers for Change and Collaboration

The need for collaboration between nursing education and nursing service is of paramount importance today more than ever before. Health care and its related institutions are faced with overwhelming and rapid change, and the nursing profession is being seriously challenged to respond and adapt to ensure viability and relevance in the new world being shaped. The changing nature of patient care, stimulated by advances in science, pharmacology, and technology, has changed the utilization of all resources that were central to the traditional health care system. The focus is appropriately shifting toward minimizing or avoiding illness and toward community-oriented care and improving overall health status. This shift can be attributed to the basic principle of managed care, which finances health care services for an enrolled population in a manner that rewards efforts to minimize and manage long-term financial risk, *not* just short-term costs. Society is demanding increased accountability on the part of all providers, payers, and the overall health care system. Significant effort and financial resources are being directed at improving organizational performance and defining and measuring quality and clinical outcomes. Ineffective and inefficient modes of care are gradually being discarded in favor of those that have demonstrated value. These strategies have led to the need for greater collaboration between hospital administrators, health policy makers, health professionals, schools, and the nursing community.

Early in this century, however, nursing education, in its struggle to be recognized as a profession and achieve excellence as a discipline, moved away from the dominance and control of hospitals and physicians, and rejected structural and personnel arrangements that would have kept the domains of service and education closely intertwined (Aydelotte, 1985). Those in service also turned away from educational responsibilities and focused on nursing care delivery. This created what has been referred to as the "gap" between service and academia. Reestablishing collaboration between those who educate nurses and those responsible for the direct provision of nursing care has not been easy. However, several authors suggest that it is now time for nursing service and education to rejoin forces to work on a variety of issues and matters of mutual professional interest (MacPhail, 1983; Aydelotte, 1985; Beddome et al, 1995), and the American Association of Colleges of Nursing (1993) recommends that all schools of nursing establish, maintain, and evaluate collaborative relationships with practice settings.

Relationship of Patient Outcomes to Educational Preparation of Caregiver

The basic content, methods, and approaches designed to prepare health care disciplines are in many ways disconnected from the current delivery system and are in need of retooling to ensure a product that can function effectively in the new world. Technology and methods of patient care have dramatically changed the roles and relationships of health-related disciplines. Role boundaries between professions are blurring rapidly, and defensive actions within disciplines attempt to maintain the status quo without consideration of new opportunities. Given the pace of change in the health care industry, this presents a particularly difficult challenge to academic institutions.

Over the last ten years, there has been an increasing demand to demonstrate value for the nursing care services purchased. The Institute of Medicine report (1996) identified the need for additional research to determine the impact of educational preparation of caregivers on patient care outcomes, and the American Nurses' Association (1995) included the educational level of the registered nurse in its core set of nursing indicators with a strong structural link to nursing quality. Recently, multiple studies (Hartz, 1989; Aiken et al, 1994; Harrington, Estes, 1994; Curran, Maggie, 1995) have shown the educational level of the registered nurse to be related to the achievement of lower patient mortality rates and shorter hospital stays. At the same time, however, the highly competitive health care marketplace and the growth of managed care have pressured many institutions to reduce costs, often at the expense of registered nurses. Seventy-five percent of American hospitals are engaged in restructuring plans, and many reported laying off 20% to 50% of their nursing staffs between 1994 and 1996 (Curran, Maggie, 1995), a shortsighted strategy if an educated, motivated, and supported nursing work force is more likely to bring about desired patient care outcomes.

The Current Collaborative Environment: Perspectives from Practice

Within both education and service, there is a consensus that collaboration is a highly productive and desirable behavior. While the service-academia division has been important in moving the structure of nursing education from the hospital to the collegiate environment, today it serves as a functional obstacle to constructive change. However, the consistent application of true collaborative behavior proves to be a challenge in the rapidly changing health care environment, in which each institution has its own traditions, politics, financial motivations, and entitlements. The existing inertia within these structures makes it easier to remain the same than to change.

To participate in health care redesign, nurses must be prepared to meet the identified marketplace needs. At minimum, the RN work force must gain the knowledge and skills acquired in baccaluareate and higher nursing education programs. The challenge for today's nursing leaders is to break the traditional stereotypes within and around education and practice. Table 44-1 provides a summary of needed transitions for both institutions. Collaborative efforts between education and service can create the necessary momentum to strengthen both clinical practice and the methods of educating new nurses. Opportunities for shared and aligned incentives that should be supported and championed by both education and service include memberships on academic advisory boards for those in practice and vice versa, jointly hosted educational workshops and educational programs, faculty practice arrangements, and joint appointments. In essence, nursing leaders need to recognize that more can be accomplished together than individually and that limited resources, namely time, money, and energy, can be put to more effective uses.

THE LEARNING ENVIRONMENT

The educational experience of nursing students must reflect the diverse practice settings in which nursing care is delivered today. The hospital is no longer the primary location for patient care, challenging faculty to find clinical experiences for students in diverse, nontraditional settings throughout the community. These sites will require changes in the traditional role of clinical faculty, providing an opportunity for experienced clinical nursing staff to serve as preceptors for students in lieu of the traditional faculty oversight.

New care models and systems being implemented in the practice environment also must be integrated rapidly into the educational experience to provide students with realistic and relevant exposure to the constantly evolving patient care environment. This integration requires that faculty actively engage in the practice of nursing. The acquisition of clinical skills and knowledge must also incorporate the effective coordination and utilization of other care team members. The educational program must recognize and incorporate the important role of technology, particularly changes in information management that are impacting nursing practice. Faculty must be active participants in the clinical delivery of care and demonstrate knowledge of current delivery systems, processes of care, and the administrative systems that surround and support clinical care. There need to be focused efforts to design ways to effectively and creatively integrate clinical and educational roles.

THE NEW COMPETENCIES

Given the expectations of the newly graduated registered nurse, the challenge for educational institutions has never been greater. Those in practice settings need to communicate what they believe distinguishes the exceptional nurse of today, including new competencies that will be advantageous as the health care delivery system evolves. We believe these new competencies should include:

- Organizational and interpersonal skills, ability to lead groups and facilitate teams
- Ability to assign, delegate and coach others, and accurately assess others' clinical and organizational abilities

TABLE 44-1
Transitions for Education and Practice

OLD WORLD	NEW WORLD
Clinical Experiences	
Grouped students within laboratory sections	Individual or small groups only
Clinical experience concentrated in inpatient hospital environment	Clinical experiences in diverse clinical sites, including, schools, mobile clinics, shelters, homes, assisted-living centers, hospices, outpatient centers
Dedicated faculty supervision	Loose oversight, clinicians as preceptors
Acquisition of Skill and Knowledge	
Demonstrated through technical ability	Demonstrated through cognitive ability
Plan of Care	
Nursing discipline–driven plan of care	Multidisciplinary, integrated pathway
Limited to current hospital episode	Incorporates pre-hospital and post-hospital care and targeted outcomes
Clinical "more is better" focus for patient care	
Financial and clinical aspects of care are isolated	Clinical and financial aspects integrated; care provided on basis of authorization and flexible use of benefits and avoidance of unnecessary care
Documentation of Care	
Narrative or problem list–driven documentation,	Exception charting with automated flowsheets, and graphical trend analysis with computer-driven interpretation
Care documentation at the discretion of the nurse	Care according to determined protocol
Expected Student Behaviors	
Student to comply with procedures, structure; cautious, risk avoidance; rules and policy/procedural approach	Student to demonstrate flexibility, self-directed risk taking, independence, initiative, critical thinking, creativity
Faculty Behaviors	
Faculty time focused in educational environment; has external relationship with clinical setting	Educational role and clinical role integrated
Is a spectator of current environment, and transmits interpretation to student	Lives in current environment; translates, precepts, and demonstrates to student

- Willingness to participate as an active team member in interdisciplinary teams
- Understanding of the value of research-based practice and outcomes and disease management research
- Familiarity with the performance improvement process and the ability to understand and use data appropriately
- Basic aptitude for information systems and familiarity with common health care applications, including financial accountability in the clinical care of patients
- Broad view of community health, understanding of principles of epidemiology
- Understanding of the health care system from a broad viewpoint, including the financial and business aspects of health care
- Understanding of and practical clinical experience with and exposure to the broader "continuum of care"
- Understanding of financing mechanisms in health care
- Understanding of the importance of the organizational mission under which one chooses to practice nursing and the responsibilities related to that choice

Beyond clinical competence and technical skills proficiency, these new functional competencies will best position nurses within the current health care system to be successful and have an impact on patient care delivery. Process skills are requisite if nursing is to influence the design of the health care system. Collaborative efforts between education and practice can ensure that future nurses are prepared to contribute at the bedside as well as in other settings where nursing's voice deserves to be heard.

The Current Collaborative Environment: Perspectives from Education

Professionals in nursing service and education do share many common interests, objectives, and concerns about the education and practice environment for nurses. However, the separate and distinct natures of the work encountered daily by those in service and those in academic nursing generate a different emphasis on the priority, context, and so-

lutions to professional issues and continue to be the major force retarding collaborative efforts. The following discussion explores three issues of particular concern to nurse educators.

SERVICE UTILIZATION OF GRADUATES OF NURSING EDUCATIONAL SYSTEMS

One continuing issue for nurse educators is how nursing service will use the graduates of nursing educational systems in a way that is commensurate with their levels of preparation and expected competence. In the past, many employers of nurses made little attempt to distinguish among job descriptions and clinical competencies for A.D.N., diploma, and baccalaureate nursing graduates. Nursing graduates with varying levels of preparation were used interchangeably in the practice setting, even though their educational programs differed widely in length, breadth, scope, and type of degree conferred (Montag, 1980; Kramer, 1981). This lack of differentiation was reinforced by the absence of differences in pay among the three types of graduates in most hospitals (Sortet, 1989). With the focus on efficiency and a cost-effective, productive work force in the current health care environment, nursing service and education together could implement care delivery strategies that would utilize the educational credentials, experience, and competencies of nurses through a model of differentiated nursing practice. Many models of differentiated practice exist, and their use is advanced by organizations such as the American Association of Colleges of Nursing (AACN) and the American Organization of Nurse Executives (AONE). As Koerner (1992) articulates, "A nursing community comprised of differentiated roles that are mutually valued and well integrated will position nursing as a powerful force in meeting the diversity and complexity of health care needs in contemporary society."

Because multiple entry points to professional practice are available, distinguishing between the practice roles and responsibilities of the different levels of nursing is paramount. The Pew Health Care Commission suggests ". . . focusing associate preparation on the entry level hospital setting and nursing home practice, baccalaureate on hospital based case management and community based practice, [and] master's degree for specialty practice in hospitals and independent practice as a primary care provider" (Pew, 1995). In some differentiated-practice models, the level of educational preparation is only one of the criteria used to distinguish nursing roles and functions (Koerner, 1992). The impact of a differentiated model of care delivery on the quality of patient care would represent an excellent collaborative research problem.

Related to differentiation of practice competencies is a commonly held view, documented by Ryan and Hodson (1992) in their review of the research literature, that nursing service and education hold different expectations about the performance of new graduates or the novice nurse. Even with appropriate orientation, internship, and in some instances preceptorships, there has to be time for newly educated practitioners to acquire and develop proficiency in their work roles (Benner, 1984). Once again, collaboration in defining the practice expectations of new graduates could ease the transition for nurses from novice to competent practitioner to expert.

USING GRADUATES' PRESENT KNOWLEDGE AND SKILLS TO SERVE PATIENTS

A second issue of increasing importance to nursing educators is the degree to which service uses the knowledge and skills of graduates prepared at various levels to optimally serve patients. This issue has come to the fore as hospitals have downsized, changed their skill mix of professional and support nursing staff, redesigned client care systems, instituted shorter lengths of stay, and incorporated case management systems. Combined with significant technological advances and issues of quality of patient care, the care and treatment of clients and the management of the work environment within hospitals have become increasingly more complex. These factors place increasing demands on nurses to view patients holistically, to practice critical thinking, to focus on cost containment, to implement short-term teaching strategies, and to progressively utilize coordination and management skills. Changes in the practice arena mandate that nurses retain responsibility and accountability for patient care and highly skilled tasks, while delegating and supervising other functions performed by a variety of assistive personnel. With the shortened lengths of hospital stay, to what degree will nurses be able

to provide teaching and other psychosocial support activities? The decrease in inpatient census, as well as increasing pressure to lower the costs per patient day and increase productivity, has resulted in the implementation of short-term savings measures such as reduction in the size of the nursing staff, cross-preparation among health care team members, and restructuring patient care delivery systems with the use of larger numbers of unlicensed personnel. The tension between cost containment efforts and the need for preservation of quality care is quite real and points to the urgency of examining these strategies on the basis of identified quality outcomes. If these measures prove to be effective over time, education will need to respond by examining the revised role competencies of ADN- and BSN-prepared nurses and determining what role, if any, educational institutions should have in the education of unlicensed personnel. Collaborative efforts are needed to support the exploration of these issues.

CHANGES IN ACADEMIC NURSING CURRICULA

The third issue that is of relevance to nurse educators and that is amenable to collaboration is the reshaping of the academic vision of nursing practice and education resulting from the current transformation in health care delivery. Nursing education must respond to societal demands and changes in the health care delivery system by developing curricular programs that produce graduates who can function in an ever-changing health care environment and be responsive to the demands of the work place. These transformations include changes in the work place settings, skill sets, and competencies for the health care professional, a shift from disease-oriented to health promotional care delivery, and increasing involvement in monitoring cost-effective, quality care outcomes. Frequently there are considerable lag times between the initial awareness of a need for change in practice, the concurrence of a sufficient critical mass of professionals to translate a trend into reality, the development of new and widely accepted practice strategies, and finally the integration of an innovation into a nursing curriculum. Fostering collaboration between practice and education can reduce these lag times and assist educational institutions to be more responsive to changes in the practice setting. Currently, nursing curricula should include the following*:

- Progressive emphasis on health promotion and disease prevention
- Greater focus on individual responsibility for healthy lifestyles and self-care management of chronic health conditions
- Movement away from institutionalized, acute care practice settings to community-based settings, including clinics, home, and long-term-care settings
- Health care services and professionals moving across the health care continuum to provide care to clients, rather than centralized services and personnel
- Content on managed care, various models of case management, and the fiscal aspects of the health care delivery system
- Content on planning and monitoring cost-effective, high-quality care outcomes
- Emphasis in higher degree programs on critical thinking, problem solving, decision making, and delegation skills
- Increased emphasis on patient and family assessment, health educational needs, and improvement of self-care and self-management skills
- Increased emphasis on the provision of culturally competent and psychosocially sensitive nursing interventions

Development of On-Site Educational Partnerships Between Academia and Service

Almost a decade ago, California State University at Los Angeles (CSULA) began to explore the concept of developing on-site educational partnerships with major local medical centers to provide an RN baccalaureate completion program for diploma and associate-degree full-time nurse employees. The overall purpose of these on-site partnerships is to increase the numbers of baccalaureate and higher-degree nurses in the work forces of the medical cen-

*Modified from Pew Health Professions Commission, Critical challenges: revitalizing the health professions for the twenty-first century, *The third report of the Pew Health Professions Commission,* 1995, Pew Health Professions Commission.

ters. Since the beginning of the program, four major medical centers have established on-site educational partnership arrangements with the University. In addition to the RN baccalaureate completion programs, graduate-level education is also being offered via the on-site partnerships.

ON-SITE PARTNERSHIP DESIGN

In these on-site partnership arrangements, the University and the medical center contract to offer an RN baccalaureate completion program at a medical center facility for qualified nurse employees. The design of the curriculum, prerequisite courses, and requirements for admission to the program are identical to those of the university-based RN baccalaureate completion program, but instead of the student traveling to the University, the resources of the University are made available to the student in his or her work setting. The dominant form of nursing staff preparation in many medical centers in the Los Angeles basin is associate-degree education. In the dense urban community of Los Angeles, RN baccalaureate completion programs are readily available in both state-sponsored and private universities, and most programs are available within a radius of twenty miles or less. Hospital nurses surveyed about their intention to complete baccalaureate or higher-degree education most commonly list commuting during rush hours, parking problems on campus, inflexibility of course offerings, and difficulty in manipulation of work schedules as impediments to returning to a university setting.

The design of the on-site programs eliminates most of the common impediments. The on-site courses are offered at the medical center facility, at convenient times, and by University faculty. The usual first step in establishing a partnership is a survey of staff RNs to determine interest and to begin the initial academic advisement. If sufficient interest exists, a contract between the University and the medical center is finalized and the terms of reimbursement are stipulated. All hospital employees in the on-site program must become matriculated students of the University and are subject to the requirements for admission; they must complete the prerequisite nursing and general education courses, and the required upper division course work leading to a baccalaureate degree in nursing. As matriculated students of the University, the students are subject to tuition and student fees, which in the State University system are nominal as compared with private tuition fees. Most medical center partners have a tuition reimbursement program for employees, with varying requirements in terms of compensation. Regardless of the tuition reimbursement policies of the medical center, the costs of academic advisement and program coordination and faculty salaries for the on-site courses are paid by the medical center at an agreed upon cost per unit of faculty time. When feasible, the medical centers are encouraged to identify their own employees who could qualify, on the basis of education and experience, as clinical faculty for the laboratory components of the curriculum. In most instances, University faculty are used to provide the didactic course components.

The usual class size for the on-site programs tends to be small, approximately 10 to 20 students for lecture courses and a maximum of 12 students per section for laboratory classes. Course scheduling is customized for each cohort of students, and the medical center usually adapts work schedules to class offerings. Didactic courses are usually offered in the late afternoon, one day a week, and laboratory experiences on a single day in a week. Some laboratory experiences, such as community health, are not offered on-site, but students take the majority of their nursing requirements at the medical centers. Often, selected electives and required nonnursing courses are also offered through the on-site partnerships; however, students usually complete general education requirements at the University. The academic and mutual outcomes of these partnership programs are found in Box 44-1.

COLLABORATIVE NURSING EDUCATION: HMH-CSULA PARTNERSHIP

In early 1992, Huntington Memorial Medical Center (HMH) recognized that changes occurring in the health care industry would have a significant impact on the practice of nursing. As patient care moved from the inpatient hospital into alternative settings, so would the role of registered nurses. There was a rapid decline in utilization of traditional inpatient hospital services—a trend driven by managed care, technology, and new methods of patient care. Within the existing nursing work

---

BOX 44-1

Academic and Mutual Outcomes of the Partnership Programs

Academic Outcomes

- Establishment of strong clinical affiliations within the local health care community
- Increased program enrollment and fees by use of external funding sources in an era of downswing of academic budgets
- Continued nursing program growth and capturing of larger market share of nurses interested in pursuing B.S.N. and higher degree programs
- Increased ability of academic programs, both baccalaureate and higher degree, to influence health care delivery within the local community
- Increased ability to build a strong alumni base and resource list for clinical placement and preceptor arrangements
- Increased program exposure within the local community and opportunity to develop potential clinical associates for clinical faculty assignments

Shared Practice and Academic Outcomes

- Provides an academic-service interface for the development of mutually beneficial relationships
- Provides the opportunity to develop joint appointments and faculty practice relationships
- Opens lines of communication between academia and service and provides opportunity for service on advisory boards and curriculum committees
- Increases the opportunities to develop joint educational programs and seminars for staff and faculty enrichment and ongoing learning
- Increases opportunities to develop joint research projects and grants for the betterment of both institutions

force, few staff had the education or preparation to move into new roles within home health care, case management, and advanced practice. There was a need to educate nurses as a viable alternative to lay-off. Historically, the hospital culture had not emphasized advanced education for nurses, and it had not been utilized as a criterion for leadership or career advancement.

The first step in the process of bringing education into focus was to clearly communicate the value of education and to define the role that educational credentials would play in the future. Through this communication process, all nurses in, or aspiring to be in, leadership positions understood that future career advancement would be influenced heavily by educational and experiential preparation for new roles. While the new emphasis on education created a level of concern and anxiety on the part of some nursing staff, interest in long-term career options created a high level of interest in and enthusiasm for advanced education. To respond to this interest and facilitate participation in baccalaureate and/or master's education, an on-site educational partnership was developed with California State University, Los Angeles. Staff nurses participated with senior management in choosing the on-site "partner" institution. The program was initiated in the fall of 1993, with plans to provide five separate class cohorts an opportunity to complete the program. Lists of required courses in both the BSN and MSN curricula were provided for associate-degree, diploma, and bachelor's-prepared nurses. This flexibility was attractive to staff, resulting in participants often raising their educational goal to a master's degree once they were in the program. Staff were also encouraged to take advantage of the flexibility by opting in and out of the program as personal circumstances required.

The program required a significant annual commitment of hospital resources to underwrite faculty-related expenses for the on-site feature. The program brought all required classes onto the hospital campus, utilizing hospital faculty as possible. This investment also included a dedicated classroom and a part-time faculty advisor to provide student advisement and counseling, and facilitate enrollment and advancement. Additional efforts were undertaken to upgrade the nursing-related resources within the hospital medical library. The ef-fort was accompanied by a tuition reimbursement program, an annual competitive scholarship program, and an interest-free loan program. A recognition mechanism was also developed in conjunction with annual employee recognition activities to acknowledge the educational accomplishments of participating nurses. Initially, over two hundred staff indicated interest in the on-site program, and many more have become interested as the program has continued.

OUTCOMES OF THE HMH-CSULA PARTNERSHIP

Through this focused emphasis on education, more than 70 nurses have graduated from either the on-site or other local programs in the last 5 years, resulting in a significant increase in advanced degree prepared nurses. The program has provided both a direct recruitment advantage and a retention benefit to the organization. Registered nurse turnover, which had declined steadily over the last 4 years, is now around 4%.

Participants have identified strong organizational support as key to their interest and success in the program. Beyond the participants themselves, the overall value placed on education by staff nurses has been greatly enhanced. A great deal of appreciation has been expressed to senior management regarding the value and importance of this program to individual career development as well as to the long-term view of the hospital as an employer. Most significantly, through advanced education, senior nursing staff are now able to play key roles in the development of new services and expansion of existing programs. Ironically, the challenge to hospital leadership has been to strategically time program evolution to coincide with availability of advanced practice nurses so as to capitalize on the educational investment. Most important, this has demonstrated that layoffs of registered nurses can be greatly reduced or eliminated through advanced education, efforts to transition staff internally to new roles, and changes in recruitment strategies and attrition management. The outcomes of this on-site educational partnership can be summarized as follows:

- Expanded and strengthened nurse case management
- Leadership enriched through education and clinical expert staff resources

- Improvement in the leadership skills of key managers and leaders
- Improved focus on research-based practice and staff interest in nursing and clinical research
- Increased participation in joint appointments with academic institutions
- Improved access of BSN programs to clinical settings
- Increased access of advanced practice students to a broad array of clinical areas and student exposure to more hospital staff and physicians
- Subtle changes in hiring choices, resulting in more effective recruitment of advanced-degree nurses and even entry-level employees
- Inclusion of degree-in-progress requirements for non-BSN or non-MSN candidates for key positions
- Improved faculty and student perceptions of environment, partly because of increased staff interest in students
- Restructuring of compensation for new graduates, allowing for priority to be given to candidates with BSN degrees
- Service-education partnerships provide external funding opportunities and community benefit efforts to eliminate or reduce risk of layoff for registered nurses

COLLABORATIVE NURSING EDUCATION: CSMC-CSULA PARTNERSHIP

The Cedars-Sinai Medical Center (CSMC) Collaborative Nursing Program was initiated in the fall of 1994 to support the recruitment and retention of baccalaureate-prepared registered nurses and also provide for the matriculation of entry-level staff into registered nursing programs. At the time of program initiation, availability of nursing programs to full-time working nurses was limited, and most education programs had long waiting lists and inflexible class scheduling. The on-site program was designed to meet institutional objectives identified in the CSMC Patient Care Services Strategic Plan, 1993 to 1997, including the following:

- To provide staff with accessible, quality education and career development

- To reduce the cost of recruiting staff and preparing baccalaureate nurses
- To increase the number of baccalaureate- and master's-prepared nurses
- To enhance CSMC's environment for employee enrichment and professional development
- To develop a creative, collaborative model designed to support full-time employees in their pursuit of continued professional development

To attract staff with a desire for a self-directed approach to learning, classes are provided on-site to allow full-time workers the flexibility to pursue a BSN degree. This supportive environment fosters employee commitment and demonstrates the value CSMC places on personal and professional development. Qualified medical center staff are utilized as adjunct faculty, and master's-prepared expert clinicians serve as lecturers, clinical instructors, and mentors. Students are provided with an on-site advisor/school liaison to review entry requirements, facilitate class scheduling and planning, and provide education and career advisement.

Several open forums were initially conducted to publicize the program. The goal was to select students who had met most, if not all, general education requirements and nursing prerequisites. After completion of the screening process, however, it was determined that many of the candidates needed to complete general education requirements and nursing prerequisites, making it necessary to offer these courses on-site before starting the nursing curriculum. As a result, the program completion date was delayed and additional expenses were incurred. The initial class started with thirteen students, who entered in the fall of 1994. Over the course of two years, three students dropped out of the program because of family crises. A second group, ten students, enrolled in the fall of 1995, and ten students graduated in May 1997. Currently forty students are enrolled, with 10 students preparing to graduate in May 1998. Many students choose to obtain baccalaureate or master's degrees outside of the on-site program. Approximately forty students graduate annually from other nursing programs, meeting CSMC's goal of promoting educational advancement for registered nurses.

OUTCOMES OF THE CSMC-CSULA PARTNERSHIP

The initial financial statement projected an annual budget of $48,000, with forty graduates a year, starting in 1996. Because an unexpected number of employees had to complete general education and prerequisite courses (some of which were offered on-site at an additional program cost), the actual cost of administering the program has steadily increased each year to double the annual projected budget. The first group of students graduated in May 1997. While large numbers of staff had initially expressed interest in the program, only a limited number actually enrolled, and many have not made the necessary long-term commitment to pursuing an academic degree. Some nurses who were interested did not meet the nursing program entry requirements. Also, the tuition loan forgiveness funds were decreased in 1996, at a time when the program was the most costly. Although the BSN program enhanced retention by attracting new graduates and experienced nurses interested in pursuing professional development, the savings on recruitment costs were not realized when changes in the local health care environment required CSMC to recruit more staff than projected during an unexpected period of high census and high patient acuity.

Because of lower-than-expected enrollments and resource constraints, CSMC had planned to discontinue the BSN program and delay the planned implementation of a collaborative Graduate Nurse Practitioner/Case Management program until the fall of 1998. (The cost of the graduate program is projected to be approximately $68,000 annually.) The importance of the BSN program to staff professional development was reemphasized, however, during meetings held in 1997 to develop the new Nursing Services Strategic Plan. At this time, the on-site BSN program will continue, with additional efforts to increase staff enrollment in the program. The graduate program will also be implemented next year.

An on-site collaborative nursing program has been a magnet for recruiting new graduates and experienced nurses seeking to advance their careers. The program has enhanced employee retention and commitment to the medical center and made program participants feel that the medical center values their professional development. Of the ten employees graduated from the program in 1997, two are enrolling in a nurse practitioner program. One nurse who currently works in transfusion medicine is now seeking a clinical nursing position because she is eager to begin utilizing the skills and knowledge acquired in the program. Many students have remarked that case management courses offered in the senior year have prepared them to coordinate patient care, and helped them acquire the tools necessary to become collaborative team members and to assist patients through the continuum of care. One graduate, who currently holds a management position, stated that the leadership course provided her with the tools and skills to become a more effective manager of resources. All graduates plan to remain with CSMC and express their gratitude to the medical center for the support they received. They also believe that they would not have achieved this educational milestone without the on-site BSN program, and they express confidence that they now possess the knowledge and skills needed to meet the challenges facing the health care industry.

Conclusion: Future Directions

The collaborative partnerships detailed in this chapter illustrate both the benefits and the difficulties encountered as nursing leaders take steps to bring education and practice closer together. The benefits of the on-site programs for students and the institutions involved are clearly illustrated, as are some of the costs and barriers to collaboration. Students are emerging with many of the newly identified competencies, and their new knowledge will benefit the institutions in which they work. The medical centers are also continuing their efforts to recognize appropriately the educational levels of those they employ. Much, however, remains to be done. Collaborative projects are needed to document the effects of specific practice models and differing levels of educational preparation of nurses on patient outcomes, examine the role of nursing education in preparing care teams that include unlicensed personnel, and identify changes in nursing curricula to meet the needs of the rapidly evolving practice environment. These, however, are only some of the challenges that lie ahead. Establishing ongoing service-academic partnerships will allow nursing professionals to respond rapidly and effectively to new challenges as they emerge and to ensure nursing's viability and relevance in the health care environment of the future.

References

Aiken LA, Smith HL, Lake ET: Lower medicare mortality among a set of hospitals known for good nursing care, *Medical Care* 32(8):771-787, 1994.

American Association of Colleges of Nursing: *Position statement: education and practice collaboration: mandate for quality education, practice, and research for health care reform,* AACN: Washington, DC, 1993, AACN.

American Nurses' Association: *Nursing report card for nursing care,* Washington, DC, 1995, American Nursing Publishing.

Aydelotte MK: Approaches to conjoining nursing education and practice. In J.C. McCloskey JC and Grace HK, eds: *Current issues in nursing,* ed 2, Boston, 1985, Blackwell Scientific Publications, pp 288-313.

Beddome, G, Budgen C, Hills MD, Lindsey AE, Duval PM, Szalay L: Education and practice collaboration: a strategy for curriculum development, *Journal of Nursing Education* 34(1):11-15, 1995.

Benner P: *From novice to expert,* Menlo Park, Calif, 1984, Addison-Wesley.

Curran C, Maggie S: *The effects of hospital restructuring on nursing,* Chicago, 1995, APM.

Fagin CM: Nursing value proves itself, *American Journal of Nursing* 10:17-30, 1990.

Harrington C, Estes C: *Health policy and nursing: crisis and reform in US healthcare delivery system,* Boston, 1994, Jones & Bartlett.

Hartz AJ et al: Hospital characteristics and mortality rates, *New England Journal of Medicine* 321:25, 1989.

Institute of Medicine: Nursing staff in hospitals and nursing homes: is it adequate? Washington, DC, 1996, National Academy Press.

Koerner J: Differentiated practice: the evolution of professional nursing, *Journal of Professional Nursing* 8(6):335-341, 1992.

Kramer M: Philosophical foundations of baccalaureate nursing education, *Nursing Outlook* 29:224-228, 1981.

MacPhail J: Collaboration/unification models for nursing education and nursing service. In Chaska NL, ed: *The nursing profession: a time to speak,* New York, 1983, McGraw-Hill Book Company, pp 637-649.

Montag ML: Looking back: associate degree education in perspective, *Nursing Outlook* 28:248-250, 1980.

Pew Health Professions Commission: Critical challenges: revitalizing the health professions for the twenty-first century. *The third report of the Pew Health Professions Commission,* Pew Health Professions Commission, San Francisco, 1995.

Ryan ME, Hodson KE: Employer evaluations of nurse graduates: a critical program assessment element, *Journal of Nursing Education* 31(5):198-202, 1992.

Sortet JP: Incongruence in the nursing profession, *Nursing Management* 20(5):64-68, 1989.

CHAPTER 45

Discovering Outcomes of a Wellness-Promotion Program Utilizing the Kaseman Evaluation Model

DEBORA S. SNARR, RN, MS, C-ANP, LISA M. ZERULL, RN, MSN, and DIANNE F. KASEMAN, RN, PhD

OVERVIEW

The effective management of any new program, particularly in a competitive health care market, depends heavily on frequent feedback that can document progress, detect problems, and verify expectations and outcomes.

This chapter describes a health-promotion program for older adults living in a large rural community and incorporates the Kaseman evaluation model to comprehensively show the outcomes of the program. This evaluation model was instrumental in the continuing development of the program and could easily be adapted to any program or project. ▲

An expansive rural health care environment poses special challenges even to the most comprehensive and integrated health care system. Special challenges, such as long travel distances, minimal public transportation, an aging population, and limited access to medical care, led a small group of acute care nurses from Valley Health System in Winchester, Virginia, to explore how to better meet the needs of the people served in the community.

The Health System

Valley Health System is composed of two private, not-for-profit hospitals located in the Shenandoah Valley between the Allegheny and Massanutten Mountains, and offers tertiary care services to approximately 100,000 individuals living in the tri-state region of Virginia, West Virginia, and Maryland. The Health System operates in an environment with less than 5% managed care, yet more than 50% of all inpatient admissions are from a Medicare population, with resultant capitation. With innovative and visionary leadership, as well as the basic mission of "improving health by serving the community," Valley Health System provides an array of community services across the care continuum, including home care, community nurse case management, and durable medical equipment, to name a few.

For review of needs and services offered by Valley Health System and other agencies, a community-needs assessment was completed to determine the targeted needs of the community as well as to discover what, if any, health-promotion services were being offered. The results showed that many of the individuals served by Valley Health System drive more than 150 miles to access health care. A large number of patients present with emergent acute and chronic illnesses that could have been prevented or minimized had they sought care sooner, or, ideally, had they been screened for disease or deficits prior to any exacerbation of illness. Overall, services and resources were limited, but primarily limited in the availability to older adults. Outreach was the natural choice and the most effective way to reach this population living in the region.

As a result of the community-needs assessment, five primary agencies indicated an interest in partnering with Valley Health System to increase well-

ness promotion through outreach to older adults: The Area Agency on Aging (AAA), the district Health Department, and three independent living facilities (ILFs). This followed the *Healthy People 2000* report (1990), which identified senior centers and community-based settings as ideal sites to reach people 65 years and older. With this in mind, each community partner agreed that together, services could be designed to meet the growing demand for health promotion and disease prevention. As a group, all were convinced that if these consumers had earlier access to education, screening, and intervention in the community, outcomes would be more favorable for the older adults, as well as for the community and the health care system. Each community agency was invited to have a representative sit on an advisory board that would meet regularly and provide direction to the program overall and at its specific site. All would share in the program, its responsibilities, risks, and successes.

In this collaborative community partnership, each agency brought a unique contribution to the program design table. Valley Health System offered one nurse practitioner, supplies, and education resources; the Health Department offered immunization and screening services; and the ILFs and senior centers offered the multiple, identified sites where groups of older adults already congregated. Collectively, these ideas and contributions gave form to a special community outreach program for older adults called the *Health Depot.*

Health Depot: An Outreach Wellness-Promotion Program for Older Adults

The name "Health Depot" was selected by the Health Systems' Auxiliary, a group of older adults actively involved in volunteer activities. Their reasons for selecting the name came from the program's focus on "health" and the fact that "depots" were places familiar to older adults in our industrialized nation. Depots are historically known as places where people can access many destinations, places where a service is coordinated to present the most direct and expedient route, places where connections are made to get closer to one's destination, or one's goals. Health, as defined by each older adult, was the individual's goal. Improving health by serving the community was Valley Health System's goal. These two goals, combined with the national goals of a "healthy community" and "access to care," became the foundation for the goals of the Health Depot (Box 45-1).

The initial plan was to interact with older adults in community settings, providing screening, health-promotion and disease-prevention education programs, individual consultation, and referrals to appropriate agencies. Activities such as blood pressure, glucose, and cholesterol screening, vision and hearing testing, foot inspection and nail care, medication review, and group wellness education were the predominant health-promotion activities, all presented in a nonthreatening manner by one advanced practice nurse and provided without charge at each site. A participant would choose to access the services when the Health Depot arrived at his or her site at a scheduled time, once or twice per month (Figure 45-1).

Establishing strong partnerships within the community was vital to the success of this program, but equally important was the need for a comprehensive evaluation plan that would allow effective management of this new program. In a competitive health care market, success depends heavily on frequent feedback that can document necessary resources, document progress, detect problems, and verify expectations and outcomes. This information led the Health Depot nurse to ask the following questions: What would be the best methodology for evaluation? How would data be collected? What were the ultimate expected outcomes for the Health Depot?

BOX 45-1
Goals of the Health Depot

- To meet the health care needs of residents in the service area who may not have adequate access to health services
- To identify individual health care needs and/or precipitating events that require medical attention prior to the need for crisis intervention
- To facilitate access to the health care system through a local referral system
- To decrease inappropriate use of emergency services
- To enhance quality of life and self-care intervention

ACTIVITY	JAN	FEB	MAR	APR	MAY	JUNE	JULY	AUG	SEPT	OCT	NOV	DEC
Medications review	X						X					
Blood pressure, weight, height		X						X				
Cholesterol			X						X			
Vision and hearing				X						X		
General health assessment					X						X	
Glucose (blood sugar)						X						X

Health care services provided during each health depot include: blood pressure monitoring, nail care, foot inspection, episodic physical assessment, consultation and referral services.

FIGURE 45-1 Health Depot Monthly Screenings Chart.

Application of the Kaseman Model to the Health Depot Program

A literature review was conducted to identify sample evaluation models that might assist with overall program evaluation. Finding none that met the needs of the Health Depot, the nursing school at a nearby academic institution, George Mason University (Fairfax, Virginia), was contacted for assistance. Faculty member Dianne Kaseman emerged as the natural consultant for the Health Depot, offering a comprehensive program evaluation model.

As with many measurement models, the Kaseman model (Figure 45-2) was developed out of necessity. As it evolved in the 1980s it drew heavily on systems theory and educational evaluation theory (Guba, Lincoln, 1991; Patton, 1978). While paying attention to the process, this model began to incorporate a strong link to outcome measurement and immediate and impact outcomes. With all that is currently written about outcomes, there is little written concerning the importance of being able to duplicate the results. This model attempts to answer the questions of whether a program has achieved the objectives as stated in the proposal and whether, when used appropriately, this model provides direction on how to have a successful program. In applying the Kaseman evaluation model to the Health Depot, the first tasks in the early stages were to:

1. Define those elements at each stage of the framework that were critical to the program. These are called "critical elements."
2. Devise a suitable measurement strategy for each element identified, including selecting the appropriate sources for data.

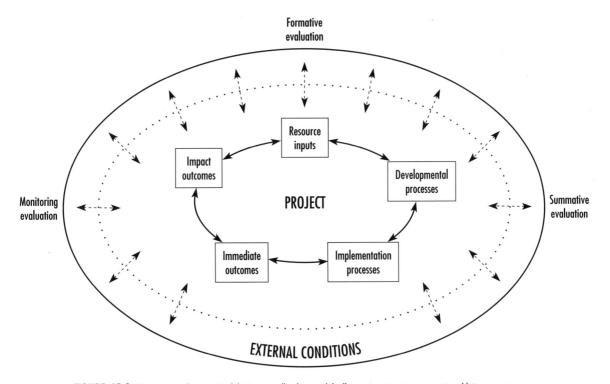

FIGURE 45-2 Kaseman Evaluation Model. Functionally this model allows attention to process in addition to outcomes. In trying to replicate conditions yielding outcomes, it is important to identify the full picture of the project, which may necessitate thinking in terms of a range of patterns rather than linear paths. Most organizations as practice systems are too complex to be limited to linear thinking processes and may have several combinations of events or patterns that produce the same or similar outcomes.

3. Identify critical points in time and select appropriate methodology for data analysis.
4. Prepare reports, including recommendations, and disseminate the information to appropriate decision makers.

In the following sections, each component of the evaluation framework is detailed and applied to the Health Depot program. Each component has the critical elements and sources of data highlighted for easy reference and application. Table 45-1 shows the components of the Kaseman evalu-

ation model and details the definition and importance of each component and the opportunity for duplication of program results.

RESOURCE INPUTS

In 1992, Valley Health System completed a community needs assessment to identify gaps in health care and availability of services. In addition, supervisors who coordinate the various activities at each senior center were interviewed. It was found that the su-

TABLE 45-1
Kaseman Evaluation Model: Components

	DEFINITION	IMPORTANCE
Resource inputs	The resources needed to accomplish the project outcomes. Include (but not limited to) initial funding, ongoing costs, the staff, staff capabilities, facilities, equipment and available community resources. Thorough cost analysis of resources is needed.	Careful documentation of resources and translation into costs and other energy sources for the project allow realistic base for the developmental phase.
Developmental process	The actions and activities that take place during the initial design and planning. The time to draw upon support literature, expert advice, and review of similar project. Time to hire staff, identify subjects or patients, get all necessary materials and equipment in place.	Careful planning and conceptual design provide the stage for project replication and modification. The objectives should be clear.
Implementation process	The action component of the project. Plans are activated. The time plans for the project activated.	This is the time to monitor what is happening with the initial plans, make adjustments as needed, and press forward to accomplish the objectives or outcomes.
Immediate outcomes	The outcomes measured are the *direct* consequences of the projects implementation processes.	Were the objectives achieved? What were the specific outcomes? What were the total costs?
Impact outcomes	The post-project measurement period—usually six months to a year or beyond to track the longer-term outcomes, such as translation of acquired learning into practice.	This component of the model allows an opportunity to observe and measure the outcomes achieved over time. Were behavioral changes maintained?
External conditions	Those external events or influences that facilitate or inhibit the achievement of outcomes.	Affords awareness of factors, such as external policy changes, that may affect project outcomes. Awareness may promote appropriate project modification.

pervisors had limited understanding of health promotion; however, they expressed a keen interest in
having these types of activities offered at their respective centers. This response, along with the results of the community assessment, confirmed the
need for outreach and wellness-promotion services
at sites where older adults gathered. Together, the
partners had the collective interest and resources to
create the Health Depot program (Box 45-2).

The resource inputs were those costs, staff capabilities, procedures, and other resources required
for the wellness-promotion program. A cost analysis of resources required for services was completed; it included the one nurse's salary and benefits, travel reimbursement, educational materials,
screening tools, and some administrative costs—a
total cost of approximately $75,000 to Valley Health
System. When the commitment from the other partners was not strong enough to ensure allocation of
resources, a breakfast was held and an invitation to
sit on an advisory board was extended. All members accepted the invitation to own a part of the
program; however, their resources were limited to
site space and indirect support. No other financial
support emerged. The limited resource inputs were
considered as the various partners began the developmental processes.

DEVELOPMENTAL PROCESSES

A literature review was conducted to evaluate existing programs in the country and to determine
predicted outcomes of such an outreach program.
The *Healthy People 2000* and *Healthy Community
2000* reports served as resources to guide the program objectives. The *Guide to Clinical Preventive Services* (1989) was used to determine appropriate
screening activities for this age group. Expert advice, in the form of nursing faculty consultation and
peer review, was sought to evaluate all screening
forms for content validity (Box 45-3). These forms
included risk assessment and education appropriate to the particular screening activity (Figure 45-3).
Forms were also designed to provide intervention
and outcome data for program evaluation, while remaining easy to use.

One particular form of interest was the Referral
Form (Figure 45-4). Special attention was given in
the development of this form, since the services of
the Health Depot were new to the regional community. Tracking the number and type of referrals
would be key to marketing and evaluating the
program. Physicians and other health care professionals who received referrals responded favor-
ably to the content of the form and often expressed surprise that wellness-promotion activities

---

BOX 45-2
Critical Elements and Sources of Data for Resource Inputs

Critical Elements
- Costs (ongoing)
- Staffing (i.e., types, qualifications, part/full-time)
- Participant characteristics
- Available community resources

Sources of Data
- Community assessment
- Agency assessment
- Salary
- Job descriptions
- Interviews

BOX 45-3
Critical Elements and Sources of Data for Developmental Processes

Critical Elements
- Number and types of staff recruitment activities
- Education program development
- Materials development
- Technical assistance plans

Sources of Data
- Literature review
- Screening tools
- Job description
- Technical support
- Contract

NAME:_____   DATE:_____
CASE NUMBER:_____   ASSESSOR:_____

QUESTION	ANSWER	EDUCATION PROVIDED
Have you ever had your blood pressure checked?	N__, Y__, U__	Define BP. Define normal BP. Explain that blood pressure and heart rate vary.
Have you ever been told that you have high blood pressure?	N__, Y__, U__	Blood pressure can be controlled with medication. Occasionally weight loss and exercise can enable a person with HTN to discontinue medications, but this is often not the case.
Has a doctor ever prescribed any medicine to lower your blood pressure? **If yes:** What is the name of the medication?	N__, Y__, U__ Med:	It is important to take medication as prescribed to control hypertension. Answer questions/concerns.
Do you have any questions/concerns about your medication?	N__, Y__, NA__	Provide information to encourage compliance with medication. Medication can control hypertension.
Do you take this medicine as prescribed? **If no**, why not:	N__, Y__, NA__ Response:	
Risk factors:		
If male, are you 45 yrs. of age or older?	N__, Y__, NA__	The following lifestyle choices can minimize hypertension: • Avoid tobacco • Maintain near-ideal body weight • Limit intake of alcohol, sodium, and saturated fat • Maintain moderate level of physical fitness—exercise (aerobic) regularly 3-5 times a week • Maintain adequate dietary potassium, calcium and magnesium intake
If female, are you 55 years of age or older *or* have hx of premature menopause without estrogen replacement?	N__, Y__, NA__	
Do you smoke cigarettes?	N__, Y__	
Do you have:		
1. A family history of heart attack or sudden cardiac death in father or brother before 55 years of age or mother or sister before 65?	N__, Y__, U__	These are risk factors that are important in predicting future cardio- and cerebrovascular problems in people with high blood pressure. African Americans are at higher risk than Caucasians. If you can control any of these risk factors, you reduce your risk of stroke and heart attack.
2. High Total-c or low HDL-c?	N__, Y__, U__	
3. Enlarged heart, angina, or atherosclerosis?	N__, Y__, U__	Uncontrolled hypertension can also damage other organs besides the heart and brain. The eyes, kidneys and extremities (peripheral vascular organs) can be damaged.
4. Diabetes mellitus?	N__, Y__, U__	
5. Kidney failure?	N__, Y__, U__	
Are you more than 20% overweight?	N__, Y__, U__	

FIGURE 45-3 Health Depot form for initial blood pressure screenings.

Stages of hypertension according to blood pressure levels:

STAGE	SYSTOLIC (mm Hg)	DIASTOLIC (mm Hg)
None	<130	<85
None or very mild	130-139	85-89
Stage 1 (mild)	140-159	90-99
Stage 2 (moderate)	160-179	100-109
Stage 3 (severe)	180-209	110-119
Stage 4 (very severe)	≥210	≥120

(Use highest level of either systolic or diastolic for staging. Isolated systolic hypertension = systolic pressure ≥140 mm Hg and diastolic pressure <90).

Take blood pressure with patient seated and the arm (the same arm for measurements at different screenings) bared, if possible, and at heart level. Clients should have had no coffee or cigarettes within 30 minutes of the reading.

Blood pressure_____ Left or right arm.
Sitting, standing, or prone.
Cuff size: Small, regular, large

Additional readings at initial screening, If applicable:_____

Refer if:

1. Stage 3 or stage 4 hypertension.

2. Stage 2, stage 3, or stage 4 hypertension with no previous history of HTN.

3. Stage 1 hypertension on three separate readings, at least a week apart, with no previous history of HTN.

4. Noncompliant hypertensive client.

5. Known hypertensive client whose blood pressure range is uncontrolled and/or unimproved.

Referral generated?   No_____, Yes_____   (Fill out referral form.)

Assessor signature:_____   Date:_____

Follow-up blood pressure readings

Date	BP	Note	Controlled?			Improved?			Referred?			Assessor
			N	Y	NA	N	Y	NA	N	Y	NA	
			N	Y	NA	N	Y	NA	N	Y	NA	
			N	Y	NA	N	Y	NA	N	Y	NA	
			N	Y	NA	N	Y	NA	N	Y	NA	
			N	Y	NA	N	Y	NA	N	Y	NA	
			N	Y	NA	N	Y	NA	N	Y	NA	
			N	Y	NA	N	Y	NA	N	Y	NA	
			N	Y	NA	N	Y	NA	N	Y	NA	

FIGURE 45-3, cont'd For legend see opposite page.

Originator: Complete the top portion and send to the appropriate referral source via mail or via client.

Client Information
    Name:_____   D.O.B.:_____
    Address:_____   Phone No.:_____
    _____   S.S. #:_____

Referred to:	Referred from:
____ Community Nurse Case Mgr	____ Community Nurse Case Mgr
____ Dentist	____ Dentist
____ Hospital Nurse Case Mgr	____ Hospital Nurse Case Mgr
____ Nurse Practitioner	____ Nurse Practitioner
____ Ophthalmologist	____ Ophthalmologist
____ Physician	____ Physician
____ Physician Referral Service WMC	____ Physician Referral Service
____ Senior Center	____ Senior Center
____ Social Worker	____ Social Worker
____ Other	____ Other

Name_____   Name_____
Address_____   Address_____
_____   _____
Phone No._____   Phone No._____

Date referral: _____ /_____ /_____

Reason for Referral:

_____
_____

Recipient: Complete the bottom portion and send to the originator of the referral in a timely manner.

Plan/Course of Action: Referral Accepted____
                                             Pt. Seen____
                                             Pt. No Show____
                                     Referral Rejected:____
                                             Pt. Not Appropriate____
                                             Pt. Not Interested____
                                             Pt. Moved____
                                             Pt. Entered a NH____
                                             Pt. Deceased____
                                             Other_____

Did this referral prevent a possible medical emergency?   No_____, Yes_____

Signature:_____   Date:_____
               White Copy: Client Record   Yellow Copy: Referral Source

FIGURE 45-4 Sample Health Depot Community Nurse Case Management Referral Form.

were being consistently offered to the older adult population.

IMPLEMENTATION PROCESSES

An introduction of the nurse and the program was the first event to occur at all sites. Blood pressure and cholesterol screenings followed, as they were activities most familiar to the older adults. Priority was given to health education topics of interest to this group. As participants became more familiar with the nurse and the screenings, other activities were introduced, such as health risk assessment and foot inspection and nail care. Monthly reports looked at the number of sites recruited, classes or talks conducted, screenings conducted, and advisory group meetings and participation. Several forms underwent revision, as they were field tested in this early stage for feasibility of use and reliability of information. Additional forms were developed, as it became obvious that the participants preferred to walk away from a screening event with something in hand, such as a pamphlet or a wallet-size blood pressure record.

Evaluation of this component of the model led to recommendations for standardization in the scheduling of screenings at each site and for highlighting a particular screening each month. The older adults know what to expect at each Depot "stop" and look forward to the nurse coming to their site—she has now become part of their social setting. The offering of services was varied and age appropriate. Community nurse case management services could often be offered on-site to individuals with medically or socially complex needs, rather than having a nurse make an individual home visit. This has proven to be acceptable to the participants, as well as cost effective for the health system (Box 45-4).

IMMEDIATE OUTCOMES

Immediate outcomes are the direct consequences of the program's activities (Box 45-5). Critical elements in this stage are primarily quantitative data on the participants accessing the Health Depots: numbers exposed to group education; changes in knowledge, behavior, and attitude; adaptation of knowledge to healthy lifestyle; and incidence and prevalence of selected diseases among the Health Depot clients.

BOX 45-4

Critical Elements and Sources of Data for Implementation Processes

Critical Elements
- Participant encounters
- Services implemented and number of sites
- Educational classes, screenings, consultation
- Advisory board meeting and participation

Sources of Data
- Identification and background information
- Sign-in sheet
- Minutes of meetings

BOX 45-5

Critical Elements and Sources of Data for Immediate Outcomes

Critical Elements
- Number and characteristic of participants being served
- Change in knowledge, behavior, and/or skill level
- Number of clients referred and compliance rate on referrals
- Number of community resources participating in screenings

Sources of Data
- Sign-in sheet
- Client survey
- Referral form
- Daily log
- Minutes of meetings

The typical Health Depot older adult is a 65-year-old white female living alone with an annual income below $10,000. Twelve percent of the people do not have a primary physician, and 10% of the participants are without insurance. Twenty-

Activity	Developmental processes	Implementation processes	Immediate outcomes	Referrals	Impact outcomes	Anecdotal note

BP SCREEN	• Develop BP screen form
	
	• Research current HTN guidelines
	
	• Schedule BP screenings
	
	• Inform clients of screen date
	
	• Review and obtain HTN information for clients
	
	• Prepare education programs about HTN
	
	• Select and requisition BP equipment for purchase
		• Assess HTN history and risk factors
		
		• Assess BP: sitting; standing prn
		
		• Provide consultation and individual instruction:
		  Normal BP
		  HTN
		  Systolic HTN
		  HTN control
		  Frequency to
		  monitor BP
		
		• Disseminate information about HTN, diet, CAD, CVD
		
		• Refer clients with BP abnormalities
		
		• Follow up with referred clients
		
		• Present group education:
		  Strokes
		  HTN, CAD
			• Total BP screenings and individual instructions:
			  1436
			
			• Clients given wallet card with BP readings
				• Total sent: 29	• Total client compliance with referrals:
					  14
					
					• Percent complying :
					  48%
						• BP found to be 186/102; was referred to free medical clinic, where she was treated for HTN

FIGURE 45-5 Sample Annual Report for Health Depot outcomes.

two percent have been seen in the emergency room in the past year.

Individuals access the Health Depot an average of ten encounters per year. Blood pressure, cholesterol, and glucose screenings are the most frequently accessed services, followed by individual consultation. Approximately eight group health-promotion talks are delivered each month. The majority of referrals are generated as a result of abnormal cholesterol and blood glucose screenings. For example, in 1995, two hundred forty referrals were made. Ninety-three percent of these referrals were made to physicians. The remaining referrals were made to community resources such as the Free Medical Clinic or the Health Depart-

ment. Total client compliance with referrals ranges from 71% for referral after a history and physical examination, to a low of 13% for referral for podiatry care. All other screening activities average a 52% referral compliance rate.

The flexibility of the evaluation tool becomes most evident in this component of the model. Every screening activity can be evaluated across the Kaseman model. Screenings for blood pressure, total cholesterol, blood glucose, vision and hearing, medication review, general health assessment, history and physical, foot inspection and nail care, individual counseling, and group education programs are reported annually in a table format—one page for each activity (Figure 45-5).

BOX 45-6
Case Studies

Mr. H

Mr. H, an 83-year-old member of his local senior center, was seen at a *Health Depot* blood pressure screening. He presented with a BP of 170/104. While discussing hypertension and lifestyle choices, he admitted to the nurse that he had stopped his medicine because it caused "sexual problems." The nurse recommended that he see his physician to report his side effects. She explained that he might not experience these side effects with a different medicine. She also provided education regarding the long-term health implications of hypertension.

Outcome: Mr. H talked to his physician and agreed to try another medication. His last three BP readings at the screenings have ranged from 130/70 to 140/80, and he denies any undesirable side effects. Mr. H is sexually active.

Lilly

Lilly is a 64-year-old, divorced female who lives alone. On her first visit to a health screening offered by the *Health Depot* at her local senior center, she reported that her "COBRA insurance policy ended" and she couldn't afford to pay her insurance premiums. She stated, "I haven't had any of my blood pressure or sugar medicines for over three months." Her blood pressure at the screening was 150/98, and her fasting blood glucose was 379 mg/dl. The nurse talked with Lilly about her options for resources in the community and urged her to explain her situation to her family physician. She referred her to the local Free Medical Clinic to obtain her medications. She also provided education regarding the effects of lifestyle factors on hypertension and diabetes.

Outcome: Lilly saw her physician, who resumed her medications and provided her with medication samples until she could visit the Free Clinic. She completed the diabetic education program and now self-monitors her blood glucose levels, and routinely attends community blood pressure screenings. At subsequent screenings, Lilly's blood pressure has ranged from 120/70 to 146/82, and her last fasting blood glucose level was 144 mg/dl.

In reporting the outcomes, the Kaseman model takes a linear form, although, conceptually, it is recognized as dynamic and interactive. Note that there have been some modifications to the reporting to meet the specific needs of the Health Depot. The resource inputs are not included in this outcome report; however, they are included in a narrative format in the annual summary report. Referrals are detailed, and anecdotal notes are included as a form of story telling in the outcome report, to bring the outcomes to life. Two case studies are presented in Box 45-6 to reflect the Health Depot interventions and immediate outcomes.

IMPACT OUTCOMES

One year after the start of the program, a Client Satisfaction Survey was conducted to evaluate each client's perception of health and quality of life after exposure to the Health Depot services (Box 45-7). This survey involved a thirteen-item questionnaire administered verbally by a master's-prepared nurse who was not involved in the program. A test-retest method was used to establish inter-rater reliability. A five-point Likert-like scale was used to indicate agreement or disagreement with the item read. A card was available to the older adult for reference to the scale. Some questions were negatively worded to avoid a response bias. Several items were included to evaluate the nurse practitioner's performance. Participation was voluntary and confidentiality was ensured. Approximately 12% (n = 130) of the population was surveyed. Over 90% of the participants agreed that the Health Depot facilitated access to the health care system, enhanced quality-of-life and self-care measures, and decreased inappropriate use of hospital and emergency services.

BOX 45-7
Critical Elements and Sources of Data for Impact Outcomes

Critical Elements
- Participants' use of new services
- Consumer perception of program impact
- Impact of intervention on professional practices
- Level of readiness in the community

Sources of Data
- Follow-up interviews at site
- Client survey
- Physician survey
- Daily log

BOX 45-8
Critical Elements and Sources of Data for External Conditions

Critical Elements
- Facilitating or inhibiting factors affecting the program
- Attitudes of participants toward the program
- Motivations of participants for participating in the program
- Community or agency interest in the project

Sources of Data
- Health system mission
- Health Depot goals
- Daily log
- Debriefing after meetings

There was an overwhelmingly high level of satisfaction with the Health Depot program.

In addition, in 1993, a survey was sent to 52 physicians to whom referrals were sent, with a response rate of 56%. The majority of physicians had no knowledge of the Health Depot; however, their comments indicated interest in and support of such a program. One such comment highlighted their overall response: "Your services facilitate and provide easier access to a select group of the population with limited transportation and appear to be greatly appreciated by the participants."

Obtaining data on emergency room utilization and access to the health care system is difficult when one is working in a large rural service area that includes multiple hospital systems—and in which there is limited access and sharing of information. The self-reported surveys are the best indicators of satisfaction and changes in behavior related to accessing health care services.

EXTERNAL CONDITIONS

The last element in the Kaseman model is external conditions. Throughout the project, attention was paid to all those external events and influences that facilitate or inhibit achievement of the outcomes

(Box 45-8). These conditions may be on an individual level, a systems level, a local level, or a national level and include entrenched attitudes and physical and financial factors affecting access to health care. In many communities, the presence of managed care and changes in health care policy are primary factors initiating and effecting change. These were not the primary motivators of change in Winchester, Virginia. Rather, the anticipation of these factors has supported the implementation of wellness-promotion programs and will certainly shape future programs in this community.

A source of data that provided rich qualitative information on external conditions was a daily log. This log was used to record events, meetings, and encounters in the early years of the Health Depot. The information was helpful in identifying events and influences that affected the program. Today the facilitating and inhibiting factors, the attitudes and interest of participants, are analyzed; and strategies and recommendations are developed, implemented, and reevaluated, as events occur.

Other Features of the Model

In addition to the distinct model components, there are overlays of ongoing evaluation phases: formative, monitoring, and summative evaluations (Box 45-9).

Formative evaluation is similar to process evaluation in that it is designed to provide information about the immediate outcomes of the developmental and implementation process components. Monitoring evaluation is designed to provide continuous information about what is being done and how well it is being done. The monitoring evaluation phase is where continuous quality improvement takes place. This phase presents an opportunity to identify and correct implementation problems and includes tracking specific information. Summative evaluation is related to the immediate outcomes and impact outcomes of the project. This is the phase in which the data are analyzed according to the previously designed measurement plan. It is the time when evidence of the project's outcomes is demonstrated. Collectively, the formative, monitoring and summative phases allow for a critical review of each stage of the Kaseman model.

Challenges and Barriers

Surprisingly, there have been few barriers in the development, implementation, and expansion phases of the Health Depot program. Initially, the older adults were slow and cautious about accessing the new wellness-promotion services brought to their sites, primarily because of their long-time belief that health care is used only when one is ill. Blood pressure and cholesterol screenings found quick popularity, and helped to establish the Health Depot nurse as a friendly and helpful presence. Over time, the older adults have welcomed the activities, choosing to participate in each wellness-promotion activity. Lack of space for private consultation at some of the sites continues to challenge the nurse; however, something as simple as the purchase and use of a mobile screen has helped to minimize these concerns.

The greatest challenge to date has been with securing the support of information systems to provide technical support in program application and outcome measurement. Most nurses are highly skilled in working with environmental factors, such as clients, organizations, and communities. Here resistant factors are easily recognized and addressed; challenges are met and barriers cease to exist. Cy-

---

BOX 45-9
Kaseman Model Evaluation Phases: Overlays of the Model

Formative
Designed to provide information about the developmental and process implementation components.
• What specific outcomes should be anticipated?
• What processes and inputs are essential to these outcomes?
• How should the outcomes be assessed or measured?
• How should data be collected and analyzed?
• What data should be collected?
• What instruments and methods should be used?
• At what point in the project or protocol should measurement be taken?
• What indices or criteria *will* represent achievement of outcomes? What are the indicators or success benchmarks?
• How will the data be used and by whom?

Monitoring
Continuous information about what is being done and how well. Time to correct problems with tracking the data.
• Data about subject, clients, staff (characteristics and qualities needed for project)
• Resource utilization, including space and equipment
• Costs and revenues
• Quality of material used
• Feedback from staff and participants concerning project
• Appropriateness of specifically designed project materials
• Time required for project activities

Summative
The immediate impact outcomes of the project.
• Data analyzed according to measurement plan
• Project data compiled and presented
• Longer-term data compiled and presented

berspace, however, is new territory to many in health care. Expert advice and direction are necessary on the front lines for successful and efficient data collection and program evaluation.

Current Status

In the five years of the program's existence, more than 1000 older adults have used Health Depot services. There are now fifteen sites, serviced by one full-time advanced practice nurse who is responsible for the coordination of the entire program, including the evaluation of immediate and impact outcomes.

Although the mission of Valley Health System and the goals and services of the Health Depot remain virtually the same, many changes have occurred. Adaptations to screening forms and program offerings, though minor and structural in nature, continue to be made to fit the needs of each new Health Depot site. The content of various screening activities has been modified to be consistent with current national recommendations (*Guide to Clinical Preventive Services*, 1994). Topics, once disease specific, have been expanded to include healthy lifestyle and self-care management initiatives, with positive response from the participants. These changes have resulted from the careful evaluation of each component of the program evaluation model. The evidence overwhelmingly and consistently supports the initial belief that the health of a population can be improved through outreach and wellness promotion, and that a program can be successful given the careful consideration of a comprehensive evaluation plan.

Plans for the Future

Each year, an annual report is written to document the progress, change, and outcomes of the Health Depot. An ongoing dialogue between the advisory group, the program nurse, and the community continues to address how to improve services and maximize outcomes. One indicator that requires follow-up intervention is referral compliance. Currently, when the nurse identifies an abnormal finding for an individual and refers him or her to the primary physician, there is no formal tracking system in place, other than asking the client if he or she accessed the physician. Why do rates for compli-

ance with referral range from 71% with some screening events to as low as 13%? What are the client factors that influence compliance? Do the current documentation forms allow for efficient tracking of referral compliance? Future plans will need to include follow-up phone calls to participants, so that reasons for noncompliance with referral can be summarized and evaluated.

The Health Depot continues to operate as a free service to the community, with the savings to Valley Health System realized at the back end. The paradigm shift from "fee for service" to "spending dollars to save dollars, instead of make dollars" is operational in this type of outreach program. Ultimate savings result from reductions in inappropriate use of emergency services and inpatient admissions over time. It is predicted that as managed care penetrates the health care environment, there will be opportunities to sell or contract the services offered by the Health Depot. With more than five years of data collection, beginning with the resource inputs and continuing to the evaluation of outcomes, it is possible to determine a cost per member per month as well as predict costs of utilization. This information will be helpful as negotiations take place between the Health System and managed care organizations. Without a doubt, the Health Depot provides cost-effective and quality-oriented services to a specific population. Further expansion of Health Depot services is anticipated, both in geographic area and to other populations. This growth will be directed by the greater community's needs, continuous monitoring of outcomes, and the needs of the changing health care environment.

Conclusion

Partnerships and outcome measurements are vital to the success and continuation of community outreach activities. In the case of the Health Depot, the partnership between Valley Health System and the other community agencies involved in supporting the older adult population allowed for more services to be provided, with minimal additional resources. Through the presence of a registered nurse in the community setting, more individuals were able to have their health status monitored to detect early signs of health problems that could threaten their independence. The predicted outcomes of better health and improved patterns of self-care management were evident in both the immediate and impact outcomes reporting.

The effective management of any new program, particularly in a competitive health care market, depends heavily on frequent feedback that can document progress, detect problems, and verify expectations and outcomes. This function is best served by considering evaluation as a key to decision making, because it supports the program planning, tracking, and refining processes needed to ensure that the program's goals are successfully accomplished. The Kaseman Evaluation model provides the framework for the ongoing evaluation of the Health Depot in its entirety.

References

American Public Health Association: *Healthy communities 2000: model standards—guidelines for community attainment of the year 2000 national health objectives,* ed 3, Washington, DC, 1991, APHA.

Fisher M, ed: *Guide to clinical preventive services: an assessment of the effectiveness of 169 interventions—report of the US Preventive Service Task Force,* Baltimore, Md, 1989, Williams & Wilkins.

Guba E, Lincoln Y: *Effective evaluation,* San Francisco, 1991, Jossey-Bass Publishers.

Himmelman A: *Communities working collaboratively for a change,* Minneapolis, 1992, The Himmelman Consulting Group.

Kaseman D: *Kaseman project evaluation tool,* unpublished manuscript, George Mason University, School of Nursing, Fairfax, Virginia, 1993.

Patton MQ: *Utilization-focused evaluation,* Beverly Hills, Calif, 1978, Sage.

US Department of Health and Human Services: *Healthy people 2000: national health promotion and disease prevention objectives,* Washington, DC, 1990, U.S. Government Printing Office (Publication No. 91-50213).

US Department of Health and Human Services, Office of Disease Prevention and Health Promotion: *Guide to clinical preventive services: report of the US Preventive Service Task Force,* ed. 2, Washington, DC, 1994, US Government Printing Office.

Epilogue

MARGARET M. MURPHY, RN, PhD

Health care is complex and difficult and is often "messy," as is most of life, inside and outside the laboratory.

An "epilogue" is not a usual part of a nonfiction work. In this instance, it is offered not so much to provide the reader with someone else's view of "so what?" as to share a perspective about what this work (i.e., the preceding chapters) brings to the discussion about the outcomes of health care.

Several consistent themes are played over and over within this book. The importance of partnership and the effect of values on the selection of outcomes to pay attention to are principles that are either directly or indirectly repeated in every chapter. The context in which outcomes are evoked is also developed and becomes the overriding challenge we all face.

Partnership

It is clear that all of these authors have experienced the importance of partnership to producing the best outcomes possible in health care. This reflects the true acceptance of health care as an offering of service that can be realized only when all affected parties are directly involved in the process. Health care is personal, whether the client is an individual or a community. Unless the partners (i.e., the client and the health care provider) are in agreement and willing to do what is necessary, the desired outcomes cannot be achieved. The power in health care lies with the consumer. If the client is not engaged in the process and does not consciously and knowledgeably decide to accept the health care provider as a partner in his or her health care, whatever benefit might have been achieved is minimized at best and negated at worst. Whether the selected outcomes measure "quality" (e.g., functional status, symptom status, immediate and after-care self-management capacity, personal goal achievement, satisfaction, quality-of-life status, perception) or "cost" (e.g., time, equipment and treatment, length of stay, loss of income, money spent and/or saved, effectiveness), the condition of the partnership between the consumer and/or client and the health care provider affects the final data generated to make a judgment regarding the outcomes.

Values

Values are another elemental factor in the examination of outcomes. Values dictate the outcomes that are deemed worthy of examination. In most in-

stances the issues related to the selection of outcomes to be examined are not "clean"; they are often fraught with the risk of bipolar thinking—that is, the "either/or" questions, such as the following:
- Can the questions of quality be asked independently of the issues of cost or vice versa?
- Can any discipline, system, or person demonstrate complete effectiveness on all measures?

To the detriment of other considerations, however, the data are often weighted in one way. This reflects the limitations of time, energy, money, and talent that force the people who would examine outcomes to select from all the possible outcomes those that *they* believe are the most important at a given time. Most obviously, the chapters that deal with ethics, legal issues, and leadership emphasize the tie of values to outcomes. Each chapter reflects the values questions that the authors have confronted and have needed to address in their own experiences with health care. After all, there is no "one way" to do anything in this business; therefore, everyone engaged in the business of health care is involved in the discussions and decisions that revolve around values.

The values issues are plainly affected by the continuing laments related to the ongoing need to deal with the shift from what some would call "the good old days," a transition from a time characterized as having little shared responsibility and apparently endless money in health care to the "new days" in which responsibility is delegated to everyone—that is, consumers, providers, institutions, staff, policy making groups, and all those referred to as payers. The orientation toward "accountability for all" complicates the values questions and the partnership arrangements that need to be made; and yet, as the authors have demonstrated, agreements can be forged and outcomes can be examined from many interest points.

Context

Perhaps the most startling observation that can be made about the writing contained within these covers is that, in contrast to the "Outcomes/ Effectiveness Research" segment provided almost every month in the Agency for Health Care Policy and Research (AHCPR) publication *Research Activities*, the discussions held here about outcomes are made within a *context* that is greater than technol-

ogy and technique. Technology and technique are important, especially to the recipient of health care; however, they are only part of the story for the recipient. The rest of the story:
- Involves the context in which the technique or technology is or is not applied
- Includes the environment and circumstances surrounding the recipient and the providers of care, as well as the people and policies that affect them both
- Includes those components of "health care" that are not yet amenable to "cure" or are aimed at the achievement of a better state of health rather than the cure or avoidance of disease

The authors of this book have focused on outcomes in context. This context includes the present time in the history of health care, health care data and data elements that inform health care policy, the legal system, ethics, service, systems, providers, payers and intermediaries, communities, popula-tions, individual and collective consumers of health care, and leadership. It is rare to have an opportunity to examine an issue in health care from so many and such diverse viewpoints. Although a number of research and measurement instruments and techniques are shared, these too are described within the context of a large picture of the client and service intention.

End Note

This is a provocative work. It raises questions about the meaning of outcomes in the abstract and in the concrete of everyday health care practice. Having read this book, one can surely believe that identifying and evaluating outcomes in health care is a rich quagmire of differing priorities and perspectives. Health care is complex and difficult and is often "messy," as is most of life, inside *and* outside the laboratory.

Index